Psychiatric
Treatment
of the
Medically Ill

Medical Psychiatry

Series Editor

William A. Frosch, M.D.

Cornell University Medical College
New York, New York

ADDITIONAL VOLUMES IN PREPARATION

Psychiatric Treatment of the Medically Ill

edited by

Robert G. Robinson

University of Iowa College of Medicine
Iowa City, Iowa

William R. Yates

University of Oklahoma Health Sciences Center
Tulsa, Oklahoma

MARCEL DEKKER, INC.   NEW YORK · BASEL

ISBN: 0-8247-1958-1

This book is printed on acid-free paper.

Headquarters
Marcel Dekker, Inc.
270 Madison Avenue, New York, NY 10016
tel: 212-696-9000; fax: 212-685-4540

Eastern Hemisphere Distribution
Marcel Dekker AG
Hutgasse 4, Postfach 812, CH-4001 Basel, Switzerland
tel: 41-61-261-8482; fax: 41-61-261-8896

World Wide Web
http://www.dekker.com

The publisher offers discounts on this book when ordered in bulk quantities. For more information, write to Special Sales/Professional Marketing at the headquarters address above.

Current printing (last digit):
10 9 8 7 6 5 4 3 2 1

PRINTED IN THE UNITED STATES OF AMERICA

Series Introduction

The post–World War II burgeoning interest in psychiatry and psychoanalysis, spurred by the experience of treating physically wounded and psychologically traumatized soldiers and civilians, reinforced medicine's interest in the borderlines of mind and brain. While it had an older history in the work of William James, Hughlings Jackson, and Paul Schilder, the new focus on "psychosomatic illness," on "the mysterious leap from the mind to the body," made us acutely aware of the impact of affect and fantasy on bodily function. Gastric and duodenal ulcers, ulcerative colitis, rheumatoid arthritis, and asthma were thought to have important psychogenetic origins in repressed memories, fantasies, and conflicts. Unfortunately, many of these older theories and the practices derived from them have proven to be either in error or too simplistic.

The positive aspects of these misguided notions included the research into mechanisms that resulted, and which played an important role in introducing biological research into psychiatry, and the reinforced continuing interest in the mind–brain interface. The consequent development of consultation, and particularly of liaison psychiatry, turned our attention back to the problems of living with medical illness, acute or chronic, of adapting to disabilities, of accommodation to disease and to approaching death. Being physically ill is stressful and can produce psychiatric symptoms and syndromes either directly or indirectly, and the treatments we use can also create psychiatric difficulties and disorders.

Recovery-room deliria, the wish to discontinue renal dialysis, poststroke depression or denial of disability, and anticholinergic confusional states are commonplaces in medical practice. Drs. Robinson and Yates present us with a well-organized, scholarly review of the multiple ways in which patients experience illness, the impact of being sick, the things a disordered physiology can do to the mind, and a comprehensive course on the psychopharmacology of the medically ill. While many of the authors are from Dr. Robinson's own distinguished department in Iowa, the chapter authors represent distinguished institutions in New York, Maryland, Oklahoma, Rhode Island, and Connecticut, as well as Canada, England, Argentina, Israel, and Germany. The result is a nonparochial view of the current state of our knowledge, of both our science and our art.

William A. Frosch, M.D.

Preface

Medical illnesses induce psychological as well as physical distress. This relationship has been known for many years but has only recently been systematically documented by studies of the epidemiology of psychiatric disorders in various medical disorders. Studies of community and clinical populations demonstrate that medical and psychiatric disorders occur together much more commonly than would be expected by chance. Both primary care physicians and psychiatrists are likely to find that a significant number of their patients have both a medical and a psychiatric diagnosis.

Acute and chronic medical illnesses produce significant psychological distress and may contribute to the production of psychiatric symptoms and psychiatric disorders. Patients with medical illness are frequently dealing with psychological threats created by the illness. These come in many forms, such as a threat to physical integrity and body image, to social and occupational functioning, or to financial self-sufficiency. Handling these psychological stressors can be crucial in a physician's overall patient-management plan.

Patients with psychiatric disorders frequently suffer physical symptoms such as pain, fatigue, dyspnea, and headache. These physical symptoms are often produced as part of the psychiatric illness and will resolve once the psychiatric illness is successfully treated. However, patients are often unaware of the source of their physical symptoms and seek relief from primary care physicians rather than a specialist in mental health care. This psychiatric link to physical symptoms is responsible for a significant number of visits to primary care physicians.

Both medical and psychiatric treatments can produce adverse effects, some of which cross the domain of treatment. A significant number of medical drugs can have psychiatric effects on mood, anxiety, or cognition. Primary care physicians often need to determine if a patient's new psychiatric symptoms are a result of the intervention they have initiated so that a proper adjustment to the treatment program can be made. Likewise, psychiatric medications can produce physical symptoms and interact with medical illnesses. A psychiatrist prescribing a tricyclic antidepressant needs to be familiar with elements of cardiac conduction and the toxic effects of tricyclic medications on the heart and the brain. The mind–body dualism is no longer valid. We now understand better that it is impossible to provide adequate care for the mind and brain without attention to and knowledge of the body.

This book is divided into three parts: an introduction, description of specific medical disorders, and discussion of psychopharmacological treatment in the medically ill. In the introductory section, issues of screening for psychiatric illness in medical patients provides a framework for psychiatric assessment. A discussion of the specificity of psychiatric symptoms then leads into a review of the epidemiology of psychiatric disorders in medical populations.

The section on specific disorders includes 18 chapters targeted to the most common medical disorders as well as those in which psychiatric issues play a key role: organ transplantation, HIV infection, and neuropsychiatric disorders. These chapters provide the clinician with a ready reference addressing the issues related to psychiatric treatment in these medical conditions.

The final section focuses on specific psychopharmacological treatment issues found in medically ill populations, including absorption and metabolism, the role of serum-level monitoring, and the effects of aging and psychotropic drug interactions. This section provides clinicians with information relevant to the pharmacology of psychotropic drug use in the medically ill.

We hope that this volume will provide both primary care physicians and psychiatrists with a resource for managing the patient with both a medical and a psychiatric disorder. The shift to increased managed care has placed pressure on primary care physicians to handle common psychiatric disorders. Psychiatrists are encountering forces targeting their work and reimbursement to areas in which their medical training and background are required. Both these forces encourage a better understanding of the interface of medicine, surgery, and psychiatry. This book seeks to provide a timely and comprehensive review of this interface.

Robert G. Robinson
William R. Yates

Contents

Psychopharmacological Treatment in the Medically Ill

Contributors

Bruce Alexander, Pharm.D., B.C.P.P.   Clinical Pharmacist Specialist, Departments of Pharmacy and Psychiatry, Department of Veterans Affairs Medical Center, Iowa City, Iowa

Gabriele M. Barthlen, M.D.*   Center for Sleep Medicine, Mount Sinai Medical Center, New York, New York

Bernard D. Beitman, M.D.   Chairman, Department of Psychiatry and Neurology, University of Missouri–Columbia, Columbia, Missouri

Kristine A. Bever, Pharm.D.   Psychopharmacology Research Fellow, Division of Clinical and Administrative Pharmacy, University of Iowa College of Pharmacy, Iowa City, Iowa

Caroline Carney, M.D.   Assistant Professor of Psychiatry and Internal Medicine, University of Iowa College of Medicine, Iowa City, Iowa

C. Lindsay DeVane, Pharm.D.   Professor, Department of Psychiatry and Behavioral Sciences, Medical University of South Carolina, Charleston, South Carolina

Vicki L. Ellingrod, Pharm.D., B.C.P.P.   Associate, Division of Clinical and Administrative Pharmacy, University of Iowa College of Pharmacy, Iowa City, Iowa

---

* *Current affiliation*: Neurologist, Department of Pulmonary and Internal Medicine, Freiburg University Medical Center, Freiburg, Germany.

Marc Fishman, M.D.   Assistant Professor, Department of Psychiatry and Behavioral Sciences, Johns Hopkins University School of Medicine, Baltimore, Maryland

Richard P. Fleet, Ph.D.   Department of Psychosomatic Medicine, Montreal Heart Institute, Montreal, Quebec, Canada

Richard J. Goldberg, M.D.   Psychiatrist in Chief, Rhode Island Hospital and Women & Infants' Hospital, Providence, Rhode Island

Michael G. Goldstein, M.D.   Associate Professor, Department of Psychiatry and Human Behavior, Brown University School of Medicine, and Center for Behavioral and Preventive Medicine, The Miriam Hospital, Providence, Rhode Island

Susan R. Johnson, M.D.   Professor, Department of Obstetrics and Gynecology, University of Iowa College of Medicine, Iowa City, Iowa

Ricardo E. Jorge, M.D.   Associate Research Scientist, Department of Psychiatry, University of Iowa College of Medicine, Iowa City, Iowa

Joel N. Kline, M.D.   Assistant Professor, Division of Pulmonary, Critical Care, and Occupational Medicine, Department of Internal Medicine, University of Iowa College of Medicine, Iowa City, Iowa

Norman B. Levy, M.D.   Director, Consultation—Liaison Psychiatry, Coney Island Hospital, and Clinical Professor of Psychiatry and Adjunct Professor of Medicine, State University of New York Health Science Center at Brooklyn, Brooklyn, New York

Constantine G. Lyketsos, M.D.   Associate Professor, Department of Psychiatry and Behavioral Sciences, Johns Hopkins University School of Medicine, Baltimore, Maryland

Jill I. Mattia, Ph.D.   Investigator, Department of Psychiatry and Human Behavior, Brown University School of Medicine and Rhode Island Hospital, Providence, Rhode Island

Paul R. McHugh, M.D.   Henry Phipps Professor and Director, Department of Psychiatry and Behavioral Sciences, Johns Hopkins University School of Medicine, Baltimore, Maryland

James R. Merikangas, M.D., F.A.C.P., F.A.P.A.   Lecturer in Psychiatry, Yale University School of Medicine, New Haven, Connecticut

Kathleen R. Merikangas, Ph.D.   Professor of Epidemiology and Psychiatry and Director, Genetic Epidemiology Research Unit, Yale University School of Medicine, New Haven, Connecticut

Del D. Miller, Pharm.D., M.D.   Associate Professor, Department of Psychiatry, University of Iowa College of Medicine, Iowa City, Iowa

Charles B. Nemeroff, M.D., Ph.D.   Reunette W. Harris Professor and Chairman,

Department of Psychiatry and Behavioral Sciences, Emory University School of Medicine, Atlanta, Georgia

Raymond Niaura, Ph.D.   Associate Professor, Department of Psychiatry and Human Behavior, Brown University School of Medicine, and Division of Behavioral and Preventive Medicine, The Miriam Hospital, Providence, Rhode Island

Michael W. O'Hara, Ph.D.   Professor and Chair, Department of Psychology, University of Iowa, Iowa City, Iowa

Sergio Paradiso, M.D., Ph.D.   House staff, Department of Psychiatry, University of Iowa College of Medicine, Iowa City, Iowa

Paul J. Perry, Ph.D.   Professor of Psychiatry and Pharmacy, Department of Psychiatry, University of Iowa College of Medicine, and Division of Clinical and Administrative Pharmacy, University of Iowa College of Pharmacy, Iowa City, Iowa

Gustavo Petracca, M.D.   Neuropsychiatrist, Department of Neuropsychiatry, Raul Carrea Institute of Neurological Research–FLENI, Buenos Aires, Argentina

Neal G. Ranen, M.D.*   Department of Psychiatry, Jefferson Medical College, Thomas Jefferson University, and Wills Geriatric Psychiatry Program, Philadelphia, Pennsylvania

Howard A. Ring, M.D., M.R.C.Psych.   Academic Department of Psychological Medicine, St. Bartholomew's and the Royal London School of Medicine, London, England

Robert G. Robinson, M.D.   The Paul W. Penningroth Professor and Head, Department of Psychiatry, University of Iowa College of Medicine, Iowa City, Iowa

Steven P. Roose, M.D.   Professor of Clinical Psychiatry, Department of Psychiatry, Columbia University College of Physicians & Surgeons, New York, New York

Barry W. Rovner, M.D.   Professor, Department of Psychiatry, Jefferson Medical College, Thomas Jefferson University, and Wills Geriatric Psychiatry Program, Philadelphia, Pennsylvania

Susan K. Schultz, M.D.   Assistant Professor, Department of Psychiatry, University of Iowa College of Medicine, Iowa City, Iowa

Joseph M. Schwartz, M.D.   Assistant Professor, Department of Psychiatry and Behavioral Sciences, Johns Hopkins University School of Medicine, Baltimore, Maryland

Peter A. Shapiro, M.D.   Associate Professor of Clinical Psychiatry, Department of

---

* *Current affiliation:* Medical Director, Health Pathways of Albright Care Services, York, and Clinical Associate Professor of Psychiatry, Penn State College of Medicine, Hershey, Pennsylvania.

Psychiatry, Columbia University College of Physicians & Surgeons, New York, New York

Sergio E. Starkstein, M.D., Ph.D. Director, Department of Neuropsychiatry, Raúl Carrea Institute of Neurological Research–FLENI, Buenos Aires, Argentina

Denise J. Stevens, Ph.D. Associate Research Scientist, Department of Epidemiology and Public Health, Yale University School of Medicine, New Haven, Connecticut

Scott Stuart, M.D. Assistant Professor, Department of Psychiatry, University of Iowa College of Medicine, Iowa City, Iowa

Glenn J. Treisman, M.D., Ph.D. Associate Professor, Department of Psychiatry and Behavioral Sciences and Department of Medicine, Johns Hopkins University School of Medicine, Baltimore, Maryland

Simon Wein, M.D.* Department of Psychiatry, Memorial Sloan-Kettering Cancer Center, New York, New York

Catherine L. Woodman, M.D. Assistant Professor, Department of Psychiatry, University of Iowa College of Medicine, Iowa City, Iowa

William R. Yates, M.D. Professor and Chair, Department of Psychiatry, University of Oklahoma Health Sciences Center, Tulsa, Oklahoma

Mark Zimmerman, M.D. Department of Psychiatry and Human Behavior, Brown University School of Medicine, and Director of Outpatient Psychiatry, Rhode Island Hospital, Providence, Rhode Island

---

* *Current affiliation:* Physician, Pain and Palliative Care Unit, Department of Oncology, Shaare Zedek Medical Center, Jerusalem, Israel.

1

Screening for Psychiatric Disorders in Medical Patients

Mark Zimmerman and Jill I. Mattia
*Brown University School of Medicine
and Rhode Island Hospital
Providence, Rhode Island*

INTRODUCTION

Psychiatric diagnoses are based on a patient's history and mental status examination. A psychiatrist today uses essentially the same methods that Kraepelin used 100 years ago to make a diagnosis—questioning, observation, and clinical acumen. In other disciplines of medicine, modern technology assists the clinician in the diagnostic process. There is much hope and desire that this technology will also result in specific diagnostic laboratory tests in psychiatry, and when one is suggested it receives much attention (e.g., the dexamethasone suppression test). Although diagnostic laboratory tests have not, as yet, been recommended for routine clinical use in making psychiatric diagnoses, there is a "technology" that can aid the diagnostic process—the self-administered paper-and-pencil questionnaire. These tests do not reveal anything about the patient that the clinician could not otherwise ascertain, and they do not provide clues about underlying pathophysiology. However, as will be reviewed below, their ability to screen for and/or "diagnose" certain psychiatric disorders is quite respectable.

Since the publication of specified diagnostic criteria for psychiatric disorders, there has been increased interest in using self-administered scales as screening and diagnostic instruments. Measures have been developed to identify major depressive disorder (1), panic disorder (2), alcohol use disorders (3), posttraumatic stress disorder (4), dysthymia and cyclothymia (5), bulimia (6), and all of the personality disorders (7). These instruments represent the second generation of measures. Prior to them, the first generation of measures nonspecifically identified individuals who were psychiatric cases regardless of the type of pathology (8). Most recently, in the past 3 years a third generation of instruments has emerged that screens for multiple, specific psychiatric disorders (9–11).

By far the most frequently studied disorder in medical patients has been major depressive disorder. Not only have many more studies been conducted regarding the performance of depression screening instruments in medical patients, but there are also many more studies of clinical detection and unrecognition of depression in medical patients, the financial and psychosocial morbidity attributed to depression, the impact of depression on the course of medical disorders, the effectiveness of treating depression in medical patients, and the ability of screening programs for depression to improve outcome. Because of this, and because depression is the most frequent psychiatric disorder in medical patients, this chapter will emphasize screening for depression in medical patients.

GOALS OF SCREENING

The provision of preventive services is one of the cornerstones of primary care, and periodic screening is a major component of providing preventive care. There are two major reasons for medical screening: (1) to detect a disease early in its natural course when it may be easier to treat, and (2) to detect factors that increase an individual's risk of developing a disease, with the goal of modifying the risk factor and thereby preventing disease. An example of the first type of screening is the use of mammography to detect breast cancer in an early stage (secondary prevention), and an example of the second type of screening is cholesterol or blood pressure determinations to lower the risk of future cardiac or cerebrovascular disease (primary prevention). Successful screening efforts modify the natural history of the disorder by virtue of early intervention.

The World Health Organization (WHO) (12) suggested that six conditions be met before routine screening can be recommended:

1. The condition must have a significant effect on the quality of life.
2. Acceptable methods of treatment must be available.
3. The condition must have an asymptomatic or unrecognized period during which detection and treatment significantly reduce morbidity and/or mortality.
4. Treatment in the asymptomatic phase must yield a therapeutic result superior to that obtained by delaying treatment until symptoms appear.
5. Tests that are acceptable to patients must be available at reasonable cost to detect the condition in the asymptomatic period.
6. The incidence of the condition must be sufficient to justify the cost of screening.

With respect to psychiatric disorders it is more appropriate to speak of case-finding than screening (13). Case-finding refers to testing and detecting symptomatic individuals, whereas screening generally refers to evaluating healthy persons. Thus,

WHO's fourth condition is not relevant to psychiatric screening. In addition, for the purposes of psychopathology screening, WHO's third and fifth conditions should be reworded to refer to an *unrecognized* (rather than *asymptomatic*) period of illness. In contrast to some medical illnesses, which can be detected in an occult asymptomatic phase, psychiatric disorders can be diagnosed only when symptoms are manifested.

REASONS TO SCREEN FOR DEPRESSION AND OTHER PSYCHIATRIC DISORDERS

Psychiatric Disorders Are Prevalent in Medical Patients

The first study to examine the prevalence of a range of specific mental disorders in primary care was conducted by Hoeper and colleagues (14) using the Research Diagnostic Criteria (15). They found that the overall prevalence of any psychiatric disorder was 26.7%, with major depression (5.8%) and phobic disorders (5.8%) as the most prevalent. Schulberg and Burns (16) summarized the results of nine studies that estimated the prevalence of current psychiatric disorders using standardized research interviews and concluded that approximately 25% of primary care patients have a current psychiatric disorder.

Recently, two screening/diagnostic systems have been developed for use in primary care settings—the Primary Care Evaluation of Mental Disorders (PRIME-MD) and the Symptom Driven Diagnostic System (SDDS). In the PRIME-MD 1000 study (10), 1000 primary care patients completed a brief multidimensional screening questionnaire covering mood, anxiety, alcohol, and eating disorders, and then patients were administered a semistructured diagnostic interview by the primary care physician for those disorders that were screen-positive. Twenty-six percent of the patients met DSM-III-R criteria for a current disorder. The most frequent disorders were major depression (12%), dysthymia (8%), and generalized anxiety disorder (7%). Another 13% of patients had "subthreshold" disorders such as anxiety disorder not otherwise specified (9%) or major depression in partial remission (6%). Of note, several disorders found to be prevalent in community-based epidemiological surveys such as phobic disorders, posttraumatic stress disorder, and obsessive-compulsive disorder were not evaluated (17,18). Another recent study of the prevalence of current DSM-III-R disorders in a rural primary care practice using the PRIME-MD found that 19% of patients had a threshold level disorder and another 15% had a subthreshold diagnosis (19).

The SDDS is also limited in the range of disorders covered (alcohol abuse/dependence, generalized anxiety disorder, major depression, obsessive-compulsive disorder, and panic disorder) (9). In the initial validity studies of the SDDS, the prevalence of any disorder was 22% in one study and 26% in another (9,20).

The literature thus suggests that psychiatric disorders occur in approximately 25–35% of medical patients depending on the threshold used to define a case and the range of disorders evaluated. Psychiatric disorders are therefore sufficiently prevalent to warrant screening.

Psychiatric Disorders Are Underrecognized in Medical Patients

Docherty (21) recently reviewed 34 studies of the recognition of depression in primary care and found that detection rates ranged from 7 to 70%, with most rates of accurate diagnosis falling in the 30–40% range. Many of the studies included in the review defined depression broadly to include major and nonmajor depression. In a recent study by Schwenk et al. (22) two-thirds of patients with major depression were undetected by the primary care doctor. Importantly, detection was strongly related to the severity of depression—only 27% of mild and moderate major depression was recognized, whereas 73% of severe major depression was identified.

Rates of alcohol use/abuse in medical patients vary between 5 and 29.1% (23–27), and alcohol problems are reported to be present in 7–27% of inpatient general medical and surgical admissions (28–33). Evidence suggests that the recognition of alcohol difficulties in outpatient medical settings is a persistent problem. Isaacson et al. (25) reported physicians' recognition rate of DSM-III-R alcohol abuse/dependence to be 44%. Similarly, Buchsbaum et al. (34) found that physicians detected 49% of patients with current alcohol problems, and Johnson et al. (35) reported that 58% of their alcohol abusing patients were identified by physicians. Schorling et al. (27) recently reported data suggesting that rates of alcohol abuse detection can be related to type of medical practice, even when controlling for physician attitudes and perceptions. Primary care, family medicine, and categorical medicine residents were compared regarding detection of alcohol abuse in their patients. Of those primary care patients identified by independent structured interview and questionnaire as abusing alcohol, 71% were questioned or screened by their physician (blind to the interview and questionnaire results) for alcohol problems, and chart documentation was present for only 38% of patients. Forty-seven percent of family medicine patients were screened by their physician, and chart documentation occurred for only 15% of patients. Sixty-five percent of categorical medicine patients were screened by their physician, and 24% of patients' charts documented these difficulties. In a study of treatment of alcohol use disorders in primary care, Cleary et al. (24) reported that although physicians were aware of serious alcohol problems in 77% of their patients who met DSM-III-R criteria for alcohol abuse/dependence, physicians addressed these problems in only 67% of these patients.

Psychiatric Disorders Negatively Impact on Psychosocial Functioning and Quality of Life

A large literature has established that psychopathology is associated with impaired functioning and poorer perceived quality of life in both epidemiological and medical patient samples. Data from the Epidemiologic Catchment Area (ECA) study (36) indicate that disability and depression frequently co-occur. Individuals with major depression in the community, compared to nondepressed individuals, had a 4.78 times greater risk of disability days and days lost from work, and individuals with minor depression had a 1.55 times greater risk of disability and days lost from work. Minor depression, because of its greater prevalence, accounted for 51% of the total number of disability days in the community. Medical patients with comorbid depressive, anxiety, and substance use conditions reported extensive functional impairment, even after controlling for general health factors (37,38). Primary care patients with depression also report substantial physical, psychological, and social functioning impairments unrelated to the severity of baseline medical comorbidity (39). Individuals diagnosed with hypertension or diabetes who have a comorbid anxiety disorder report poorer quality of life than their non-anxious counterparts (40). Depressed patients in comparison to individuals with chronic medical illnesses like diabetes, hypertension, recent myocardial infarction, and congestive heart failure indicate that they have similar, if not worse, long-lasting decrements in multiple domains of functioning and well-being (41–43). Medical patients who use alcohol also report poorer health and functioning, but it is uncertain if this is a direct result of the substance use per se or due to the presence of other psychiatric disorders that are frequently comorbid with substance use (35). Nevertheless, children of drinkers are at substantially higher risk for injury than children of nondrinkers (44).

The presence of psychiatric disorders has a significant negative effect on the course of medical illnesses. Elderly medical patients with depression are more likely to die during their medical hospitalization than their nondepressed counterparts (45). Elderly hypertensives are at increased risk for stroke (46), and older patients on antihypertensive therapy who manifest increasing depressive symptoms over time are at greater risk of death and stroke or myocardial infarction (47). Elderly individuals without hypertension at baseline, but with anxiety and depression, are at increased risk for hypertension during the subsequent 16 years (48).

Baseline depression predicts follow-up mortality in post–myocardial infarction patients (49,50) and rehospitalization among patients with coronary artery disease (51). Individuals with depressed mood following stroke are 3.4 times more likely to have died during follow-up, even after controlling for age, gender, social class, type of stroke, lesion location, and level of social functioning (52). Baseline depression also predicts poorer discharge medical outcome for stroke patients (53), and depression in HIV-infected men is associated with greater mortality versus HIV men without depression (54). Overall, individuals who have life-threatening illnesses (myocardial infarction, subarachnoid hemorrhage, pulmonary embolism, and acute upper gastrointestinal hemorrhage) are almost five times more likely to die or have life-threatening complications within 28 days than nondepressed individuals with the same illnesses (55).

Psychiatric Disorders Are Costly

Evidence suggests that the economic cost of depression can be substantial. Individuals with both a medical illness and depression tend to use more health care resources than nondepressed medical patients (56). Elderly depressed medical patients use more services after discharge than nondepressed elderly medical patients (45), and psychiatric comorbidity increases the average length of stay among hospitalized AIDS patients (57). Based on 1990 U.S. population data, depression has been estimated to cost a total of

$43.7 billion annually (58). The majority of that figure is estimated to be derived from the indirect costs of depression (lost days from work, decreased productivity at work, lost income due to premature death, etc.). The direct cost of treating depression represents only one-quarter of its costs. Depressive disorders, only a piece of the much larger mental illness price tag, is comparable to the cost of illnesses such as coronary heart disease ($43 billion) and arthritis ($38 billion) (59). Of note, these numbers underestimate the true cost of depression because they do not include the cost of treatment delivered in primary care settings (60). Primary care patients with depression have twice the annual health care cost as primary care patients without depression. Depressed individuals rack up higher bills in every type of care (primary care, medical specialty, medical inpatient, pharmacy, laboratory), even after controlling for medical morbidity (61). In fact, the cost of increased medical care utilization is greater than the cost of treating the depression directly (61–63).

Although the body of evidence is smaller, a similar cost pattern emerges for medical patients with anxiety disorders. Primary care patients with anxiety disorders have almost twice the annual health care costs as their nonanxious counterparts. These individuals are substantially more expensive to treat because they utilize more services, a reflection of greater general medical services utilization rather than mental health service utilization (61). Panic disorder, the anxiety disorder that is most associated with health care utilization (emergency room visits, cardiac stress tests, etc.) can be very expensive, though the ultimate cost of treating the panic disorder is offset by savings realized by increasing individuals' functionality and therefore productivity (64). In fact, anxiety disorders cost approximately $46.6 billion annually, and less than one-quarter of the total expense is calculated to be a direct cost of treatment (65). The majority of the anxiety price tag is estimated to be associated with the morbidity of the syndrome.

This pattern of increased health services utilization stands for individuals who use alcohol; current alcohol use leads to increased outpatient doctor visits while mental health visits are decreased (66,67). Individuals admitted to the emergency room for trauma who are also intoxicated are 2.5 times more likely to be readmitted for another trauma than individuals not intoxicated at admission (67). The 1985 cost of alcohol use disorders was estimated to have been $13.9 billion—$9.4 billion in private costs and an additional $4.5 billion in government costs (68).

Psychiatric Disorders Are Treatable

There is little doubt that psychiatric disorders are effectively treated. Whether the research demonstrating the efficacy of treatment in psychiatric settings generalizes to medical settings has been the subject of increasing discussion during the past 5 years. Recently, studies have begun to appear in the literature demonstrating that treatment for depression is also effective in medical patients (69–71). Placebo-controlled studies have established the efficacy of antidepressants in patients with chronic obstructive pulmonary disease (72), diabetes (73), cancer (74), and stroke (75). Miranda and Munoz (76) found that 8 weeks of cognitive-behavioral therapy for medical patients with minor depression was associated with reduced depression, lowered somatic symptomatology, and fewer missed appointments with primary care providers. In a randomized control trial of problem-solving therapy, amitriptyline plus routine clinical management, and pill placebo plus routine clinical management, problem solving resulted in significantly greater benefits than the other two conditions (77). More recently, Lynch et al. (78) reported brief (6 weeks) telephone therapy for minor depression decreased symptoms of depression and improved functioning. In general, it appears that standardized protocol treatment for primary care patients with psychiatric disorders is associated with greater improvement in more domains of functioning than usual physician's care (39), and pharmacotherapy and psychotherapy specifically are more effective than routine care (70% vs. 20% response rate) (79). Treatment for alcohol use disorders demonstrates similar benefits for primary care patients. Brief physician intervention (advice, written contract, self-help booklet, diaries) results in a significant decrease in alcohol use, length of hospital stay, and episodes of binge drinking (80–82).

THE COSTS OF MENTAL HEALTH SCREENING

Psychiatric disorders are prevalent, underrecognized, impairing, costly, and treatable. However, widespread screening can only be recommended when the potential benefits outweigh the costs. The costs of screening for medical disorders include the financial cost of the procedure, the discomfort caused by the procedure, the financial cost, discomfort and risks of the follow-up tests, and the consequences of false-positive results. The adverse consequences of false positives include the unnecessary discomfort, costs, and risks associated with the follow-up testing, as well as the psychological burden of believing that a serious, potentially life-threatening illness is present (83). Mental health screening, in stark contrast to medical screening, yields a negligible financial burden because many instruments are currently available from pharmaceutical companies free of charge.

Surveys of primary care physicians have found that physicians believe that their patients are uncomfortable discussing mental health–related issues; thus, there may be an emotional cost of psychiatric screening. In a national survey of family practitioners, two thirds of the respondents reported that patients' resistance to psychiatric diagnosis and treatment was an obstacle in providing service or making treatment referral (84). Main and colleagues (85) recently found that primary care physicians' belief that their patients do not want inquiry about depression accounted for one third of the variance in physicians' belief of whether depression is an important clinical problem, and it was strongly associated with the clinician's discomfort in assessing depression. To avoid stigmatizing patients, some physicians substitute technical sounding euphemisms such as "limbic system dysfunction" (86) or deliberately do not make the diagnosis of depression (87).

In fact, research on patients' attitudes toward mental health screening has failed to support primary care physicians' beliefs about patient discomfort. Frowick and colleagues (88) found that more than 90% of family practice patients want their physician's involvement with psychological problems. Brody et al. (89) found that the majority of primary care patients, and almost all patients who screened positive for depression, indicated that it was at least somewhat important to receive help from their primary care physician for emotional problems. Similarly, other studies in primary care have indicated that the majority of patients want their doctor to address their psychological distress (90–92).

Zimmerman and colleagues conducted the only direct comparison of patient and physician attitudes towards mental health screening in primary care (93–95). The survey consisted of more than 1600 primary care patients in four settings: a general medical clinic at a Veterans Affairs (VA) medical center, a faculty general internal medicine practice in Philadelphia, and two private practice internal medicine practices in Rhode Island. At each site patients completed two questionnaires. The first measure was a brief self-administered questionnaire that covered a broad range of psychopathology including DSM-IV mood, anxiety, eating, substance use, and somatoform disorders. The second questionnaire assessed patients' attitudes toward completing the first measure. After these patient studies were completed, Zimmerman and colleagues conducted two surveys of family practice and internal medicine physicians (95). The physicians were shown the screening questionnaire and asked to predict patients' attitudes towards completing the screening questionnaire. The discrepancy between the physicians' predictions and actual patient attitudes was dramatic. Only 10–15% of patients indicated that they were at least minimally annoyed, embarrassed, upset, or uncomfortable by completing the screening questionnaire, whereas the physicians predicted that 80–90% of patients would be so affected.

The literature therefore fails to support primary care physicians' perceptions of patient resistance to psychiatric assessment and treatment. It is possible that the cause of physicians' mistaken belief about patient attitudes is that physicians have generalized from rare, but salient, examples of patient resistance to receiving a psychiatric diagnosis or a mental health referral. There is concern that physicians' beliefs will become self-fulfilling prophecies resulting in continued minimization of mental health issues (96). This is at odds with research that indicates that patients are more satisfied with their care if their physicians address psychosocial matters (97,98).

For most medical screening tests a major cost result of false-positive tests are more expensive, invasive follow-up procedures, as well as the emotional distress of waiting for the results of the more definitive test to rule out a serious illness. With mental health screening these risks are not present because the purpose of the "screening" is really case identification rather than detection of occult illness. The principal cost of false-positive results will be the more thorough follow-up diagnostic evaluation that is difficult to fit into a busy physician's schedule.

THE STATISTICS OF SCREENING

There are several excellent articles describing the descriptive statistics of test performance (99–101). Despite these, in several studies of the performance of self-administered screening tests, incorrect definitions and miscalculations of these statistics were found (102); therefore, we present a brief overview of this area.

The diagnostic performance of self-report scales relies on interviewer-derived diagnoses as the "gold standard." *Sensitivity* refers to a test's ability to correctly identify individuals with the illness, whereas *specificity* refers to a test's ability to identify nonill persons. Studies of test performance are typically presented as in Figure 1. Sensitivity, also called the true positive rate, is the percentage of ill persons who are identified by the test as ill (a/a + c). Specificity, the true negative rate, is the percentage of nonill persons identified by the test as nonill (d/b + d).

Sensitivity and specificity provide useful psychometric information about a test; however, the clinically more meaningful conditional probabilities are positive and negative predictive values. These values indicate the probability that an individual is ill or nonill given that the test identifies them as ill or nonill. Accordingly, *positive predictive value* is the percentage of individuals classified ill by the test who truly are ill (a/a + b), whereas *negative predictive value* is the percentage of individuals classified not ill by the test who truly are not ill (d/c + d).

Sensitivity, specificity, and positive and negative predictive values are not invariant properties of a test—they are a function of the cutoff point used to distinguish cases from noncases, they are influenced by disease prevalence, and they are related to each other. Four axioms characterize these relationships.

1.   Lowering a test's threshold to identify cases increases the test's sensitivity and decreases its specificity. Referring to Figure 1, when the cutoff score (above which individuals are designated cases and below which they are classified as noncases) is lowered, some persons in cells c and d of the 2 × 2 matrix will be redistributed into

Disease/Diagnosis

		Present	Absent	Total
	Positive	a	b	a + b
Test				
	Negative	c	d	c + d
	Total	a + c	b + d	a + b + c + d

Figure 1   Presentation of test data. Sensitivity = a/a + c; specificity = d/b + d; positive predictive value = a/a + b; negative predictive value = d/c + d.

cells a and b, respectively. Sensitivity (a/a + c) increases because cell a increases while the sum of a + c remains the same (the true disease prevalence is unaffected by the test threshold). Analogously, specificity (d/b + d) decreases when the threshold is lowered because d decreases and b + d remains the same.

2. Raising the test threshold to identify cases decreases the test's sensitivity and increases its specificity. Following the same logic as above, when the threshold to identify cases increases, sensitivity decreases because the size of cell a decreases (while a + c remains the same) and specificity increases because d increases (while b + d remains the same).

3. A test's positive predictive value is higher in samples where disease prevalence is greater. This postulate assumes that test sensitivity and specificity are fixed across samples and independent of prevalence. Consider two studies with samples of equal size but different illness prevalence rates. If test sensitivity (a/a + c) is to remain constant, then in the sample with the higher prevalence rate (a + c) both cells a and c must be greater. Likewise, for specificity (d/b + d) to remain constant, when wellness (b + d) decreases then both cells b and d must be lower. Positive predictive value (a/a + b) is greater in the sample with a higher prevalence rate because b is smaller. Vecchio and Baldessarini et al. (99,103) illustrated the direct relationship between positive predictive value and prevalence.

4. A test's negative predictive value is higher in samples where disease prevalence is lower. When disease prevalence (a + c) decreases, for sensitivity (a/a + c) to remain constant, both a and c must decrease. Specificity (d/b + d) will remain constant when more individuals are not ill (b + d) only when b and d both increase. Negative predictive value (d/c + d) is higher in samples with lower rates of disorder because c is smaller.

In studies of the ability of self-report scales to identify depressed individuals, investigators have manipulated both disease prevalence and questionnaire thresholds to identify cases. Disease prevalence is not usually considered to be under the control of the investigator. However, in the study of depression, prevalence is a function of the number of disorders considered under the depression rubric. Most investigators included only major depressive disorder. However, some used a broader definition and included dysthymic disorder, atypical depression (depressive disorder not otherwise specified), minor depression, and adjustment disorder with depressed mood.

HOW EFFECTIVE ARE SCREENING INSTRUMENTS?

Most studies of screening have examined the performance of scales detecting depressive or alcohol use disorders. Mulrow et al. (104) recently summarized the results of 18 studies conducted in primary care settings of the utility of self-administered questionnaires for detecting depression. Across all 18 studies, involving more than 15,000 patients, the overall sensitivity for detecting major depression was 84% and the overall specificity was 72%. Screening for alcohol abuse/dependence can achieve sensitivity and specificity levels comparable to those for depression (see Ref. 105 for a specific discussion of screening performance of certain instruments).

Up until recently almost all studies of screening instruments focused on one disorder. In 1994, Zimmerman and colleagues (11) published an article questioning the practice of screening only for a single psychiatric disorder. They suggested that because comorbidity among psychiatric disorders is high, screening efforts limited to only one disorder such as depression might be too narrow. In their study, 508 medical outpatients completed a broad-based self-administered questionnaire that screens for DSM disorders in five domains—eating, depressive, anxiety, substance, and somatoform disorders. As predicted, 85% of the patients who screened positive for depression also screened positive for a nondepressive disorder. Moreover, compared with patients who only screened positive for depression, patients who screened positive for both depression and a nondepressive disorder rated their physical and emotional health more poorly and made more visits to the doctor. A limitation of their study was the failure to validate the screening measure against research diagnostic interviews.

Since then two other research groups have published multidimensional screening instruments that simultaneously assess several DSM disorders. Spitzer and colleagues developed the PRIME-MD (10), and Broadhead (9) and Weissman and colleagues (106) developed the SDDS.

Both systems have two components—a brief self-administered questionnaire that is followed up by a clinician administered semi-structured interview to make a diagnosis. The brief questionnaire is conceptualized as a screening tool to alert the clinician to which interview modules to administer. In the PRIME-MD study (10) the diagnostic efficiency statistics for the screening instrument were presented for broad categories of mood, anxiety, alcohol, and eating disorders rather than specific diagnoses. Only the alcohol scale had a specificity above 90%, and the specificity for detecting any disorder was 48%. Three of the scales had sensitivities above 80% (alcohol—81%; anxiety—94%; eating—86%), whereas the specificity for mood disorder was 69%. Recently, Whooley et al. (107) examined the test characteristics of the two-question PRIME-MD depression screen in 536 medical outpatients who were interviewed with the Diagnostic Interview Schedule. The sensitivity of the two-question screen was excellent (96%) but the specificity was poor (57%). Overall, though, the two-question PRIME-MD screen did almost as well as longer instruments.

The screening questionnaire component of the SDDS began as a 62-item measure that covered alcohol abuse/dependence, generalized anxiety disorder, major depression, obsessive-compulsive disorder, panic disorder, suicidal ideation, agoraphobia, drug abuse, social phobia, and somatization. After the initial validity study the scale was abbreviated to a 16-item version, and agoraphobia, drug abuse, social phobia, and somatization were eliminated because the sensitivities and positive predictive values of the screen questions were low (9). (The authors did not report the results for these four disorders. It was unclear, however, why the generalized anxiety and obsessive-compulsive disorder scales were retained because their positive predictive values were below 10% in both the derivation and cross-validation studies.) A year later this group published a cross-validation study of a revised 26-item screening questionnaire covering the same six disorders covered by the 16-item scale plus drug dependence (108). The sensitivities of the scales ranged from 50% (drug dependence) to 80% (suicidal ideation), and the positive predictive values ranged from 15% (obsessive-compulsive disorder) to 75% (suicidal ideation).

The initial results in these studies of the screening questionnaire components of these new broad-based screening instruments are hopeful, albeit modest. It is our belief that it is not possible for a scale to screen for so many disorders with so few items and achieve both good sensitivity and specificity for every diagnosis-specific subscale. A minimum of four or five items is probably necessary for a subscale to achieve adequate diagnostic properties, and more items (up to a limit) should improve a scale's screening performance. Scale developers have to strike a balance between scale length, which if too long may not be practical for clinical utility, and reliability and validity. Multidimensional screening scales should also be subject to rigorous psychometric analyses including assessments of internal consistency, test-retest reliability, and discriminant and convergent validity. Neither the PRIME-MD nor the SDDS screening scales have been examined in this way.

DOES SCREENING IMPROVE CASE DETECTION?

Nine controlled studies have examined the impact of informing primary care physicians of the results of a mental health screening measure on case detection or treatment. Johnstone and Goldberg (109) administered the General Health Questionnaire (GHQ) to nearly 1100 patients in Dr. Johnstone's practice and found that knowledge of GHQ results increased the frequency of psychiatric treatment and consultation.

Moore and colleagues (110) notified family practice residents of their patients' results on the Zung Self-Rated Depression Scale (SDS) (111). If a patient scored above 50 on the SDS, a note was placed in half of the patients' charts indicating that the patient screened positive for depression. The control subjects had a note placed in their chart indicating that they had been screened, but the results of the screening were withheld. Feedback of the screening results more than doubled the recognition of depression noted in the patients' charts (from 22% to 56%).

Linn and Yager (112) conducted a study similar to that of Moore et al. (110) and also found that screening increased detection of depression as determined by physician chart notation. There was a nonsignificant increase in the frequency of treatment for depression in the feedback group.

Two other studies that used the SDS found that feedback significantly increased the detection of depression (113,114), whereas two studies using the GHQ failed to find evidence of improved detection (115,116). Magruder-Habib and colleagues (113) found that increased detection of depression was associated with increased depression treatment.

In the only study focusing on anxiety disorders, Mathias et al. (117) found that screening feedback increased recognition and treatment of anxiety. And in the only study of the new generation of multidimensional measures, the influence of types of staff support on implementation of the PRIME-MD assessment tool was examined in more than 2000 patients attending the general medicine clinic at a Veterans Affairs Medical Center (118). When support staff were given responsibility for distributing and collecting the screening questionnaire and putting it in patients' charts, more patients were newly diagnosed with psychiatric disorders and providers were more likely to intervene for a psychiatric condition.

In sum, screening increased detection in seven of nine studies. The only two negative studies used nonspecific measures of symptoms, whereas all six studies using assessments of specific symptom domains found that screening improved case detection. Thus, measures that are more closely tied to specific diagnostic syndromes such as depression and anxiety might have a greater likelihood of modifying physician behavior.

DOES SCREENING IMPROVE OUTCOME?

Regular screening can be recommended only if it improves clinical outcomes (i.e., reduced symptom levels, improved functioning, or improved quality of life) or reduces health care costs. If undetected pathology is resistant to treatment or resolves spontaneously without treatment, then screening might improve recognition and increase treatment delivery yet not improve outcome. Five controlled studies have examined the impact of screening on symptoms, functioning, or general health care utilization.

In the Johnstone and Goldberg study (109) patients completed the GHQ at the index visit and at 3-month intervals for a year. For half the patients the results of the GHQ were revealed to the practitioner. The authors found that patients whose high GHQ scores were known had a better outcome than patients whose high GHQ scores were kept hidden.

Zung and colleagues (114) administered the SDS to 1086 family practice patients who had not been previously diagnosed with depression. Two thirds of the patients who screened positive were identified to the family physician, and one third was not. Outcome was examined in three groups: patients who were identified and treated, patients who were identified but not treated, and patients who were not identified to the primary care physician. One month after the index visit 64% of the identified treated patients had improved, in contrast to 28% of the identified untreated and 18% of the unidentified patients.

Magruder-Habib et al. (113) attempted to replicate Zung et al.'s study (114) in a Veterans Affairs medical center. They used the same depression scale and reassessed patients 3, 6, 9, and 12 months after the index visit. As noted above, notification of the patients' depression score increased detection and treatment of depression, but there was no difference in depression symptom levels at the follow-up assessments.

Mathias and coworkers (117) studied the impact of screening for anxiety (but not specific anxiety disorders) on outcome and found that informing primary care physicians about anxiety levels significantly increased the number of patients who reported improvement in anxiety symptoms and functional status 5 months after the index visit. Identified patients were also significantly more likely to report that their physicians spent more time with them talking about their feelings. No differences between the groups were found on questionnaire assessments of anxiety and functional status.

Finally, Reifler et al. (119) administered the 16-item SDDS to 358 patients of two internal medicine practices. One group of physicians received the results of the screening and was given the SDDS second-stage diagnostic modules to administer. The other group of physicians was not informed of the screening findings. At baseline and 3-month follow-up patients completed the SF-36, the SDS, the Sheehan anxiety scale, and questionnaire assessments of satisfaction with care and health care utilization. Interestingly, physician compliance with the diagnostic interview modules was a modest 55%. Physicians were much more likely to administer the depression module (76.4%) than the general anxiety (52.3%), panic disorder (45.7%), substance abuse (25.0%), and obsessive-compulsive disorder (32.0%) modules. Patients in the experimental group used significantly fewer health care resources during the follow-up interval than the patients in the control group. Specifically, experimental group patients made fewer outpatient visits to non–mental health clinicians (there was no difference in visits to mental health professionals), received fewer x-rays, and were less likely to be hospitalized. There were no differences between the groups on the measures of symptoms, functioning, and patient satisfaction.

So, how does one interpret these studies? Different authors have come to varying conclusions when reviewing this literature. Higgins (120) discounted the study by Johnstone and Goldberg (109) because it included only one physician, and he minimized the significance of the study of Zung and colleagues (114) because the follow-up interval was too short (4 weeks). Higgins (120) consequently concluded that "no large study of notification to physicians of patients' psychiatric symptoms had a positive outcome." Reifler and colleagues (119), in the discussion of their paper, concluded "the evidence is mixed regarding improvements in patient function, with some studies showing improvement and some showing no change." Finally, Leon and colleagues (108), after alluding to this literature, recommended the routine screening of all primary care patients for mental health problems.

Certainly mental health screening does not have a profound effect on outcome; however, a profound effect perhaps should not be expected. Although primary care physicians underdiagnose major depression by 50%, it is important to remember that appropriate recognition is being made in 50% of patients. Thus, at best, screening will improve outcome by a factor of two. Other factors that need to be taken into consideration is that treatment for depression results in improvement rates of approximately 75%, that a percentage of patients who are untreated improve without treatment, and that even when screen positive cases are brought to the attention of the primary care physician, many will not be adequately treated. Figure 2 illustrates the potential effect of screening on the outcome of depression. An analysis of the potential impact on

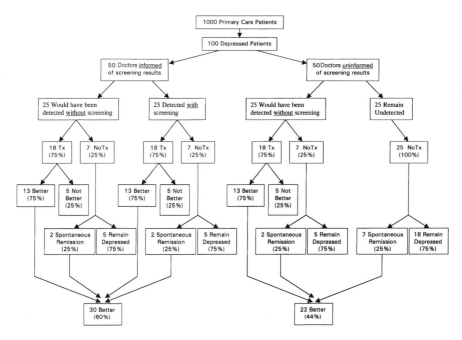

Figure 2 Potential benefit of screening. Tx = treated; NoTx = untreated.

outcome of screening is based on estimates of four parameters: frequency of disorder underdetection in routine clinical practice, likelihood of a positive treatment outcome when adequate levels of treatment are delivered, likelihood that adequate treatment will be administered upon recognition, and spontaneous remission rate. Based on some estimates of these parameters, we found that mental health screening will improve outcome by only about 15%.

In the model it is estimated that 50% of individuals with major depression are detected without the benefit of a screening program. The research supporting this estimate is reviewed above. Second, adequate treatment for depression is estimated to result in a 75% improvement rate. Third, it is estimated that primary care providers, upon recognizing major depression, will provide adequate care in 75% of patients. This may be an overly generous estimate of treatment adequacy. Several studies have questioned the adequacy of treatment provided by primary care providers (121–123), though these studies were conducted before the widespread use of the selective serotonin-reuptake inhibitors (SSRIs). Because of the relative simplicity and safety of prescribing the SSRIs, it is more likely that pharmacotherapy will achieve minimally acceptable standards. It should be realized that if our estimate is high, then we have overestimated the potential impact of screening. (For example, if only 40% of depressed primary care patients received adequate treatment, then the improvement rates in the informed and uninformed groups would drop to 44% and 36%, respectively.) Finally, we estimated a 25% spontaneous remission rate. This estimate may be too low. Studies of the untreated course of depression in medical patients have demonstrated significant levels of improvement (79,124–127). Again, if we underestimated the spontaneous remission rate, this would result in our overestimating the potential benefit of screening. (For example, if the spontaneous remission rate estimate were increased to 50%, then the improvement rates in the informed and uninformed groups would be 66% and 58%, respectively.) Another important factor not included in our model is the difference between depressed patients who are and are not detected in routine clinical practice. Depressed patients who are detected by the primary care provider are more severely ill than the depressed patients who are undetected (22,62,124,128), and milder symptom severity may be associated with a greater response to placebo (and possibly a greater spontaneous remission rate).

Our analysis suggests that the impact of screening will not be robust; consequently, it will be important to use sensitive research methods to detect these differences. Compared to the methods used in longitudinal studies in the psychiatry literature, the methods used in follow-up studies of the impact of screening interventions in primary care have been relatively crude. Outcome evaluations in primary care follow-up studies are usually cross-sectional, assessing symptoms and functioning at a single time point, rather than longitudinal, in which the outcome variables are assessed over the entire follow-up interval. Because disorders such as depression often remit without treatment, the beneficial effect of screening and improved detection might be to shorten the length of the depressive episode rather than increase the long-term remission rate. It is noteworthy that the most robust demonstration of the beneficial impact of screening for depression was found in a study that assessed outcome 4 weeks after the index visit. A cross-sectional outcome evaluation 6 or 12 months after a randomized screening trial would not detect differences in symptom levels, days missed from work, work efficiency, and quality of life during the first month or two after patients were screened.

CONCLUSIONS

Substance use and other mental disorders are highly prevalent in medical patients, result in significant morbidity and economic cost, and are treatable. Primary care physicians do not identify a large percentage of patients with these disorders. It is therefore reasonable to expect that the use of sensitive and specific screening instruments would uncover hidden psychiatric disorders, increase case detection, thereby improving outcomes. Our review of the literature suggests that the routine use of screening instruments improves outcome in primary care patients, albeit modestly. More than a modest effect should perhaps not be expected.

Much needed are longitudinal studies of the impact of screening that use measures such as the Longitudinal Interval Follow-up Evaluation (129) to comprehensively track the course of symptomatology, psychosocial functioning, and health services utilization. It is reasonable to hypothesize that the impact of screening will be to reduce the duration of symptoms rather than the long-term recovery rate because psychiatric disorders such as major depression often remit spontaneously. Just as it would be inappropriate to examine the impact of screening on the outcome of headache by conducting a cross-sectional follow-up assessment one month after the screening, it may be inappropriate to limit the assessment of outcome of depression to 6 or 12 months after screening.

Naturalistic follow-up studies have shown that the outcome of detected and undetected patients differs little; however, this is not inconsistent with data suggesting that screening improves outcome. The outcome of undetected psychopathology is heterogeneous; improved detection could alter the natural history of those patients whose symptoms would not remit spontaneously. Perhaps screening will improve the outcome of only 1% of all patients screened, and only 10% of patients who are cases. The incremental degree of improvement in outcome necessary to justify routine screening is a value judgment. We leave it to others to judge if this is a sufficiently large enough effect size to pursue.

REFERENCES

1. Zimmerman M, Coryell W. The Inventory to Diagnose Depression (IDD): A self-report scale to diagnose major depressive disorder. J Consulting Clin Psychol 1987; 55:55–59.
2. Norton GR, Dorward J, Cox BJ. Factors associated with panic attacks in nonclinical subjects. Behav Ther 1986; 17:239–252.
3. Selzer ML. The Michigan Alcoholism Screening Test: the quest for a new diagnostic instrument. Am J Psychiatry 1971; 127:1653–1658.
4. Foa EB, Riggs DS, Dancu CV, Rothbaum BO. Reliability and validity of a brief instrument for assessing post-traumatic stress disorder. J Traumatic Stress 1993; 6:459–473.
5. Depue RA, Krauss S, Spoont MR, Arbisi P. General behavior inventory identification of unipolar and bipolar affective conditions in a nonclinical university population. J Abnorm Psychol 1989; 98:117–126.
6. Thelan MH, Farmer J, Wonderlich S, Smith M. A revision of the Bulimia Test: The BULIT-R. Psychological Assessment. J Consulting Clin Psychol 1991; 3:119–124.
7. Hyler SE, Rieder RD, Williams JBW, Spitzer RL, Hendler J, Lyons M. The Personality Diagnostic Questionnaire: development and preliminary results. J Personality Disorders 1988; 2:229–237.
8. Goldberg DP. The Detection of Psychiatric Illness by Questionnaire: A Technique for the Identification and Assessment of Nonpsychotic Psychiatric Illness. London: Oxford University Press, 1972.
9. Broadhead WE, Leon AC, Weissman MM, Barrett JE, Blacklow RS, Gilbert TT, Keller MB, Olfson M, Higgins ES. Development and validation of the SDDS-PC screen for multiple mental disorders in primary care. Arch Fam Med 1995; 4:211–219.
10. Spitzer RL, Williams JB, Kroenke K, Linzer M, DeGruy III FV, Hahn SR. Utility of a new procedure for diagnosing mental disorders in primary care. The PRIME-MD 1000 study. JAMA 1994; 272:1759–1756.

11. Zimmerman M, Lish JD, Farber NJ, Hartung J, Lush D, Kuzma MA, Plescia G. Screening for depression in medical patients: Is the focus too narrow? Gen Hosp Psychiatry 1994; 16:388–396.

12. Wilson JMG, Jungner G. Principles and Practice of Screening for Disease. Geneva: World Health Organization, 1968.

13. Coulehan JL, Schulberg HC, Block MR. The efficiency of depression questionnaires for case finding in primary medical care. J Gen Intern Med 1989; 4:541–547.

14. Hoeper EE, Nycz GR, Cleary PD, Regier DA, Goldberg ID. Estimated prevalence of RDC mental disorder in primary medical care. Int J Mental Health 1979; 8:6–15.

15. Spitzer RL, Endicott J, Robins E. Research diagnostic criteria: rationale and reliability. Arch Gen Psychiatry 1978; 35:773–782.

16. Schulberg HC, Burns BJ. Mental disorders in primary care: epidemiologic, diagnostic, and treatment research directions. Gen Hosp Psychiatry 1987; 10:79–87.

17. Kessler RC, McGonagle KA, Zhao S. Lifetime and 12-month prevalence of DSM-III-R psychiatric disorders in the United States: results from the National Comorbidity Survey. Arch Gen Psychiatry 1994; 51:8–19.

18. Robins LN, Locke BZ, Regier DA. An overview of psychiatric disorders in America. In: Robins LN, Regier DA, eds. Psychiatric Disorders in America: The Epidemiologic Catchment Study. New York: The Free Press, 1991; 13:328–386.

19. Philbrick JT, Connelly JE, Wofford AB. The prevalence of mental disorders in rural office practice. J Gen Intern Med 1996; 11:9–15.

20. Leon AC, Olfson M, Broadhead WE, Barrett JE, Blacklow RS, Keller MB, Higgins ES, Weissman MM. Prevalence of mental disorders in primary care. Arch Fam Med 1995; 4:857–861.

21. Docherty JP. Barriers to the diagnosis of depression in primary care. J Clin Psychiatry 1997; 58(suppl):5–10.

22. Schwenk TL, Coyne JC, Fechner-Bates S. Differences between detected and undetected patients in primary care and depressed psychiatric patients. Gen Hosp Psychiatry 1996; 18:407–415.

23. Beresford TP, Blow FC, Hill E, Singer K, Lucey MR. Comparison of CAGE questionnaire and computer-assisted laboratory profiles in screening for covert alcoholism. Lancet 1990; 336:482–485.

24. Cleary PD, Miller M, Booker T. Prevalence and recognition of alcohol abuse in a primary care population. Am J Med 1988; 85:466–471.

25. Isaacson JH, Butler R, Zacharek M, Tzelepis A. Screening with the Alcohol Use Disorders Identification Test (AUDIT) in an inner-city population. J Gen Intern Med 1994; 9: 550–553.

26. Jones TV, Lindsey BA, Yount P, Soltys R, Farani-Enayat B. Alcoholism screening questionnaires: Are they valid in elderly medical outpatients? J Intern Gen Med 1993; 8:674–678.

27. Schorling JB, Klas PT, Willems JP, Everett AS. Addressing alcohol use among primary care patients: differences between family medicine and internal medicine residents. J Gen Intern Med 1994; 9:248–254.

28. Arolt V, Driessen M. Alcoholism and psychiatric comorbidity in general hospital inpatients. Gen Hosp Psychiatry 1996; 18:271–277.

29. Curtis JR, Geller G, Stokes EJ, Levine DM, Moore RD. Characteristics, diagnosis, and treatment of alcoholism in elderly patients. J Am Geriatr Soc 1989; 37:310–316.

30. Mayou R, Hawton K. Psychiatric disorder in the general hospital. Br J Psychiatry 1986; 149:172–190.
31. Moore RD, Bone LR, Geller G, Mamon JA, Stokes EJ, Levine DM. Prevalence, detection, and treatment of alcoholism in hospitalized patients. JAMA 1989; 261:403–407.
32. Sherin KM, Piotrowski ZH, Panek SM, Doot MC. Screening for alcoholism in a community hospital. J Fam Practice 1982; 15:1091–1095.
33. Smals GLM, van der Mast R. Alcohol abuse among general hospital inpatients according to the Munich Alcoholism Test (MALT). Gen Hosp Psychiatry 1994; 16:125–130.
34. Buchsbaum DG, Buchanan RG, Poses RM, Schnoll SH, Lawton MJ. Physician detection of drinking problems in patients attending a general medicine practice. J Gen Intern Med 1992; 7:517–521.
35. Johnson JG, Spitzer RL, Williams JBW, Linzer M, deGruy F, Kroenke K, Brody D, Hahn S. Psychiatric comorbidity, health status, and functional impairment associated with alcohol abuse and dependence in primary care patients: findings of the PRIME MD-1000 study. J Consulting Clin Psychol 1995; 63:133–140.
36. Broadhead WE, Blazer DG, George LK, Tse CK. Depression, disability days, and days lost from work in a prospective epidemiologic survey. JAMA 1990; 264:2524–2528.
37. Olfson M, Fireman B, Weissman MM, Leon AC, Sheehan DV, Kathol RG, Hoven C, Farber L. Mental disorders and disability among patients in a primary care group practice. Am J Psychiatry 1997; 154:1734–1740.
38. Marcus SC, Olfson M, Pincus HA, Shear MK, Zarin DA. Self-reported anxiety, general medical conditions, and disability bed days. Am J Psychiatry 1997; 154:1766–1768.
39. Coulehan JL, Schulberg HC, Block MR, Madonia MJ, Rodriguez E. Treating depressed primary care patients improves their physical, mental, and social functioning. Arch Intern Med 1997; 157:1113–1120.
40. Sherborne CD, Wells KB, Meredith LS, Jackson CA, Camp P. Comorbid anxiety disorder and the functioning and well-being of chronically ill patients of general medical providers. Arch Gen Psychiatry 1996; 53:889–895.
41. Hays RD, Wells KB, Sherbourne CD, Rogers W, Spritzer K. Functioning and well-being outcomes of patients with depression compared with chronic general medical illnesses. Arch Gen Psychiatry 1995; 52:11–19.
42. Schonfeld WH, Verboncoeur CJ, Fifer SK, Lipschutz RC, Lubeck DP. The functioning and well-being of patients with unrecognized anxiety disorders and major depressive disorder. J Affect Disord 1997; 43:105–119.
43. Wells KB, Stewart A, Hayes RD, Burnam MA, Rogers W, Daniels M, Berry S, Greenfield S, Ware J. The functioning and well-being of depressed patients: results from the Medical Outcomes Study. JAMA 1989; 262:914–919.
44. Bijur PE, Kurzon M, Overpeck MD, Scheidt PC. Parental alcohol use, problem drinking, and children's injuries. JAMA 1992; 267:3166–3171.
45. Koenig HG, Shelp F, Goli V, Cohen HJ, Blazer DG. Survival and health care utilization in elderly medical inpatients with major depression. J Geriatr Soc 1989; 37:599–606.
46. Simonsick EM, Wallace RB, Blazer DG, Berkman LF. Depressive symptomatology and hypertension-associated morbidity and mortality in older adults. Psychosom Med 1995; 57:427–435.
47. Wassertheil-Smoller S, Applegate WB, Berge K, Chang CJ, Davis BR, Grimm Jr. R, Kostis J, Pressel S, Schron E. Change in depression as a precursor of cardiovascular events. Arch Intern Med 1996; 156:553–561.

48. Jonas BS, Franks P, Ingram DD. Are symptoms of anxiety and depression risk factors for hypertension? Longitudinal evidence from the National Health and Nutrition Examination Survey I Epidemiologic Follow-up Study. Arch Fam Med 1997; 6:43–49.

49. Frasure-Smith N, Lespérance F, Talajic M. Depression following myocardial infarction. JAMA 1993; 270:1819–1825.

50. Lespérance F, Frasure-Smith N, Talajic M. Major depression before and after myocardial infarction: Its nature and consequences. Psychosom Med 1996; 58:99–110.

51. Levine JB, Covino NA, Slack WV, Safran C, Safran DB, Boro JE, Davis RB, Buchanan GM, Gervino EV. Psychological predictors of subsequent medical care among patients hospitalized with cardiac disease. J Cardiopulmonary Rehabil 1996; 16:109–116.

52. Morris PLP, Robinson RG, Andrzejewski P, Samuels J, Price TR. Association of depression with 10-year poststroke mortality. Am J Psychiatry 1993; 150:124–129.

53. Dunham NC, Sager MA. Functional status, symptoms of depression, and the outcomes of hospitalization in community-dwelling elderly patients. Arch Fam Med 1994; 3:676–681.

54. Mayne TJ, Vittinghoff E, Chesney MA, Barrett DC, Coates TJ. Depressive affect and survival among gay and bisexual men infected with HIV. Arch Intern Med 1996; 156:2233–2238.

55. Silverstone PH. Depression increases mortality and morbidity in acute life-threatening medical illness. J Psychosom Res 1990; 34:651–657.

56. Johnson J, Weissman MM, Klerman GL. Service utilization and social morbidity associated with depressive symptoms in the community. JAMA 1992; 267:1478–1483.

57. Uldall KK, Koutsky LA, Bradshaw DH, Hopkins SG, Katon W, Lafferty WE. Psychiatric comorbidity and length of stay in hospitalized AIDS patients. Am J Psychiatry 1994; 151:1475–1478.

58. Greenberg PE, Stiglin LE, Finkelstein SN, Berndt ER. The economic burden of depression in 1990. J Clin Psychiatry 1993; 54:405–417.

59. Greenberg PE, Stiglin LE, Finkelstein SN, Berndt ER. Depression: a neglected major illness. J Clin Psychiatry 1993; 54:419–423.

60. Reiger DA, Narrow WE, Rae DS, Manderscheid RW, Locke BZ, Goodwin FK. The de facto US mental and addictive disorders service system: epidemiological Catchment Area prospective 1-year prevalence rates of disorders and services. Arch Gen Psychiatry 1993; 50:85–94.

61. Simon G, Ormel J, VonKorff M, Barlow W. Health care costs associated with depressive and anxiety disorders in primary care. Am J Psychiatry 1995; 152:352–357.

62. Simon G, VonKorff M, Barlow W. Health care costs of primary care patients with recognized depression. Arch Gen Psychiatry 1995; 52:850–856.

63. Unützer J, Patrick DL, Simon G, Grembowski D, Walker E, Rutter C, Katon W. Depressive symptoms and the cost of health services in HMO patients aged 65 years and older. JAMA 1997; 277:1618–1623.

64. Salvador-Carulla L, Seguí J, Fernández-Cano P, Canet J. Costs and offset effect in panic disorders. Br J Psychiatry 1995; 166:23–28.

65. DuPont RL, Rice DP, Miller LS, Shiraki SS, Rowland CR, Harwood HJ. Economic costs of anxiety disorders. Anxiety 1996; 2:167–172.

66. Jackson CA, Manning Jr. WG, Wells KB. Impact of prior and current alcohol use on use of services by patients with depression and chronic medical illnesses. Health Serv Res 1995; 30:687–705.

67. Rivara FP, Koepsell TD, Jurkovich GJ, Gurney JG, Soderberg R. The effects of alcohol abuse on readmission for trauma. JAMA 1993; 270:1962–1964.
68. Heien DM, Pittman DJ. The external costs of alcohol abuse. J Stud Alcohol 1993; 54: 302–307.
69. Brown C, Schulberg HC, Madonia MJ, Shear KM, Houck PR. Treatment outcomes for primary care patients with major depression and lifetime anxiety disorders. Am J Psychiatry 1996; 153:1293–1300.
70. Cohen-Cole SA, Kaufman KG. Major depression in physical illness: diagnosis, prevalence, and antidepressant treatment (a ten year review: 1982–1992). Depression 1993; 1:181–204.
71. Rickels K, Schweizer E, Clary C, Fox I, Weise C. Nefazodone and imipramine in major depression: a placebo-controlled trial. Br J Psychiatry 1994; 164:802–805.
72. Borson S, McDonald GJ, Gayle T, Deffebach M, Lakshminarayan S, Van Tuinen C. Improvement in mood, physical symptoms, and function with nortriptyline for depression in patients with chronic obstructive pulmonary disease. Psychosomatics 1992; 33:190–201.
73. Lustman PJ, Griffith LS, Clouse RE, Freedland KE, Eisen SA, Rubin EH, Carney RH, McGill JB. Effects of nortriptyline on depression and glycemic control in diabetes: results of a double-blind, placebo-controlled test. Psychosomatics 1997; 59:241–250.
74. vanHeeringen K, Zivkov M. Pharmacological treatment of depression in cancer patients. A placebo-controlled study of mianserin. Br J Psychiatry 1996; 169:440–443.
75. Anderson G, Vestergaard K, Lauritzen L. Effective treatment of poststroke depression with the selective serotonin reuptake inhibitor citalopram. Stroke 1994; 25:1099–1104.
76. Miranda J, Munoz R. Intervention for minor depression in primary care patients. Psychosom Med 1994; 56:136–142.
77. Mynors-Wallis LM, Gath DH, Lloyd-Thomas AR, Tomlinson D. Randomised controlled trial comparing problem solving treatment with amitriptyline and placebo for major depression in primary care. Br Med J 1995; 310:441–445.
78. Lynch DJ, Tamburrino MB, Nagel R. Telephone counseling for patients with minor depression: preliminary findings in a family practice setting. J Fam Practice 1997; 44: 293–298.
79. Schulberg HC, Block MR, Madonia MJ, Scott CP, Rodriguez E, Imber SD, Perel J, Lave J, Houck PR, Coulehan JL. Treating major depression in primary care practice. Arch Gen Psychiatry 1996; 53:913–919.
80. Fleming MF, Barry KL, Manwell LB, Johnson K, London R. Brief physician advice for problem alcohol drinkers: a randomized controlled trial in community-based primary care practices. JAMA 1997; 277:1039–1045.
81. Scott E, Anderson P. Randomized controlled trial of general practitioner intervention in women with excessive alcohol consumption. Drug Alcohol Rev 1990; 10:311–322.
82. Wallace R, Cutler S, Haines A. Randomized controlled trial of general practitioner intervention in patients with excessive alcohol consumptions. Br Med J 1988; 297:663–668.
83. Feldman W. How serious are the adverse effects of screening? J Gen Intern Med 1990; 5(suppl):S50–S53.
84. Orleans CT, George LK, Houpt JL, Brodie HKH. How primary care physicians treat psychiatric disorders: a national survey of family practitioners. Am J Psychiatry 1985; 142:52–57.
85. Main DS, Lutz LJ, Barrett JE. The role of primary care clinician attitudes, beliefs, and

training in the diagnosis and treatment of depression: a report from the Ambulatory Sentinel Practice Network Inc. Arch Fam Med 1993; 2:1061–1066.

86. Reynolds RD. Practice commentary. Arch Fam Med 1993; 1993:84.
87. Rost K, Smith GR, Matthews DB, Guise B. The deliberate misdiagnosis of major depression in primary care. Arch Fam Med 1994; 3:333–337.
88. Frowick B, Shank JC, Doherty WJ, Powell TA. What do patients really want? Redefining a behavioral science curriculum for family physicians. J Fam Practice 1986; 23:
141–146.
89. Brody DS, Khaliq AA, Thompson TL. Patients' perspectives on the management of emotional distress in primary care settings. J Gen Intern Med 1997; 12:403–406.
90. Clark CH, Schewenk TL, Plackis CX. Patients' perspectives of behavioral science care by
family practice physicians. J Med Educ 1983; 58:954–961.
91. Hansen JP, Bobula J, Meyer D, Kusher K, Pridham K. Treat or refer: patients' interest
in family physician involvement in their psychosocial problems. J Fam Practice 1987; 24:
499–503.
92. Schwenk TL, Clark CH, Jones GR, Simmons RC, Coleman ML. Defining behavioral
science curriculum for family physicians: What do patients think? J Fam Practice 1982;
15:339–345.
93. Zimmerman M, Farber NJ, Hartung J, Lush DT, Kuzma MA. Screening for psychiatric
disorders in medical patients: a feasibility and patient acceptance study. Med Care 1994;
32:603–608.
94. Zimmerman M, Lush DT, Farber NJ, Hartung J, Plescia G, Kuzma MA, Lish J. Primary
care patients' reactions to mental health screening. Int J Psychiatry Med 1996; 26:431–
441.
95. Zimmerman M, Horowitz B, Mattia J. Patient Acceptance and Physician Reluctance to
Screen for Psychiatric Disorders in Primary Care. Association for the Advancement of
Behavior Therapy, New York, 1996.
96. Williamson P, Beitman BD, Katon W. Beliefs that foster physician avoidance of psychosocial aspects of health care. J Fam Practice 1981; 13:999–1003.
97. Bertakis KD, Roter D, Putnam SM. The relationship of physician medical interview style
to patient satisfaction. J Fam Practice 1981; 32:175–181.
98. Brody DS, Miller SM, Lerman CE, Smith DG, Lazaro CG, Blum MJ. The relationship
between patients' satisfaction with their physicians and perceptions about interventions
they desired and received. Med Care 1989; 27:1027–1035.
99. Baldessarini RJ, Finklestein S, Arana GW. The predictive power of diagnostic tests and
the effect of prevalence of illness. Arch Gen Med 1983; 40:569–573.
100. Glaros AG, Kline RB. The sensitivity, specificity, and predictive value model. J Clin Psychol 1988; 44:1013–1023.
101. Griner PF, Mayewski RJ, Mushlin AI, Greenland P. Selection and interpretation of diagnostic tests and procedures: principles and applications. Ann Intern Med 1981; 94:553–
600.
102. Kessel JB, Zimmerman M. Reporting errors in studies of the diagnostic performance of
self-administered questionnaires: extent of the problem, recommendations for standardized presentation of results, and implications for the peer review process. Psychol Assess
1993; 5:395–399.
103. Vecchio TJ. Predictive value of a single diagnostic test in unselected populations. N Engl
J Med 1966; 274:1171–1173.

104. Mulrow CD, Williams JW, Gerety MB, Ramirez G, Montiel OM, Kerber C. Case-finding instruments for depression in primary care settings. Ann Intern Med 1995; 122:913–921.

105. Bohn MJ, Babor TF, Kranzler HR. The Alcohol Use Disorders Identification Test (AUDIT): validation of a screening instrument for use in medical settings. J Stud Alcohol 1995; 56:423–432.

106. Weissman MM, Olfson M, Leon AC, Broadhead WE, Gilbert TT, Higgins ES, Barrett JE, Blacklow RS, Keller MB, Hoven C. Brief diagnostic interviews (SDDS-PC) for multiple mental disorders in primary care: a pilot study. Arch Fam Med 1995; 4:220–227.

107. Whooley MA, Alvins AL, Miranda J, Browner WS. Case-finding instruments for depression. J Gen Intern Med 1997; 12:439–445.

108. Leon AC, Olfson M, Weissman MM, Portera L, Fireman BH, Blacklow RS, Hoven C, Broadhead WE. Brief screens for mental disorders in primary care. J Gen Intern Med 1996; 11:426–430.

109. Johnstone A, Goldberg D. Psychiatric screening in general practice: a controlled trial. Lancet 1976; i:605–608.

110. Moore JT, Silimperi DR, Bobula JA. Recognition of depression by family medicine residents: the impact of screening. J Fam Practice 1978; 7:509–513.

111. Zung WWK. A self-rating depression scale. Arch Gen Psychiatry 1965; 12:63–70.

112. Linn LS, Yager J. Recognition of depression and anxiety by primary physicians. Psychosomatics 1984; 24:593–600.

113. Magruder-Habib K, Zung WWK, Feussner J, Alling C, Saunders WB, Stevens HA. Management of general medical patients with symptoms of depression. Gen Hosp Psychiatry 1989; 11:201–207.

114. Zung WWK, Magill M, Moore JT, George DT. Recognition and treatment of depression in a family medicine practice. J Clin Psychiatry 1983; 44:3–6.

115. Hoeper EW, Nycz GR, Kessler LG, Burke JJ, Pierce WE. The usefulness of screening for mental illness. Lancet 1984; i:33–35.

116. Shapiro S, German PS, Skinner EA, VonKorff M, Turner RW, Klein LE, Teitelbaum ML, Kramer M, Burke Jr. JD, Burns BJ. An experiment to change detection and management of mental morbidity in primary care. Med Care 1987; 25:327–339.

117. Mathias SD, Fifer SK, Mazonson PD, Lubeck DP, Buesching DP, Patrick DL. Necessary but not sufficient: the effect of screening and feedback on outcomes of primary care patients with untreated anxiety. J Gen Intern Med 1994; 9:606–615.

118. Valenstein M, Dalack G, Blow F, Figueroa S, Standiford C, Douglass A. Screening for psychiatric illness with a combined screening and diagnostic instrument. J Gen Intern Med 1997; 12:679–685.

119. Reifler DR, Kessler HS, Bernhard EJ, Leon AC, Martin GJ. Impact of screening of mental health concerns on health service utilization and functional status in primary care patients. Arch Intern Med 1996; 156:2593–2599.

120. Higgins ES. A review of unrecognized mental illness in primary care. Arch Fam Med 1994; 3:908–917.

121. Katon W, Von Korff M, Lin E. Adequacy and duration of antidepressant treatment in primary care. Med Care 1992; 30:67–76.

122. Strum R, Wells KB. How can care for depression become more cost-effective? JAMA 1995; 273:51–55.

123. Wells KB, Katon W, Rogers WH. Use of minor tranquilizers and antidepressant medication by depressed outpatients: results from the Medical Outcome Study. Am J Psychiatry 1994; 151:694–700.
124. Dowrick C, Buchan I. Twelve month outcome of depression in general practice: Does detection or disclosure make a difference? Br Med J 1995; 311:1274–1276.
125. Ronalds C, Creed F, Stone K, Webb S, Tomenson B. Outcome of anxiety and depressive disorders in primary care. Br J Psychiatry 1997; 171:427–433.
126. Simon GE, VonKorff M. Recognition, management, and outcomes of depression in primary care. Arch Fam Med 1995; 4:99–105.
127. Kathol RG, Wenzel RP. Natural history of symptoms of depression and anxiety during inpatient treatment on general medicine wards. J Gen Intern Med 1992; 7:287–293.
128. Tiemens BG, Ormel J, Simon GE. Occurrence, recognition, and outcome of psychological disorders in primary care. Am J Psychiatry 1996; 153:636–644.
129. Keller MB, Lavori PW, Friedman B, Nielsen E, Endicott J, McDonald-Scott NC, Andreasen NC. The Longitudinal Interval Follow-Up Evaluation: a comprehensive method for assessing outcome in prospective longitudinal studies. Arch Gen Psychiatry 1987; 44: 540–548.

2

Specificity of Psychiatric Symptoms in the Medically Ill

Robert G. Robinson
University of Iowa College of Medicine
Iowa City, Iowa

INTRODUCTION

In Chapter 1, Zimmerman and Mattia discussed the use of screening instruments for the detection of specific psychiatric disorders in general medical populations. They pointed out that the "gold standard" against which screening instruments are measured is the structured or semi-structured psychiatric interview used in conjunction with defined diagnostic criteria such as Diagnostic and Statistical Manual IV (DSM-IV). This constitutes the standard of practice in psychiatry and forms the basis for much of our knowledge about success rates in the identification and treatment of psychiatric disorders in the medically ill.

A more fundamental question than whether screening instruments accurately identify psychiatric disorders in the medically ill, however, is whether the "gold standard" is applicable to the diagnosis of psychiatric disorder in patients with comorbid medical illness. The psychiatric disorder that has received the most attention in this regard is depression. In evaluating depression associated with medical illness, one must determine whether a reliable and valid diagnosis of depression can be made when symptoms fundamental to the diagnosis of depression (e.g., disturbance of sleep or appetite) may be produced by the medical illness itself independent of the depressive disorder. If a valid diagnosis cannot be made in a medically ill population using existing diagnostic criteria, the next question is whether the method of assessment of depressive disorder could be altered so that nonspecific symptoms related to the physical illness were eliminated and only symptoms specific to the depressive disorder would be used.

This issue has been examined in a number of studies (1–3), and several alternative methods for handling the problem have been proposed. Some investigators suggested that psychological symptoms of depression should be substituted for vegetative symptoms because psychological symptoms are less likely to be influenced by physical illness than vegetative symptoms (1). Another method proposed to address this problem of diagnosis in the medically ill is to make a "clinical judgment" about whether symptoms are due to physical illness or to depression and to only count symptoms that are believed to be specifically related to depression (2). Another method for the diagnosis of depression in the medically ill is to use only those depressive symptoms that have been demonstrated to be specific for depression in that population (3). According to this line of reasoning, symptoms that are significantly more frequent in patients with depressed mood compared to patients without depressed mood, when all other factors are comparable, are considered to be specific for depression. Finally, unaltered diagnostic criteria may be used if it can be shown that these criteria do not falsely elevate the number of cases based on nonspecific symptoms.

In addition to the problem of including nonspecific symptoms related to the medical illness leading to the overdiagnosis of depression, medical illness may also lead to the underdiagnosis of depression. Patients with a serious medical illness may deny the existence of depression due to unawareness of their own mood state (i.e., anosognosia of mood, a general unawareness of physical illness) or they may be unable to comprehend the questions that they are asked (e.g., fluent or global aphasia).

Given the current state of our research into psychiatric disorders associated with medical illnesses, these are difficult issues in diagnosis and the answers are probably different for each medical illness. Symptoms that are specific for the diagnosis of depression in patients with Parkinson's disease, for example, may be different from those in multiple sclerosis. Thus, there is an enormous amount of work to be done determining whether our existing psychiatric diagnostic criteria are applicable to psychiatric diagnoses in a wide range of medical illnesses. Robinson et al. have examined this issue in depression associated with several medical disorders (4–6). The results of these studies are described below and suggest that symptoms of depressive disorder, although sometimes nonspecific, are not widespread in patients with acute physical illnesses and that the standard diagnostic criteria contained in DSM-III and DSM-IV (7,8) can be used to diagnose major depression in several medical illnesses.

DIAGNOSTIC ISSUES

Before addressing the specificity of the symptoms of psychiatric disorder, a brief review of applicable diagnoses is appropriate. Beginning with the DSM-IV classification, psychiatric disorders associated with medical conditions may now be classified as "due" to a specified medical condition. The diagnostic criteria for several of the major conditions are shown in Table 1.

These diagnoses require (1) that there be evidence from the history, physical examination, or laboratory findings that the disturbance is the direct physiological consequence of the general medical condition, (2) that the disturbance is not better ac-

Table 1 Mental Disorders Due to
General Medical Condition

Cognitive disorders
   Delirium
   Dementia
   Amnestic disorder
Psychotic disorders
   Catatonic disorder
   Psychotic disorder with delusion
   Psychotic disorder with hallucinations
Mood disorders
   with depressive features
   with major depressive-like episode
   with manic features
   with mixed features
Anxiety disorders
   with generalized anxiety
   with panic attacks
   with obsessive-compulsive symptoms
Sexual dysfunctions
Sleep disorders
Personality change
Mental disorder NOS

counted for by another mental disorder, and (3) that the disturbance does not occur exclusively during the course of a delirium.

There are specific diagnostic criteria for each of these disorders, although generally they do not require the same specificity of syndromic presentation as does the corresponding mental disorder without associated medical illness. For example, mood disorder with depressive features only requires that the predominant mood is depressed, but no other specific symptoms of major depression are required. Similarly, anxiety disorder with obsessive-compulsive symptoms only requires that the obsessions or compulsions are dominant in the clinical presentation.

If the mental disorder is not believed to be the direct physiological consequence of the general medical condition, the diagnostic criteria for the mental disorder not associated with a medical illness are used. Thus, adjustment disorders with depressed mood or anxiety may be appropriate diagnostic conditions, or psychological factors affecting the medical condition may be appropriate diagnoses. An adjustment disorder is defined as the development of clinically significant emotional or behavioral symptoms in response to an identifiable psychosocial stressor or stressors. The symptoms must develop within 3 months after the onset of the stressors and must resolve within 6 months of determination of the stressor. The symptoms, however, may persist for a prolonged period if they occur in response to a chronic stressor. The stressor may be a single event or multiple stressors.

The criteria for a mental disorder affecting a general medical condition requires the presence of one or more specific psychological or behavioral factors that adversely affect the general medical condition. The factors may influence either the course of the general medical condition or the treatment. These diagnoses include a mental disorder affecting a general medical condition, psychological symptoms affecting the general medical condition, personality traits or coping style affecting the medical condition, maladapted health behaviors affecting the medical condition, or stress-related physiological responses affecting the medical condition.

In summary, the psychiatric disorders associated with a comorbid medical condition include the entire spectrum of psychiatric disorders with the exception of the somatoform disorders. The major difficulty in relating psychiatric disorders to associated medical conditions is a determination of whether or not the psychiatric disorder is a direct physiological consequence of the medical disorder or whether it represents a response to the stress of the medical disorder or is an independent or comorbid condition. Conditions that are independent but comorbid to the medical disorders are no less important clinically than those that result from the medical condition. In general, however, we do not treat these conditions differently than they would be treated without the medical condition with the exception of contraindicated treatments based on the medical condition, such as use of tricyclic antidepressants in depressed patients with cardiac conduction disease. The ultimate validation that a mental disorder is the direct physiological consequence of a medical disorder is dependent upon the identification of the mechanism of that mental disorder. In the meantime, demonstration of temporal associations, clinical correlations, or differences in the course of the disorder may help to validate these mental conditions as being due to the associated medical disorder. The validation of diagnostic entities in psychiatry as well as other fields of medicine is an ongoing process, however, requiring numerous studies, and it ends only when the etiology and pathophysiology of these disorders are identified.

STUDIES OF SYMPTOMS SPECIFIC TO DEPRESSION IN PATIENTS WITH MEDICAL ILLNESSES

One study of the specificity of depressive symptoms in patients following stroke was conducted by Fedoroff et al. (9). The study included 205 patients with acute stroke, excluding only patients with a decreased level of consciousness or moderate-to-severe comprehension deficit. The 205 patients meeting the criteria for inclusion in this study were divided into those who reported a depressed mood (85 patients or 41%) and those who reported no depressed mood (120 or 59%). There were no statistically significant differences in demographic or background characteristics between the depressed and nondepressed groups in term of sex, race, socioeconomic status, marital status, personal or family history of psychiatric disorder, previous medical history, or medications taken at the time of interview. The depressive group, however, was found to be younger than the nondepressed group (mean age 56.5 ± 12 years depressed vs. 60.4 ± 14 years nondepressed). The depressed group also had more severe cognitive impairment as evidenced by lower Mini-Mental Exam scores (22 ± 5.6 vs. 24 ± 4.8) and had greater impairment in activities of daily living as evidenced by higher scores on the Johns Hopkins Functioning Inventory (7.3 ± 5.7 vs. 5.3 ± 5.8).

The frequency of 8 autonomic (vegetative) symptoms and 13 psychological symptoms of depression between the depressed and nondepressed groups was compared. The autonomic symptoms as identified by Davidson and Turnbull (10) were autonomic anxiety, anxious foreboding, morning depression, weight loss, delayed sleep, subjective anergia, early morning awakening, and loss of libido. The 13 psychological symptoms included worrying, brooding, loss of interest, hopelessness, suicidal plans, social withdrawal, self-depreciation, lack of confidence, simple ideas of reference, guilty ideas of reference, pathological guilt, and irritability. The depressed patients had an average of 3.6 ± 2.1 SD autonomic symptoms and 4.1 ± 2.8 SD psychological symptoms compared to the nondepressed group, which had an average of 0.9 ± 1.1 SD autonomic and 0.9 ± 1.1 SD psychological symptoms ($p < 0.001$ for both comparisons). Differences in the frequency of these symptoms between the depressed and nondepressed groups are shown in Figures 1 and 2.

Although almost all psychological and vegetative symptoms were significantly more frequent in the depressed than the nondepressed group, it might be construed that the autonomic symptoms in the nondepressed patients represent nonspecific effects of acute medical illness. In order to determine whether the inclusion of these additional nonspecific symptoms significantly influenced the rate of diagnosis of major depression, the rates of major depression were compared with and without one additional depressive symptom required for the diagnosis of major depression. This resulted in a change of diagnosis (i.e., failure to meet diagnostic criteria) in 3 of 46 patients with major depression (7%). The requirement of two additional depressive symptoms reduced the frequency of major depression by 5 patients (11%). Thus, in the overall population, a reduction in the number of patients meeting criteria for major depression from 46 to 43 would have resulted in a change in the frequency of major depression from 24% to 22.5%.

Fedoroff et al. (9) then determined whether patients might be underdiagnosed for major depression because they were unable or unwilling to acknowledge their depressed mood. Using the same population of 205 patients with acute stroke, the number of patients who failed to meet diagnostic criteria for major depression only because they denied having a depressed mood was determined. There were 10 such patients of the 205 with acute stroke. Although there were no differences in demographic or clinical characteristics between the patients who acknowledged depression and those who did not (even though they otherwise met criteria for major depression), the patients who acknowledged depression had a higher frequency of left hemisphere lesions (54% vs. 10%). Thus, if these 10 patients were added to those with major depression who acknowledged depressed mood, the frequency of major depression would have increased

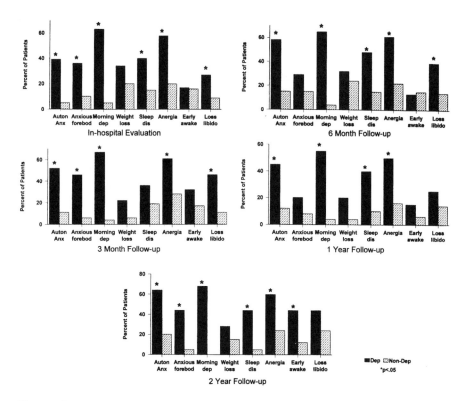

Figure 1   The frequency of vegetative symptoms of depression in patients with and without depressed mood following stroke. Symptom frequency is shown over the 2-year follow-up. Morning depression (i.e., diurnal mood variation) and anergia were associated with depression throughout the entire 2-year period. Loss of libido was seen only early in the follow-up, whereas early-morning awakening was seen only late in the follow-up. These findings suggest changes over time in both the effects of chronic medical illness and the phenomenology of depression following stroke. (Adapted from Ref. 6.)

from 24% to 29%. It should be pointed out, however, that all of the patients who denied a depressed mood acknowledged the presence of other psychological symptoms of depression such as loss of interest, feelings of hopelessness, etc. Fedoroff concluded from this study that altered diagnostic criteria that accounted for the rate of nonspecific autonomic symptoms in nondepressed patients would have decreased the rate of major depression by 1.5% and similarly that the rate of masked depressions due to processes such as denial may have underestimated the rate of depression by 5%. This is not a very large change from the rate of depression diagnosed using standard criteria. Therefore, standard diagnostic criteria were useful for the diagnosis of poststroke major depression.

A subsequent follow-up study including 142 of these 205 patients who were

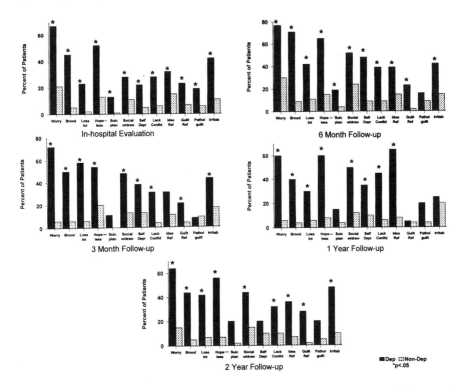

Figure 2 The frequency of psychological symptoms of depression in patients with depressed mood and without depressed mood following stroke. Symptom frequency is shown over the 2-year follow-up. Most symptoms (i.e., worrying, brooding, loss of interest, hopelessness, social withdrawal, lack of self-confidence, self-depreciation, ideas of reference, and irritability) were more frequent in depressed patients throughout the 2 years following stroke. Feelings of self-blame (self-depreciation and pathological guilt) were less common after the first year poststroke. (Adapted from Ref. 6.)

available for longitudinal study over 2 years examined changes in the specificity of these depressive symptoms associated with medical illness over time (6). Changes in the frequency of the autonomic (vegetative) and psychological depressive symptoms over time are shown in Figures 1 and 2. At 3 months follow-up, all of the vegetative symptoms were more common in the patients with depressed mood than those without depressed mood except for weight loss, delayed sleep, and early morning awakening. At 6 months follow-up, depressed patients had a higher frequency of all vegetative symptoms except weight loss and early awakening. At one year, depressed patients had a higher frequency of all symptoms except anxious foreboding, weight loss, early awakening, and loss of libido. At 2 years follow-up, depressed patients had a higher frequency of all vegetative symptoms except weight loss and loss of libido.

The frequency of psychological symptoms in the depressed compared to the nondepressed patients are shown in Figure 2. At the initial evaluation, all psychological symptoms were significantly more frequent in the depressed than the nondepressed group. At 3 months follow-up, the depressed group showed higher frequency of all psychological symptoms except suicidal plans, simple ideas of reference, and pathological guilt. At 6 months follow-up, depressed patients had a higher frequency of all psychological symptoms except pathological guilt. At one year follow-up, depressed patients had higher frequency of all psychological symptoms except suicidal plans, guilty ideas of reference, pathological guilt, and irritability. At 2 years follow-up, depressed patients had significantly greater frequency of all psychological symptoms except self-depreciation and pathological guilt.

Paradiso et al. (6) then examined the various alternative means of diagnosing depression for its impact on the frequency of major depression. The initial inpatient evaluation used only specific symptoms (i.e., excluding weight loss), meaning that 3 of 27 patients with major depression were excluded. If specific symptoms were regarded as the gold standard, unmodified DSM-IV criteria had a 100% sensitivity and 98% specificity. When DSM-IV criteria were modified to substitute a psychological symptom that was not included in the DSM-IV criteria but was one of the 13 assessed in this study for a vegetative symptom, none of the 27 major depressed patients were excluded. At 3 months follow-up, requiring only specific symptoms eliminated 2 of 12 patients (16%) with major depression. Unmodified DSM-IV criteria had 100% sensitivity and 97% specificity. The substitution of a psychological symptom allowed all 12 patients to maintain the diagnosis of major depression.

At 6 months follow-up, the requirement that all symptoms be specific led to 3 out of 15 patients being excluded. This resulted in 100% sensitivity and 96% specificity for the original DSM-IV criteria. Using the psychological symptoms method, none of the 15 patients were excluded. At one year follow-up, requiring specific symptoms led to the exclusion of 3 of 7 patients with major depression; unmodified DSM-IV criteria had a 100% percent sensitivity and 95% specificity at this time point. The substitution of psychological symptoms did not exclude any of the patients with major depression. At 2 years follow-up, the requirement of specific symptoms led to 2 of 16 patients with major depression being excluded. Unmodified DSM-IV criteria had 100% sensitivity and 96% specificity at this time point. The substitution method led to 1 of 16 patients being excluded from a major depression diagnosis.

There were several significant findings from this study. First, all vegetative as well as psychological symptoms were significantly more common among patients with depressed rather than nondepressed mood throughout the 2 years following stroke. Three vegetative symptoms—autonomic anxiety, morning depression, and subjective anergia—were significantly more frequent in depressed than in nondepressed patients throughout the 2-year follow-up period. The vegetative symptom of loss of libido was no longer significantly more common in depressed than nondepressed patients after 6 months. Self-depreciation was no longer more common after one year. In contrast, early morning awakening was more frequent in the depressed group only at 2 years. Weight loss was the only symptom that was not significantly more frequent in depressed than nondepressed patients over the entire 2-year period. Anxiety symptoms, including autonomic anxiety, anxious foreboding, and worrying, were significantly associated with depression throughout the entire 2-year follow-up. Although the pattern of symptoms specific for depression changed over the course of the 2-year follow-up, vegetative symptoms as well as psychological symptoms tended to be significantly associated with depression throughout the entire 2-year period.

Another finding from this study was that unmodified DSM-IV criteria consistently had a sensitivity of 100% for major depression, while the specificity ranged from 95% to 98% compared to modified criteria. The modified DSM-IV criteria that included enlarged numbers of psychological symptoms (substitution method) yielded almost the same diagnostic results as unmodified DSM-IV criteria. Thus, this study suggests that attempts at clinical differentiation between nonspecific symptoms that are secondary to the hospital routine or to the patient's comorbid medical illness and symptoms that are related to depression are probably unnecessary. There may be a few patients with "masked depressions" as well as a few patients who are overdiagnosed based on nonspecific symptoms. These false-positive and false-negative cases, however, do not constitute a significant portion of the patients, and it is unclear whether the substitutive method would lead to the diagnosis of major depression in an even larger group of patients than currently diagnosed by DSM-IV.

Starkstein et al. (4) conducted a similar study examining the specificity of psychological and vegetative symptoms of depression in patients with Parkinson's disease. This study included 33 patients who reported a depressed mood compared with an identical number of nondepressed patients who are matched for Hoehn and Yahr stage of Parkinson's disease, duration of illness (± 2 years), age (± 2 years), and education (± 2 years). All patients were attending an outpatient follow-up clinic and the mean duration of illness was 10.6 years. There were no significant between-group differences in the severity of symptoms of Parkinson's disease, levodopa dosage, or frequency of on-off phenomena. Using the Present State Examination to elicit autonomic and psychological symptoms of depression in the same way as the Fedoroff (9) paper, it was found that depressed patients did not have more psychological than autonomic symptoms and that they showed a significantly higher frequency of all autonomic and psychological symptoms of depression compared to nondepressed patients with the exception of early morning awakening, anergia, and retardation. Thus, among patients with chronic Parkinson's disease almost all depressive symptoms, including vegetative symptoms, were more common in depressed than nondepressed patients. With the exception of early morning awakening and loss of energy, depression was associated with an increased frequency of both depressive vegetative and psychological symptoms. It is not surprising in this population that anergia and retardation might be as frequent in the nondepressed as the depressed patients because of the akinesia of Parkinson's disease. Thus, although there were some differences between stroke and Parkinson's disease, the same general finding held true. Symptoms using unmodified DSM-III or DSM-IV criteria for the diagnosis of major depression in patients with concomitant physical illness did not produce a significant number of false-positive or false-negative cases. Although patients may have physical illnesses, these illnesses do not produce a marked number of symptoms that we associate with depressive disorder.

Another study that used similar methodology to examine this issue was conducted by Jorge et al. in patients with traumatic brain injury (TBI). This study included 66 patients with acute TBI, 58 of whom were followed up during a one-year period for symptoms and diagnosis of depressive disorder. Using the same instrument as the other two studies (i.e., the Present State Examination) to elicit autonomic and psychological symptoms of depression, at the initial evaluation, all autonomic and psychological symptoms were significantly more frequent in depressed than nondepressed patients except for anxious foreboding, early awakening, and loss of libido. At 3 months follow-up, all symptoms were more frequent in the depressed mood group except for early morning awakening, delayed sleep, and morning depression. At 6 months follow-up, all symptoms were significantly more frequent except morning depression, weight loss, delayed sleep, and loss of libido. At one year follow-up, all symptoms were significantly more frequent in the depressed compared to the nondepressed group except autonomic anxiety, anxious foreboding, morning depression, weight loss, and delayed sleep.

If the diagnostic criteria were modified to require only specific symptoms, two of the original 17 major depressed patients (12%) would have been excluded. Compared to the diagnoses made using only specific symptoms, standard criteria had 100% sensitivity and 94% specificity. At 3 months follow-up, modification of diagnostic criteria to require only specific symptoms would still lead to all 10 of the patients originally diagnosed with major depression continuing to receive this diagnosis. If we required patients to have three of six specific symptoms for the diagnosis of major depression, the sensitivity of DSM-III standard criteria would be 88% and the specificity 94%.

At 6 months follow-up, if two specific symptoms in addition to depressed mood were required for a diagnosis of major depression, all 11 of the patients originally diagnosed with major depression would continue to be such. If three specific symptoms were required, one of the original 11 patients with a major depression diagnosis would be excluded. This would lead to a 91% sensitivity and 96% specificity for standard criteria. At one year follow-up if depressed mood and three specific symptoms were required for the diagnosis of major depression, all 8 patients with a diagnosis of major depression would remain classified as such. The sensitivity using three specific symptoms was 80%, and the specificity was 100%. We did not examine the substitution method, but based on the findings from the study of patients with stroke, it is likely that all of the originally diagnosed patients would continue to have major depression if a psychological symptom could have been substituted.

This study found that psychological symptoms that discriminated depressed from nondepressed patients at both the initial evaluation and one year follow-up were symptoms related to changes in self-attitude (feelings of hopelessness, suicidal ideation, loss of interest, self-depreciation, lack of self-confidence). The only vegetative symptom that held up over the one-year follow-up was lack of energy (anergia). Anxiety symptoms were significantly associated with depression during the first 6 months. At one-year follow-up, however, the frequency of anxiety symptoms was not significantly different between patients with and without depressed mood. Autonomic symptoms such as decreased appetite and weight loss, difficulty falling asleep, and diurnal mood variation appeared to be significantly associated with depression only during the initial or 3-month evaluation but not at one-year follow-up. On the other hand, early morning awakening, loss of libido, difficulty concentrating, and inefficient thinking distinguished depressed from nondepressed patients only after 6 months or a year had elapsed. Finally, increased appetite, weight gain, and hypersomnia did not differentiate between depressed and nondepressed groups at any time point. The median frequency of psychological and vegetative symptoms was three times the rate found among nondepressed patients. Thus, vegetative (autonomic) symptoms were not rampant even among patients with acute traumatic brain injury.

It should be noted that standard DSM-III-R criteria identified almost the same group of patients as modified criteria that included only specific symptoms for depression. Sensitivity ranged from 100% at the acute phase to 80% at one-year follow-up, while specificity increased slightly from 94% in the initial stage to 100% at one-year follow-up. This study, like the study in patients with stroke, found that symptoms that were specific to depression varied with time following injury. Some vegetative symptoms (e.g., poor appetite and weight loss, diurnal mood variation) were significantly associated with depression only during the first 3 months of follow-up. In contrast, other symptoms such as terminal insomnia, difficulty concentrating, and inefficient thinking were significantly more frequent in the depressed group only at one-year follow-up. Within the first few months following TBI, the etiological mechanism of major depression may be different than the etiological mechanism of major depression at one-year follow-up. These findings suggested that the nature of posttraumatic brain injury depressions may change over time.

The most important finding, however, from these studies in three different types of physical illnesses is that standard DSM-III or DSM-IV diagnostic criteria identify the great majority of patients with major depression without any need for modification of the criteria even in an acutely physically ill population. Without evidence that these modified criteria (e.g., using only specific symptoms) would define a population of patients with a more uniform syndrome, more consistent prognostic outcome, or more predictable response to treatment, the available data suggest that the use of current diagnostic criteria is appropriate for patients with medical illnesses. Each condition, however, needs to be studied separately to determine whether the findings that held up in these three medical conditions would also hold true with other disorders.

DIAGNOSIS OF MENTAL DISORDER

Although the specificity of symptoms in patients with acute medical illness does not appear to be significantly altered by a physical disorder, the issue of how the treating physician should go about making a diagnosis in patients with acute medical illnesses remains. As indicated by the studies presented, depressive symptoms were not affected greatly by the existence of chronic Parkinson's disease, acute stroke, or traumatic brain injury. Thus, the way to determine the existence of depressive disorder in patients with stroke or traumatic brain injury is to conduct a mental status examination in which the symptoms of major depressive disorder are assessed as well as their duration and effect on daily activities. Patients should be asked specifically about the existence of each symptom included in the diagnostic criteria for that mental disorder. Patients who meet the diagnostic criteria for mental disorders would be expected to respond to treatment shown to be effective for patients without associated medical illness.

Although they are often convenient and may be an adjunct to diagnosis, rating scales are not a substitute for a systematic mental status examination that leads to a diagnosis based on meeting specified diagnostic criteria. Depression rating scales are probably most widely used to assess mental disorders. They are useful in determining the severity of depression and can be used as screening instruments to determine the likelihood of the existence of a depression. Although a number of depression scales have been used with cutoff scores to define the presence or absence of depression, a score above an arbitrary cutoff point can only be considered suggestive that a depression may exist. The "gold standard" for the existence of depression or other mental disorders remains the established diagnostic criteria elicited through clinical interview.

Studies evaluating depression based on depression rating scale scores have found cases of major or minor depression that would not meet the cutoff criteria on rating scales for depression. Similarly, cases may meet the cutoff criteria on the depression rating scale but not fulfill the diagnostic criteria for major depression. Among patients with comorbid physical illness, Parikh et al. (11) examined patients with depression following stroke and compared scores on the Center for Epidemiological Scale for Depression (CES-D) (12) with the presence of DSM-III–defined major depression based on findings from a semi-structured psychiatric interview. Of the 180 patients given the CES-D and the semi-structured psychiatric interview, a cutoff score of 16 on the CES-D had a 90% specificity for major depression and a 86% sensitivity with a positive predictive value of 80%. Increasing the cutoff score to 21 increased the specificity to 94% but decreased the sensitivity to 72% with a positive predictive value of 85%. The correlation between DSM-III diagnosis of major or minor depression and CES-D in-hospital score was 0.53 using a Spearman rank correlation coefficient. These findings demonstrate that cutoff scores on depression rating scales are not a sufficient substitute for the diagnosis of depression based on clinical interview and defined diagnostic criteria.

Depressions may be missed by depression rating scales because some symptoms evaluated by the depression rating scale are not used in the diagnostic criteria and, therefore, may falsely elevate the depression score. In addition, symptoms that are essential to the diagnosis of major depression may not be significantly more frequent in depressed compared with nondepressed patients. Thus, the inclusion of symptoms in a rating scale that did not differentiate depressed from nondepressed patients may falsely elevate the scale score leading to misdiagnosis.

Some of the most widely used depression rating scales include the Hamilton Depression Scale (13), an interviewer-rated scale, the Beck Depression Inventory (14), a self-rated questionnaire, the Zung Depression Scale (15), a self-rated scale, the General

Health Questionnaire (16), a self-rated scale that involves several areas of assessment besides depression, the CES-D, another self-rated scale described previously, and the Montgomery-Asberg Depression Rating Scale (17), an interviewer-rated scale.

An example of how these rating scales may interfere with assessment of patients with comorbid physical illnesses is the question on the Hamilton Depression Scale that evaluates the patient's capacity to carry on usual work and activities. The most severe rating for depression (rating of 4) is based on the patient's stopping working because of the present illness. Rating this item in a patient with an associated medical illness that has produced a physical impairment requires some judgment. Similarly, the Hamilton Depression Scale evaluates the severity of psychomotor retardation, which involves slowness of thought and speech. In patients with aphasia or bradykinesia due to Parkinson's disease, this assessment is difficult. This problem of the applicability of depression rating scale in patients with physical illness is also true for the assessment of psychological symptoms of depression. For example, the Beck Depression Inventory includes a question about self-appearance where the most severe rating (rating of 3) is based on the patient's belief that they "look ugly." This obviously could be complicated by physical impairments produced by a physical illness. Similarly, ratings of capacity to work and worries about health may also be influenced by the existence of a comorbid physical illness. Decisions about scoring each of the items on the rating scales must be interpreted in relationship to the physical or cognitive effects of the physical disorder. Thus, although some modifications of the rating scales can be made to minimize the effect of associated physical illnesses, these rating scales may not accurately reflect the severity of depression.

In summary, rating the presence and severity of mental disorders in patients with concomitant physical illness is dependent, in part, upon identifying the extent of overlap between symptoms that may be attributed to the physical illness and symptoms associated with a mental disorder. In the disorders that have been studied, including depression in stroke, Parkinson's disease, and traumatic brain injury, standard diagnostic criteria for depressive disorder appear to be applicable because the physical illness has not produced a high frequency of any major depression symptoms. Rating scales may be helpful in determining severity of mental disorder, although they are complicated by the interaction between physical illness and symptoms rated by the standard rating scales. The only satisfactory way of determining the existence of a mental disorder is to determine that the physical illness produced a significant number of "depressive-like" symptoms and then to conduct a mental status examination to determine whether the type and duration of symptoms meet the diagnostic criteria for that condition.

ETIOLOGY OF MENTAL DISORDERS

A discussion about diagnosis in patients with concomitant mental and physical disorders would not be complete without a consideration of the issue of etiology. Since the DSM-IV diagnostic criteria for "a condition due to a physical illness" requires that the clinician believe that the mental disorder is a direct physiological consequence of the physical illness, this requires some judgment about etiology. For example, depressions that are seen as understandable psychological responses to an acute physical illness or to the change in life circumstances associated with a chronic physical or cognitive impairment may be regarded as an "adjustment disorder with depression" that will improve within several months or require psychotherapeutic intervention to deal with the underlying psychological issue. On the other hand, depression that is felt to be the consequence of a physiological change produced by a physical illness such as stroke may be regarded as a "biochemical" depression, which requires pharmacological or other physical treatment. While these kinds of considerations are helpful in directing therapeutic efforts, one should remember that we do not know the etiological mechanism of any depressive disorder at the present time. This is also true of other mental disorders, and our judgments about the relationship between physical illness and mental illness are based on clinical conjecture or perhaps simply bias. Patients with physical illnesses are likely to have an understandable psychological explanation for their depression or other mental disorders. The hypothesis on the part of the physician that anyone would be depressed in that circumstance has an empathetic appeal and may sometimes be valid. That kind of explanation, however, may lead the clinician to overlook a disorder that could respond to antidepressant treatment or may be the result of physiological changes produced by the physical illness. In general, treatment of mental disorders associated with physical illness should not be dependent upon the physician's judgment of the etiology of that condition but should be dependent upon the clinical manifestations of the mental disorder. Major depressions, panic disorder, and cognitive impairment associated with depression are likely to respond to pharmacological intervention. Patients presenting with these conditions should be treated based on the clinical manifestations of the mental disorder and only modified by contraindications associated with the physical illness.

CONCLUSIONS

The diagnosis of mental disorder in patients with associated physical illnesses requires a clinical mental status examination that specifically elicits the symptoms relevant to that mental disorder. As demonstrated by the studies of patients with chronic physical illnesses and depression, depressive symptoms are not rampant among nondepressed patients with either acute or chronic Parkinson's disease, stroke, or traumatic brain injury. The specificity of depressive and other symptoms needs to be investigated for each physical illness. Studies thus far have indicated that the physical illness does not dramatically alter the presentation or the applicability of standard diagnostic criteria for the mental disorder. Rating scales should be used with caution and recognition that they are not a substitute for specifically eliciting the symptoms associated with each mental disorder. Preconceptions about the etiology of mental disorders tend to inhibit the examination of patients for specific syndromes of mental disorder because an explanation is already identified. Patients should, however, be evaluated for the existence of a syndromic cluster and treatment based on the clinical presentation rather than judgments about presumed etiology. The chapters that follow will provide detailed descriptions of the kinds of conditions in which psychiatric disorders are associated with physical illnesses. Each of these may touch on the special issues relevant to the understanding and evaluation of psychiatric symptoms in patients with physical illness.

REFERENCES

1. Endicott J. Measurement of depression in patients with cancer. Cancer 1984; 53 (suppl): 2243–2248.
2. Magni G, Schifano F, deLeo D. Assessment of depression in an elderly medical population. J Affect Disord 1986; 11:121–124.
3. Cohen-Cole SA, Kauffman KG. Major depression in physical illness: diagnosis, prevalence, and antidepressant treatment. Depression 1993; 2:281–294.
4. Starkstein SE, Preziosi TJ, Forrester AW, Robinson RG. Specificity of affective and autonomic symptoms of depression in Parkinson's disease. J Neurol Neurosurg Psychiatry 1990; 53:869–873.
5. Jorge RE, Robinson RG, Arndt SV. Are depressive symptoms specific for a depressed mood in traumatic brain injury? J Nerv Ment Dis 1993; 181:91–99.
6. Paradiso S, Ohkubo T, Robinson RG. Are DSM-IV criteria for major depression useful following stroke? The specificity of depressive symptoms for depressed mood over the first two years after stroke. Int J Psychiatry Med 1997; 27:137–157.
7. American Psychiatric Association. Diagnostic and Statistical Manual of Mental Disorders, Revised Third Edition (DSM-III-R). Washington, DC: American Psychiatric Press, Inc., 1987.
8. American Psychiatric Association. Diagnostic and Statistical Manual of Mental Disorders—DSM-IV. Washington, DC: American Psychiatric Press, Inc., 1994.
9. Fedoroff JP, Starkstein SE, Parikh RM, Price TR, Robinson RG. Are depressive symptoms non-specific in patients with acute stroke? Am J Psychiatry 1991; 148:1172–1176.
10. Davidson J, Turnbull CD. Diagnostic significance of vegetative symptoms in depression. Br J Psychiatry 1986; 148:442–446.
11. Parikh RM, Eden DT, Price TR, Robinson RG. The sensitivity and specificity of the Center for Epidemiologic Studies depression scale as a screening instrument for post-stroke depression. Int J Psychiatry Med 1988; 18:169–181.
12. Radloff LS. The CES-D Scale, a self-report depression scale for research in the general population. Appl Psychol Meas 1977; 1:385–401.
13. Hamilton M. A rating scale for depression. J Neurol Neurosurg Psychiatry 1960; 23:56–62.
14. Beck AT, Ward CH, Mendelson M, Mock J, Erbaugh J. An inventory for measuring depression. Arch Gen Psychiatry 1961; 4:551–571.
15. Zung WWK: A self-rating depression scale. Arch Gen Psychiatry 1965; 12:377–395.
16. Goldberg DP, Hiller VF. A scaled version of the General Health Questionnaire. Psychol Med 1979; 9:139–198.
17. Montgomery SA, Asberg M. A new depression scale designed to be sensitive to change. Br J Psychiatry 1979; 134:383–389.

3

Epidemiology of Psychiatric Disorders in the Medically Ill

William R. Yates

University of Oklahoma Health Sciences Center
Tulsa, Oklahoma

Epidemiology forms the basis for the understanding of clinical disorders in both medicine and psychiatry. This volume focuses on understanding the issues involved in the diagnosis and treatment of patients with both medical and psychiatric disorders. The term *comorbidity* in this chapter will be defined as the presence of a psychiatric and a medical illness in the same individual. This is to be distinguished from the term *psychiatric comorbidity*, which usually denotes more than one psychiatric illness within an individual patient. A *secondary* illness is defined as an illness that occurs chronologically after the primary illness. There may be a pathophysiologic relationship between a primary and secondary disorder, or there may not be any such relationship.

Psychiatric illnesses occur in the medically ill at rates higher than expected by chance. The reasons for high rates of comorbidity can be explained using models for relationships between two illnesses (Fig. 1).

Medical illnesses can result in a variety of psychiatric disorders, including mood disorders, anxiety disorders, psychotic disorders, cognitive impairment disorders, and sleep and sexual disorders (Model 1). One example of this pathway to comorbidity is the development of depression following stroke. There is good evidence to support the pathophysiologic relationship between stroke and depression, particularly when stroke involves those localized brain structures felt to modulate mood. Another example of a Model 1 relationship would be depression associated with Huntington's disease.

A second model that explains a portion of the increased risk for comorbidity designates psychiatric illnesses that increase the rate for certain medical illnesses (Model 2). An example of this would be alcohol dependence leading to alcoholic cirrhosis. Obviously alcohol consumption is required for the development of alcoholic cirrhosis. The majority of patients with alcoholic cirrhosis do meet criteria for alcohol abuse/

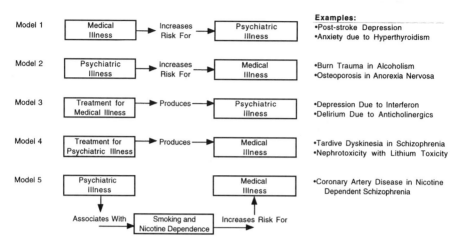

Figure 1   Models of association to explain high rates of medical and psychiatric illness comorbidity.

dependence, although not all would do so. Another example of a psychiatric disorder directly increasing the risk for a medical disorder is the medical morbidity associated with suicide attempts. Here affective disorder, personality disorder, and other psychiatric illnesses increase the risk for suicide attempts and suicide contributing to a significant number of admissions to medical intensive care units for management of intentional overdose and self-inflicted trauma. Also noted in the figure is the relationship of high rates of burn trauma in alcoholism and osteoporosis secondary to the starvation effects seen in anorexia nervosa.

Medical treatments for medical illnesses can produce significant psychiatric symptomatology and disorders (Model 3). Here the psychiatric comorbidity occurs due to the adverse effect of treatment for the medical illness. An example of this mechanism is the development of depression with interferon for the treatment of hepatitis C or the development of delirium in a geriatric patient treated with an anticholinergic medication for sedation. Often the development of a psychiatric adverse effect from medication used to treat a medical disorder is unpredictable. Certain drugs and drug classes present higher risks. Nevertheless, when medical and psychiatric illness occur simultaneously, a medication-induced psychiatric syndrome should be considered.

Another mechanism for comorbidity is the development of medical complications related to the treatment for psychiatric illness (Model 4). Although psychotropic drug use is usually safe, the risk of significant medical morbidity due to psychotropic adverse effects and toxicity is present. An example of this mechanism would be the development of tardive dyskinesia associated with long-term antipsychotic use for schizophrenia. In this example, the psychiatric illness requires a treatment that increases risk for a medical disorder. Another example consistent with this mechanism would be the renal complications linked to lithium therapy. Lithium can produce significant polyuria and with lithium toxic episodes renal insufficiency.

A final mechanism that might explain some of the increased risk for medical and psychiatric comorbidity is the possibility of a link between psychiatric illnesses and behaviors or habits that increase risk for medical illness (Model 5). One behavioral problem that is increased in psychiatric disorders is smoking and nicotine dependence. The medical complications associated with cigarette use are well documented. Breslau (1) conducted an epidemiologic survey of the psychiatric correlates of nicotine dependence in a sample of over 1000 young adults in Michigan. DSM-III-R diagnoses including nicotine dependence were made using the Diagnostic Interview Schedule. The lifetime nicotine dependence prevalence rate was 20%. People with nicotine dependence were compared to those without dependence in regard to rates of other psychiatric disorders.

Nicotine dependence was associated with a variety of psychiatric disorders. People with nicotine dependence were three times more likely to suffer from a major depressive disorder than those without nicotine dependence. Additionally, nicotine dependence associated with a 2.6 odds ratio for any anxiety disorder, a 4.0 odds ratio for drug abuse or dependence, and a 2.6 odds ratio for alcohol abuse or dependence.

The reason for increased rates of psychiatric disorders in nicotine dependence is unclear. Gilbert and Gilbert (2) proposed several mediators of the genetic risk for smoking. Personality, psychopathology, and individual nicotine response might mediate the genetic risk for smoking. Nicotine dependence appears to be linked to neurotic traits (e.g., depression, anxiety, anger), social alienation, and low achievement/socioeconomic status. Nicotine may also be used by people with psychopathology to self-medicate for psychiatric symptoms. Regardless of the mechanism involved, high rates of nicotine dependence in psychiatric disorder is likely to increase the risk for smoking-related medical illness in the population at large with mental disorders.

Studies of the prevalence of psychiatric illnesses in the medically ill provide the basis for understanding medical psychiatric comorbidity. The next sections focus on general population and clinical studies of medical-psychiatric comorbidity.

PREVALENCE STUDIES

General Population Studies

Few general population studies for psychiatric comorbidity in the general population have been completed. One exception to this lack of data is the National Institute of Mental Health's Epidemiological Catchment Area (ECA) study (3). This multicenter population-based study targeted DSM-III disorders and utilized a structured interview—the Diagnostic Interview Schedule. The prevalence of psychiatric disorders in subjects with general medical conditions was compared to the prevalence of psychiatric disorders in subjects without general medical conditions (4). The eight medical disorder categories were arthritis, cancer, lung disease, neurological disorder, heart disease, physical handicap, hypertension, and diabetes.

Thirty-four percent of approximately 2500 persons in the ECA general population sample reported the presence of one of the eight medical disorders. Twenty-one percent endorsed current treatment for their medical disorder. The most common medical conditions were arthritis (14.8%) and hypertension (10.4%). The least common medical conditions were cancer (1.3%) and neurological disorder (1.3%). Presence of a medical condition significantly increased the rate of lifetime psychiatric disorder for any psychiatric disorder, mood disorders, substance abuse/dependence disorders, and anxiety disorders. The extent of the increase ranged from a 54% increase for lifetime mood disorder, to a 47% increase for lifetime anxiety disorder, to a 34% increase for substance abuse/dependence, to a 28% increase for any psychiatric disorder. Psychiatric disorders were increased also for the period of 6 months prior to the interview for the medically ill population. This was particularly true for anxiety disorders. Recent anxiety disorders occurred in 11.9% of the chronically medically ill compared to 6.0% of the population without a chronic medical illness. This represents a 98% increase for the chronically medically ill group.

When specific medical conditions were examined, Wells et al.'s study (4) reported that most of the chronic medical conditions were associated with increased rates of psychiatric disorder. The two exceptions were hypertension and diabetes, neither of whose diagnoses predicted increased rates of psychiatric disorder. Any recent psychiatric disorder rates were highest for heart disease (46%), arthritis (43%), physical handicap (40%), chronic handicap (32%), and neurological condition (32%). These rates contrasted with the 18% rate for any psychiatric disorder found in subjects with none of the general medical conditions. The authors of the study concluded that psychiatric disorders are increased in a variety of general medical conditions. They emphasized the need to also pay attention to anxiety disorders when studying the epidemiology of psychiatric conditions in medically ill populations.

One weakness of the ECA study of medical and psychiatric conditions is the lack of information about timing and sequencing of the two disorders. It is impossible to tell the mechanism for the development of the two disorders. Did the medical condition cause the increased rate of psychiatric disorder? Did the psychiatric disorder lead to an increased risk for the medical disorder? Did treatment for either disorder lead to the other? More general population studies of the relationship between medical and psychiatric conditions are necessary with attention paid to sequencing, timing, and causality in the two conditions.

Clinical Population Studies

Multiple Psychiatric Disorder Studies

A recent study of DSM-IV psychiatric illness demonstrates the heterogeneity of psychiatric disorders in medical inpatients (5). Three hundred and thirteen consecutive medical patients admitted for a medical illness participated in a study of DSM-IV diagnosis. This study examined the rate of illness in the 7 days after admission compared to the rate of psychiatric illness prior to admission. Twenty-seven percent of the patients met criteria for a DSM-IV diagnosis. The most frequent diagnoses were adjustment disorder (14%), anxiety disorder (6%), alcohol abuse/dependence (5%), and major depressive disorder (5%). Most of the cases of depression were present prior to admission. An important insight uncovered in this study focused on the medical staff knowledge of psychiatric illness. When medical staff and nursing staff were blindly asked to identify patients with psychiatric illness, nurses outperformed the medical staff by recognizing 61% of the cases compared to 41% recognized by the medical staff.

Barrett et al. (6) conducted a well-designed two-stage study of the prevalence of mental disorders in a primary care practice. The population sampled included adult members of an internal medicine group practice. More than 1000 patients were screened, with patients demonstrating high screening scores receiving a direct psychiatric interview. The prevalence for all psychiatric disorder diagnoses was 26.5%. The majority of psychiatric disorders in this primary care setting were depressive disorders or anxiety disorders.

Mood Disorders

Depression commonly develops following the onset of many different medical illnesses (7). Depression secondary to medical illness appears to have some distinct clinical features compared to primary major depression (depression without medical illness). Winokur et al. (8) summarized the differences in depression secondary to medical illness compared to primary major depression. Depression secondary to medical illness is more likely than primary depression to have a later age of onset, respond to electroconvulsive therapy (ECT), and present with impaired cognition. Depression secondary to medical illness is less likely than primary depression to be associated with a family history of alcoholism or a family history of depression and less likely to result in suicide (9).

Many prevalence studies of depression in specific medical illnesses have been completed. Although the methodologies often differ, depression appears to be common in a variety of disorders. Several studies of patients with coronary artery disease estimate the rate of major depression at 16–19% (10–13). Rates of depression in patients with cancer appear slightly higher, with estimates in the 25–38% range (14,15). The highest estimated rates of secondary depression in the medically ill occur in patients with neurological disorders such as Parkinson's disease (16), epilepsy (17), and Huntington's disease (18). Estimated rates of depression in these conditions range from 40 to 55%. Haskett (19) observed one of the highest rates of depression in a series of patients with Cushing's syndrome—67%.

Katon and Schulberg (20) summarized the findings of the literature for depression in primary care populations. Rates of major depression in the community have been estimated to be between 2 and 4%. Primary care studies of ambulatory patients estimate the rates in these populations to be between 5 and 10%. For medical inpatients, the rates appear even higher, with estimates in the range of 10–14%. The authors report that two to three times as many primary care patients exhibit depressive symptoms that fall short of criteria for major depressive disorder. These findings support a high rate of major depression and depression symptoms in the primary care populations; many of these patients will have comorbid medical illness.

Geriatric populations tend to have the highest rates of medical disorders and also appear to have significant psychiatric comorbidity. Lish et al. (21) examined a series of geriatric and nongeriatric patients attending a Veterans Administration hospital general medical clinic. Geriatric patients had high rates of a variety of psychiatric disorders including mood disorders (primarily depression), anxiety disorders, substance use disorders, and somatoform disorders. The authors concluded that screening for depression alone in geriatric populations will only identify approximately one half of all geriatric patients with psychiatric disorders. Physicians need to expand their screening and assessment methods to include substance abuse, anxiety disorders, somatoform disorders, and cognitive impairment disorders in the general medical population.

SPECIFIC PSYCHIATRIC CONDITIONS

Anxiety Disorders

Sherbourne et al. (22) examined the prevalence rates for anxiety disorders in a series of family practice patients. Nearly 2500 adult patients with hypertension, diabetes, heart disease, or depression received a structured interview for panic disorder, phobia, and generalized anxiety disorder. Depending on the type of presenting problem, 14–66% of the family practice patients had one concurrent anxiety disorder. Anxiety disorder was more common among the depressed patients than among patients with a primary medical illness.

Anxiety disorders including panic disorder have been increasingly recognized as important components of psychiatric illness in medically ill populations. Gerdes et al. (23) examined the prevalence of panic disorder in a series of patients referred for psychiatric consultation for the years 1980, 1985, and 1990. Over that decade, medical physicians referred an increasing number of patients for evaluation of anxiety symptoms, increasing from 10.6% of all consultation requests in 1980 to 14.9% in 1990. Panic disorder consultation rates increased from 2.5% to 5.1% of all consultations during the same period. Referring physicians identified panic attacks as a key feature in panic disorder at a much higher rate in 1990 than in 1980. Only 5% of patients with panic disorder in 1980 had panic attacks identified in the consultation request. The rate of identification of panic attacks increased to 59% of all panic disorder patients in 1990. The development of DSM-III and DSM-III-R along with increased psychiatric training for medical physicians probably contributed to the increase in identification of panic disorder.

Primary care populations appear to have a significant rate of mixed anxiety and depression in the distribution of psychiatric disorders. Pure major depression or pure anxiety disorder may be the exception rather than the rule for the majority of patients with psychiatric disorder in primary care. Stein et al. (24) studied a series of patients from a primary care outpatient setting. Seventy-eight of 798 patients (9.8%) screened demonstrated evidence of an anxiety disorder or a depressive disorder. Of those with a mood or anxiety disorder, only 20% had a depressive disorder alone and 25% had an anxiety disorder alone. The majority (55%) had evidence of both an anxiety disorder and a mood disorder or significant anxiety in the context of depression that met ICD-10 criteria for mixed affective disorder. This study confirms the need to consider the contribution of anxiety disorder in the clinical presentation of psychiatric illness among medically ill populations.

Although anxiety disorders can produce physical symptoms mimicking medical illness, it is possible that some anxiety disorders are more common in specific medical conditions. A recent study of the prevalence of medical illness in patients with anxiety disorder demonstrated a link between panic disorder and peptic ulcer disease, angina, and thyroid conditions (25). Somatic complaints in patients with psychiatric illness cannot be ignored but need to be examined carefully to rule out significant medical illness.

Alcohol and Drug Abuse

Alcohol abuse and dependence contribute directly to significant morbidity and mortality in the United States and throughout the world. An estimated 200,000 deaths per year in the United States are alcohol-related (26). About 25,000 of these deaths are due to alcohol-related motor vehicle accidents. Adolescents and young adults appear most vulnerable to the behavioral complications of drinking such as alcohol-related trauma, alcohol-related legal problems, and high-risk sexual behaviors while intoxicated. Medical complications like cirrhosis tend to occur following a long career of heavy drinking.

An estimated 25% of general hospital inpatients and 20% of medical outpatients have alcohol-related disorders (27–29). Seppa and Makela (30) studied the prevalence of heavy drinking in a series of patients hospitalized in a university hospital in Finland. Heavy drinking was defined as drinking greater than 280 grams of alcohol per week for men and greater than 140 grams of alcohol per week for women. Using this cutoff, 27% of male admissions and 11% of women met the criteria for heavy drinking. Physicians identified only 43% of men and only 26% of women with alcohol problems. Psychiatrists and neurologists had the highest identification rates in this study, while internal medicine specialists had lower rates of correctly identifying alcohol problems.

This study confirms that a significant percentage of medical patients with alcoholism go unrecognized by their physicians. Several factors may contribute to this under-recognition. Patients may be reluctant to discuss their drinking and drinking-related problems. Physicians may not ask about the patient's drinking history or may not collect information from family members that might be diagnostic for alcoholism.

Alcoholism contributes to a significant number of medical illnesses in various

Table 1 Alcohol-Attributable Fractions for
Medical Disorders

Alcoholic cirrhosis	1.00
Esophageal cancer	0.80
Homicide	0.46
Fire deaths	0.45
Motor vehicle accidents	0.42
Suicide	0.28
Stroke	0.07

body systems. The extent of alcohol's contribution to specific medical conditions has been designated as the alcohol-attributable fraction. Table 1 lists the alcohol-attributable fraction for a variety of medical conditions.

Drugs other than alcohol also contribute to medical disorders. Cocaine use has been linked to a variety of medical disorders, including nasal septal necrosis, seizures, myocardial infarction, cardiac arrhythmias, and significant weight loss with long-term use. Intravenous use of cocaine and other drugs increases the risk of complications related to self-injection: endocarditis, septicemia, HIV infection, hepatitis B and C, pulmonary embolus, and local cellulitis and vasculitis.

Amphetamine use appears to be on the increase in the United States. A recent psychiatric consultation series found that 15.6% of patients referred for psychiatric consultation in a general hospital had used amphetamine (31). Amphetamine use was documented by urine drug screens and verbal reports. Patients with amphetamine use had high rates of suicide attempts with medical morbidity and were more likely to be encountered in consultation requests from the departments of infectious disease, obstetrics and gynecology, and trauma surgery.

The use of alcohol and/or drugs in pregnancy increases the risk for fetal and neonatal disorders. Heavy alcohol consumption during pregnancy increases the risk of premature labor and delivery and low birth weight. Cocaine use during pregnancy results in an increased risk for abruptio placenta and behavioral abnormalities in infants (32).

Personality Disorders

The personality disorders have received relatively little attention in medically ill populations. Several contributing factors probably have influenced the limited study in this area. First, the development of reliable and valid personality disorder instruments trailed the development of reliable and valid axis I disorders. Second, personality disorders often are incorrectly assumed to be less prevalent and less important than the major axis I psychiatric disorders. Several community studies of the prevalence of personality disorder have been completed (33,34). These studies estimate the community prevalence rate of personality disorder to be between 5 and 12%. Some studies find significant correlations between personality psychopathology and use of medical services (35,36). Cluster B personality scores in women correlated highly with the number of outpatient visits to a primary care physician. These studies point to the need for further exploration of how personality affects somatic symptoms and medical care utilization.

Personality disorder appears common in some medical disorders in the few studies in clinical populations available. This is particularly true for patients with chronic pain disorders and patients with substance abuse problems. Polatin et al. (36) interviewed 200 chronic low back pain patients entering a rehabilitation program. Fifty-one percent of the low back pain patients met criteria for at least one personality disorder. Personality disorder, anxiety disorder, and substance abuse disorders in this study tended to emerge prior to the onset of back pain, while depression occurred both before and after the onset of back pain. Personality disorders develop early in life and tend to be chronic conditions, potentially influencing a variety of medical conditions.

Personality disorders associate with a variety of chronic medical conditions and with a variety of presenting complaints. A high percentage of a series of patients with chronic insomnia demonstrated personality disorder characterized by internalization of stress with an anxious-depressed reaction style (37).

Somatoform Disorders

Kirmayer and Robbins (38) surveyed 685 patients attending two family practice clinics. Using the Diagnostic Interview Schedule, three measures of somatization were described: (a) high levels of functional somatic distress, (b) hypochondriasis, defined as high levels of illness worry in the absence of serious medical illness, and (c) somatic presentations alone in patients with current major depression or anxiety. One percent of the subjects met the criteria for somatization disorder, 16.6% met abridged criteria for subsyndromal somatization disorder (significant functional somatic symptoms without meeting criteria for somatization disorder), and hypochondriacal worry was present in 7.7% of the patients. A pure somatic presentation for patients with major depression or anxiety disorder occurred in 8% of the sample. This survey underscores the variety of manifestations of somatic distress in primary care and the high prevalence rates in a common clinical outpatient setting.

General practice attendees in England have also demonstrated high rates of somatization disorder and other somatic presentations of psychiatric disorder. Using the General Health Questionnaire (GHQ), Weich et al. (39) surveyed a series of consecutive general practice patients. Pure somatization was defined as a medical consultation for somatic symptoms that were judged to be attributable to a psychiatric disorder unrecognized by the patient. Twenty-five percent of patients were identified as somatic presenters. Four percent of attenders met criteria for pure somatization. The majority of the remainder of somatic presenters were GHQ probable psychiatric cases. Somatic presentation of psychiatric disorder resulted in lower rates of accurate psychiatric diagnosis than for psychiatric presentation. This survey documents the tendency of somatic presentation to confuse physicians about the presence of psychiatric morbidity.

Other Psychiatric Disorders

Sleep disorders and complaints of chronic insomnia commonly present with comorbid mental disorders. In a large series of more than 2500 general practice attenders, patients with complaints of chronic insomnia were interviewed for the presence of mental disorders including personality disorder (37). One hundred and five patients reported chronic insomnia, and 66 of these patients met the DSM-III-R criteria for suffering from chronic insomnia. For those meeting DSM-III-R criteria for chronic insomnia, 50% of the patients had at least one axis I or II diagnosis. Mood disorders and substance abuse disorders ranked highest in prevalence in this group.

SPECIFIC MEDICAL POPULATIONS

Seizure Disorder

Seizure disorder has been noted to be associated with psychiatric symptoms and psychiatric disorder for many years. A recent study evaluated 97 consecutive patients admitted with seizures for neurodiagnostic imaging completed psychiatric evaluations (40). Sixty-five percent of the patients were in need of psychiatric treatment. Mood disorders ranked first in prevalence at 34%, followed by conversion disorder, pseudoseizure type at 22% and other psychiatric diagnoses at 9%.

Traumatic Brain Injury

A recent well-designed survey examined the prevalence of psychiatric comorbidity in a series of 50 outpatients with traumatic brain injury (41). Thirteen (26%) of the subjects demonstrated current major depression, and an additional 28% reported post-traumatic depression that had resolved. Generalized anxiety was noted in 24% of the sample, and 8% reported current substance abuse. Comorbid depression or anxiety was associated with significantly more impairment and self-reported more severe injury and more cognitive impairment. These self-reports were not validated by objective measures of illness severity and cognitive function. This effect has been noted in other medical illnesses. Medically ill patients with psychiatric illness tend to overestimate the severity of their medical illness.

Stroke

Stroke provides a model for understanding psychiatric disorders produced by lesions in various brain sites. Several psychiatric disorders occur at high rates in patients following stroke. The most extensive work has focused on depression following stroke (42). Depression complicates recovery from stroke in up to 30–50% of stroke patients. Depression may occur immediately after stroke or develop in a more delayed presentation in the year following stroke. The risk for depression following stroke appears to be related to lesion location. Strokes involving the left frontal region of the brain produce depression more frequently than strokes in other brain sites. In addition to depression, stroke can in rare circumstance also induce mania (43). Generalized anxiety disorder also appears to occur in some poststroke patients. (44).

Respiratory Disease

Psychiatric illnesses, particularly anxiety disorder and panic disorder, frequently complicate chronic respiratory diseases such as asthma and chronic obstructive pulmonary disease. Some patients with panic disorder seek evaluation for possible pulmonary causes for their respiratory symptoms related to panic disorder. In a series of patients referred for pulmonary testing, 41% reported panic attacks and 17% met screening criteria for panic disorder (45).

Among patients with chronic obstructive pulmonary disease, the prevalence of panic disorder has been estimated at 8–24%—a rate 10 times higher than that found in community studies of panic disorder (46–48). Similar high rates of panic disorder have been described for asthma (49). Dyspnea is a common symptom in anxiety disorders, and the interaction between pulmonary disease and subjective breathing complaints may explain some of the reason for higher rates of anxiety disorders in the pulmonary disease population (50).

Cancer

A multicenter study of the prevalence of psychiatric disorders in cancer patients confirmed clinicians' impressions of high rates of mental disorders in this population (51). Forty-seven percent of a series of patients with various types of cancer met criteria for a psychiatric diagnosis when interviewed with a structured psychiatric interview. The most common psychiatric disorder identified was adjustment disorder with a prevalence rate of 32%, followed by major depression with 6%, organic mental disorder with 4%, personality disorder with 3%, and anxiety disorder with 2%. Estimated rates of depression have been higher in other clinical samples of cancer patients. Pancreatic cancer appears to be particularly likely to be complicated by depression (52). Several mechanisms may explain this association. One hypothesis is that pancreatic cancers may produce an antibody or autoantibody that crosses the blood-brain barrier and interferes with serotonin synaptic functioning (53).

Gastrointestinal Disease

Gastrointestinal complaints and gastrointestinal disease are common physical problems. Psychiatric disorders occur with a variety of gastrointestinal conditions at rates higher than chance. Irritable bowel syndrome appears to have a particularly high rate of psychiatric comorbidity. A general population survey of gastrointestinal complaints, depression, and anxiety has been published from the ECA data set (54). Medically unexplained gastrointestinal symptoms were noted in 6–25% of the general population. Subjects with one medically unexplained gastrointestinal complaint had about a threefold increase in major depression, panic disorder, and agoraphobia. When subjects with two or more medically unexplained gastrointestinal complaints were examined, their rate of major depression, panic, and agoraphobia was increased four- to fivefold.

Diabetes and Other Endocrine Disorders

Insulin-dependent diabetes mellitus often represents a lifelong serious, progressive, and disabling condition. Like other chronic diseases, patients with diabetes are reminded daily of their illness with insulin injections and measurement of blood glucose levels. Gavard et al. (55) reviewed studies of the prevalence of depression among clinical populations with diabetes. The prevalence range for depression in diabetes was 8.5–27.3%, an estimated threefold increase in risk of depression compared to the rate in the general population. Death by suicide also appears to be increased among diabetic patients. Kyvik et al. (56) studied a cohort of Danish men born between 1949 and 1964 with diabetes. Compared to the general population, male diabetics demonstrated a 60% increase in completed suicide.

Psychiatry Consultation Series

Wallen et al. (57) reviewed 19 studies of the epidemiology of psychiatric consultation. These studies utilized hospitalized medical samples from the United States, Canada, and Great Britain. The size of the consultation series generated from total admissions ranged from 230 to over 29,000. The percentage of admissions receiving a psychiatric consultation ranged from 0.6 to 10.3%, with an average of about 3% of all hospital admissions. Most consultation series report that the most frequent psychiatric diagnosis encountered is depression. An exception to this finding is the report of hysteria being the most common psychiatric consultation diagnosis in a pediatric consultation series reported by Monnelly et al. (58).

After reviewing the literature for psychiatric consultation, Wallen reported the results of a study of consultation in general hospitals using a base of 263,000 medical admissions. This sample came from a national data set in the United States. The rate of psychiatric consultation in this large series was 0.9%. Medical and psychiatric diagnoses were coded from discharge abstracts classified according to the Hospital Adaptation of the International Classification of Diseases (H-ICD) (59). This system of classification was a precursor to ICD-9.

The principal ICD medical diagnoses that had the highest rates of psychiatric consultation included (1) accidents, poisoning, and violence, (2) endocrine, nutritional, and metabolic diseases, and (3) symptoms and ill-defined conditions. Principal ICD medical diagnoses that had the lowest rates of psychiatric illness included (1) genitourinary system diseases, (2) neoplasms, and (3) respiratory diseases. The most frequent ICD mental disorders in this psychiatric consultation series included (1) neurosis,

(2) psychosis, (3) alcoholism, and (4) organic brain syndrome. Somatoform disorders probably made up a significant percentage of those classified in the neurosis group.

University of Iowa Psychiatry Consultation Series

To better understand the epidemiology of psychiatric illness in the medical setting, a series of psychiatric consultation patients at the University of Iowa Hospitals and Clinics were reviewed. This consultation service sees patients referred from medical and surgical physicians and performs about 1200 new consultations per year. Approximately two thirds of these consultations occur in the medical or surgical inpatient, while about one third of the consultations are performed in the outpatient setting.

A database for July 1, 1993 to June 30, 1995 provides information on psychiatric diagnosis rates for approximately 2400 patients referred for consultation. This academic consultation service included family practice and psychiatry residents. All consultation patients were staffed and seen by a psychiatrist with expertise in diagnosis in the consultation setting. Diagnoses were made based on DSM-III-R or DSM-IV criteria. When multiple psychiatric diagnoses were present, the one diagnosis most predominant or most related to the consultation request was coded.

For the purposes of analysis, 200 consults from internal medicine, 200 consults from neurology, and 200 consults from surgery were reviewed. All consults were selected randomly from the series, with half coming from female patients and half coming from male patients. Additionally, the series was stratified by referral site, with half of each group seen while inpatients and half seen as outpatients.

Table 2 outlines the distribution of major psychiatric diagnostic categories according to referral source and site of consultation. Mood disorders rank first on the prevalence list for all specialties and in both inpatient and outpatient settings. Mood disorders make up about one third of all consultation diagnoses. After mood disorders, some variability in the prevalence of diagnosis develops. Seven diagnostic categories rank closely together after mood disorders, with prevalence rates of 5–10% in the consultation series. These seven diagnostic categories are substance use disorders, adjustment disorders, personality disorders, anxiety disorders, cognitive impairment disorders, somatoform disorders, and psychotic disorders. Most diagnostic categories have similar prevalence rates in inpatient and outpatient settings. One significant exception to this distribution are the cognitive impairment disorders, including dementia and delirium. These disorders occur much more commonly in the inpatient series than in the outpatient series. The outpatient series includes more patients with personality disorder and anxiety disorder diagnoses.

Distribution of psychiatric diagnosis varies somewhat by referring specialty group. Surgical consultation inpatients display the highest rates of cognitive impairment disorders. Neurology inpatient consultations rate highest in somatoform disorder frequency. Substance abuse diagnoses are seen in all groups, with rates slightly lower in the obstetrics and gynecology series.

Table 3 displays the gender distribution of the psychiatric disorders split by

Table 2 Distribution of Psychiatric Consultation Diagnoses by Referring Specialty and Site of Contact

Disorder category	Internal medicine IP	OP	Neurology IP	OP	Surgery IP	OP	OBGYN IP	OP	Combined sample IP	OP	Total	% Total
Mood	31	41	38	46	25	25	10	15	104	127	231	34.7
Personality	7	3	5	17	7	14	3	6	22	40	62	9.3
Alcohol/Drug	12	9	5	8	13	11	1	2	31	30	61	9.2
Adjustment	8	13	6	3	10	10	5	4	29	30	59	8.9
Cognitive impairment	15	2	13	1	23	1	0	0	51	4	55	8.3
Anxiety	6	14	5	10	4	13	1	2	16	39	55	8.3
Somatoform	9	6	12	7	2	6	3	0	26	19	45	6.8
Psychotic	8	6	5	1	11	6	5	2	29	15	44	6.6
None	2	5	4	3	4	9	4	0	14	17	31	4.7
Other psychiatric	2	1	7	4	1	5	1	2	11	12	23	3.5
Total	100	100	100	100	100	100	33	33	333	333	666	

Table 3 Distribution of Psychiatric Consultation Diagnoses by Referring Specialty and Gender

Disorder category	Internal medicine		Neurology		Surgery		OBGYN	Combined sample			
	Female	Male	Female	Male	Female	Male	Female	Female	%	Male	%
Mood	30	42	43	41	28	22	25	126	34.4	105	35.0
Anxiety	16	4	8	7	9	8	9	42	11.5	19	6.3
Somatoform	11	4	15	4	3	5	9	38	10.4	13	4.3
Adjustment	9	12	6	3	13	7	3	31	8.5	22	7.3
Cognitive impairment	9	8	9	5	13	11	0	31	8.5	24	8.0
Personality	5	5	5	17	10	11	3	23	6.3	33	11.0
Alcohol/Drug	4	17	4	9	8	16	7	23	6.3	42	14.0
None	6	1	5	2	8	5	3	22	6.0	8	2.7
Psychotic	8	6	1	5	6	11	4	19	5.2	22	7.3
Other psychiatric	2	1	4	7	2	4	3	11	3.0	12	4.0
Total	100	100	100	100	100	100	66	366		300	

referring service. Mood disorders are common across both genders, and the rates do not reflect the higher rates of mood disorder in women in the general population. However, like the general population, substance abuse diagnoses are more common in the male consultation series. Anxiety disorders, adjustment disorders, and somatoform disorders were diagnosed at higher rates in the female series.

This consultation series provides a view of the spectrum of psychiatric illnesses in the medically ill population. Although the distribution of psychiatric disorders may vary by referring source, eight groups of disorders make up the majority of all diagnoses. In this series these eight groups make up over 90% of the consultation diagnoses and form the core group of psychiatric disorders important in the medically ill population. The next section will address some the risk factors for the development of psychiatric illness in medical populations.

RISK FACTORS

Costello et al. (60) conducted one of the few studies of risk factors for psychiatric disorders among pediatric primary care populations. Children between the ages of 7 and 11 received the Diagnostic Schedule for Children interview with 22% meeting criteria for at least one psychiatric diagnosis. Oppositional defiant disorder and conduct disorder were associated with male gender. Additionally, risk for oppositional defiant disorder was increased in lower socioeconomic classes, in children who had repeated a grade, and in children without a father in the home. Parents reporting significant stress for their child were more likely to have a child with a behavior, anxiety, or mood disorder.

There has been limited study of the risk factors for psychiatric comorbidity among medical patients in general adult medical populations. In general, psychiatric illness appears more common in more severe medical illness and in medical illness that results in significant impairment in daily functioning.

COURSE AND OUTCOME

Depression

Wells et al. (61) studied the course of comorbid depression in patients with hypertension, diabetes, and myocardial infarction. More than 600 patients with depression from general medical practices received follow-up interviews 1–2 years following an index interview. These follow-up interviews were done by phone using the Diagnostic Interview Schedule. High rates of persistence of depressive symptoms occurred in patients with and without medical comorbidity. History of myocardial infarction appeared to predict a more severe chronic course for depression. Myocardial infarction comorbidity in depression predicted more episodes of depression, more total depressive symptoms in the second following year, and more depressive symptoms at the time of each follow-up interview. Comorbid hypertension and diabetes did not predict a poorer outcome for depression.

Patients hospitalized for depression exhibit extended lengths of stay when concurrent medical illness is present. Depressed patients with medical illness were hospitalized nearly twice as long as depressed patients without physical illness (20.1 days vs. 10.5 days) (62). The authors of this study suggest that several mechanisms might explain the increased length of stay in depression associated with comorbid medical illness. These mechanisms may include a tendency for depression to mask physical illness and a tendency for mood symptoms to result in neglect of physical symptoms.

Winokur et al. (8) compared the clinical presentation and outcome of depression secondary to medical illness to those of depression secondary to psychiatric illness in a series of over 400 patients. Patients with depression secondary to medical illness demonstrated an older age of onset with higher rates of cognitive impairment. However, the prognosis for depression secondary to medical illness appeared to be better. A higher percentage of patients with depression secondary to medical illness were improved after discharge from an index admission. Also, fewer patients in the medically ill group relapsed during the follow-up period, and fewer in this group had suicide as a cause of death.

Depression secondary to medical illness can be split into two groups. In one group, the medical illness can be a direct contributor to pathophysiologic changes in the brain that can induce depression. Examples of secondary depression of this type include depression following stroke in the central nervous system sites felt to be important in the control and modulation of mood. A second group of secondary depressions would include those that do not seem to be due to a direct contribution to pathophysiologic changes in the brain. Examples of the second type of secondary depression would be depression in diabetes or in coronary artery disease. The clinical presentation and outcome may be different in these two types of secondary depression.

Yates et al. (63) contrasted the clinical presentation and outcome for these two groups of secondary depression. Subjects in this study were identified from a series of psychiatric consultations in a university hospital population. Fifty subjects were identified with what was felt to be an "organic" depression due to a direct physiologic effect on the brain. The most common medical illnesses in this group included depression following stroke, seizure disorder, and corticosteroid use. A second group of secondary illnesses occurred in a group not felt to have a direct pathophysiologic effect. The most common medical illnesses in this group include diabetes mellitus, hypertension, and coronary artery disease. Groups were matched by age and sex and compared on a variety of clinical and outcome measures.

The type of DSM-III-R symptoms noted in the two groups did not differ. The secondary depressions due to an "organic" etiology displayed significant differences from secondary depressions without an "organic" etiology in other areas. Patients with organic depression demonstrated a higher severity of axis IV stress and were receiving more total numbers of medication for their illnesses. They were also more likely to be in their initial episode of a mood disorder and to show evidence on cognitive testing of cognitive impairment. Despite similar exposure to adequate antidepressant treatment, fewer subjects in the organic secondary depression group were recovered during the year of follow-up. This study supports a poorer outcome and response to treatment in secondary depressions felt to come from an "organic" cause. The authors suggest that these differences contribute to the validity of considering two types of secondary depression in medically ill populations.

Other studies support that depression complicated by comorbid medical illness appears to have a poorer prognosis than depression without medical illness. Several studies examined the longitudinal course of depression among primary care patients (64,65). Initial severity of depression predicts the outcome of depression—those with the highest severity at an index interview tend to have the poorest prognosis. Chronic medical illness appears to predict a poorer psychiatric outcome compared to acute medical conditions. Chronic medical illness may produce a long-term psychological burden that prohibits complete recovery from depression. Further studies of the treatment of depression in the chronically medically ill are needed to determine if this poor prognosis can be improved.

Anxiety Disorders

Up to 25–30% of patients develop generalized anxiety following a stroke. Generalized anxiety disorder can occur early or late in the course of recovery. Astrom (66) found that early development of generalized anxiety predicted a poor functional outcome for patients with stroke. Only 23% of patients with early generalized anxiety disorder following stroke recovered by one year. Generalized anxiety disorder developing at any time associated with dependence in daily activities and reduced social functioning.

Personality Disorder

Personality disorder in primary care settings can contribute to increased medical morbidity, increased medical and psychiatric service utilization, and high rates of psychotropic drug use. Seivewright et al. (67) studied 357 patients identified in a primary care practice with psychiatric illness identified with a structured interview. Personality disorder predicted morbidity, psychiatric service use, and psychotropic drug use in this medical setting. Rural primary care patients with personality disorder received more consultation for medical illnesses than those without personality disorder. This study emphasizes the need for more study of the role of personality disorder in primary care settings.

Alcohol and Drug Abuse

The use of alcohol or drugs appears to complicate the course of many medical disorders. Alcohol plays a key role in the etiology of many medical conditions including hypertension, heart disease, peptic ulcer disease, alcoholic liver disease, pancreatitis, and cancer.

Jackson et al. (68) studied the effect of current alcohol consumption on a series of family practice outpatients with hypertension, diabetes, heart disease, and major depression. Alcohol consumption predicted increased outpatient utilization of medical services in this primary care group.

In another study of alcohol disorder in primary care, Sherbourne et al. (69) examined 2296 patients from a family practice. Subjects in the study had one of four illnesses: diabetes, hypertension, heart disease, or depressive disorder. Both medical disorders and depression were associated with high rates of lifetime alcohol disorder (14% vs. 19%). Depressed patients with current alcohol problems were more likely to report need for help with their drinking problem. Many patients in this primary care setting reported an unmet need for care for alcohol or drug problems in the medical care setting. This study points to the need for both accurate assessment and treatment protocols for alcohol and drug abuse problems in primary care settings.

Medical Illnesses

Psychiatric disorders appear to influence the outcome of medical complaints and medical disorders. Clark et al. (70) examined factors that predicted the persistence of fatigue in a series of patients followed for 30 months. Seventy-eight patients who reported fatigue for 6 months or more were reevaluated $2^{1}/_{2}$ years after an index psychiatric examination. Fatigue symptom persistence was associated with DSM-III-R dysthymia at index interview. Other factors associated with symptom persistence included more than eight medically unexplained symptoms not associated with chronic fatigue syndrome, duration of symptoms longer than $1^{1}/_{2}$ years at index evaluation, less than 16 years of formal education, and age greater than 38 years. This well-designed study emphasizes the negative effects that comorbid psychiatric illness can have on medical outcome.

Several studies in insulin-dependent diabetes suggest psychiatric factors contribute to poor compliance and adverse diabetic outcomes. Orlandini et al. (71) studied a series of 77 diabetic patients with a structured self-report DSM-III-R personality inventory. Elevated dramatic-dependent personality scores predicted high glycosylated hemoglobin levels (poor diabetic control).

Economic Effects of Psychiatric Illness in Primary Care

Psychiatric comorbidity can have significant effects on length of hospital stay for medical inpatients. Saravay and Lavin (72) reviewed the studies of the effect of psychiatric comorbidity on hospital length of stay. More than 26 studies had been completed at the time of the review. The majority of studies in the United States found a significantly increased length of stay for patients in general hospitals. Psychiatric disorders associated with prolonged length of stay included major depression, dementia, delirium, and personality disorder. The reviewers concluded that further well-designed research could provide better understanding of the mechanisms for increased length of stay and provide strategies for accurate psychiatric assessment and prevention.

The World Health Organization (WHO) recently published results of a study of mental disorders and disability in general practice populations (73). More than 25,000 patients from 14 countries received a two-stage interview starting with the General Health Questionnaire followed by the Composite International Diagnostic Interview. Psychopathology was a significant contributor to disability among this medical population, even when effects of medical illness on disability were controlled. Disability was most significant in major depression, panic disorder, generalized anxiety, and neurasthenia. This study underscores the importance of psychiatric factors in disability among medical populations throughout the world.

SUMMARY

Psychiatric disorders occur more commonly in persons with medical illness than in persons without medical illnesses. Several mechanisms promote the increased rate of comorbidity. Comorbidity may develop when a primary psychiatric illness increases the risk for medical complications and when primary medical illness increases the risk of a psychiatric illness. Treatment for medical and psychiatric illness can induce comorbidity. Psychiatric illnesses are associated with behaviors such as smoking and nicotine dependence, which increase rates of medical complications.

Clinical population studies of medical-psychiatric comorbidity are more common than general population studies. However, clinical populations are subject to various biases. For example, if psychiatric comorbidity increases the risk of seeking medical attention, clinical population studies would overestimate the extent of comorbidity. The Epidemiological Catchment Area (ECA) study provided evidence of true increased rates of medical-psychiatric comorbidity in excess of that expected by chance.

Clinical population studies of medical and psychiatric patients do support increased psychiatric comorbidity for a variety of medical conditions. Medical disorders that are chronic, disabling, and associated with significant pain appear to most increase the rates of psychiatric comorbidity. In studies of patients receiving psychiatric consultation, mood disorders such as major depression and dysthymia rank highest among all psychiatric conditions. The vast majority of psychiatric disorders found in medical patients come from seven categories: mood disorders, personality disorders, adjustment disorders, substance abuse disorders, anxiety disorders, somatoform disorders, and psychotic disorders. Studies of psychiatric patients also document a high rate of medical comorbidity.

Medical-psychiatric comorbidity predicts important aspects of clinical outcome and health services utilization. Medical disorders accompanied by serious psychiatric illness frequently have poorer outcomes including increased rates of mortality. Medical-psychiatric comorbidity increases the length and cost of hospitalization and increases the utilization of ambulatory medical care.

The epidemiology of psychiatric illness in the medically ill underscores the need for further studies of the mechanisms of comorbidity and further study of the treatment of psychiatric illness in specific medical populations. Such studies will address an important public health issue, reduce significant morbidity and mortality, and provide strategies for the prevention of comorbid illness.

REFERENCES

1. Breslau N. Psychiatric comorbidity of smoking and nicotine dependence. Behav Genet 1995; 25:95–101.
2. Gilbert DG, Gilbert BO. Personality, psychopathology, and nicotine response as mediators of the genetics of smoking. Behav Genet 1995; 25:133–147.
3. Robins LN, Helzer JE, Weissman MM, et al. Lifetime prevalence of specific psychiatric disorders in three sites. Arch Gen Psychiatry 1984; 41:949–958.
4. Wells KB, Golding JM, Burnam MA. Psychiatric disorder in a sample of the general population with and without chronic medical conditions. Am J Psychiatry 1988; 145:976–981.
5. Silverstone PH. Prevalence of psychiatric disorders in medical inpatients. J Nerv Ment Dis 1996; 184:43–51.
6. Barrett JE, Barrett JA, Oxman TE, Gerber PD. The prevalence of psychiatric disorders in a primary care practice. Arch Gen Psychiatry 1988; 45:1100–1106.
7. Rouchell AM, Pounds R, Tierney JG. Depression. In: Rundell JR, Wise MG, eds. Textbook of Consultation Liaison Psychiatry. Washington, DC: American Psychiatric Press Inc., 1996.
8. Winokur G, Black D, Nasrallah A. Depressions secondary to other psychiatric illness and medical illnesses. Am J Psychiatry 1988; 145:233–240.
9. Winokur G. The concept of a secondary depression and its relationship to comorbidity. Psychiatr Clin North Am 1990; 123:567–583.
10. Carney RM, Rich MW, Tevelde A, et al. Major depressive disorder in coronary artery disease. Am J Cardiol 1987; 60:1273–1275.
11. Forrester AW, Lipsey JR, Teitelbaum ML, et al. Depression following myocardial infarction. Int J Psychiatry Med 1992; 22:33–46.
12. Schleifer SJ, Macari-Hinson MM, Coyle DA, et al. The nature and course of depression following myocardial infarction. Arch Intern Med 1989; 149:1785–1789.
13. Frasure-Smith N, Lesperance F, Talajic M. Depression following myocardial infarction impact on 6-month survival. JAMA 1993; 270:1819–1825.
14. Massie MJ, Holland JC. Depression and the cancer patient. J Clin Psychiatry 1990; 51(suppl 7):12–17.
15. Kathol RG, Mulgi A, Williams J, et al. Diagnosis of major depression in cancer patients according to four sets of criteria. Am J Psychiatry 1990; 147:1021–1024.
16. Sano M, Stern Y, Williams J, et al. Coexisting dementia and depression in Parkinson's disease. Arch Neurol 1989; 46:1284–1286.
17. Mendez MF, Cummings JL, Benson F. Depression in epilepsy: significance and phenomenology. Arch Neurol 1986; 43:766–770.
18. Folstein SE, Abbott MH, Chase GA, et al. The association of affective disorder with Huntington's disease in a case series and in families. Psychol Med 1983; 13:537–542.

19. Haskett RF. Diagnostic categorization of psychiatric disturbance in Cushing's syndrome. Am J Psychiatry 1985; 142:911–916.
20. Katon W, Schulberg H. Epidemiology of depression in primary care. Gen Hosp Psychiatry 1992; 14:237–247.
21. Lish JD, Zimmerman M, Farber NJ, Lush D, Kuzma MA, Plescia G. Psychiatric screening in geriatric primary care: Should it be for depression alone? J Geriatr Psychiatry Neurol 1995; 8:141–153.
22. Sherbourne CD, Jackson CA, Meredith LS, Camp P, Wells KB. Prevalence of comorbid anxiety disorders in primary care outpatients. Arch Fam Med 1996; 5:27–34.
23. Gerdes T, Yates WR, Clancy G. Increasing identification and referral of panic disorder over the last decade. Psychosomatics 1995; 36:480–486.
24. Stein MB, Kirk P, Prabhu V, Grott M, Terepa M. Mixed anxiety-depression in a primary-care clinic. J Affect Disord 1995; 84:79–84.
25. Rogers MP, White K, Warshaw MG, Yonkers KA, Rodriguez-Villa F, Chang G, Keller MB. Prevalence of medical illness in patients with anxiety disorders. Int J Psychiatry Med 1994; 24:83–96.
26. U.S. Department of Health and Human Services. Seventh Special Report to the United States Congress on Alcohol and Health. Rockville, MD: National Institute on Alcohol Abuse and Alcoholism, 1990.
27. Franklin JE, Frances RJ. Substance-related disorders. In: Rundell JR, Wise MG, eds. Textbook of Consultation Liaison Psychiatry. Washington DC, American Psychiatric Press Inc, 1996.
28. Cleary PD, Miller M, Bush BT, et al. Prevalence and recognition of alcohol abuse in a primary care population. Am J Med 1988; 85:466–471.
29. Moore RD, Bone LR, Geller G, et al. Prevalence, detection and treatment of alcoholism in hospitalized patients. JAMA 1989; 261:403–407.
30. Seppa K, Makela R. Heavy drinking in hospitalized patients. Addiction 1993; 88:1377–1382.
31. Baberg HT, Nelesen RA, Dimsdale JE. Amphetamine use: return of an old scourge in a consultation psychiatry setting. Am J Psychiatry 1996; 153:789–793.
32. Chasnoff IJ, Burns WJ, Scholl SH. Cocaine use in pregnancy. N Engl J Med 1985; 813:666–669.
33. Reich J, Yates W, Nduaguba M. Prevalence of DSM-III personality disorders in the community. Soc Psychiatry Psychiatr Epidemiol 1989; 24:12–16.
34. Samuels JF, Nestadt G, Romanoski AJ, Folstein MF, McHugh PR. DSM-III personality disorders in the community. Am J Psychiatry 1994; 151:1055–1062.
35. Reich J, Boerstler H, Yates W, Nduaguba M. Utilization of medical resources in persons with DSM-III personality disorders in a community sample. Int J Psychiatry Med 1989; 19:1–9.
36. Polatin PB, Kinney RK, Gatchel RJ, Lillo E, Mayer TG. Psychiatric illness and chronic low-back pain. The mind and the spine—which goes first? Spine 1993; 18:66–71.
37. Schramm E, Hohagen F, Kappler C, Grasshoff U, Berger M. Mental comorbidty of chronic insomnia in general practice attenders using DSM-IIIR. Acta Psychiatr Scand 1993; 91:10–17.
38. Kirmayer LJ, Robbins JM. Three forms of somatization in primary care: prevalence, co-occurrence, and sociodemographic characteristics. J Nerv Ment Disord 1991; 179:647–655.

39. Weich S, Lewis G, Donmall R, Mann A. Somatic presentation of psychiatric morbidity in general practice. Br J Gen Pract 1993; 45:143–147.

40. Blumer D, Montouris G, Hermann B: Psychiatric morbidity in seizure patients on a neurodiagnostic monitoring unit. J Neuropsychiatry Clin Neurosci 1995; 7:445–456.

41. Fann JR, Katon WJ, Uomoto JM, Esselman PC. Psychiatric disorders and functional disability in outpatients with traumatic brain injuries. Am J Psychiatry 1995; 152:1493–1499.

42. Robinson RG, Starkstein SE. Current research in affective disorders following strokes. J Neuropsychiatry Clin Neurosci 1990; 2:1–14.

43. Starkstein SE, Robinson RG, Honig MA, et al. Mood changes after right hemisphere lesion. Br J Psychiatry 1989; 155:79–85.

44. Starkstein SE, Robinson RG. Neuropsychiatric aspects of cerebral vascular disorder. In: Yudofsky SC, Hales RE, eds. The American Psychiatric Press Textbook of Neuropsychiatry. 2d ed. Washington, DC: American Psychiatric Press, 1992:449–472.

45. Pollack MH, Kradin R, Otto MW, Worthington J, Gould R, Sabatino S, Rosenbaum JF. Prevalence of panic in patients referred for pumonary fuction testing at a major medical center. Am J Psychiatry 1996; 53:110–113.

46. Yellowlees PM, Alpers JH, Bowden JJ, et al. Psychiatric morbidity in patients with chronic airflow obstruction. Med J Aust 1985; 146:305–307.

47. Yellowlees PM, Haynes S, Potts N, et al. Psychiatric morbidity in patients with chronic life-threatening asthma: initial report of a controlled study. Med J Aust 1988; 149:246–249.

48. Karajgi B, Rifkin A, Doddi S, et al. The prevalence of anxiety disorders in patients with chronic obstructive pulmonary disease. Am J Psychiatry 1990; 147:200–201.

49. Shavitt RG, Gentil V, Mandetta R. The association of panic/agoraphobia and asthma: contributing factors and clinical implications. Gen Hosp Psychiatry 1992; 14:420–423.

50. Klein DF. False suffocation alarms, spontaneous panics, and related conditions: an integrative hypothesis. Arch Gen Psychiatry 1993; 50:306–317.

51. Derogatis LR, Morrow GR, Fetting J, et al. The prevalence of psychiatric disorders among cancer patients. JAMA 1983; 249:751–157.

52. Holland JC, Korzun AH, Tross S, et al. Comparative psychological disturbance in patients with pancreatic and gastric cancer. Am J Psychiatry 1986; 143:982–986.

53. Lesko LM, Massie MJ, Holland J. Oncology. In: Stoudemire A, Fogel B, eds. Psychiatric Care of the Medical Patient. New York: Oxford Press, 1993:565–590.

54. Walker EA, Katon KJ, Jemelka RP, Roy-Bryne PP. Comorbidity of gastrointestinal complaints, depression, and anxiety in the Epidemiologic Catchment Area (ECA) study. Am J Med 1992; 92:26S–30S.

55. Gavard JA, Lustman PJ, Clouse RE. Prevalence of depression in adults with diabetes. An epidemiological evaluation. Diabetes Care 1993; 16:1167–1178.

56. Kyvik KO, Stenager EN, Green A, Svendsen A. Suicides in men with IDDM. Diabetes Care 1994; 17:210–212.

57. Wallen J, Pincus HA, Goldman HH, Marcus SE. Psychiatric consultation in short-term general hospitals. Arch Gen Psychiatry 1987; 44:163–168.

58. Monnelly EP, Ianzito BM, Stewart MA. Psychiatric consultations in a children's hospital. Am J Psychiatry 1993; 130:789–792.

59. Commission on Professional and Hospital Activities. Hospital Adaptation of ICDA. 2d ed. Ann Arbor, MI: Commission on Professional and Hospital Activities, 1983.

60. Costello EJ, Costello AJ, Edelbrock C, Burns BJ, Dulcan MK, Brent D, Janiszewski S.

Psychiatric disorders in pediatric primary care. Prevalence and risk factors. Arch Gen Psychiatry 1988; 45:1107–1116.

61. Wells KB, Rogers W, Burnam MA, Camp P. Course of depression in patients with hypertension, myocardial infarction, or insulin-dependent diabetes. Am J Psychiatry 1993; 150: 632–638.

62. Schubert DS, Yokley J, Sloan D, Gottesman H. Impact of the interaction of depression and physical illness on a psychiatric unit's length of stay. Gen Hosp Psychiatry 1995; 17: 326–334.

63. Yates WR, Wesner RB, Thompson R. Organic mood disorder: a valid psychiatry consultation diagnosis? J Affect Disord 1991; 22:37–42.

64. Parker G, Holmes S, Manicavasagar V. Depression in general practice attenders. "Caseness," natural history and predictors of outcome. J Affect Disord 1986; 10:27–35.

65. Mayou R, Hawton K, Feldman E. What happens to medical patients with psychiatric disorder? J Psychosom Res 1988; 32:541–549.

66. Astrom M. Generalized anxiety disorder in stroke patients. A 3-year longitudinal study. Stroke 1996; 27:270–275.

67. Seivewright H, Tyrer P, Casey P, Seivewright N. A three-year follow-up of psychiatric morbidity in urban and rural primary care. Psychol Med 1991; 21(2):495–503.

68. Jackson CA, Manning WG Jr, Wells KB. Impact of prior and current alcohol use on use of services by patients with depression and chronic medical illnesses. Health Serv Res 1995; 80:687–705.

69. Sherbourne CD, Hays RD, Wells KB, Rogers W, Burnam MA. Prevalence of comorbid alcohol disorder and consumption in medically ill and depressed patients. Arch Fam Med 1993; 2:1142–1150.

70. Clark MR, Katon W, Russo J, Kith P, Sintay M, Buchwald D. Chronic fatigue: risk factors for symptom persistence in a 2½-year follow-up study. Am J Med 1995; 98:187–195.

71. Orlandini A, Pastore MR, Fossati A, Clerici S, Sergi A, Balini A, Parlangeli MA, Maffei C, Secchi A, Pozza G. Effects of personality on metabolic control in IDDM patients. Diabetes Care 1995; 18:206–209.

72. Saravay SM, Lavin M. Psychiatric comorbidity and length of stay in the general hospital. A critical review of outcome studies. Psychosomatics 1994; 35(3):233–252.

73. Ormel J, VonKorff M, Ustun TB, Pini S, Korten A, Oldehinkel T. Common mental disorders and disability across cultures. Results from the WHO Collaborative Study on Psychological Problems in General Health Care. JAMA 1994; 272:1741–1748.

4

Hypertension

Raymond Niaura and Michael G. Goldstein
Brown University School of Medicine
and the Miriam Hospital
Providence, Rhode Island

HISTORICAL BACKGROUND

The link between hypertension and psychiatric illnesses has its roots in the genesis of American psychosomatic medicine. Indeed, hypertension has been considered one of the "holy seven" psychosomatic disorders: i.e., asthma, peptic ulcer, hypertension, ulcerative colitis, anorexia nervosa, rheumatoid arthritis, and hyperthyroidism (1). The influences of studies and reports by Helen Flanders Dunbar and Franz Alexander, in particular, were, and to a large degree still are, extremely influential in shaping the view that hypertension is related to certain personality profiles and to regulation of emotions.

Dunbar, summarizing the results of her studies, suggested that hypertensives show a desire to please but are chronically rebellious; are ambitious but afraid of failure; and are afraid to show anger because they want to be liked (2). In contrast to Dunbar's more empirically based personality view of the psychosomatic roots of hypertension, Alexander's views were shaped more from a psychoanalytic perspective (3,4). However, his and Dunbar's conclusions are remarkably similar. For example, Alexander viewed hypertension as related to repressed hostility, especially in interpersonal contexts, and that this repressed hostility was related to unresolved childhood conflicts. Moreover, hypertensives were also seen often to be anxious and depressed compared to nonhypertensives. Alexander further postulated that repression of hostile or threatening impulses and anxiety related to potentially antagonistic interpersonal interactions contributed to tonic physiological arousal, which, over time, induced the pathophysiological changes associated with hypertension. Others described hypertensives as exhibiting a disorder of neurotic personality, such that they are thought to be characteristically tense individuals given to states of anxiety and depression (5).

These and many other early psychosomatic conceptions of hypertension gave rise to a multitude of studies, which, over time, became increasingly sophisticated as technology for assessing psychological traits and states, and physiological functioning, steadily improved. Current psychosomatic views of hypertension suggest that it is a multifaceted disorder, both psychologically and physiologically. Personality theories of hypertension have fallen out of favor, but there is still some consensus that suppressed hostility or internalized anger is associated with hypertension (6–8). In addition, numerous studies have documented a link between excessive stress-induced pressor reactivity, increased resting blood pressure, and hypertension (9). Moreover, suppressed anger or hostility has also been associated with increased pressor reactivity, suggesting a physiological mechanism whereby suppressed hostility might be related to hypertension (10,11). However, it may be premature to view these associations as causal; some have suggested that pressor reactivity may be epiphenomenal or, at best, only a marker for some other physiological process implicated in the pathogenesis of hypertension (12).

A recent meta-analytic review examined the relationship between three constructs derived from Alexander's psychosomatic theory and elevated blood pressure. The constructs included affect-anger expression, negative affectivity (including such measures as anxiety and depression), and defensiveness (13). The analyses confirmed expectations that blood pressure and hypertension were inversely related to affect expression and positively related to negative affectivity and defensiveness. The strongest associations occurred for defensiveness and measures of anger and affect expression linked to interpersonal contexts. However, these relationships were moderated to a significant degree by such factors as awareness of blood pressure status, gender, and occupation, supporting the view that psychological variables interact with other psychosocial variables to influence blood pressure and hypertension.

The relationship between suppressed anger or hostility and blood pressure may also be influenced to a significant degree by type of hypertensive disorder. Increasingly, essential hypertension is recognized as a hetereogeneous disease state, with different pathophysiologic profiles. Some studies have demonstrated, for example, that hypertensives with high circulating levels of plasma renin may be more prone to psychosomatic traits than others. In one study, hypertensives with high plasma renin exhibited a raised plasma norepinephrine concentration and suppressed hostility compared to normal plasma renin hypertensives (14). In a similar study, compared to normal-renin hypertensives, high-renin hypertensives were found to be significantly less assertive, to fail to externalize their aggression, to perceive frustration less and to try to please others more, and they had a stronger need to solve problems immediately yet tended to deny social conflicts (15). The results of these studies underscore the need to control for the biological heterogeneity of hypertension, lest important relationships be obscured. In addition, although not examined in this paper, other important psychosocial influences on hypertension must be examined to determine the true relationship between psychological factors/psychiatric disorders and hypertension. Among these are age, sex, socioeconomic status (SES), lifestyle factors (e.g., smoking, lack of physical activity, obesity), workplace and other environmental stressors, and the effects of being labeled as hypertensive (16,17).

More modern psychosocial views of hypertension also suggest the interesting possibility that the personality/behavior of the hypertensive patient is a consequence of the hypertension rather than the cause (18). In this view, hypertension, through unknown mechanisms, affects an individual's neurocognitive performance and thus the ability to cope with certain environmental stimuli and interpersonal relationships that are potentially antagonistic or unpleasant. For example, hypertensives may be more aware of their "hyperactivity" during interpersonal interactions and may then learn to shy away from these interactions or perhaps learn to inhibit strong emotional reactions and avoid confrontations.

PREVALENCE, CLINICAL MANIFESTATIONS AND CLINICAL CORRELATES OF PSYCHIATRIC DISORDERS AMONG HYPERTENSIVE PATIENTS
Prevalence of Psychiatric Disorders

Studies have shown that hypertension is positively associated with psychiatric comorbidity. For example, Johnson (19) found in a nationally representative sample of black adults that subjects experiencing a high level of overall psychiatric symptomatology were more likely to have been physician diagnosed with a variety of disorders, including hypertension, compared to those with fewer psychiatric symptoms. These results were statistically independent of sociodemographic factors, smoking, and alcohol use. However, this study did not differentiate the association of hypertension with specific psychiatric disorders or their symptoms. Recently, Hayward (20) reviewed the results of several studies providing support for a relationship between anxiety disorders, depression, mania, and hypertension. He concluded that the association was strongest for hypertension and anxiety disorders, slightly more equivocal for depression and hypertension, and only one study found a relationship between mania and hypertension (21). Although not exhaustive, Table 1 lists these and several other, including more recent, powerful, prospective studies, which shed further light on this issue.

Depression

Associations between depression and high blood pressure have anecdotally been noted since the turn of the century (22). More recent cross-sectional studies that assessed depression using DSM-III or DSM IIIR criteria have, in general, supported a relationship between depression and elevated blood pressure and/or hypertension. For example, Rabkin et al. (23) noted a nearly threefold increase in prevalence of depression among psychiatric outpatients with hypertension as compared to those without, independent of effects of age, sex, other chronic medical illness, and current use of antihypertensive medications. In a study of more than 11,000 consecutive psychiatric outpatients, patients who were primarily depressed were about 30% more likely to be currently hypertensive compared to psychiatric outpatients who were not diagnosed as depressed (24).

Table 1   Studies Examining the Relationship Between Hypertension and Selected
Psychiatric Disorders or Symptoms of Psychiatric Disorders

Disorder	Study	Relationship?
Mood disorders		
	Heine et al., 1969 (66)	Yes
	Heine, 1970 (67)	Yes
	Wheatley et al., 1975 (68)	No
	Friedman and Bennet, 1977 (69)	No
	Lyketsos et al., 1982 (70)	Yes
	Rabkin et al., 1983 (23)	Yes
	Reus and Miner, 1985 (71)	Yes
	Mezzich et al., 1987 (24)	Yes
	Fuller, 1988 (25)	No
	Wells et al., 1989 (27)	Yes
	Wells et al., 1989 (28)	Yes
	Wells et al., 1991 (59)	Yes
	Jonas et al., 1997 (29)	Yes
Anxiety disorders		
	Wheatley et al., 1975 (68)	Yes
	Friedman and Bennet, 1977 (69)	Yes
	Noyes et al., 1980 (72)	Yes
	Lyketsos et al., 1982 (70)	Yes
	Sparrow et al., 1982 (73)	No
	Katon, 1984 (35)	Yes
	Dunner, 1985 (74)	No
	Charney and Heninger, 1986 (75)	No
	Wells et al., 1989 (27)	Yes
	Wells et al., 1989 (28)	Yes
	Davidson et al., 1991 (36)	Yes
	Markovitz et al., 1991 (39)	Yes
	Markovitz et al., 1993 (38)	Yes
	Jonas et al., 1997 (29)	Yes
Substance abuse disorders		
	Wells et al., 1989 (27)	?
	Wells et al., 1989 (28)	Yes
Mania		
	Yates and Wallace, 1987 (21)	Yes

Source: Adapted from Ref. 20.

Another study failed to find a relationship between depression and hypertension (25), but this may have been due to numerous factors including lack of standardization of diagnostic assessment and measurement of blood pressure and sociodemographic differences in outpatient samples. However, in a comprehensive study of adult medical and mental health outpatients, prevalence of hypertension was found to be almost twice as high among depressed patients seen in a general medical setting compared to those seen in a psychiatric setting or a household sample (26). Moreover, the results remained significant after adjusting for age, sex, marital status, and race.

A series of recent population-based studies lends further support to the notion that hypertension and depression are positively associated. In one study, prevalence of lifetime diagnosis of depression assessed using the Diagnostic Interview Survey (DIS) was significantly greater (24.4%) among respondents with a lifetime history of depression compared to subjects with a negative lifetime depression history (16%) (27). However, the strength of this association diminished when recent (past 6 months) diagnosis of depression was considered. In another, similar study, compared to subjects with no history of chronic illness prevalence rates for both lifetime (16.4% vs. 6.9% for hypertensives vs. no medical history) and recent (11.3% vs. 4.4% for hypertensives vs. no medical history) depression remained elevated among hypertensives, even after adjustment for sex and age (28).

In a recent prospective investigation, a cohort of almost 3000 men and women without evidence of hypertension at baseline were followed for 7–16 years (29). Incident hypertension was defined as blood pressure of 160/95 mmHg or more or prescription of antihypertensive medication. Depressive symptoms were measured at baseline using the four-item General Well-Being depression subscale (30). For both whites and blacks, high depressive symptoms at baseline predicted both incident hypertension and treated hypertension, controlling for age, sex, education, cigarette smoking, body mass index (a measure of obesity), alcohol use, history of diabetes, stroke, coronary heart disease, and baseline blood pressure.

Hypotheses concerning the association between hypertension and depression were summarized succinctly by Fuller (25): as follows: (1) a common physiological factor underlies both disorders; (2) depression results from side effects of some antihypertensive medications; (3) depression is secondary to experiencing a chronic illness (hypertension); (4) depression results from treatment that lowers blood pressure such that it causes cerebral insufficiency (especially in the elderly); and (5) this association is coincidental. The preponderance of evidence suggests that the association between depression and hypertension is more than coincidental. The results of the population-based and prospective studies are particularly convincing in this regard. It is entirely possible, however, that depression in some hypertensives is associated with the use of antihypertensive medications, but it is unlikely that this accounts completely for the association, as depressive symptoms predict both incident treated and untreated hypertension (29). Likewise, cerebral insufficiency secondary to antidepressant treatment could be a culprit in some cases, especially in the elderly, but again studies have suggested that the association is independent of age and treatment. It is also possible that depression is a result of experiencing a chronic illness; this possibility has only been explored to a limited extent (e.g., the effects of being labeled a hypertensive) (31).

Finally, it is highly likely that depression and hypertension are related to some common underlying physiological mechanism(s). Some forms of depression have been characterized as syndromes of neurotransmitter dysregulation (32), where failure in regulation of noradrenergic and related systems results in loss of responsivity to environmental stimuli and delayed homeostasis when stressful stimuli are withdrawn. Chronic pressor hyperreactivity to stressful stimuli combined with a delay in return to baseline could contribute to sustained elevations in blood pressure and, eventually, hypertension. Hypercortisolemia is also associated with some forms of depression and also with visceral obesity (possibly in response to prolonged stressful stimulation). In turn, visceral obesity is associated with the metabolic syndrome, a constellation of symptoms including insulin resistance, dyslipidemias, and hypertension, which is associated with cardiovascular disease risk (33). It is also important to recognize that depression is strongly associated with other risk factors for hypertension including cigarette smoking and a sedentary lifestyle (20). One should also bear in mind the possibility raised indirectly by Shapiro (18) that depression is secondary to hypertension, mediated perhaps by the effect of blood pressure on neurocognitive functioning.

Anxiety

The association between anxiety and depression appears to be somewhat more consistent than that observed between depression and hypertension. The population-based studies reported by Wells and colleagues illustrate this point. In one study (27), bivariate analyses revealed that lifetime diagnosis of anxiety disorders was significantly more prevalent among hypertensives (25.9%) compared to medical outpatients without a chronic medical condition (16%). Similarly, recent diagnosis of anxiety disorder was significantly associated with hypertension (18.2%) compared to controls (10.2%). In the other study reported by Wells and colleagues (28), both lifetime and recent diagnoses of depression and anxiety disorders were significantly more prevalent among hypertensives than subjects with no lifetime chronic medical conditions (21.7% vs. 10.5% and 15.1% vs. 5.3% for lifetime and recent anxiety disorder, respectively).

To our knowledge no study has directly compared prevalence of specific anxiety disorders between hypertensives and individuals who do not suffer from chronic medical conditions. However, a recent observational study provides some estimates of specific prevalence rates (34). Adult outpatients of primary care providers were assessed for anxiety disorders using a screening version of the DIS. Lifetime prevalence rates among hypertensives were as follows: panic disorder—2.2%; phobia—9.7%; generalized anxiety disorder—22.6%; and any anxiety disorder—28%. Rates for panic disorder appear to be similar to those observed in the general population, so the relationship between anxiety disorders and hypertension is probably accounted for mostly by generalized anxiety disorder. However, this hypothesis has not been formally tested. In addition, at least one study (35) noted significantly increased prevalence of hypertension (15%) in patients with panic disorder compared to adult primary care patients (9%).

At least one study has documented an association between hypertension and posttraumatic stress disorder (PTSD) (36). The DIS was administered to almost 3000 community respondents, who were also asked about a variety of chronic diseases. Those diagnosed with PTSD had a significantly greater prevalence of hypertension than those without PTSD (31.4% vs. 18.5%). This is consistent with other studies reporting greater basal blood pressure levels in patients with PTSD (37).

Two recent well-controlled prospective studies examined the relationship between symptoms of anxiety and incident hypertension. The study reported by Jonas et al. (29) (reviewed above), which showed that baseline depressive symptoms predicted incident hypertension, also found that baseline symptoms of anxiety predicted new onset hypertension over a period of 7–16 years, independent of sex, education, smoking, body mass index, alcohol use, history of diabetes, stroke, coronary heart disease, and baseline systolic blood pressure. As with depression, positive associations were found between symptoms of anxiety at baseline and incidence of both untreated and treated depression.

Markovitz and colleagues (38) tested the hypothesis that heightened anxiety measured at baseline in the Framingham Heart Study would increase the risk of developing subsequent hypertension. Anxiety was measured using a seven-item anxiety symptoms scale, and incident hypertension was defined as taking medication for hypertension or blood pressures higher than 160/95 mmHg at a follow-up examination. Over a period of 18–20 years, baseline anxiety symptoms predicted incident hypertension over and above initial blood pressure and heart rate, relative weight, age, hematocrit, alcohol intake, smoking, education, and glucose intolerance. This relationship was observed among middle-aged men but not among older men or women at any age. However, in another prospective study, these investigators did find that anxiety predicted incident hypertension among women (39). Methodological and sampling differences between the two studies may explain the discrepant findings for women.

As with depression, the preponderance of evidence suggests that anxiety and hypertension are related. Moreover, this relationship appears to extend to the general population, and it may be causal, as evidenced by the results of the prospective studies. The mechanisms whereby anxiety and hypertension are linked may be entirely similar to those enumerated above for depression (e.g., alterations in central and peripheral noradrenergic functioning). Indeed, anxiety and depression are often so closely related (34) that it might be impossible to tease apart their separate influences (if any) on hypertension and consequently to describe different etiologic mechanisms for each disorder.

Substance Abuse

The two studies by Wells and colleagues provide some estimate for the prevalence of substance abuse disorders among hypertensives, although actual prevalence of specific substance abuse disorders is not provided. In the first study, hypertensives had a significantly higher (22.9%) lifetime substance abuse prevalence rate compared to subjects with no chronic medical conditions (16%) (27). Curiously, when recent substance abuse was considered, hypertensives had a significantly lower rate (3.4%) compared to controls (10.2%). The authors speculated that the difference could be accounted for by the possibility that persons with hypertension may have been advised to stop drinking. In the second study, however, both lifetime and recent substance abuse were positively associated with hypertension (28). Thirty percent of hypertensives had a lifetime history of substance abuse as compared to 17.3% of those with no chronic medical condition (rates were 12.7% vs. 6.0% for recent substance abuse). Because the majority of substance abuse involves alcohol and alcohol is known to exacerbate hypertension (40), this could explain the higher prevalence rates of substance abuse among hypertensives.

Mania

One study found that bipolar, but not unipolar, depression was associated with increased prevalence of hypertension (21). It is unclear why no relationship was observed for unipolar depression, but the study contained a small sample of subjects and may have limited its ability to detect this association.

Clinical Manifestations and Correlates

There is no reason to suspect that the clinical manifestation of psychiatric disorders among hypertensives would differ from that of other subpopulations, nor are there data to address this point. It is worth commenting briefly, however, about possible clinical correlates that may be important in treating both psychiatric disorders and hypertension. Hypertensives are at risk for cardiovascular diseases and, consequently, tend to suffer from these diseases (e.g., coronary heart disease with angina; stroke). They also are more likely to suffer from disorders that contribute to their hypertension (e.g., prediabetic state insulin resistance; non–insulin-dependent diabetes; hyperthyroidism).

As noted earlier, there may also be lifestyle correlates related to hypertension such as smoking and physical inactivity. Smoking is potentially a very important correlate in that it is related to depression and anxiety disorders. Quitting smoking may exacerbate symptoms of anxiety and depression. However, pharmacologic agents such as clonidine may help to control symptoms of nicotine withdrawal, with the added benefit of being an antihypertensive. Bupropion hydrochloride, an antidepressant recently approved for smoking cessation, may also prove to be useful as a smoking cessation tool among depressed hypertensives. Hypertension also appears to be associated, as are psychiatric disorders such as depression, with lower socioeconomic status (SES). Thus, hypertensives with psychiatric disorders may tend to be overrepresented among those with lower income, fewer years of education, blue-collar work status, etc. These factors may play a role in psychiatric treatment in that low-SES hypertensives may be less able to access and afford sustained contact with the health care system, compromising continuity of care and effective management of both psychiatric disorders and hypertension.

CASE STUDY

A 42-year-old male was evaluated by his internist for a long overdue general physical evaluation. He was married, with two preadolescent children, and worked as a typesetter at a local newspaper. His physical was unremarkable except for the presence of hypertension (160 mmHg systolic blood pressure; 105 mmHg diastolic blood pressure). The patient was mildly obese, largely sedentary, and consumed alcohol on a daily basis (several drinks in the evening). He had smoked regularly for almost 20 years, but had quit about 6 months previously because of increased shortness of breath upon exertion. Both his mother and one brother were also hypertensive. Because the patient's blood pressure was significantly elevated, his physician prescribed propranolol (150 mg bid). In addition, the physician recommended reducing alcohol intake and increasing physical activity. The patient responded that he had been drinking a little more than usual lately because of the stress of marital problems and dissatisfaction with his job. At this point, the physician referred the patient for a psychiatric evaluation, suspecting alcohol abuse and/or depression. The patient reluctantly agreed to the referral.

The psychiatric evaluation revealed a moderate major depressive disorder, with depressed mood, anhedonia, insomnia, fatigue, feelings of worthlessness, and difficulty concentrating. The depressive episode had persisted for 3 months and was related to ongoing marital difficulties (he and his wife were considering a trial separation). In addition, the patient revealed that his job was characterized by considerable time pressure and deadlines and often required that he work overtime during evenings and weekends. He felt he was stuck in a dead-end job but could do nothing because he had to support his family and had no other job prospects. The patient did not meet the criteria for alcohol abuse or dependence. His past psychiatric history was significant for a bout of major depression during his twenties when he had attended but then dropped out of college. At that time he had received several sessions of counseling with a psychologist, and his depression resolved as a result. Further interviews revealed that the patient had been excessively shy as a child and that he still had difficulties in interpersonal contexts, especially meeting new people. This was a source of some contention between him and his wife; she liked to socialize, whereas he tended to avoid dinner parties and other social gatherings. The psychiatrist noted that the patient also had difficulty maintaining eye contact. The patient was prescribed fluoxetine, 20 mg/day, to treat his symptoms of depression. This choice was informed partly because of its lack of effect on blood pressure. Additional psychotherapy was offered by the psychiatrist, but the patient declined.

Over the course of the next several weeks, the patient noticed that his anhedonia and feelings of worthlessness improved. His mood had improved somewhat, but not as much as he had hoped. Moreover, he continued experiencing insomnia, and feelings of fatigue and difficulty concentrating had worsened. The patient's blood pressure was well controlled. At a follow-up psychiatric visit, the patient complained of ongoing symptoms. The psychiatrist suspected that propranolol might be complicating his treatment for depression. In consultation with the internist, the patient was switched from propranolol to captopril (150 mg bid) with good effect. The patient's vegetative symptoms improved considerably. In time, he and his wife agreed to seek marriage counseling.

IMPACT OF PSYCHIATRIC ILLNESS ON MEDICAL MANAGEMENT OF HYPERTENSION

Effects of Psychiatric Illness

Table 2 presents the most common psychiatric disorders that, directly or indirectly, affect the medical management and/or course of hypertension and some of the mechanisms by which psychiatric disorders impinge upon hypertension. As noted above, to the extent that mood and anxiety disorders influence noradrenergic functioning, in

Table 2   Psychiatric Disorders That May Affect Medical Management of Hypertension and/or Its Course

Disorder	Possible mechanisms	
	Noradrenergic	Lifestyle
Mood disorders		
Major depression	X	X
Bipolar disorder	?	?
Anxiety disorders		
Generalized anxiety	X	?
PTSD	X	X
Panic	X	?
Organic mental disorders		
Delirium/Agitation	X	—
Dementia	X	—
Substance Intoxication/ Withdrawal/Dependence		
Alcohol	X	X
Amphetamine	X	—
Caffeine	X	—
Cocaine	X	—
Nicotine	X	X
Opiates	X	?
Sedatives/Anxiolytics	X	—
Sleep disorders		
Nonorganic parasomnias	?	—
Organic hypersomnia	—	?

X = Definite or highly probable; ? = possible; — = unlikely/unknown.

particular regulation of central and peripheral norepinephrine and epinephrine, they may also elevate blood pressure acutely and, perhaps, chronically. However, debate continues as to whether depression, for example, can be characterized as a disorder primarily of adrenergic functioning. However, it is probably true that, for a subset of depressives, activity of the hypothalamic-pituitary-adrenocortical (HPA) axis is heightened, which manifests in part as elevated blood pressure. In addition, hypercortisolemia, which is characteristic of some forms of depression, is also associated with hypertension through its influence on visceral adiposity and insulin resistance (41). Arguably, anxiety disorders are more likely to be associated with HPA dysregulation, especially panic disorder and PTSD. To the extent that dysregulation of HPA functioning is involved in depression, anxiety and hypertension, then severity of depression or anxiety may also influence severity of hypertension.

Depression and perhaps anxiety may also indirectly influence hypertension through their influence on lifestyle factors. For example, history of depression and symptoms of depression/anxiety are strongly associated with cigarette smoking and, to some degree, a sedentary lifestyle (20). Most military veterans with PTSD smoke (37). These factors are important determinants of blood pressure.

Mood and anxiety disorders also present a diagnostic and clinical challenge in terms of managing hypertension. For example, it is presently unclear that knowledge of HPA functioning can guide effective treatment of either depression or hypertension, although this knowledge may prove useful someday. Antihypertensive agents with pressor effects may exacerbate hypertension. While most antidepressants do not suffer from this problem, there is a risk of elevated blood pressure with some agents (e.g., bupropion, protriptyline). Other agents such as selective serotonin-reuptake inhibitors (SSRIs) probably do not have much, if any, effect on blood pressure, while certain tricyclics may display pressor effects that are essentially canceled out by their anticholinergic effects. Depression and anxiety also present a challenge in terms of treatment of hypertension insofar as some antihypertensive medications may exacerbate depression (more likely) and anxiety (less likely). Effects of antihypertensive medications on psychiatric symptoms are reviewed in more detail below.

Organic mental disorders are also commonly associated with increased blood pressure. For example, delirium and agitation can cause acute increases in blood pressure, which may not be especially problematic in the nonhypertensive, but which may increase risk of cerebrovascular events in the hypertensive patient. Neuroleptics or sedatives used to treat delirium/agitation should decrease the acute increase in blood pressure associated with the delirious state, but they are unlikely to return blood pressure to normal levels in the hypertensive patient.

Dementia may also be associated with increased blood pressure, and the association may follow two paths. For example, on the one hand dementia may be secondary to hypertension that has contributed indirectly to cerebral infarction (e.g., multi-infarct dementia). Degenerative dementias, on the other hand, may cause hypertension as neuroregulatory systems that control blood pressure are progressively eroded.

An important category of psychiatric disorders in terms of blood pressure management are the substance use disorders, including dependence, intoxication, and withdrawal. Alcohol is probably the most important example. Alcohol use has acute pressor effects, and its chronic use is associated with hypertension or exacerbation of hypertension (40). Moreover, alcohol use diminishes the effectiveness of some antihypertensive agents. Alcohol withdrawal is also associated with acute elevations in blood pressure, related to increased sympathetic drive (42). Most alcoholics smoke (43), and they are also less likely to engage in healthy lifestyle practices compared to nonalcoholics (e.g., poor diet). For all of these reasons, the alcoholic patient is at great risk for exacerbation and/or failure to manage effectively their hypertension. Therefore, it is important to acknowledge that treatment for alcoholism must become a priority if hypertension is to be managed successfully.

It is less clear that chronic use of other substances is associated with elevated blood pressure and hypertension. However, those substances with acute pressor effects (i.e., stimulants) could conceivably contribute to hypertension with extended use, or at least exacerbate it. However, with sedatives/anxiolytics, pressor effects are seen during acute withdrawal from the substance. The implications for managing hypertension are severalfold. It is clear that the nature of the substance being used must be taken into account. Moreover, it is important to distinguish between acute effects during intoxication (e.g., alcohol and stimulants), effects of chronic use (alcohol and possibly nicotine), and the effects of withdrawal (alcohol and sedatives/anxiolytics). Blood pressure in hypertensives both before and during treatment should be assessed after acute intoxication and withdrawal have dissipated. However, it is unclear whether repeated, frequent episodes of acute intoxication with stimulants and acute withdrawal do, in fact, contribute to sustained hypertension. It is also unclear what peripheral vascular damage is inflicted by repeated acute intoxication and withdrawal-induced pressor reactivity short of sustained hypertension, especially over years of use and abuse.

Sleep disorders may be related to hypertension in at least two ways. First, to the extent that sleep disorders, in particular dysomnias, are related to other nonorganic disorders, such as mood or anxiety disorders, they may be indirectly linked to hypertension. It is unclear, however, whether primary dysomnias (insomnia and hypersomnia) in the absence of nonorganic mental disorders are related to hypertension. Second, hypersomnia may be related to a known organic factor, such as a physical condition, substance use disorder, or use of certain medications (e.g., sedatives or anxiolytics). About 50% of hypersomnias related to a known organic factor are associated with sleep apnea. Obstructive sleep apnea is associated in turn with obesity and systemic hypertension and tends to begin in middle age, becoming increasingly common with advanced age.

Psychiatric Treatments Influencing Blood Pressure

As noted above, some antidepressants (e.g., bupropion, protriptyline) may have pressor effects that can affect blood pressure. Tricyclic antidepressants may have mild antihypertensive effects, as well as the potential to exacerbate orthostatic hypotension (44). In addition, tricyclics may antagonize the antihypertensive effects of centrally acting anti-hypertensive agents (45). Use of monoamine oxidase inhibitors can lead to hypotension, but an acute hypertensive crisis can be provoked if foods rich in tyramine are consumed or if the patient is concurrently administered stimulant medications or meperidine (44). Selective serotonergic reuptake inhibitors appear to have little or no effect on blood pressure (46). Psychostimulants such as methylphenidate can increase blood pressure and should be used with caution in hypertensive patients (47). Neuroleptics also tend to have hypotensive effects; however, hypertensive episodes associated with neuroleptic use may be a sign of neuroleptic malignant syndrome (48). To the extent that with-drawal from sedatives or anxiolytics are related to increased noradrenergic activity, then blood pressure may also be increased, albeit transiently.

Electroconvulsive therapy (ECT) increases blood pressure acutely. Moreover, the patient with uncontrolled hypertension is likely to have marked fluctuations in blood pressure during anesthesia for ECT (49). Therefore, it is recommended that, prior to receiving ECT, hypertensive patients' blood pressure first be stabilized medically. During ECT, brief-acting antihypertensive agents should be used to stabilize blood pressure (e.g., bolus and infusion of esmolol or labetolol). Blood pressure should be monitored frequently both during ECT and afterwards to ensure stability.

Psychiatric illness and compliance with medications

Although this is an infrequently studied issue, studies have demonstrated that medica-tion noncompliance occurs among as many as one third to one half of all psychiatric outpatients (50). This obviously has direct implications for the pharmacologic manage-ment of hypertension. Recently, however, Kelly et al. (51) demonstrated that two brief interventions with psychiatric outpatients—engaging families as active participants in the aftercare process and training patients to become effective health care consumers—significantly improved medication compliance. Thus, brief and readily implemented interventions such as these should be considered seriously in the pharmacologic treat-ment of hypertension among psychiatric patients.

EFFECTS OF HYPERTENSION AND ITS TREATMENT ON MANIFESTATION OF PSYCHIATRIC DISORDERS

Psychiatric Side Effects of Antihypertensive Agents

The literature on psychiatric side effects of antihypertensive agents has recently been summarized (48,52). Table 3 presents a summary of probable psychiatric side effects associated with various antihypertensive agents, and these results are briefly summarized below.

Ganglionic agents are not widely used because of their poor efficacy and side effects. Among the side effects is depression, estimated to be as high as 14% (53). Of the centrally acting agents, reserpine is no longer used as an antihypertensive agent. Its

Table 3 Psychiatric Side Effects of Antihypertensive Medications

Agent	Psychosis	Anxiety	Depression	Cognitive	Sleep
Ganglionic					
Guanethidine	—	—	?	—	—
Central					
Reserpine	X	—	X	—	X
Methyldopa	?	—	X	X	—
Clonidine	—	—	X	—	X
Diuretics					
Thiazides	—	—	X	—	—
Vasodilators					
Hydralazine	?	?	?	—	—
Prazosin	—	?	X	—	?
Beta-blockers	—	—	X	?	X
Calcium-channel blockers	—	—	?	—	—
ACE inhibitors	—	—	—	—	—

X = Definite or highly probable; ? = possible; — = unlikely/unknown.

psychiatric side effects include a low incidence of psychosis and a somewhat higher incidence of depression (up to 15%) (45). Methlydopa also has been associated with depression rates between 4 and 21% (53). Clonidine, an α_2-agonist, is a more widely used centrally acting agent. Its use has been associated with depression in 1–11% of patients (45), and delirium and psychosis have been anecdotally reported, but are probably rare. Although use of clonidine as an antihypertensive is not very popular, it has been used in treating alcohol and opiate withdrawal (48). Therefore, to the extent that blood pressure increases significantly during drug withdrawal, clonidine may be an ideal drug for use in the drug-dependent hypertensive patient. Use of diuretics has been associated with episodes of depression and delirium, although these are thought to occur relatively infrequently and are probably secondary to electrolyte imbalances (48). Vasodilators, such as hydrazaline and prazosin, have been associated anecdotally with depression, delirium, psychosis, anxiety, and sleep disturbances. However, these effects probably occur infrequently.

Beta blockers remain among the most popular antihypertensives in current use, and there are too many to enumerate separately here. Their neuropsychiatric side effects have been reviewed extensively elsewhere (54). Collectively, use of beta blockers has most often been associated with depression and sleep disturbance. However, this belies the fact that beta blockers differ in their pharmacologic properties, which may influence incidence of such side effects. For example, beta blockers differ in their selectivity (B-1 and/or B-2), with B-1 agents being considered more cardioselective. It is conceivable that the less selective agents would have more psychiatric side effects, although this has not been demonstrated definitively. Beta blockers also differ in terms of their lipophilicity, which refers to the degree to which they penetrate a cell's lipid membrane. Conceivably, beta blockers that are more lipophylic should have more access to the central nervous system, and therefore may cause more neuropsychiatric side effects. However, the evidence on this point is mixed (54,55).

Calcium channel blockers are currently among the most widely prescribed antihypertensive agents. Their use has been associated anecdotally with depression and delirium, but, given widespread and lengthy experience with these agents, the incidence of these effects is probably exceedingly low. Moreover, calcium channel blockers have also been used to treat unipolar depression and panic disorder (48). ACE inhibitors also currently enjoy widespread popularity. The use of these agents has not been significantly associated with psychiatric comorbidity.

Short of frank psychiatric side effects, several studies have examined effects of antihypertensive agents on quality of life, including such domains as general perceived health, vitality, health status, sleep, and emotional control (56). Comparative studies suggest that, despite similar efficacy in terms of controlling hypertension, antihypertensive agents differ in their effects on quality of life. For example, Croog et al. (57) compared the effects of methyldopa, propranolol, and captopril (an ACE inhibitor) on quality of life and found that, while global ratings of quality of life decreased with methyldopa and propranolol treatment, ratings improved with captopril. More recently, Testa et al. (56) compared the effects of two ACE inhibitors, captopril and enalapril, and found that the drugs were indistinguishable in terms of clinical efficacy and safety. However, patients treated with captopril had more favorable changes in overall quality of life, general perceived health, vitality, health status, sleep, and emotional control, compared to patients treated with enalapril. Of interest was the finding that the changes varied according to quality of life at baseline: patients with low quality of life remained stable or improved with either drug, whereas those with a high baseline quality of life remained stable with captopril, but worsened with enalapril. These results underscore the complex and sometimes subtle effects these medications may have on psychological functioning, the variability in response to medications even within the same drug class, and the need for further research to better understand the effects of antihypertensive medications on all aspects of quality of life so that physicians and patients can match their choice of medications to patients' particular psychological vulnerabilities and needs.

Table 4, adapted from Rauch et al. (48), presents some guidelines for prescribing antihypertensive medications in patients with comorbid psychiatric disorders.

Effects of Hypertension on Psychiatric Symptoms

There is no evidence to suggest that hypertension per se influences development and course of psychiatric disorder, with the possible exception of dementias by virtue of cortical and subcortical morphological changes and microvascular damage. However, recent studies have suggested that deficits in neuropsychological functioning in hypertensives relative to nonhypertensives are manifest across a wide age range. The most

Table 4 Suggested Antihypertensive Agents in Patients with Comorbid Psychiatric Disorders

	Antihypertensive agent	
Disorder	Preferred	Contraindicated
Anxiety	Beta- and calcium-channel blocker	None
Delirium	ACE inhibitor and calcium blocker	Beta-blocker and central agents
Dementia	ACE inhibitor and calcium blocker	Beta-blocker and central agents
Depression		
bipolar	Calcium-channel blocker	Beta-blocker and central agents
unipolar	Calcium-channel blocker and ACE inhibitor	Beta-blocker and central agents
Impulsivity	Beta- and calcium-channel blocker	None
Mania	Beta- and calcium-channel blocker	ACE inhibitor
Psychosis	Calcium-channel blocker	Central agents
Drug withdrawal	Clonidine and beta-blocker	None

Source: Ref. 48.

pronounced hypertension-related deficits appear on tests of memory, abstract reasoning, and attention. Hypertension is also associated with deficits in perception, visuospatial skills, and psychomotor speed, although the evidence here is more mixed. One would expect that hypertension-related deficits would become more apparent among older hypertensives, as elevated blood pressure has produced cumulative cortical damage over several years, yet such deficits are apparent in hypertensives as young as 25 years of age (58). Moreover, one study demonstrated that visuoperceptive learning and memory deficits in hypertensives relative to controls were independent of the effects of antihypertensive medications, age, education, socioeconomic status, alcohol consumption, medical or neurologic disorders, knowledge of hypertensive status, depression, and anxiety (59). The investigators concluded that the deficits were most likely a consequence of elevated blood pressure per se, but the mechanism(s) responsible for the deficits are poorly understood. It is possible that, even at relatively young ages, elevated blood pressure is associated with subtle structural changes in brain morphology that produce neuropsychological deficits. In turn, these deficits may contribute to difficulties in learning, academic, and job performance or perhaps even contribute to attention deficit disorders that are manifest in adulthood.

COGNITIVE-BEHAVIORAL TREATMENTS FOR HYPERTENSION

The effects of psychotherapy, relaxation, and biofeedback on blood pressure in hypertensives are modest, and there is little evidence to suggest that effects are sustained after treatment has been discontinued (60). In one study, relaxation training decreased blood pressure among hypertensives as assessed in the laboratory, but this effect was not evident when blood pressure was assessed in the real world via 24-hour ambulatory monitoring (61). Moreover, in a comparison with hypertensive medications, relaxation training produced smaller decreases in blood pressure. Conflicting evidence also exists. For example, one study demonstrated that relaxation training over a prolonged period produced blood pressure decreases that persisted over 4 years (62). Yet another study showed that the combination of relaxation therapy and medication was more effective in achieving blood pressure control than medication alone (63). A report by Glasgow and colleagues (64) showed that, as compared to a usual care group, hypertensives assigned to a behavioral stepped-care condition, which involved blood pressure monitoring, self-employed blood pressure biofeedback, and relaxation in sequence as needed, resulted in greater decreases in blood pressure and a reduction in doses of antihypertensive medications. A recent meta-analysis of cognitive-behavioral treatments for blood pressure (biofeedback, meditation, relaxation, stress management, combinations) showed that, compared to no treatment, cognitive-behavioral treatments significantly reduced systolic and diastolic blood pressures, but the effect was smaller than that seen with medications (65). However, the cognitive-behavioral treatments did not outperform "placebo" interventions (e.g., sham biofeedback; pseudo meditation). Moreover, there was no evidence that any single intervention outperformed any other. The results confirm the efficacy of cognitive-behavioral treatments for hypertension, but call into question the mechanisms of action, which appear to be largely unspecified, given the lack of differences between the active and "placebo" treatments.

Cognitive-behavioral treatments for hypertension probably have a place in the comprehensive management of the hypertensive patient, and they probably work best in combination with pharmacotherapy and with other lifestyle interventions that address hypertension (e.g., dietary changes, exercise). Cognitive-behavioral treatments may be particularly useful in cases where patients are unable or unwilling to use medications to control their blood pressure. However, such treatments are costly both in terms of therapists' and patients' time and suffer from problems of adherence, as do any complex treatments. Their efficacy in treating hypertension in psychiatric populations has not been systematically evaluated.

SUMMARY

Hypertension has long been viewed as a disorder with associated psychosomatic features. Recent research has discounted the importance of personality or psychoanalytic formulations of hypertension, but there remains support for the notion that hypertension is associated inversely with negative affective (particularly anger) expression and is positively associated with negative affect, defensiveness, and acute pressor responsivity to behavioral challenges. Hypertension appears to be associated with depressive, anxiety, and substance abuse disorders, but there is less evidence that it is associated with other psychiatric disorders. Medical management of hypertension may be influenced by psychiatric disorders such as anxiety and depression and substance withdrawal, to the extent they influence noradrenergic function. In addition, some antidepressant medications may have pressor effects. Psychiatric illness may also interfere with antihypertensive medication compliance. Psychiatric side effects of antihypertensive agents are far-ranging, but well documented, so antihypertensive therapy among psychiatric patients must be guided by this knowledge. In general, though, use of calcium channel blockers or angiotensin-converting enzyme (ACE) inhibitors is not associated to a significant degree with psychiatric side effects. Efficacy of cognitive behavioral treatments for hypertension (e.g., relaxation therapies) has not been systematically evaluated in psychiatric populations.

REFERENCES

1. Levenson D. Mind, Body, and Medicine: A History of the American Psychosomatic Society. New York: Susan O'Donnell, 1994.
2. Dunbar HF. Psychosomatic Diagnosis. New York: Paul Hoeber, 1943.
3. Alexander F. Psychoanalytic study of a case of hypertension. Psychosom Med 1939; 1: 139–152.
4. Alexander F. Psychosomatic Medicine. London: Allen & Unwin, 1952.
5. Binger CAL. On so-called psychogenic influences in essential hypertension. Psychosom Med 1951; 13:273–276.
6. Dimsdale JE. Research links between psychiatry and cardiology: hypertension, type A behavior, sudden death, and the physiology of emotional arousal. Gen Hosp Psychiatry 1988; 10:328–338.
7. Sommers-Flanagan J, Greenberg RP. Psychosocial variables and hypertension: a new look at an old controversy. J Nerv Ment Dis 1989; 177:15–24.
8. Schneider RH, Egan BM, Johnson EH, Drobny H, Julius S. Anger and anxiety in borderline hypertension. Psychosom Med 1986; 48:242–248.
9. Fredrikson M, Matthews KA. Cardiovascular response to behavioral stress and hypertension: a meta-analytic review. Ann Behav Med 1990; 12:30–39.
10. Perini C, Muller FB, Buhler FR. Suppressed aggression accelerates development of essential hypertension. J Hypertension 1991; 9:499–503.
11. Perini C, Mailer FB, Rauchfleish U, Battegay R, Hobi V, Buhler FR. Psychosomatic factors in borderline hypertensive subjects and offspring of hypertensive parents. Hypertension 1990; 16:627–634.
12. Pickering TG, Gerin W. Cardiovascular reactivity in the laboratory and the role of behavioral factors in hypertension: a critical review. Ann Behav Med 1990; 12:3–16.
13. Jorgensen RS, Johnson BT, Kolodziej ME, Schreer GE. Elevated blood pressure and personality: a meta-analytic review. Psychol Bull 1996; 120:293–320.
14. Esler M, Julius S, Zweifler A, Randall O, Harburg E, Gardiner H, DeQuattro V. Mild high-renin hypertension: neurogenic human hypertension? N Engl J Med 1977; 296:405–411.
15. Perini C, Rauchfleisch U, Buhler FR. Personality characteristics and renin in essential hypertension. Psychother Psychosom 1985; 43:44–48.

16. Krantz DS, DeQuattro V, Blackburn H, Eaker E, Haynes S, James S, Manuck SB, Myers H, Shekelle RB, Syme SL, Tyroler HA, Wolf S. Psychosocial factors in hypertension. Circulation 1987; 76(suppl I):84–88.

17. Shapiro AP, Alderman MH, Clarkson TB, Furberg CD, Jesse MJ, Julius S, Miller RE, Pitt B. Behavioral consequences of hypertension and antihypertensive therapy. Circulation 1987; 76(suppl I):101–103.

18. Shapiro AP. Psychological factors in hypertension: an overview. Am Heart J 1988; 116: 632–637.

19. Johnson EH. Psychiatric morbidity and health problems among black Americans: a national survey. J Natl Med Assoc 1989; 81:1217–1223.

20. Hayward C. Psychiatric illness and cardiovascular disease risk. Epidemiol Rev 1995; 17: 129–38.

21. Yates WR, Wallace R. Cardiovascular risk factors in affective disorder. J Affect Disord 1987; 12:129–134.

22. Bruce LC, Alexander H. The treatment of melancholia. Lancet 1901; ii:516–518.

23. Rabkin JG, Charles E, Kass F. Hypertension and DSM-III depression in psychiatric outpatients. Am J Psychiatry 1983; 140:1072–1074.

24. Mezzich JE, Fabrega H, Jr., Coffman GA. Multiaxial characterization of depressive patients. J Nerv Ment Dis 1987; 175:339–446.

25. Fuller BF. DSM-III depression and hypertension in two psychiatric outpatient populations. Psychosomatics 1988; 29:417–423.

26. Wells KB, Rogers W, Burnam A, Greenfield S, Ware JE, Jr. How the medical comorbidity of depressed patients differs across health care settings: results from the Medical Outcomes Study. Am J Psychiatry 1991; 148:1688–1696.

27. Wells KB, Golding JM, Burnam MA. Chronic medical conditions in a sample of the general population with anxiety, affective, and substance use disorders. Am J Psychiatry 1989; 146:1440–1446.

28. Wells KB, Golding JM, Burnam MA. Affective, substance use, and anxiety disorders in persons with arthritis, diabetes, heart disease, high blood pressure, or chronic lung conditions. Gen Hosp Psychiatry 1989; 11:320–327.

29. Jonas BS, Franks P, Ingram DD. Are symptoms of anxiety and depression risk factors in hypertension? Arch Fam Med 1997; 6:43–49.

30. Fazio AF. A concurrent validational study of the NCHS General Well-Being Schedule. Vital Health Statistics 2. Vol 73, 1977.

31. Robbins MA, Elias MF, Schultz NR. The effects of age, blood pressure, and knowledge of hypertensive diagnosis in anxiety and depression. Aging Res 1990; 16:199–207.

32. Siever LJ, Davis KL. Overview: toward a dysregulation hypothesis of depression. Am J Psychol 1985; 142:1017–1031.

33. Kissebah AH, Krakower GR. Regional adiposity and morbidity. Physiol Rev 1994; 74: 761–811.

34. Sherbourne CD, Jackson CA, Meredith LS, Camp P, Wells KB. Prevalence of comorbid anxiety disorders in primary care outpatients. Arch Fam Med 1996; 5:27–34.

35. Katon W. Panic disorder and somatization. Review of 55 cases. Am J Med 1984; 77:101–106.

36. Davidson JR, Hughes D, Blazer DG, George LK. Post-traumatic stress disorder in the community: an epidemiological study. Psychol Med 1991; 21:713–721.

37. McFall ME, Murburg M, Roszell DK, Veith RC. Psychophysiologic and neuroendocrine

findings in posttraumatic stress disorder: a review of theory and research. J Anxiety Disord 1989; 3:243–257.

38. Markovitz JH, Matthews KA, Kannel WB, Cobb JL, D'Agostino RB. Psychological predictors of hypertension in the Framingham study: Is there tension in hypertension? JAMA 1993; 270:2439–2443.

39. Markovitz JH, Matthews KA, Wing RR, Kuller LH, Meilahn EN. Psychological, biological and health behavior predictors of blood pressure changes in middle-aged women. J Hypertension 1991;9:399–406.

40. Beilin LJ. Epidemiology of alcohol and hypertension. Adv Alcohol Subst Abuse 1987; 6: 69–87.

41. Bjorntorp P. Visceral fat accumulation: The missing link between psychosocial factors and cardiovascular disease? J Intern Med 1991; 230:195–201.

42. Swift RM. Alcohol and drug abuse in the medical setting. In: Stoudemire A, Fogel BS, eds. Psychiatric Care of the Medical Patient. New York: Oxford University Press, 1993.

43. Burling TA, Ziff DC. Tobacco smoking: a comparison between alcohol and drug abuse inpatients. Addict Behav 1988; 13:185–190.

44. Risch SC, Groom GP, Janowsky DS. Interfaces of psychopharmacology and cardiology. Part 1. J Clin Psychiatry 1981; 42:23–34.

45. Stoute JA, Hall WD. Treatment of essential hypertension in the psychiatric patient. Emory Univ J Med 1990; 4:19–24.

46. Cooper GL. The safety of fluoxetine: an update. Br J Psychiatry 1988; 153(suppl 3):77–86.

47. Satel SL, Nelson JC. Stimulants in the treatment of depression: a critical overview. J Clin Psychiatry 1989; 50:241–249.

48. Rauch SL, Stern TA, Zusman RM. Neuropsychiatric considerations in the treatment of hypertension. Int J Psychiatry Med 1991; 21:291–308.

49. Knos GB, Sung YF. ECT anesthesia strategies in the high risk medical patient. In: Stoudemire A, Fogel BS, eds. Psychiatric Care of the Medical Patient. New York: Oxford University Press, 1993.

50. Andur MA. Medication compliance in outpatient psychiatry. Compr Psychiatry 1979; 20: 339–345.

51. Kelly GR, Scott JE, Mamon J. Medication compliance and health education among outpatients with chronic mental disorders [published erratum appears in Med Care 1991; 29(9): 889]. Med-Care 1990; 28:1181–1197.

52. Levenson JL. Cardiovascular disease. In: Stoudemire A, Fogel BS, eds. Psychiatric Care of the Medical Patient. New York: Oxford University Press, 1993.

53. Paykel ES, Fleminger R, Watson JP. Psychiatric side effects of drugs other than reserpine. J Clin Psychopharmacol 1982; 2:14–39.

54. Dimsdale JE, Newton RP, Joist T. Neuropsychological side effects of beta-blockers. Arch Intern Med 1989; 149:514–525.

55. Gengo FM, Fagan SC, DePadova A, et al. The effect of B-blockers on mental performance in older hypertensive subjects. Arch Intern Med 1988; 148:779–784.

56. Testa MA, Anderson RB, Nackley JF, Hollenberg NK. Quality of life and antihypertensive therapy in men: a comparison of captopril with enalapril. The Quality-of-Life Hypertension Study Group [see comments]. N Engl J Med 1993; 328: 907–913.

57. Croog SH, Levine S, Testa MA, et al. The effects of antihypertensive therapy on the quality of life. N Engl J Med 1986; 314:1657–1664.

58. Waldstein SR, Manuck SB, Ryan CM, Muldoon MF. Neuropsychological correlates of hypertension: review and methodologic considerations. Psychol Bull 1991; 110:451–468.

59. Waldstein SR, Ryan CM, Manuck SB, Parkinson DK, Bromet EJ. Learning and memory function in men with untreated blood pressure elevation. J Consult Clin Psychol 1991; 59:513–517.

60. Niaura R, Goldstein MG. Psychological factors affecting physical condition Part II: Coronary artery disease, sudden death, and hypertension. Psychosomatics 1992; 33:146–155.

61. Jacob RG, Shapiro AP, Reeves RA, et al. Comparison of relaxation therapy for hypertension with placebo, diuretics, and beta-blockers. Arch Intern Med 1986; 146:2335–2340.

62. Patel C, Marmot MG, Terry DJ, et al. Trial of relaxation in reducing coronary risk: four year follow-up. Br Med J 1985; 290:1102–1106.

63. Agras WS, Southam MA, Taylor CB. Long-term persistence of relaxation-induced blood pressure lowering during the working day. J Consult Clin Psychol 1983; 51:792–794.

64. Glasgow MS, Engel BT. A controlled trial of a standardized behavioral stepped treatment for hypertension. Psychosom Med 1989; 51:10–26.

65. Eisenberg DM, Delbanco TL, Berkey CS, Kaptchuk TJ, Kupelnick B, Kuhl J, Chalmers TC. Cognitive behavioral techniques for hypertension: are they effective? Ann Intern Med 1993; 118:964–972.

66. Heine BE, Sainsbury P, Chynoweth RC. Hypertension and emotional disturbance. J Psychiatr Res 1969; 7:119–130.

67. Heine BE. Psychogenesis of hypertension. Proc Royal Soc Med 1970; 63:1267–1270.

68. Wheatley D, Balter M, Levine J, Lipman R, Bauer ML, Bonato R. Psychiatric aspects of hypertension. Br J Psychiatry 1975; 127:327–336.

69. Friedman MJ, Bennet PL. Depression and hypertension. Psychosom Med 1977; 39:134–142.

70. Lyketsos G, Arapakis G, Psaras M, Photiou I, Blackburn IM. Psychological characteristics of hypertensive patients. J Psychosom Res 1982; 26:255–262.

71. Reus VI, Miner C. Evidence for physiological effects of hypercortisolemia in psychiatric patients. Psychiatry Res 1985; 14:47–56.

72. Noyes RJ, Clancy J, Hoenk PR, et al. The prognosis of anxiety neurosis. Arch Gen Psychiatry 1980; 37:173–178.

73. Sparrow D, Garvey AJ, Rosner B, Thomas HE. Factors in predicting blood pressure change. Circulation 1982; 65:789–794.

74. Dunner D. Anxiety and panic: relationship to depression and cardiac disorders. Psychosomatics 1985; 26(11 suppl):18–22.

75. Charney DS, Heninger DR. Abnormal regulation of noradrenergic function in panic disorders: effects of clonidine in healthy subjects and patients with agoraphobia and panic disorder. Arch Gen Psychiatry 1986; 43:1042–1054.

5

Psychological State, Arrhythmias, and Cardiac Mortality

Peter A. Shapiro and Steven P. Roose
Columbia University College of Physicians & Surgeons
New York, New York

INTRODUCTION

This chapter reviews the many dimensions of the clinically significant relationship between the emotions and cardiac function. To consider whether psychological states (brain events) affect the heart, four questions are addressed:

1. What is the effect of normal excitatory emotions on the normal heart?
2. What is the effect of normal excitatory emotions on the person with manifest or occult heart disease?
3. What is the impact of abnormal psychological states, i.e., mood or anxiety disorders, on the function of the normal heart?
4. What is the impact of mood or anxiety disorders on the patient with pre-existing heart disease?

Finally, this chapter considers the effect of cardiac function on emotions, specifically which psychiatric problems can develop in patients with cardiac arrhythmias.

DO EMOTIONS CAUSE CARDIOVASCULAR EFFECTS IN HEALTHY PEOPLE?

The most common cardiovascular effect of fear, excitement, or anxiety is increased heart rate, due primarily to sympathetic nervous system activation and secondarily to withdrawal of parasympathetic tone. This sinus tachycardia is generally of no pathological significance, but it may precipitate myocardial ischemia in the presence of coronary artery disease. Paroxysmal supraventricular tachycardia is occasionally induced in states of emotional excitement. This condition results from activation of an ectopic atrial pacemaker. It may be associated with chest discomfort and shortness of breath.

DO EMOTIONS PRODUCE ARRHYTHMIA AND DEATH?

More important are the severe cardiovascular reactions to emotional stress, instances captured in the common expression "scared to death." In studies of "voodoo death," Walter Cannon, a pioneer in the investigation of the effects of psychological stimuli on the heart, proposed that these deaths were attributable to sustained sympathetic nervous system and adrenal activation in the face of fear, which resulted in circulatory collapse (1). Subsequent studies have helped to define the circumstances and elaborate the mechanisms by which emotion and affect lead to malignant rhythm disturbances.

Cardiac arrhythmia is the mechanism of most cases of sudden cardiac death, which is the leading cause of death in patients who have had myocardial infarction and a frequent cause of death even in those without evidence of heart disease. While brady-cardic arrest occurs occasionally, the usual arrhythmia in sudden cardiac death is ventric-ular tachycardia-ventricular fibrillation. In this condition, a rapid heart rate originating in the ventricle from one or more ectopic foci of rhythmic electrical depolarization drives the heart at a rate incompatible with effective pumping function, and the elec-trical disturbance ultimately degenerates into chaotic, unsynchronized depolarization throughout the myocardium, resulting in cessation of blood flow, immediate loss of consciousness, and brain death within minutes. An overwhelming body of evidence links acute emotional stress with precipitation of ventricular ectopic activity and sudden cardiac death (2,3).

EVIDENCE FROM ANIMAL MODELS

Bernard Lown, in a series of studies utilizing a dog model, demonstrated the effect of emotional factors on ventricular arrhythmia (2,4–6). Lown combined methods of in-ducing ventricular arrhythmias through electrical stimulation with classical condition-ing paradigms. Dogs aversively conditioned to a restraining sling were more easily pro-voked to arrhythmia by electrical stimulation in the presence of this stimulus than in its absence. Increased circulating catecholamines were noted in association with the stressful stimulus. These arrhythmias were blocked by pretreatment with beta-adrener-gic blocking agents or by cardiac sympathectomy. Lown concluded that the effect of emotional excitement on ventricular arrhythmias was mediated by sympathetic nervous system activation (2,7).

Skinner found similar effects of familiar versus unfamiliar environments on the risk of ventricular fibrillation in pigs with experimentally produced acute coronary oc-clusion. He demonstrated that stimulation of sympathetic cardiac efferents increases susceptibility to ventricular fibrillation and that stimulation of hypothalamic nuclei can increase the profibrillatory effect of acute myocardial ischemia. Sympathetic blockade, stellate ganglion ablation, and cardiac sympathectomy block these effects. Intracerebral injection of beta-adrenergic blockers or ablation of frontal cortico-thalamic pathways reduced the incidence of sudden death (8–15).

Vagal stimulation, which reduces heart rate and reduces ventricular irritability, tends to offset the effects of sympathetic nervous activation, but protective parasympathetic vagal effects are demonstrable only in the setting of enhanced sympathetic drive and disappear if beta-blockade is employed. Vagal antagonism of augmented sympathetic drive is due to muscarinic inhibition of norepinephrine release from sympathetic nerve terminals (16–18).

EVIDENCE FROM HUMAN STUDIES

The role of sympathetic activation is further underscored in clinical populations, where Schwartz et al. demonstrated the effectiveness of ablation of the stellate ganglion or other means of cardiac sympathectomy in many cases of treatment-refractory recurrent ventricular tachycardia (19–22).

Reich and colleagues (23) examined 117 patients with life-threatening ventricular arrhythmias. They found that 25 had experienced severe acute emotional distress in the 24 hours before their episode of arrhythmia; compared to patients without such an emotional stressor, these patients had less severe structural heart disease. However, Reich cautioned against an overinvocation of stress-related factors in precipitating arrhythmias and overenthusiastic interventions for "stress reduction," noting relative lack of evidence for the effect of interventions and the risk of psychological disability incurred by pathologizing normal daily stress responses (24).

Follick and colleagues (25) examined the correlation of the SCL-90 general distress score after acute myocardial infarction with subsequent ventricular ectopy in 125 patients. Over one year of follow-up, 59 patients had ventricular ectopy and 66 did not. After adjusting for gender, smoking, in-hospital complications, age, use of beta-blockers, and prior myocardial infarction, distress remained a significant predictor of ectopic activity.

Leor and colleagues studied deaths in the aftermath of the Northridge, California, earthquake of 1994 (26). They found a steady daily rate of sudden cardiac deaths in the weeks preceding the earthquake. On the day of the earthquake, beginning several hours after the event, there was a dramatic upsurge in sudden cardiac deaths. Over the next several days, sudden cardiac death occurred at a lower than normal rate, then gradually returned to its usual daily level. Their investigation excluded deaths occurring in the presence of extreme physical exertion. Twenty-four of 25 sudden cardiac deaths witnessed on the day of the earthquake occurred in individuals with risk factors for or a definite history of atherosclerotic coronary artery disease. Chest pain was the most frequent premonitory symptom, and the age and sex distribution of the victims—75%

male with a mean age of 64 years, 25% female with a mean age of 80 years—resembled those of other atherosclerotic heart disease fatalities in the same region at other times. These results suggest that the acute psychological stress created by the devastating effects of the earthquake triggered disturbances in autonomic cardiac control, which stimulated the onset of lethal ventricular arrhythmias, but only in susceptible individuals—namely, those with the preexisting physiological substrate for lethal arrhythmia.

DO DEPRESSION AND ANXIETY ASSOCIATE WITH ARRHYTHMIAS AND/OR SUDDEN CARDIAC DEATH?

Recent studies have demonstrated unequivocally that both anxiety and depression are associated with sudden cardiac death. Effects are seen both in community samples of individuals without preexisting heart disease and in clinical samples of heart-diseased patients.

Kawachi et al. examined the relationship between anxiety and heart disease in the Normative Aging Study, a prospective epidemiological follow-up of 2280 men from the Boston area aged 21–80 years who were screened at entry and found to be free of chronic diseases (27). A five-item anxiety scale was constructed from items of the Cornell medical index, which was completed by the cohort at baseline. On the five-item anxiety scale, 89.3% scored zero, 8.8% scored one, and 1.9% scored two or more. In a 32-year follow-up there were 132 cases of incident coronary artery disease, including 131 fatal coronary heart disease (CHD) (26 sudden cardiac death, 105 nonsudden death), whereas 1869 subjects did not develop coronary disease. Compared to men with no anxiety symptoms, men with two or more symptoms had elevated risk of fatal CHD (age-adjusted OR = 3.20; 95% CI 1.27–8.09) and sudden death (age-adjusted OR = 5.73; 95% CI 1.26–26.1). Multivariate OR after adjusting for potential confounding variables was 1.94 (95% CI 0.70–5.41) for fatal CHD and 4.46 (95% CI 0.92–21.6) for sudden death. No excess risk was found for angina or nonfatal myocardial infarction (MI). These data suggest an association between anxiety and fatal CHD, in particular sudden cardiac death. This finding is bolstered by the results of a second epidemiological study, the Health Professionals Follow-Up Study, in which Kawachi and colleagues found an association between sudden cardiac death and elevated scores on a scale measuring anxiety and propensity to phobic and panic reactions (28). For this study, 33,999 male health professionals aged 42–77 years completed an anxiety questionnaire along with a health history screening. At 2-year follow-up there were 168 new cases of CHD, including 128 cases of nonfatal MI and 40 coronary disease deaths. Age-adjusted relative risk of fatal CHD for men in the highest phobic anxiety level was 3.01 compared to those in the lowest anxiety group. Risk of fatal CHD increased with level of phobic anxiety ($p < 0.02$). The excess risk was limited to cases of sudden death (RR = 6.08). No association was found between phobic anxiety and nonfatal MI.

Follick and colleagues (29) studied post-MI patients with frequent PVCs enrolled in the Cardiac Arrhythmia Pilot Study (CAPS). Ventricular ectopy was not related to any measures of psychological state or trait measured (trait and state anxiety, depression, anger, type A behavior pattern) or to blood pressure or heart rate reactivity to a standardized video game stressor at baseline. In placebo-treated patients, PVCs were not correlated with psychosocial measures or stress reactivity at follow-up. Suppression of PVCs over the course of the 12 month study was also unrelated to psychosocial or reactivity measures. Baseline biobehavioral variables were related to subsequent mortality, however (30). Of 502 patients, 353 completed questionnaires and 341 completed psychophysiological reactivity testing (265 patients completed both). Type B behavior pattern, depression, and low heart rate reactivity to video game stress were associated with increased risk of death or cardiac arrest after adjustment for other known risk factors. The mean Beck Depression Inventory score in the 27 nonsurvivors was 12.15, compared to 8.13 in the 324 survivors. (A score of 10 or more is frequently considered a criterion for clinically significant depressive illness.)

There has been a longstanding clinical belief that patients with depression have a higher than expected rate of sudden cardiovascular death. The first systematic study supporting this clinical observation compared the mortality rate of patients hospitalized for melancholia to the mortality rate of the general population (31). The effect of age was controlled by constructing 5-year age cohorts for both the patients and the general population and then comparing the mortality rate for each cohort; e.g., the death rate of patients aged 60–64 was compared to the death rate in the general population for same age group. Overall the death rate was 6 times greater in patients with melancholia compared to the general population, and this was consistent in all age groups. Cardiac disease accounted for almost 40% of deaths reported in patients, and the rate of cardiac death in patients was eight times greater than the corresponding rate in the general population. This study was published in 1937 and remains both influential and unique because the data were collected in an era when there were no specific somatic treatments for depression, and thus the findings reflect the natural course of the illness.

The observation that depressed patients have a higher cardiovascular mortality than the general population has been replicated by a number of different investigators in both the United States and Europe (32–35). One of the most informative studies compared mortality rates in adequately versus inadequately depressed patients; in a sample of 519 patients, 301 were classified as having received adequate treatments (defined as a certain minimum dose of tricyclic or electroconvulsive therapy [ECT]) and 191 as having received inadequate treatment (36). Cardiac mortality was significantly greater in the inadequately versus the adequately treated patients.

The mechanism underlying the increased cardiac mortality in medically healthy depressed patients is unclear, but a recent line of investigation suggests that changes in the ratio between sympathetic and parasympathetic tone may make depressed patients more vulnerable to ventricular fibrillation (37–39). As previously discussed, it has been established that increased sympathetic input to the heart can lower the threshold for ventricular fibrillation, whereas increased parasympathetic tone (which is generally transmitted through vagal activity) raises the threshold and therefore reduces the risk of ventricular fibrillation (22). Measurements of heart rate variability have been used to illuminate a possible relationship between depression and the development of ventricular fibrillation. Heart rate variability is the standard deviation of successive R to R intervals in sinus rhythm and reflects the interplay and balance between sympathetic and parasympathetic input on the cardiac pacemaker. A healthy heart with normal function is characterized by a high degree of heart rate variability, whereas heart rate variability can be significantly decreased in patients with severe coronary artery disease or congestive heart failure. Furthermore, in a study of mortality following myocardial infarction, reduced heart rate variability emerged as the most significant predictor of death during a 31-month follow-up of 808 post-MI patients (40).

Heart rate variability components measured in depressed patients were not found to be significantly different compared to normal controls (41). However, assessment of the high-frequency component of heart rate variability, defined as the absolute difference between successive normal R to R intervals that are greater than 50 msec expressed as a percentage of all heart periods, a measurement that represents exclusively parasympathetic tone, was found to be significantly decreased in depressed patients. This implies that depressed patients may have reduced parasympathetic activity compared to normal controls. Insofar as decreased parasympathetic tone lowers the threshold of ventricular fibrillation, it is possible that decreased high-frequency variability in depressed patients reflects part of the mechanism that leads to the increased rate of cardiovascular death in this group.

The relationship between heart rate variability measurements and predisposition to ventricular fibrillation may also shed light on the occasional reports of sudden cardiovascular death in children being treated with tricyclic antidepressants (42). Walsh et al. reported that in children treatment with tricyclic antidepressants induces a significant increase in the heart rate, possibly mediated by blockade of parasympathetic input as a consequence of the anticholinergic properties of the tricyclics (43). In the same tricyclic-treated children a substantial reduction in the high-frequency component of heart rate variability was also observed. It has been established that parasympathetic input to the heart declines substantially with age, and therefore the significant anticholinergic effect of the tricyclics will produce a relatively greater decrease in parasympathetic tone in younger compared to older patients. This decrease in parasympathetic tone may contribute to the development of ventricular fibrillation in some children, although reduction in parasympathetic tone alone cannot be an adequate explanation for these cases of unexpected cardiac death in tricyclic-treated children.

Another illuminating approach to this topic is to consider the impact of depression on cardiac rhythm in patients with manifest heart disease. Carney and colleagues (44) studied 103 patients found to have coronary artery disease on diagnostic catheterization using psychiatric diagnostic interviews and ambulatory ECG monitoring. Twenty-one patients (20%) met the criteria for major or minor depression. Depressed patients did not differ from nondepressed patients with respect to the severity of coronary disease or ventricular function, but five (23%) of the depressed patients, compared to only three (4%) of the nondepressed patients, had episodes of ventricular tachycardia on 24-hour monitoring. This was a significant difference even after adjusting for other ventricular tachycardia risk factors.

Frasure-Smith and colleagues identified cases of major depressive disorder and patients with elevated depressive symptom scores in the first 2 weeks following myocardial infarction and examined the relationship of depression to subsequent mortality (45). This study was especially important for a number of reasons. It was designed as a prospective study with the primary objective of testing the depression–mortality relationship, which permitted it to avoid a number of limitations occurring when such analyses are conducted as secondary objectives of other studies. It included both men and women, and had a large sample size. Standardized structured diagnostic interviews were used to establish the diagnosis of depression, and the patients were representative of the full range of severity of myocardial infarction. Thirty-five of 222 patients (16%) studied met criteria for major depressive disorder, and 68 patients (31%) had elevated depressive symptoms (Beck Depression Inventory score greater than 10). A diagnosis of major depressive disorder was associated with an almost fourfold increased mortality rate at 6 months, after adjustment for other prognostic factors, and elevated depressive symptoms conferred an eightfold increased risk of death by 18 months. After statistical adjustment for other prognostic variables, elevated depressive symptoms remained a significant predictor of mortality (adjusted OR = 6.64; 95% CI = 1.76–25.09; p = 0.0026). Patients with frequent PVCs on 24-hour ambulatory electrocardiography shortly after myocardial infarction are generally recognized as being at increased risk of subsequent sudden cardiac death. In this study, such patients were present in the same proportion among those with high and low depressive symptoms. In those with low depressive symptoms, the presence of premature contractions was not associated with increased sudden cardiac death during the 18-month follow-up period, while in the high depression group, those with frequent PVCs had an almost 80% mortality due to sudden death. Deaths were concentrated among depressed patients with PVCs (OR = 29.1; 95% CI 6.97–122.07; $p < 0.00001$). This result is compatible with literature suggesting an arrhythmic mechanism linking psychological factors and sudden cardiac death. Major depression, depressive symptoms, anxiety, and history of major depression all significantly predicted cardiac events, independent of each other and of measures of cardiac disease severity (46). Acute coronary syndromes were related to elevated depressive symptoms, history of major depression, and gender, and marginally to ACE inhibitor use. Arrhythmias were linked to elevated anxiety symptoms and anger held in, but not to anxiety.

Moser and Dracup (47) found that anxiety and depression ratings in acute MI patients still in the cardiac care unit were significantly associated with arrhythmias as well as reinfarction and other cardiac events during the remainder of the hospital stay. They measured anxiety within the first 48 hours of hospitalization in 86 patients with acute MI and followed the rate of complications including reinfarction, new onset ischemia, ventricular fibrillation, sustained VT, and in-hospital death. All patients received thrombolytic therapy. Patients completed the Brief Symptom inventory, which includes six items in its anxiety subscale. High anxiety levels (above the median) were associated with more complications than low anxiety (19.6% vs. 6%; $p = 0.001$). Higher anxiety level was associated with a relative risk of 4.9 for subsequent complications.

PSEUDO-ARRHYTHMIAS (PALPITATIONS IN THE ABSENCE OF RHYTHM DISORDER) AND PSYCHIATRIC DISORDERS

While depression and anxiety, as well as acute emotional distress, appear to be related to ventricular arrhythmias, they also, along with somatization disorder and panic disorder, appear to bear a significant relationship to pseudo-arrhythmias, the perception of irregular heart beats in the absence of clinically significant arrhythmia.

Orth-Gomer and colleagues (48) identified a population of 51 men with ischemic heart disease and comparison groups of 50 men with cardiac risk factors but no established CAD and 50 healthy men, all employed in a company of 4000. Subjects completed ambulatory ECG monitoring, psychological measures, and diaries of cardiac activity during monitoring as well as questionnaires regarding history of arrhythmic sensations. Symptoms and ECG findings were unrelated. Symptomatic patients without arrhythmias tended to be free of organic heart disease, less trustful, and more aggressive.

Lochen (49) reported on a community survey of 19,222 male and female community-dwelling subjects in Tromso, Norway, in 1986–87. Arrhythmia was self-reported by 17% of women and 12% of men, with the same prevalence in healthy subjects. Self-reported arrhythmia was strongly associated with sleep disturbance, mental depression, and contact problems and with self-rated overall health. In males, frequency of alcohol intoxication was also associated with self-report of arrhythmias.

In another study, Lochen and Rasmussen (50) surveyed 10,497 residents of Nordland, Norway, aged 40–42. In 6436 subjects, the prevalence of palpitations was 15% in men and 25% in women. Palpitations were associated with coffee consumption, smoking, alcohol intoxication, physical inactivity, depression, and poor self-rated health. In a logistic regression analysis, significant predictors were depression and poor self-rated health in both sexes, coffee drinking and physical inactivity in men, and alcohol intoxication in women.

Mayou and colleagues (51) assessed a series of 94 consecutive referral cases to cardiology clinic for complaints of chest pain and/or palpitations. In 39 (41%) a definite or probable cardiac diagnosis was established, in 4 cases other specific somatic diagnoses were established, and in 51 (54%) no somatic diagnosis was identified. Eight of the cardiac disease group had paroxysmal arrhythmias. Four of the 39 cardiac patients had major depressive disorder, and 5 had various anxiety disorders. Noncardiac pain patients were generally younger, more likely to be female, and less likely to have a family history of heart disease.

Weber and Kapoor (52) reported a series of 190 consecutive patients presenting with a chief complaint of palpitations. The etiology was cardiac disease in 43%, psychiatric disorder in 31%, miscellaneous other disorders in 10%, and unknown in 16%. One-year mortality was 1.6%. One-year incidence of stroke was 1.1%. Panic attack or panic disorder plus anxiety was considered the etiology in 10%, panic attack alone in 9%, panic disorder alone in 7%, anxiety alone in 3%, and panic plus anxiety plus somatization in 1%. Co-morbid depression occurred in 15%. Psychiatric illness was associated with the highest rate of recurrent symptoms at 3-month follow-up (61%). A history of heart disease of any kind, advanced age, symptom duration over 5 minutes, and a chief complaint of irregular heart beat were associated with increased likelihood of a cardiac etiology of palpitations.

Barsky and colleagues (53) compared 145 ambulatory patients referred for ambulatory ECG monitoring to evaluate palpitations with 70 asymptomatic control subjects. Recognition of resting heart rate was accurate in 20% of palpitation subjects and only 5% of control subjects. Accuracy was unrelated to measures of somatosensory amplification, somatization, hypochondriasis, psychiatric morbidity, or ECG findings. Thirty-four percent of palpitation patients consistently reported symptoms coinciding with documented arrhythmias. These patients had lower scores on somatization, somatosensory amplification, hypochondriasis, and psychiatric morbidity. Accuracy of symptom reports was not correlated with accuracy of resting heartbeat detection. Among the palpitations patients, 40 (28%) were found to have lifetime panic disorder, and 27 (19%) had current panic disorder (54). Panic disorder cases did not have more arrhythmias, and their symptom reports were less well correlated with Holter abnormalities than the other patients. They were not better heartbeat detectors, but scored higher on measures of hypochondriasis, somatization, and somatosensory amplification.

In a follow-up study, Barsky and colleagues (55) studied 125 consecutive medical outpatients referred for ambulatory electrocardiographic monitoring due to a chief complaint of palpitations. Forty-three percent had significant arrhythmias. Twenty-four of the remaining 82 patients (29%) had current psychiatric disorder, including 20 with major depression or panic disorder. Patients with psychiatric disorder had increased emergency room visits, more recurring symptoms, more hypochondriacal concerns, and more impairment in daily activity. Though their physicians were more likely to ascribe their symptoms to a psychiatric disorder, few were treated or referred for treatment of this disorder. Patients with psychiatric disorder had more severe palpitations, were younger, more often had symptoms lasting longer than 15 minutes, and had more accompanying somatic symptoms. The interaction of somatosensory amplification and self-rated daily life stress was a significant predictor of persistence of palpitations and of unscheduled medical visits over 3-month follow-up; in contrast, ventricular premature contractions were not a predictor of recurring palpitation symptoms (55).

Katon and colleagues have performed a series of investigations in the primary care setting over the past 15 years delineating the extent of covert psychiatric disorder among individuals, particularly high utilizers of general medical services, with palpitations and related somatic complaints. For example, in a large community-based health maintenance organization sample, only about one in 10 visits to the primary care physician for chest pain, and only about one in 5 visits for dizziness, can be attributed to a definable somatic disorder (56). Palpitations were prominent among the presenting symptoms of 25% of a sample of 55 patients referred by their primary care physicians to psychiatrists for evaluation of anxiety or panic disorder (57). The lifetime prevalence of panic disorder was 21.8% and of somatization disorder 20.2% in a sample of 767 "distressed high utilizers" of primary care (58). In another study, patients with medically unexplained dizziness had a 13% prevalence of panic disorder (59).

MOOD AND ANXIETY DISORDERS IN PATIENTS WITH CARDIAC ARRHYTHMIAS

The prevalence and incidence of psychiatric disorders in patients with cardiac arrhythmias has not been extensively studied. Adjustment disorders, generalized anxiety, and mood disorders would be expected as psychiatric morbidity, as for other serious general medical conditions. In addition, patients who have experienced ventricular tachycardia-ventricular fibrillation may have posttraumatic stress symptoms associated either with the circumstances of the occurrence of the arrhythmia itself or with the experience of being defibrillated. Prevailing thinking about the treatment of depression in arrhythmia patients has changed in recent years because of evidence of increased mortality with Type 1A antiarrhythmic agents in ischemic heart disease patients. This will be discussed below.

Discussions of the psychiatric aspects of the arrhythmia patient's experience (60,61) emphasize the psychological stress of repeated trials of drugs and electrophysiological studies, the stress of confinement in the cardiac care unit, and the experience of overdrive pacing and defibrillation and of surgery for implantation of an automated defibrillator. Patients experience anxiety and a sense of loss of control and may fear sleep or separation from cardiac monitoring. Hypervigilance and insomnia may be observed. Near-death experiences may be perceived as traumatic and lead to fear of recurrent cardiac arrest, fear of dying, and fear of being left alone (62). Treatment of anxiety in this setting includes providing information while conveying hope and acknowledging possible frustrations; supportive psychotherapy with ventilation of affect and shoring up of adaptive defenses; medication with benzodiazepines and beta-blockers; and behavioral techniques such as progressive muscle relaxation, meditation or self-hypnosis. Depression often accompanies a sense of loss of independence and role transition with concerns about provision for self and family, burdening the family, or abandonment. Delirium and psychosis are unusual problems except as side effects of antiarrhythmia therapy. Defibrillator-related panic, agoraphobia, and posttraumatic stress symptoms may be managed with benzodiazepines, supportive reassurance, and understanding and behavioral management. Anxiety about defibrillator discharges can be disabling in its own right (63,64). Arrhythmia patients may experience intensification of previously present panic disorder symptoms or somatization.

PSYCHIATRIC SEQUELAE TO CARDIAC ARREST

Kolar and Dracup (65) evaluated 19 cardiac arrest survivors and 21 patients with recurrent ventricular tachycardia for psychological adjustment using the Psychosocial Adjustment to Illness Scale. Unmarried marital status, more episodes of dysrhythmia, and more severe heart failure were associated with poorer psychosocial adjustment.

In general, cerebral hypoxia and anoxia are associated with subsequent cognitive impairment. Especially affected functions include short-term memory and laying down of new memory as well as capacity to perform complex operations. Roine et al. (66) prospectively followed a group of consecutive patients resuscitated from out-of-hospital cardiac arrest. Three months after resuscitation, 41 of 68 patients (60%) had moderate to severe cognitive deficits. Twelve months after resuscitation, 26 of 54 survivors (48%) still had significant deficits. Severe depression occurred in 24% of these survivors. The most common residual deficit was impaired delayed memory; speech, reading, writing, and visual perception were relatively spared. More severe depressive symptoms correlated with more neuropsychological impairment at the 12-month follow-up.

PSYCHIATRIC DISORDERS ASSOCIATED WITH ARRHYTHMIA TREATMENT

Antiarrhythmia drug therapy also causes psychiatric morbidity. Lidocaine is a first-line drug for treatment of ventricular tachycardia in intensive care settings. It is associated with significant central nervous system behavioral toxicity, including obtundation, seizures, psychosis, and delirium, even at blood levels within the therapeutic range. Procainamide, mexilitene, and other agents may also cause delirium or psychosis. These adverse effects may occur even at levels within the therapeutic range for these agents. Digoxin, sometimes used in the treatment of atrial fibrillation, causes visual hallucinations at supertherapeutic blood levels. Amiodarone has become increasingly important as a treatment for ventricular tachycardia, especially in the setting of congestive heart failure, as an alternative to Type 1A antiarrhythmic agents. However, amiodarone induces a transient thyroiditis and subsequent hypothyroid state. Patients may develop a depressive disorder secondary to this hypothyroid state.

Arteaga and Windle (67) evaluated 75 patients treated with amiodarone or an automatic implantable cardioverter defibrillator (AICD) for life-threatening ventricular arrhythmias and 29 comparison subjects with heart disease but without arrhythmias. In contrast to Kolar and Dracup, they found no relationship between marital status and quality of life, although higher NYHA heart failure class and younger age were correlated with lower quality of life. Amiodarone- and AICD-treated patients did not differ in measures of quality of life and psychological distress.

Implanted automatic pacemaker-defibrillators have grown in importance in the treatment of ventricular tachycardia-ventricular fibrillation. New generations of these devices detect the cardiac rhythm and are programmed to respond to excessive ventricular rate by delivering overdrive pacing or defibrillating shocks in escalating dosage if the rhythm fails to convert. While defibrillators are effective at preventing cardiac arrest and reducing mortality, they induce a psychiatric morbidity associated with reactions to anticipation of being shocked. Patients may experience shocks as painful thumps or blows to the chest, sometimes associated with restoration of consciousness and sometimes occurring in long series. Defibrillator discharges may be hard to anticipate and may interfere in their own right with activities of daily living. Moreover, despite the capacity to restore sinus rhythm in cases of VT/VF, defibrillators may not prevent the patient from losing consciousness when the arrhythmia commences, and therefore driving and some other activities may be curtailed. Consequently, anxiety and depression appear to be common but relatively untreated in patients with defibrillators (63). While Keren and colleagues (68) found that anxiety and depression in AICD-treated patients were no more severe than in arrhythmia patients treated with medication guided by electrical stimulation studies, Morris and colleagues (69) found that half of AICD-treated patients evaluated 3–21 months after device implantation had psychiatric disorders, including adjustment disorders, major depression, and panic disorder. Early perioperative shocks were associated with increased risk of subsequent psychiatric disturbance. In addition, posttraumatic stress symptoms appear in a small number of defibrillator patients who have experienced multiple, consecutive, painful discharges without losing consciousness and without warning in the course of ordinary activities of daily living, such as showering, recreational sports, and sexual relations. Such patients may become highly fearful and autonomically aroused if placed in the environment associated with their previous episode and may be preoccupied with intrusive recollections of this event to the exclusion of other interests. Heller and colleagues (70) sent 135 AICD patients questionnaires and received responses from 58 (43%). Most respondents (76%) were moderately or very positive about the AICD at follow-up. More than five shocks correlated with increased fatigue, sadness, stress, health concern, and nervousness. Other psychiatric-behavioral syndromes have also been described in defibrillator patients, including abuse of the defibrillator and psychological dependence on it (64). Morris and colleagues (69) and Teplitz and colleagues (71) have described beneficial effects of group therapy for AICD patients.

CARDIOVASCULAR EFFECTS OF ANTIDEPRESSANT MEDICATION IN PATIENTS WITH ARRHYTHMIAS

Tricyclic antidepressants have been by far the most extensively studied class of psychotropic agents in patients with heart disease. Tricyclic agents may cause ventricular arrhythmias in overdose, but at therapeutic levels have Type 1A antiarrhythmic properties, similar to quinidine or procainamide. Their main cardiovascular effects at therapeutic blood levels are orthostatic hypotension and slowing of cardiac conduction. Unfortunately, however, the CAST study demonstrated that Type 1 antiarrhythmic agents increase mortality for MI patients with PVCs (72–74). The increased mortality appears to be predominantly due to a proarrhythmic effect with an increased rate of sudden cardiac death. This effect appears to occur in the setting of myocardial ischemia (75). Since tricyclic agents also have Type I antiarrhythmic effect, caution has been urged in using them for ischemic heart disease patients (76).

Desipramine has been associated with several cases of sudden cardiac death in children (77,78). Whether these deaths were due to desipramine-induced arrhythmias cannot be determined from the available data. Modest ECG changes appear with desipramine treatment but are not correlated with dose or blood level of desipramine or its metabolites (79–81). QT interval prolongation on medication may indicate increased risk for sudden death (82).

Serotonin reuptake inhibitors appear to have a generally benign cardiovascular profile even in the presence of heart disease (83–85). Their main cardiovascular effect is slowing of heart rate by 2–3 beats per minute. In rare instances, bradycardia has been reported, and combinations of beta-adrenergic blockers with paroxetine or fluoxetine have led to isolated case reports of bradycardic syncope (86–88). They may increase left ventricular ejection fraction in patients with impaired left ventricular function (84). They do not have a pro-arrhythmia effect.

Antiarrhythmic drugs are metabolized through the hepatic cytochrome P450 system, and possible drug-drug interactions should be appreciated in decisions about prescription of psychotropic agents in arrhythmia patients. Fluoxetine, paroxetine, and, to a lesser extent, sertraline all inhibit the CYP2D6 isoenzyme, which metabolizes encainide, flecainide, mexilitene, and propafenone, as well as tricyclic antidepressants, some antipsychotic agents, and metoprolol, propranolol, and timolol. Fluvoxamine inhibits the CYP1A2 isoenzyme, another system involved in imipramine metabolism. The 3A4 isoenzyme is primary in metabolism of lidocaine, as well as quinidine, propafenone, and the short-acting benzodiazepines midazolam and triazolam. Fluoxetine, fluvoxamine, nefazodone, and sertraline may inhibit this system, leading to potential lidocaine toxicity. Nefazodone may increase serum digoxin levels.

CONCLUSION

The association between psychological states and cardiac function has been recognized since antiquity. However, it is only recently that we have appreciated the bidirectional nature of this relationship and illuminated some of the physiological mechanisms that mediate its clinical manifestations. Awareness of the prevalance and prognostic implications of comorbid depression, anxiety, and arrhythmias is essential for both the medical and psychiatric clinician.

REFERENCES

1. Cannon WB. "Voodoo" death. Psychosom Med 1957; 19:182.
2. Lown B, De Silva RA, Reich P, Murawski BJ. Psychophysiologic factors in sudden cardiac death. Am J Psychiatry 1980; 137:1325–1335.
3. Hartel G. Psychological factors in cardiac arrhythmias. Ann Clin Res 1987; 19:104–109.
4. Lown B, Verrier R, Corbalan R. Psychologic stress and threshold for repetitive ventricular response. Science 1973; 182:834–836.
5. Lown B, Verrier R. Neural activity and ventricular fibrillation. N Engl J Med 1976; 294: 1165–1170.
6. Lown B. Role of higher nervous activity in sudden cardiac death. Jpn Circ J 1990; 54: 581–602.
7. DeSilva RA. Central nervous system risk factors for sudden cardiac death. J S C Med Assoc 1983; 561–572.
8. Skinner JE, Lie JT, Entman ML. Modification of ventricular fibrillation latency following coronary artery occlusion in the conscious pig. Circulation 1975; 51:656–667.
9. Skinner JE, Reed JC. Blockade of a frontocortical-brainstem pathway prevents ventricular fibrillation of the ischemic heart in pigs. Am J Physiol 1981; 240:H156–H163.
10. Skinner JE. Regulation of cardiac vulnerability by the cerebral defense system. J Am Coll Cardiol 1985; 5:88B–94B.
11. Skinner JE, Martin JL, Landisman CE, Mommer MM, Fulton K, Mitra M, Burton WD, Saltzberg B. Chaotic attractors in a model of neocortex: dimensionalities of olfactory bulb surface potentials are spatially uniform and event related. In: Basar E, Bullock TH, eds. Chaos is Brain Function. New York: Springer-Verlag 1990:158–173.
12. Skinner JE. Brain control of cardiovascular dynamics. Event-Related Brain Res EEG 1991; 42(suppl):270–283.
13. Skinner JE, Carpeggiani C, Landisman CE, Fulton KW. Correlation dimension of heartbeat intervals is reduced in conscious pigs by myocardial ischemia. Circ Res 1991; 68: 966–976.
14. Skinner JE. Interrupting neural pathways that transduce stressful information into physiological responses. Integrative Physiol Behav Sci 1991; 26:330–334.
15. Skinner JE, Molnar M, Vybiral T, Mitra M. Application of chaos theory to biology and medicine. Integrative Physiol Behav Sci 1992; 27:39–53.
16. DeSilva RA, Verrier RL, Lown B. The effects of psychological stress and vagal stimulation with morphine on vulnerability to ventricular fibrillation (VF) in the conscious dog. Am Heart J 1978; 95:197–203.
17. DeSilva RA. Cardiac arrhythmias and sudden cardiac death. In: Stoudemire A, Fogel BS, eds. Medical-Psychiatric Practice. Washington, DC: American Psychiatric Press, 1993: 199–236.
18. Fukudo S, Lane JD, Anderson NB, Kuhn CM, Schanberg SM, McCown N, Muranaka M, Suzuki J, Williams RB. Accentuated vagal antagonism of β-adrenergic effects on ventricular repolarization: evidence of weaker anatagonism in hostile type A men. Circulation 1992; 85:2045–2053.
19. Schwartz PJ, Motolese M, Pollavini G, Lotto A, Ruberti U, Trazzi R, Bartorelli C, Zanchetti A, The Italian Sudden Death Prevention Group. Prevention of sudden cardiac death after a first myocardial infarction by pharmacologic or surgical antiadrenerigic interventions. J Cardiovasc Electrophysiol 1992; 3:2–16.

20. Schwartz PJ. Stress and sudden cardiac death: the role of the autonomic nervous system. JCP Monograph 1984; 2:7–13.
21. Schwartz PJ, De Ferrari GM. The influence of the autonomic nervous system on sudden cardiac death. Cardiology 1987; 74:297–309.
22. Schwartz PJ. The autonomic nervous system and sudden death. Eur Heart J 1998; 19(suppl F):F72–F80.
23. Reich P, DeSilva RA, Lown B, Murawski BJ. Acute psychological disturbances preceding life-threatening ventricular arrhythmias. JAMA 1981; 246:233–235.
24. Reich P. Psychological predisposition to life-threatening arrhythmias. Ann Rev Med 1985; 36:397–405.
25. Follick MJ, Gorkin L, Capone RJ, Smith TW, Ahern DK, Stablein D, Niaura R, Visco J. Psychological distress as a predictor of ventricular arrhythmias in a post-myocardial infarction population. Am Heart J 1988; 116:32–36.
26. Leor WJ, Poole WK, Kloner RA. Sudden cardiac death triggered by an earthquake. N Engl J Med 1996; 334:413–419.
27. Kawachi I, Sparrow D, Vokonas PS, Weiss ST. Symptoms of anxiety and risk of coronary heart disease. The Normative Aging Study. Circulation 1994; 90:2225–2229.
28. Kawachi I, Colditz GA, Ascherio A, Rimm E, Giovannucci E, Stampfer M, Willett WC. Prospective study of phobic anxiety and risk of coronary heart disease in men. Circulation 1994; 89:1992–1997.
29. Follick MJ, Ahern DK, Gorkin L, Niaura RS, Herd JA, Ewart C, Schron EB, Kornfeld DS, Capone RJ, CAPS Investigators. Relation of psychosocial and stress reactivity variables to ventricular arrhythmias in the Cardiac Arrhythmia Pilot Study (CAPS). Am J Cardiol 1990; 66:63–67.
30. Ahern DK, Gorkin L, Anderson JL, Tierney C, Hallstrom A, Ewart C, Capone RJ, Schron E, Kornfeld D, Herd JA, Richardson DW, Follick MJ, for the CAPS Investigators. Biobehavioral variables and mortality or cardiac arrest in the Cardiac Arrhythmia Pilot Study (CAPS). Am J Cardiol 1990; 66:59–62.
31. Malzberg B. Mortality among patients with involution melancholia. Am J Psychiatry 1937; 93:1231–1238.
32. Black DW, Warrack G, Winokur G. The Iowa record-linkage study: III. Excess mortality among patients with "functional" disorders. Arch Gen Psychiatry 1985; 42:82–88.
33. Weeke A, Vaeth M. Excess mortality of bipolar and unipolar manic-depressive patients. J Affect Disord 1986; 11:227–234.
34. Murphy JM, Monson RR, Olivier DC, Sobol AM, Leighton AH. Affective disorders and mortality. A general population study. Arch Gen Psychiatry 1987; 44:473–480.
35. Rabins PV, Harvis K, Koven S. High fatality rates of late-life depression associated with cardiovascular disease. J Affect Disord 1985; 9:165–167.
36. Avery D, Winokur G. Mortality in depressed patients treated with electroconvulsive therapy and antidepressants. Arch Gen Psychiatry 1976; 33:1029–1037.
37. Carney RM, Rich MW, Tevelde A, Saini J, Clark K, Freedland KE. The relationship between heart rate, heart rate variability and depression in patients with coronary artery disease. J Psychosom Res 1988; 32:159–164.
38. Yeragani VK, Pohl RB, Balon R, et al. Heart rate variability in patients with major depression. Psychiatry Res 1991; 37:35–46.
39. Roose SP, Dalack GW. Treating the depressed patient with cardiovascular problems. J Clin Psychiatry 1992; 53(suppl):25–31.

40. Kleiger RE, Miller JP, Bigger JT, Moss AJ, the Multicenter Post-Infarction Research Group. Decreased heart rate variability and its association with increased mortality after acute myocardial infarction. Am J Cardiol 1987; 59:256–262.
41. Roose SP, Dalack GW, Woodring S. Death, depression, and heart disease. J Clin Psychiatry Supp 1991; 52:34–39.
42. Biederman J. Sudden death in children treated with a tricyclic antidepressant. J Am Acad Child Adolesc Psychiatry 1991; 30:495–498.
43. Walsh BT, Giardina EGV, Sloan RP, Greenhill L, Goldfein J. Effects of desipramine on autonomic control of the heart. J Am Acad Child Adolesc Psychiatry 1994; 33:191–197.
44. Carney RM, Freedland KE, Rich MW, Smith LJ, Jaffe AS. Ventricular tachycardia and psychiatric depression in patients with coronary artery disease. Am J Med 1993; 95:23–28.
45. Frasure-Smith N, Lesperance F, Talajic M. Depression and 18-month prognosis following myocardial infarction. Circulation 1995; 91:999–1005.
46. Frasure-Smith N, Lesperance F, Talajic M. The impact of negative emotions on prognosis following myocardial infarction: Is it more than depression? Heath Psychol 1995; 14:388–398.
47. Moser DK, Dracup K. Is anxiety early after myocardial infarction associated with subsequent ischemic and arrhythmic events? Psychosom Med 1996; 58:395–401.
48. Orth-Gomer K, Edwards M-E, Erhardt LR, Sjogren A, Theorell T. Relation between arrhythmic sensations, cardiac arrhythmias and psychological profile. Acta Med Scand 1981; 210:201–205.
49. Lochen M-L. The Tromso Study: associations between self-reported arrhythmia, psychological conditions and lifestyle. Scand J Prim Health Care 1991; 9:265–270.
50. Lochen M-L, Rasmussen K. Palpitations and lifestyle: impact of depression and self-rated health: the Nordland Health Study. Scand J Soc Med 1996; 24:140–144.
51. Mayou R, Bryant B, Forfar C, Clark D. Non-cardiac chest pain and benign palpitations in the cardiac clinic. Br Heart J 1994; 72:548–553.
52. Weber BE, Kapor WN. Evaluation and Outcomes of Patients with Palpitations. Am J Med 1996; 100:138–148.
53. Barsky AJ, Cleary PD, Brener J, Ruskin JN. The perception of cardiac activity in medical outpatients. Cardiology 1993; 83:304–315.
54. Barsky AJ, Cleary PD, K. SM, Ruskin JN. Panic disorder, palpitations, and the awareness of cardiac activity. J Nerv Ment Dis 1994; 182:63–71.
55. Barsky AJ, Delamater BA, Clancy SA, Antman EM, Ahern DK. Somatized psychiatric disorder presenting as palpitations. Arch Intern Med 1996; 156:1102–1108.
56. Katon W. Panic disorder: relationship to high medical utilization, unexplained physical symptoms, and medical costs. J Clin Psychiatry 1996; 57(suppl 10):11–18.
57. Katon W. Panic disorder and somatization. Am J Med 1984; 77:101–106.
58. Katon W, Von Korff M, Lin E, Lipscomb P, Russo J, Wagner E, Polk E. Distressed high utilizers of medical care: DSM-III-R diagnoses and treatment needs. Gen Hosp Psychiatry 1990; 12:355–362.
59. Katon WJ, Von Korff M, Lin E. Panic disorder: relationship to high medical utilization. Am J Med 1992; 92 (suppl 1A):7S–11S.
60. Fricchione GL, Vlay SC. Psychiatric aspects of patients with malignant ventricular arrhythmias. Am J Psychiatry 1986; 143:1518–1526.

61. Baker B, Dorian P, Woloshyn N, Kazarian S, Lanphier C. Psychiatric treatment strategies for patients at risk of dying suddenly. Psychother Psychosom 1991; 56:242–246.

62. Druss RG, Kornfeld DS. Survivors of cardiac arrest. JAMA 1967; 201:75–80.

63. Fricchione GL, Vlay LC, Vlay SC. Cardiac psychiatry and the managment of malignant ventricular arrhythmias with the internal cardioverter-defibrillator. Am Heart J 1994; 128: 1050–1059.

64. Fricchione GL, Olson LC, Vlay SC. Psychiatric syndromes in patients with the automatic internal cardioverter defibrillator: anxiety, psychological dependence, abuse, and withdrawal. Am Heart J 1989; 117:1411–1414.

65. Kolar JA, Dracup K. Psychosocial adjustment of patients with ventricular dysrhythmias. J Cardiovasc Nurs 1990; 4:44–55.

66. Roine RO, Dajaste S, Kaste M. Neuropsychological sequelae of cardiac arrest. JAMA 1993; 269:237–242.

67. Arteaga WJ, Windle JR. The quality of life of patients with life-threatening arrhythmias. Arch Intern Med 1995; 155:2086–2091.

68. Keren R, Aarons D, Veltri EP. Anxiety and depression in patients with life-threatening ventricular arrrhythmias: impact of the implantable cardioverter-defibrillator. PACE 1991; 14:181–187.

69. Morris PL, Badger J, Chmielewski C, Berger E, Goldberg RJ. Psychiatric morbidity following implantation of the automatic implantable cardioverter defibrillator. Psychosomatics 1991; 32:58–64.

70. Heller SS, Ormont MA, Lidagoster LC, Sciacca RR, Steinberg JS. Psychosocial outcome after ICD implantation: a current perspective. PACE 1998; 21:1207–1215.

71. Teplitz L, Egenes KJ, Brask L. Life after sudden death: The development of a support group for automatic implantable cardioverter-defibrillator patients. J Cardiovasc Nurs 1990; 4: 20–32.

72. Echt DS, Liebson PR, Mitchelle LB, Peters RW, Obias-Manno D, Barker AH, Arensberg D, Baker A, Friedman L, Greene L, Huther ML, Richardson DW. Mortality and morbidity in patients receiving encainide, flecainide or placebo. N Engl J Med 1991; 324:781–788.

73. CAST II Investigators. Effect of the antiarrhythmic agent moricizine on survival after myocardial infarction. N Engl J Med 1992; 327:227–233.

74. Epstein AE, Hallstrom AP, Rogers WJ, Leibson PR, Seals AA, Anderson JL, Cohen JD, Capone RJ, Wyse DG. Mortality following ventricular arrhythmia suppression by encainide, flecainide, and moricizine after myocardial infraction. JAMA 1993; 270:2451–2456.

75. Lynch JJ, Dicarlo LA, Montgomery DG, Lucchesi BR. Effects of flecainide acetate on ventricular tachyarrhythmia and fibrillation in dogs with recent myocardial infarction. Pharmacology 1987; 35:181–193.

76. Glassman AH, Roose SP, Bigger JT Jr. The safety of tricyclic antidepressants in cardiac patients. Risk-benefit reconsidered. JAMA 1993; 269:2673–2675.

77. Riddle MA, Nelson C, Kleinman CS, Rasmusson A, Leckman JF, King RA, Cohen DJ. Sudden death in children receiving norpramin: a review of three reported cases and commentary. J Am Acad Child Adolesc Psychiatry 1991; 30:104–108.

78. McClellan J. Case study: two additional sudden deaths with tricyclic antidepressants. J Am Acad Child Adolesc Psychiatry 1997; 36:390–394.

79. Johnson A, Giuffre RM, O'Malley K. ECG changes in pediatric patients on tricyclic antidepressants, desipramine, and imipramine. Can J Psychiatry 1996; 41:102–106.

80. Leonard HL, Meyer MC, Swedo SE, Richter D, Hamburger SD, Allen AJ, Rapoport JL,

Tucker E. Electrocardiographic changes during desipramine and clomipramine treatment in children and adolescents. J Am Acad Child Adolesc Psychiatry 1995; 34:1460–1468.

81. Flood JG. Electrocardiographic effects of desipramine and 2-hydroxydesipramine in children, adolescents, and adults treated with desipramine. J Am Acad Child Adolesc Psychiatry 1993; 32:798–804.

82. Alderton HR. Tricyclic medication in children and the QT interval: case report and discussion. Can J Psychiatry 1995; 40:325–329.

83. Shapiro PA, Lespérance F, Frasure-Smith N, O'Connor C, Jiang JW, Baker B, Dorian P, Harrison W, Glassman AH. An open label preliminary trial of sertraline treatment of major depression after acute myocardial infarction (the "SADHAT" study). Am Heart J. In press.

84. Roose SP, Glassman AH, Attia E, Woodring S et al. Cardiovascular effects of fluoxetine in depressed patients with heart disease. Am J Psychiatry 1998; 155:660–665.

85. Roose SP, Laghrissi-Thode F, Kennedy JS. Comparison of paroxetine and nortriptyline in depressed patients with ischemic heart disease. JAMA 1998; 279:287–291.

86. Feder R. Bradycardia and syncope induced by fluoxetine. J Clin Psychiatry 1991; 52:138–139.

87. Ellison JM, Milofsky JE, Ely E. Fluoxetine induced bradycardia and syncope in two patients. J Clin Psychiatry 1990; 51:385–386.

88. Walley T, Pirmohamed M, Proudlove C, Maxwell D. Interaction of metoprolol and fluoxetine. Lancet 1993; 341:967–968.

6

Noncardiac Chest Pain

Richard P. Fleet
Montreal Heart Institute
Montreal, Quebec, Canada

Bernard D. Beitman
University of Missouri–Columbia
Columbia, Missouri

Peter is a 43-year-old assistant accountant who presented to the emergency department with a chief complaint of chest pain. His pain was substernal yet unrelated to effort and was not quickly relieved with rest. Peter's first "recent" episode of chest pain occurred at work, "out of the blue" while in his weekly meeting 6 months prior to his emergency visit. The chest pain was accompanied by palpitations, sweating, hyperventilation, dizziness, and fear of losing control and dying. The episode had a rapid onset (within 1–4 minutes to reach its full intensity) and was partially relieved approximately 10 minutes after Peter rushed out of the meeting and relaxed in the men's room. Since this first recent episode, Peter reported at least two to five daily episodes of similar symptoms. Medical history was negative for coronary artery disease. A series of cardiac tests, conducted 5 years previous to his visit, did not show any significant stenosis or electrical abnormalities. Peter's chest pain at the time had essentially resolved after the finalization of his divorce. In the emergency department, the EKG revealed nonspecific abnormalities. A stress EKG conducted the next day was clinically positive but electrically normal. Because of the patient's family history of coronary artery disease (father had died at age 69 of sudden cardiac death), an angiogram was ordered. The results were normal indicating less than 35% stenosis in the major coronary arteries. The patient was referred to a gastroenterologist, who conducted esophageal motility studies, acid perfusion tests, as well as a 24-hour pH monitoring. Results were normal. The patient was then referred to psychosomatics and received a diagnosis of panic disorder with mild agoraphobia. Both pharmacological and cognitive-behavioral treatment were provided. Peter was free of chest pain and related symptoms after 3 months of weekly psychotherapy.

Pharmacotherapy consisted of paroxetine 10 mg daily for 1 week. The dose was increased to 20 mg for the 2 following weeks and increased to 30 mg, and the medication remained at that level thereafter for 4 months. The medication was progressively tapered off over a 2-month period of weekly visits.

INTRODUCTION

The above case history describes the complex, highly prevalent clinical problem of noncardiac chest pain. Few medical complaints involve as many medical specialties as noncardiac chest pain. Primary care physicians, specialists in emergency medicine, cardiology, cardiac surgery, gastroenterology, and internal medicine, and psychiatrists are all consulted by patients with chest pain eventually found to be noncardiac. In this chapter, we will review the literature on the subject of noncardiac chest pain. The medical and psychosocial costs of this syndrome will be examined. Special emphasis will be placed on psychiatric disorders, primarily panic disorder (PD), the most psychiatric common condition in noncardiac chest pain patients. We will review studies that examined the prevalence and characteristics of patients with noncardiac chest pain with psychiatric disorders. We will also discuss the problematic issue of the low rates of physician recognition of PD in these patients and its related consequences. We will briefly describe detection instruments that have been developed to improve physician recognition of this disorder. Finally, we will review recent literature on the management of the noncardiac chest pain patient.

Noncardiac Chest Pain: A Disabling and Costly Syndrome

Chest pain, a cardinal feature of a potentially lethal coronary artery disease (CAD), is a symptom that commands attention from both the patient and physician. However, in more than 50% of patients consulting for chest pain, the pain does not have a clear cardiac cause (1–3). More than 500,000 angiograms are performed yearly in the United States; of these, 10–30% are normal. Since the cost of an angiogram is over $2,000, it can be estimated that more than $10,000,000 is spent annually to exclude a CAD (4). Follow-up research of patients with normal angiograms suggests that despite an excellent survival prognosis, as many as 70% of patients continue to complain of chest pain, report significant psychosocial disability, and repeatedly consult medical services for their symptoms (5,6). A decade ago, the costs to manage noncardiac chest pain were approximately $4,000 per year per patient. This estimate included an average of 1.2 prescriptions per month, 2.2 emergency room or physician visits per year, and one hospitalization per year for further evaluation of the pain (7). Thus, noncardiac chest pain is a common and costly phenomenon in medicine.

A Definition of Noncardiac Chest Pain

Noncardiac chest pain is defined as chest pain with normal cardiac findings. The definitive test of normal coronary status is the angiogram. Angiographic tests are generally interpreted as normal when there is less than 50% stenosis in one of the major coronary arteries. Because the angiogram is an invasive and costly procedure, it is not conducted on all patients. Less invasive tests, such as resting and exercise EKGs as well as blood enzymes and nuclear medicine myocardial perfusion studies, are used along with the clinical examination to establish the probability of CAD for most patients. Hence, although the definitive diagnosis of noncardiac chest pain is made through angiographic testing, many patients receive diagnoses of probable noncardiac chest pain based on noninvasive tests. Moreover, some patients who have a history of CAD can also have noncardiac chest pain. These patients may have suffered a myocardial infarction or may have undergone coronary bypass surgery or angioplasty, and despite optimal cardiac therapy their pain remains unexplained by their current cardiac status. Noncardiac chest pain in CAD patients remains understudied regardless of the fact that it is a also a major clinical problem. In this chapter we will focus on noncardiac chest pain in patients with and without a history of CAD who are diagnosed using both invasive angiography as well as the less invasive tests described above.

Physical Causes of Noncardiac Chest Pain

Chronic noncardiac chest pain can be caused by several other physical abnormalities. The most commonly reported physical causes are esophageal motility disorders, gastroesophageal reflux disease, mitral valve prolapse, microvascular angina, and abnormal visceral nociception. A multidisciplinary review of the subject concluded that although several individual or combined physical abnormalities can be found in noncardiac patients, the majority of patients do not have a distinct physical cause for their pain (8). Moreover, even when a physical disorder is found, treatment for a subgroup of chest pain patients is suboptimal. Finally, psychiatric disorders are common in a significant proportion of patients with any of the above-mentioned medical conditions (9–11). Yet, it is unclear if psychiatric disorders cause, result from, or simply parallel these conditions.

PSYCHOLOGICAL CORRELATES OF NONCARDIAC CHEST PAIN

History

Psychological factors have been suspected as a cause for chest pain for over a century (12). During the nineteenth century, there were several reports of a pain syndrome different from Heberden's angina pectoris, described in 1772 (13). This novel pain syndrome, described by Da Costa in 1871 (14), was particularly common in soldiers of the American Civil War. Although unsure of the causes of this pain, DaCosta suggested that it was due to a disordered innervation, and, with a few exceptions, his patients were "functional." In 1892, Osler (15) also acknowledged the difficulty of differentiating pain caused by a cardiac condition from that attributable to noncardiac factors. He described two distinct categories of chest pain: true angina and pseudoangina. In the latter category he found that the patient population was comprised mainly of women in whom pain was characteristically periodic, nocturnal, and accompanied by nervous symptoms and vasomotor disturbances. He stated that treatment must be directed to the general nervous condition. With time, DaCosta's pain syndrome was increasingly documented in the civilian population. In 1941, Wood (16) compared patients with heart disease to normal controls and concluded that a proper psychiatric diagnosis was almost always available. He believed that the cause of the pain was usually psychological, due to "misinterpretation of emotional symptoms, certain vicious circular patterns, the growth of a conviction that the heart is to blame, consequent fears of sudden death on exertion, conditioning, and hysteria." Today, various labels, partially based on the above evidence, are still used to describe pain of noncardiac origin including neurocirculatory asthenia, DaCosta's syndrome, irritable heart syndrome, and soldier's heart.

Recent studies of the specific psychological aspects of noncardiac chest pain appeared much later in the literature. They first used self-report measures to examine psychological distress. Elias et al. (17) found an inverse correlation between the degree of coronary stenosis and measures of neuroticism (anxiety, depression, and somatic complaints) in 136 men and women awaiting arteriography. Similarly, Channer et al. (18) found that a significant number of chest pain patients with notable levels of depression and anxiety had negative exercise stress tests.

These psychological and somatic differences between cardiac and noncardiac patients led investigators to suspect specific psychiatric disorders in these patients. In fact, Sheehan (19) indicated that the symptomatology of the "diseases of yesteryear" (DaCosta's pain syndrome, etc.) are embodied in the DSM III criteria of PD. Hence because of the similarity with the symptoms of PD, investigators examined in the most recent studies the prevalence of PD in noncardiac chest pain patients.

Panic Disorder Prevalence in Noncardiac Chest Pain Patients

We are aware of seven original published PD prevalence studies in patients with primarily noncardiac chest pain that used structured interview protocols (standard criterion for psychiatric diagnoses). Katon et al. (20) examined the prevalence of PD in 74 consecutive patients with chest pain without a previous CAD who were referred for coronary arteriography. Of patients with normal angiograms, 43% (12/28) met DSM III criteria for PD, compared with 6.5% (3/46) of patients with positive coronary arteriographies. Beitman et al. (21), in a larger sample of patients with normal angiograms, reported a PD prevalence of 34% (32/94).

Because patients with PD tended to present with atypical or nonanginal chest pains, Beitman et al. (22) examined the prevalence of PD in these patients. They found that 59 of 103 (57%) cardiology outpatients with atypical chest pain met DSM III-R criteria for PD. In a similar study conducted in an emergency department, Wulsin et al. (23) found that 11 of 35 (31%) consenting patients with atypical chest pain met DSM III-R criteria for PD.

Carter et al. (24) hypothesized that many chest pain patients admitted to the coronary care unit (CCU) for suspected myocardial infarction may suffer from PD and estimated its prevalence in this setting. They found that one third of 62 consecutive patients met criteria for PD. Seventy-nine percent of patients did not have clear evidence of CAD. Carter et al. (25) recently examined the prevalence of PD in consecutive referrals of patients with chest pain without previous evidence of CAD to a nuclear medicine department for cardiac stress scintigraphy. Fifty patients (82%) participated; 28 patients (56%) met DSM III-R criteria for PD. Of the patients with PD, one had a positive stress scintigram.

The studies described above presented certain methodological problems that complicated interpretation. First, all studies had small samples (between 35 and 104 patients). Second, two of these reports (22,23) had low subject participation rates (up to 70% refusal), contributing to possible selection bias. Finally, in half of these studies, psychiatric interviewers were not blinded to the patients' medical diagnoses (21–23), and investigators failed to report interrater reliability ratings in this same proportion of studies (23–25).

Attempting to improve upon the methodological aspects of these pioneering studies, researchers from the Montreal Heart Institute examined the prevalence of PD in a sample of 441 consecutive walk-in patients of the emergency department for a chief complaint of chest pain (26). Approximately 25% (108/441) met DSM III-R criteria for PD (with or without agoraphobia). Although 44% of the patients with PD had a documented history of CAD, 80% had atypical or nonanginal chest pain and 75% were discharged from the hospital with a final diagnosis of noncardiac chest pain. This study strengthens the findings of previous research suggesting a high prevalence of PD in chest pain patients, as in addition to its large sample of consecutive patients with a high participation rate (84%), interviewers were blinded to the patients' medical diagnoses as well as to the study's specific hypotheses. Moreover, interrater agreement on the PD diagnoses was high (Kappa = 0.81). Finally, physicians were also unaware of the psychiatric diagnoses limiting experimenter expectancy effects.

In summary, between 25 and 57% of noncardiac or atypical chest pain patients in various cardiology settings and emergency departments of North America suffer from PD (see Table 1). Despite the limitations of these studies, results suggest that a broad range of physicians who treat chest pain are likely to be confronted with PD. Of particular interest is that the prevalence of PD in chest pain patients is far in excess of the 1–4% rates reported in the general population. The clinical characteristics of PD in chest pain patients will now be described.

Table 1 Panic Disorder Prevalence Studies Using Structured Interview Protocols in Noncardiac/Atypical Chest Pain Patients

Year	Investigators (Ref.)	Patients	Sample size	Panic disorder prevalence
1988	Katon et al. (20)	Referred for angiographic testing with no previous history of CAD	74	15/74 (20%) in total sample 3/46 (6.5%) in CAD+ patients 12/28 (43%) in CAD− patients
1989	Beitman et al. (21)	With normal angiograms (CAD−)	94	32/94 (34%)
1987	Beitman et al. (22)	With atypical or nonanginal chest pain referrred to study by cardiologists	103	59/103 (57%)
1991	Wulsin (23)	With atypical chest pain consulting the ED	35	11/35 (31%)
1992	Carter et al. (24)	Consecutive admissions to the coronary care unit	62	19/62 (31%)
1994	Carter et al. (25)	Consecutive referrals for cardiac stress scintigraphy with no previous history of CAD	50	28/50 (56%)
1996	Fleet et al. (26)	Consecutive patients consulting an ED of a cardiology hospital with chief complaint of chest pain	441	108/441 (24.5%)

ED = Emergency department.

Characteristics of Noncardiac Chest Pain Patients with Panic Disorder

Patients with noncardiac or atypical chest pain with PD range in age from 45 to 54 years (20–26). Although they tend to consist of proportionately more women across most studies, this difference was not significant where analyzed. Finally, there is generally no difference in marital or socioeconomic status between patients with or without PD.

The fact that patients with PD presenting for chest pain are over 40 years of age is of interest. This finding contrasts with those of psychiatric settings where patients are generally younger, ranging from their early twenties to the late thirties. Since PD patients in psychiatric settings usually report onset of their disorder in their early twenties, Beitman et al. (27) conducted a more detailed analysis of age and onset of PD in noncardiac chest pain patients to further understand this peculiarity. They concluded that PD may have an older age of onset in these patients. This finding probably reflects the normal distribution of the disorder, with older patients more likely to consider heart disease as the cause.

Levels of Self-Reported Psychological Distress

Patients with noncardiac chest pain and PD have higher levels of psychological distress than noncardiac patients without PD. Although the studies reporting these results have used different self-report instruments, which somewhat complicates cross-study comparisons, this finding is consistent and suggests higher and possibly clinically significant levels of distress in patients meeting interview criteria for PD (26). Specifically, patients with PD report higher scores on measures of general anxiety, somatization, fear of bodily sensations, and agoraphobic avoidance as well as depression compared to noncardiac chest pain patients without PD (21,24,26). Moreover, the levels of psychological distress are not explained by the cardiac status of the patient (24,26).

The most prevalent psychiatric diagnosis in noncardiac chest pain patients across studies is PD. Yet, because PD often co-occurs with other axis I disorders, a few studies have examined co-morbidity. Beitman et al. (28) examined co-morbidity with current major depression and reported that 9 of 43 patients (21%) with PD had major depression. Carter et al. (24), in their CCU study, found that 68% (13/19) of noncardiac patients with PD had agoraphobia and 32% (6/19) major depression. Fleet et al. (26) found in their emergency patients a slightly lower prevalence of these disorders in PD patients, with 11% (12/108) meeting criteria for major depression and 14.8% agoraphobia (16/108). However, this study found high rates of co-morbidity with generalized anxiety disorder (33%, 36/108) and dysthymia (13%, 14/108). This study also found that these co-morbid psychiatric disorders were significantly more common in patients with PD than those without this diagnosis. These findings are consistent with data from mental health settings, suggesting that 50% or more of patients with an anxiety disorder have additional disorders (29).

Suicidal Ideation

Suicidal ideation in patients with PD is an important yet controversial issue. Fleet et al. (26) reported that 25% of chest pain patients with PD had thoughts of killing themselves in the week previous to their emergency department visit compared to 5% of patients without PD. In a series of logistic regression analyses, adjusting for demographic, medical, and psychiatric co-morbidity, PD was found to be an independent risk factor for suicidal ideation in these primarily noncardiac chest pain patients presenting to the emergency department (30).

Although the above study (26,30) was the first to examine suicidal ideation in chest pain patients, its results were consistent with Weissman et al.'s (31) controversial study suggesting that PD was a significant risk factor for suicidal ideation and attempt. Investigators reported that patients with a lifetime diagnosis of PD were at twice the risk of ever having thoughts of killing themselves or attempting suicide compared to patients with other psychiatric disorders. These findings were not replicated in at least two reports (32,33) from psychiatric settings, which found that suicidal ideation and attempts are relatively uncommon in PD outpatients without a mood or a borderline personality disorder.

The differences in the findings may be attributed to the different methods used to assess suicidal ideation as well as to the differences between psychiatric and medical/community patients with PD. For example, psychiatric setting patients, at the time at which their suicidal ideation is assessed, may be less distressed because they have knowledge of their disorder and have been promised a proven-effective treatment. In contrast, medical and community patients may not know they have PD and therefore ignore the possibility that effective therapy exists.

Nonfear Panic Disorder

Researchers have found that a subgroup of noncardiac chest pain patients with PD have nonfear PD. A person can meet DSM III-R (and DSM IV) criteria for PD when suffering from panic attacks without reporting fear. The contemporary concept of nonfear PD arose from Beitman et al.'s (34) observations of atypical/noncardiac chest pain patients. In these studies, nonfear PD was defined in the following way: it meets DSM III-R criteria for PD, except that attacks involve discrete periods of intense discomfort without fear and the last bad attack did not include symptoms that involve a subjective element of fear (i.e., fear of dying, going crazy, or losing control).

Using these criteria Beitman et al. (34) found that of the 104 patients interviewed, of which 38 met criteria for current PD, 12 patients (31.6%) also met criteria for nonfear PD. Carter reported an identical proportion of CCU patients with nonfear PD (6 of 19 patients; 31.6%) (24).

These research teams (24,34) have compared these two types of PD patients in the areas of demographic, psychological, family history of PD as well as on responses to biological panic challenges. Nonfear PD patients were not different from PD patients in terms of age, gender, marital status, or social class. Moreover, the panic subtypes do not differ in terms of age of onset of the disorder, duration of PD, or number of attacks during the week preceding the interview. Nor do these groups differ on self-reported measures of depression, anxiety, or agoraphobic symptoms. Furthermore, both fear and nonfear PD patients report a family history of PD in 17% of their first-degree relatives. Finally, nonfear PD patients experience attacks when infused with sodium lactate and exhibit marked improvement when treated with antipanic medication (34).

The concept of nonfear PD is important for several reasons. First, it is a common subtype of PD in cardiology settings that must be recognized because of its similarities with fear PD. Second, nonfear PD may be one of the reasons why this disorder often goes unrecognized in medicine, and consequently it may hint to the fact that epidemiologic studies not using this criterion may underestimate the prevalence of PD.

Panic as a Risk Factor for Cardiovascular Mortality

Although most studies of PD have focused on noncardiac patients, there is a growing body of evidence suggesting that panic or phobic anxiety is associated with higher than expected risk of cardiovascular mortality. In two retrospective follow-up reports of psychiatric in- and outpatients, Coryell et al. (35,36) found that men with probable PD were at twice the risk of mortality from cardiovascular causes relative to age-, period- and sex-specific vital statistics. Results of these retrospective reports were supported by the findings of three prospective studies (37–39), which found that patients with high levels of self-reported phobic anxiety were at two to three times higher risk of cardiovascular death, particularly sudden death, relative to patients with initially low levels of anxiety.

These studies point to the intriguing link between panic-like anxiety and cardiovascular death in noncardiac patients, yet certain methodological limitations must lead us to cautiously interpret the findings. Although most investigators suggest that PD is the psychiatric condition that confers the higher risk of cardiovascular death, no study has specifically examined this association using both structured diagnostic interviews and thorough medical evaluations in prospective designs. Moreover, clinical relevance of the findings is unclear, because cardiovascular death in panic-like patients occurred late in the lives of the participants and at a relatively low base rate. Finally, the association was exclusively studied in men, whereas PD is two to four times more common in women.

These results are nevertheless interesting in light of recent research suggesting that laboratory-induced mental stress in CAD patients causes ischemia (40). It is thus possible that a subgroup of CAD patients with PD and atypical/noncardiac chest pain can have ischemia-related panic attacks. Although per-panic ischemia in PD patients without CAD has not been found (41), it remains unstudied in patients with both CAD and PD. Future research should study the possibility of per-panic attack ischemia in CAD patients with noncardiac chest pain.

Low Rates of Physician Recognition of PD

The fact that some chest pain patients with PD undergo expensive and extensive cardio-logic tests suggests that this disorder is not suspected as a cause for chest pain. The largest panic prevalence study to date that also examined physician recognition uncovered that 98% of the 108 patients found to meet DSM III-R criteria for PD were not specifically recognized by physicians as having this specific disabling disorder (26). Of particular interest in this study is that it included all of the physicians ($n = 28$) (cardiologists) that cover the hospital's emergency department on rotating schedules.

Since a label of noncardiac chest pain is often insufficient to reassure the patient with PD, efforts to improve physician recognition of this disorder are important. Without a specific explanation or treatment, the patient may suffer chronically. A 3- to 4-year follow-up of patients with normal coronary arteries showed that those with PD report more continuing chest pain, worsening of health, greater reduction in exertional capacity, poorer social adjustment, more anxiety symptoms, and more psychological distress than do those without PD (42). This finding, in the context that treatments are effective for psychiatric patients, supports the need to detect and treat these patients. Furthermore, early recognition of PD, especially in emergency settings, may help prevent suicidal behavior.

Detection Instruments to Improve Physician Recognition of PD

Because of the low rates of physician recognition and the availability of proven effective treatments, there has been a pressing need for detection instruments. Fleet et al. (43) developed and validated a model to improve the probability of recognizing PD in chest pain patients. Through logistic regression analysis, demographic, self-report psychological, and pain variables were explored as factors predictive of the presence of PD in 180 consecutive emergency department chest pain patients. The detection model was then prospectively validated in a sample of 212 patients recruited following the same procedure. Panic-agoraphobia (Agoraphobia Cognitions Questionnaire, Mobility Inventory for Agoraphobia), chest pain quality (Short Form McGill Pain Questionnaire), pain loci, and gender variables best predicted the presence of PD. The variables correctly classified 84% of chest pain patients in panic and nonpanic disorder categories. The model displayed a sensitivity of 59%; specificity: 93%; positive predictive power: 75%; negative predictive power: 87% at a PD prevalence of 26%. The model correctly classified 73% of the patients in the validation phase. The model takes approximately 10 minutes for the patient to complete and a physician or nurse to score (total time). Combined with clinical judgment, including results of medical testing and perceived severity of the panic syndrome, physicians can make decisions about patient management.

Although not specifically developed and validated in a sample of chest pain patients, the PRIME-MD (44) may also be helpful in improving physician recognition of PD. It also has the advantage of being designed to detect other common psychiatric disorders in medical patients, such as depression, general anxiety, etc. One possible problem with the PRIME-MD with respect to its ability to detect PD in chest pain patients is that the trigger question for panic—Have you had an anxiety attack (suddenly feeling fear or panic)?—may not detect the significant proportion of nonfear PD chest pain patients. Both the PRIME-MD and the Montreal Heart Panic Model should be compared in future research. Meanwhile we recommend that either instrument be used to improve the actually low rates of physician recognition in chest pain patients.

Treatments

Proven effective treatments exist for patients with PD seen in psychiatric settings. These treatments are thus potentially applicable to a significant subgroup of noncardiac chest pain patients with this disorder. Psychopharmacotherapy and cognitive-behavioral interventions bring relief fairly quickly to 70–90% of patients with PD (with or without agoraphobia). The most widely studied medications are tricyclic antidepressants (TCAs), monoamine oxidase inhibitors (MAOs) and benzodiazepine. Recently, selective serotonin-reuptake inhibitors (SSRIs) have been shown to be effective antipanic agents, and paroxetine has an FDA indication for PD (45).

A recent meta-analysis of treatments for PD (with and without agoraphobia) suggested that antidepressants were the most effective psychotrope (46). However, the side effects of TCAs—amphetamine-like stimulation in early stages of treatment and weight gain in prolonged therapy—are common reasons for treatment discontinuation. Nighttime insomnia and daytime lethargy, along with dietary restrictions, have led to possible underuse of MAOs. The more favorable side effect profile of SSRIs has made them a potential first-line pharmacologic treatment, especially for older patients at risk of cardiovascular complications. However, the antipanic action of most antidepressants takes approximately 1 month.

In contrast, benzodiazepines provide almost immediate relief for patients with PD. However, their potential for abuse and dependence does not make them the treatment of choice for long-term management of the panic patient. In order to minimize the risk of addiction, some clinicians suggest adding an antidepressant to the drug regimen several weeks after the initial symptoms have resolved with benzodiazepine treatment and then slowly tapering the benzodiazepine dose.

Cognitive-behavioral interventions are also proven effective treatments for PD, either used alone or in combination with medication. The cognitive-behavioral techniques used for PD include the following: cognitive reinterpretation of catastrophically misinterpreted bodily sensations, thought stopping, applied and deep muscle relaxation, breathing retraining, as well as exposure to panic-provoking cues. Margraf et al. (47) reviewed the most methodologically robust cognitive-behavioral panic treatment research. They concluded that approximately 80% of patients receiving this type of intervention achieved panic-free status as well as strong and clinically significant improvement in general anxiety, panic-related cognitions, depression, and phobic avoidance. Furthermore, the gains were maintained at a 2-year follow-up.

Although effective treatments exist for patients with PD in psychiatric settings, have these above-described treatments been specifically tested on noncardiac chest pain patients? We are aware of three published treatment studies for patients with atypical/noncardiac chest pain that used effective interventions for PD patients. Beitman et al. (48) reported that in a nonblind, 8-week trial of alprazolam in patients presenting with chest pain and PD, 15 of 20 patients met the single criterion for improvement: a 50% or greater reduction in panic frequency. Moreover, patients showed significant reductions in scores on physician-rated measures of anxiety (Hamilton Anxiety scale), depression (Hamilton Depression scale), and global functioning (Physician's Global Impression scale). Patients rated themselves as significantly improved in their work and social functioning. Finally, these patients reported a marginally significant drop in episodes of chest pain or discomfort. However, as suggested by the authors of this study, results must be interpreted cautiously because the trial was not placebo controlled and was conducted by a research group invested in a positive outcome. Beitman recommended that future investigations be double-blind, placebo-controlled using other effective antipanic medications.

Recently, Cannon et al. (49) conducted a randomized, double-blind, placebo-controlled 3-week trial comparing the efficacy of clonidine to imipramine and placebo for chest pain patients despite normal angiograms. Sixty patients participated in the study, with 20 in each treatment condition. During the treatment phase, the imipramine group had a mean (SD) reduction of 52% (25) in episodes of chest pain, the clonidine group had a reduction of 39% (51), and the placebo group a reduction of 1% (86), all compared with the initial placebo phase of the trial. The only statistically significant improvement was with imipramine ($p = 0.03$). The response to imipramine did not depend on the results of cardiac, esophageal, or psychiatric testing at baseline or on the change in the psychiatric profile during the course of the study, which was found to improve in all conditions. The authors concluded that imipramine improved chest pain possibly through visceral analgesic effects.

To our knowledge, Pearce et al. (50) are the only investigators to date to have examined the effectiveness of cognitive-behavioral interventions for atypical chest pain patients. Thirty-five patients were randomized to either the cognitive-behavior therapy treatment condition or to an assessment-only control group. Patients in the treatment group received 3–11 sessions of cognitive-behavior therapy, which included information, cognitive restructuring techniques aimed at teaching the patient more realistic appraisals of his or her symptomatology, breathing retraining, as well as deep muscle relaxation.

Patients in the treatment group had a significantly better outcome than the control, assessment-only group on measures of chest pain, limitation of daily activity, and use of medication. The control group in this study remained unimproved and was offered the experimental treatment. Furthermore, 35% ($n = 11$) of all patients were pain-free, and improvements were maintained at 3-month follow-up.

In summary, proven-effective treatments for PD patients seen in psychiatric settings exist, and preliminary research suggests that they may be effective for noncardiac chest pain patients. The three studies reviewed above show that two proven-effective medications for PD as well as one cognitive-behavioral treatment support this notion. Of interest is that with the exception of Beitman et al.'s (48) study with alprazolam, which consisted of PD patients only, the two other studies of noncardiac/atypical chest pain patients included patients without PD, who either had other psychiatric disorders or no psychological distress that met DSM III-R criteria for diagnoses searched (49,50). It should be mentioned that in Cannon et al.'s (49) study over 40% had PD and in Pearce et al.'s (50) study 27% had this disorder. These studies therefore suggest that these treatments are effective for patients with atypical chest pain with and without PD. The mechanisms are yet unclear. TCAs may act as analgesics in these patients, and cognitive-behavioral interventions may be effective for a wide range of psychiatric and nonpsychiatric pain syndromes.

SUMMARY

Noncardiac chest pain is a major public health issue. Although several physical disorders can explain the symptoms of several patients, many have no clear physical cause that accounts for the chest pain. Recent research suggests that roughly 30% of noncardiac or atypical chest pain patients suffer from PD. PD appears to be the most common psychiatric disorder in these patients. Patients with PD tend to be older than those seen in psychiatric settings, and at least 30% of these patients have nonfear PD. Noncardiac chest pain patients with PD tend to present more psychological distress than chest pain patients without PD and may be at risk for suicidal behavior. Moreover, patients with noncardiac chest pain are more likely to suffer from co-morbid psychiatric disorders including depression, general anxiety disorder, dysthymia, and agoraphobia than noncardiac patients without PD. Patients with PD are also more likely to display a more chronic social distress pattern. Despite the apparent distress in these noncardiac chest pain patients, up to 98% of patients with PD are undiagnosed. Recently developed instruments to improve physician recognition are now available and should help more patients suffering from this condition receive treatment.

REFERENCES

1. Karlson BW, Hellitz J, Pettersson P, Ekvall H-E, Hjalmarson Å. Patients admitted to the emergency room with symptoms indicative of acute myocardial infarction. J Intern Med 1991; 230:251–258.
2. Kroenke K, Mangelsdorff AD. Common symptoms in ambulatory care: incidence, evaluation, therapy and outcome. Am J Med 1989; 86:262–266.
3. Lee TH, Cook EF, Weisberg M, Sargent RK, Wilson C, Goldman L. Acute chest pain in the emergency room. Identification and examination of low-risk patients. Arch Intern Med 1985; 145:65–69.

4. Katon WJ, Von Korff M, Lin E. Panic disorder: relationship to high medical utilization. Am J Med 1992; 92:1A-7S–1A-11S.

5. Ockene JS, Shay MJ, Alpert JS, Weiner BH, Dalen JE. Unexplained chest pain in patients with normal coronary arteriograms. N Engl J Med 1980; 303:1249–1252.

6. Papanicolaou MN, Califf RM, Hlatky MA. Prognostic implications of angiographically normal and insignificantly narrowed coronary arteries. Am J Cardiol 1986; 58:1181–1187.

7. Richter JE, Bradley LA, Castell DO. Esophageal chest pain: current controversies in pathogenesis, diagnosis, and therapy. Ann Intern Med 1989; 110:66–78.

8. Richter JE, Beitman BD, Cannon III RO. Unexplained chest pain: differential diagnosis of chest pain with normal cardiac studies. In: Saunders WB, ed. The Medical Clinics of North America. Philadelphia: WB Saunders, 1991:1045–1223.

9. Carney RM, Freedland KE, Ludbrook PA, Saunders RD, Jaffe AS. Major depression, panic disorder, and mitral valve prolapse in patients who complain of chest pain. Am J Med 1990; 89:757–760.

10. Roy-Byrne PP, Schmidt P, Cannon RO, Diem H, Rubinow DR. Microvascular angina and panic disorder. Int J Psychiatr Med 1989; 19:315–325.

11. Clouse RE, Lustman PJ. Psychiatric illness and contraction abnormalities of the esophagus. N Engl J Med 1983; 309:1337–1342.

12. Fleet RP, Beitman BD. Unexplained chest pain: When is it panic disorder? Clin Cardiol 1997; 20:187–194.

13. Heberden W. Some account of a disorder of the breast. Med Trans R Coll Phys Lond 1772; 2:59–67.

14. DaCosta JM. On irritable heart: a clinical study of a form of functional cardiac disorder and its consequences. Am J Med Sci 1871; 61:17–52.

15. Osler W. The Principles and Practice of Medicine. Edinburgh: J Pentland Young, 1892.

16. Wood PW. DaCosta's syndrome (or effort syndrome). Br Med J 1941; i:845–851.

17. Elias MF, Robbins MA, Blow FC, Rice AP, Edgecomb JL. Symptom reporting, anxiety and depression in arteriographically classified middle aged chest pain patients. Exp Aging Res 1982; 8:45–51.

18. Channer KS, Papouchado M, James MA, Rees JR. Anxiety and depression with chest pain in patients referred for exercise testing. Lancet 1985; ii:820–822.

19. Sheehan DV, Ballenger J, Jacobsen G. Treatment of endogenous anxiety with phobic, hysterical and hypochondriacal symptoms. Arch Gen Psychiatry 1980; 37:51.

20. Katon W, Hall ML, Russo J. Chest pain: relationship of psychiatric illness to coronary arteriographic results. Am J Med 1988; 84:1–9.

21. Beitman BD, Mukerji V, Lamberti JW. Panic disorder in patients with chest pain and angiographically normal coronary arteries. Am J Cardiol 1989; 63:1399–1403.

22. Beitman BD, Basha I, Flaker G. Atypical or nonanginal chest pain. Panic disorder or coronary artery disease? Arch Intern Med 1987; 147:1548–1552.

23. Wulsin LR, Arnold LM, Hillard JR. Axis I disorders in ER patients with atypical chest pain. Int J Psychiatry Med 1991; 21:37–46.

24. Carter C, Maddock R, Amsterdam E, McCormick S, Waters C, Billette J. Panic disorder and chest pain in the coronary care unit. Psychosomatics 1992; 33:302–309.

25. Carter C, Maddock R, Zoglio M, Lutrin C, Jella S, Amsterdam E. Panic disorder and chest pain: a study of cardiac stress scintigraphy patients. Am J Cardiol 1994;74:296–298.

26. Fleet RP, Dupuis G, Marchand A, Burelle D, Arsenault A, Beitman BD. Panic disorder

in emergency department chest pain patients: prevalence, comorbidity, suicidal ideation and physician recognition. Am J Med 1996; 101:371–380.

27. Beitman BD, Kushner M. Late onset panic disorder: evidence from a study of patients with chest pain and normal cardiac evaluations. Int J Psychiatry Med 1991; 21:29–35.

28. Beitman BD, Basha I, Flaker G, DeRosear L, Mukerji V, Lamberti JW. Major depression in cardiology chest pain patients without coronary artery disease and with panic disorder. J Affect Disord 1987; 13:51–59.

29. Brown TA, Barlow DH, et al. Comorbidity among anxiety disorders: implications for treatment and DSM-IV. J Consult Clin Psychol 1992; 60:835–844.

30. Fleet RP, Dupuis G, Kaczorowski J, Marchand A, Beitman BD. Suicidal ideation in emergency department chest pain patients: panic disorder a risk factor. Am J Emerg Med 1997; 15:345–349.

31. Weissman MM, Klerman GL, Markowitz JS, Ouellette R. Suicidal ideation and suicide attempts in panic disorder and attacks. N Engl J Med 1989; 321:1209–1214.

32. Beck AT, Steer RA, Sanderson WC, Skeie TM. Panic disorder and suicidal ideation and behavior: discrepant findings in psychiatric outpatients. Am J Psychiatry 1991; 148:1195–1199.

33. Friedman S, Jones JC, Cherner L, Barlow DH. Suicidal ideation and suicide attempts among patients with panic disorder: a survey of two outpatient clinics. Am J Psychiatry 1992; 149:680–685.

34. Beitman BD, Mukerji V, Russell JL, Grafing M. Panic disorder in cardiology patients: a review of the Missouri panic/cardiology project. J Psychiatr Res 1993; 27(suppl I):35–46.

35. Coryell W, Noyes R, Clancy J. Excess mortality in panic disorder: a comparison with primary unipolar depression. Arch Gen Psychiatry 1982; 39:701–703.

36. Coryell W, Noyes R Jr, House DJ. Mortality among outpatients with anxiety disorders. Am J Psychiatry 1986; 143:508–510.

37. Haines AP, Imeson JD, Meade TW. Phobic anxiety and ischaemic heart disease. Br Med J 1987; 295:297–299.

38. Kawachi I, Colditz GA, Ascherio A, et al. Prospective study of phobic anxiety and risk of coronary heart disease in men. Circulation 1994; 89:1992–1997.

39. Kawachi I, Sparrow D, Vokonas PS, et al. Symptoms of anxiety and risk of coronary heart disease. The normative aging study. Circulation 1994; 90:2225–2229.

40. Rozanski A, Bairey CN, Krantz DS, et al. Mental stress and the induction of silent myocardial ischemia in patients with coronary artery disease. N Engl J Med 1988; 318:1005–1012.

41. Yeragani VK, Pohl R, Balon R, et al. Risk factors for cardiovascular illness in panic disorder patients. Neuropsychobiology 1990; 23:134–139.

42. Beitman BD, Kushner MG, Basha I, Lamberti J, Mukerji V, Bartels K. Follow-up status of patients with angiographically normal coronary arteries and panic disorder. JAMA 1991; 265:1545–1549.

43. Fleet RP, Dupuis G, Marchand A, Burelle D, Beitman BD. Detecting panic disorder in emergency department chest pain patients: a validated model to improve recognition. Ann Behav Med 1997; 19:124–131.

44. Spitzer RL, Williams JBW, Kroenke K. Utility of a new procedure for diagnosing mental disorders in primary care. The PRIME-MD 1000 study. JAMA 1994; 272:1749–1756.

45. Oehrberg S, Christiansen PE, Behnke K, Borup AL, Severin B, Soegaard J, Calberg H,

Judge R, Ohrstrom JK, Manniche PM. Paroxetine in the treatment of panic disorder. A randomised, double blind, placebo controlled study. Br J Psychiatry 1995; 167:374–379.
46. Clum GA, Clum GA, Surls R. A meta-analysis of treatments for panic disorder. J Cons Clin Psychol 1993; 61:317–326.
47. Margraf J, Barlow DH, Clark DM, Telch MJ. Psychological treatment of panic: work in progress on outcome, active ingredients, and follow-up. Behav Res Ther 1993; 31:1–8.
48. Beitman BD, Basha IM, Trombka LH, Jayaratna MA, Russell B, Flaker G, Anderson S. Pharmacotherapeutic treatment of panic disorder in patients presenting with chest pain. J Family Practice 1989; 28:177–180.
49. Cannon III RO, Quyyumi AA, Mincemoyer R, Stine AM, Gracely RH, Smith WB, Geraci MF, Black BC, Uhde TW, Waclawiw MA, Maher K, Benjamin SB. Imipramine in patients with chest pain despite normal coronary angiograms. N Engl J Med 1994; 330:1411–1417.
50. Pearce MJ, Mayou RA, Klimes I. The management of atypical non-cardiac chest pain. Q J Med 1990; 76:991–996.

7

Liver Disease and Transplantation

William R. Yates
University of Oklahoma Health Sciences Center
Tulsa, Oklahoma

INTRODUCTION

Psychiatric illness in the patient with liver disease or liver transplantation present significant challenges in diagnosis and management. Chronic liver disease frequently produces significant fatigue that can influence the ability of patients to carry on their daily activities and social interactions. Liver transplantation produces the need for lifetime immunosuppressive therapy. Immunosuppressive agents can induce neuropsychiatric adverse effects in some individuals. Liver disease can impair the absorption and metabolism of psychopharmacologic agents, as most of these agents undergo metabolism by the liver.

This chapter will focus on the interactions between liver disease and psychiatric disorders. Alcohol dependence and alcoholic cirrhosis represent a significant public health challenge in the United States and other countries throughout the world. The epidemiology of alcoholic liver disease will be reviewed with attention to the interaction of alcohol dependence with the liver disease and liver transplantation. The psychiatric issues involved in selection of liver transplant recipients will also be reviewed along with potential interactions of liver disease and psychotropic agents. Additionally, the psychiatric effects of medications for liver disease will also be reviewed.

Case histories can provide a method to better understand the relationship between liver disease and psychiatric disorders. Two case histories are provided to introduce this chapter.

Case 1

Mr. A, a 46-year-old man, is seen for psychiatric consultation prior to liver transplantation to evaluate for possible psychiatric contraindications to transplantation. Mr. A's primary liver diagnosis is alcoholic cirrhosis. Medical complications related to cirrhosis have included gastroesophageal varices and hemorrhage, ascites, and intermittent periods of hepatic encephalopathy.

Mr. A started drinking at about age 15. He joined the Army after high school and increased the frequency and quantity of consumption of alcohol during his period in the service. He was given an early honorable discharge from the military, but his alcohol use contributed to the early discharge. He became a daily drinker of alcohol with a usual pattern of drinking about 18 beers per day.

He continued to drink at this level for approximately 20 years. Despite his heavy consumption he was able to maintain a job as a self-employed painter. Five years ago, a physician told him he needed to stop drinking because of elevated liver enzyme levels. He checked himself into an alcoholism treatment facility and remained abstinent for 2 years before relapsing about one year ago. He now has been abstinent about one month coincident with the time of deterioration in his medical condition.

Mr. A had no history of any nonalcohol drug use, abuse, or dependence. He had no evidence of other psychiatric comorbidity. He had been married for 15 years, but his wife filed for divorce due to his drinking, and he had been living alone for many years.

The psychiatric consultant felt that the severity and acuity of alcohol dependence was a psychiatric contraindication to transplant. Mr. A was referred for outpatient substance abuse counseling, signed an agreement to remain abstinent from alcohol, and was told his candidacy could be reevaluated after 6 months of sobriety.

This case illustrates the often complex clinical relationship between alcoholic liver disease and alcohol dependence. Multiple medical, social, and psychiatric factors need to be evaluated prior to transplantation. Severe alcohol dependence and recent drinking appear to indicate an increased risk for relapse to drinking even when a severe medical complication, like cirrhosis, is present. Understanding prognostic factors in alcoholism can increase the chance that liver transplantation will be provided for those most likely to benefit from this aggressive surgical treatment.

Case 2

A 42-year-old women developed fatigue and consulted her family physician. She had developed progressive fatigue over a period of 2 years prior to her presentation. During her teenage years, she had a period of experimentation with alcohol and drug use. For a brief period, she used intravenous methamphetamine. After several years of intermittent drug use, she stopped all drug use when her boyfriend insisted that she do so.

Her family physician completed a medical workup. Blood tests revealed elevation of liver transaminase levels. She was referred to a gastroenterologist for further diagnostic workup and treatment. Serum tests and a liver biopsy confirmed a diagnosis of hepatitis C. Interferon therapy was recommended, and she was referred for psychiatric consultation prior to initiating interferon to rule out psychiatric contraindications to interferon therapy. Psychiatric consultation identified her previous drug use but showed no evidence for a history of depression or active depression. There was felt to be no psychiatric contraindication to interferon therapy.

Interferon therapy began, and the patient did well for several weeks. However, she began to notice mood lability, irritability, and sleep disturbance. Her symptoms distressed her a great deal, and she began to have difficulty with occupational and social functioning. She denied suicidal ideation. Psychiatric reevaluation resulted in a diagnosis of mood disorder due to interferon. Her initial liver response to interferon was excellent, with reduction of liver transaminase levels to normal. Since her response had been very positive to interferon, her gastroenterologist and psychiatrist elected to continue the interferon therapy while treatment with a selective serotonin-reuptake inhibitor was initiated.

Following 3 weeks of antidepressant therapy, her mood symptoms improved including a return to normal sleep patterns. She continued antidepressant therapy during the year of interferon therapy. Her mood remained normal during interferon therapy. Following completion of interferon, her antidepressant medication was tapered without recurrence of depression.

This case illustrates the potential psychiatric effects of drugs used for gastrointestinal disorders. Interferon can produce a significant mood disorder in some individuals. Since suicide has been reported during interferon therapy, mood symptoms should not be ignored. Early consultation with a psychiatrist can facilitate coordinated care. Active psychiatric treatment can allow for successful completion of medical therapy.

PSYCHIATRIC CONSULTATION IN GASTROINTESTINAL DISEASE

Patients with gastrointestinal disorders frequently require psychiatric consultation. In a series of 1250 patients referred for psychiatric consultation over a one-year period, 103 (8%) presented with a gastrointestinal disorder as their primary medical diagnosis (Table 1). This series of psychiatric consultations occurred in a tertiary care university hospital setting. Consultation requests originated from medical inpatients (55%) and medical outpatients (45%) referred from primary care internists and gastroenterologists. The majority of patients were female (56%). All consultation patients in this series were seen by a faculty psychiatrist using DSM-IV (1) criteria in diagnosis. A database of primary medical and psychiatric disorders coded for ICD-9 and DSM-IV diagnoses for these consultation patients provides some insight into the epidemiology of psychiatric illness in the gastrointestinal disorders.

Specific gastrointestinal disorders encountered in this recent series are ranked in Table 1. Hepatitis topped the rank list in this series. The majority of hepatitis patients presented with hepatitis C and were seen with mood disorders or referred for consultation prior to interferon therapy. Undiagnosed gastrointestinal symptoms of abdominal pain, diarrhea, and constipation were common, with many representing functional gastrointestinal disorders. Pancreatitis presented primarily in the inpatient setting with

Table 1 Frequency of Medical and Psychiatric Disorders in Psychiatric Consultation for Gastrointestinal Disease

Medical disorder	%	Psychiatric diagnosis	%
1. Hepatitis	25	1. Major Depression/Dysthymia	30
2. Abdominal Pain	12	2. Alcohol/Drug Dependence	17
3. Pancreatitis	12	3. Somatoform Disorder	10
4. Crohns/Ulcerative Colitis	10	4. Anxiety Disorder	7
5. Peptic Ulcer/Gastritis	8	5. Personality Disorder	7
6. Cirrhosis	7	6. Adjustment Disorder	6
7. Gastroesophageal Reflux	6	7. Bipolar Affective Disorder	5
8. Diarrhea/Constipation	6	8. Psychotic Disorder	5
9. Esophageal Disorder	5	9. Factitious Disorder	4
10. Gastroparesis	5	10. No Psychiatric Diagnosis	4

Rankings based on a series of 103 patients referred from internal medicine for psychiatry consultation. Patients had a primary diagnosis of a gastrointestinal disorder in a university hospital setting.

alcohol dependence as the primary psychiatric comorbid condition. Inflammatory bowel disease, peptic ulcer, gastritis and gastroesophageal reflux disease, esophageal disorders, and gastroparesis each represented at least 5% of the series total. The type of gastrointestinal disorders seen in consultation can vary by the site of practice, and tertiary care center distributions may not reflect the patient profiles seen in other practice settings.

Major depression and dysthymia ranked first in the psychiatric diagnosis category for this series. This is consistent with the most prevalent diagnoses seen overall in internal medicine referrals. Substance dependence and somatoform disorders each occurred in 10% or more of consultations. Anxiety disorder, personality disorder, adjustment disorder, bipolar affective disorder, and psychotic disorder occurred in at least 5% of the diagnoses. Factitious disorder, a very rare psychiatric disorder, also made the top 10 ranking for this series of patients. The results document the spectrum of psychiatric disorders seen in the gastroenterology population.

EPIDEMIOLOGY OF LIVER DISEASE AND TRANSPLANTATION

Epidemiology of Liver Disease

A variety of illnesses can involve the liver directly or secondarily. Table 2 outlines some of the common diseases of the liver. Viral infections of the liver can present a spectrum of illness severity ranging from mild, transient illnesses lasting several days to acute fulminant illnesses that can precipitate liver failure. Hepatitis A is transmitted through the fecal/oral route and is generally a mild illness that does not progress to a carrier state or chronic hepatitis. Hepatitis B is transmitted via blood, sexual activity, and the

Table 2   The Liver Diseases

Viral hepatits
  Hepatitis A
  Hepatitis B
  Hepatitis C
  Other viral agents
Toxic and drug-related liver disease
  Intrinsic hepatotoxins
  Idiosyncratic hepatotoxins
  Alcohol
  Acetaminophen
Cholestatic liver disease
  Primary biliary cirrhosis
  Primary sclerosing cholangitis
  Granulomatous hepatitis
Metabolic liver disease
  Wilson's disease
  Hemochromatosis
  α_1-antitrypsin deficiency
Primary liver cancer
Metastatic liver cancer
Miscellaneous liver disease
  Vascular disease
  Hepatic abscess
  Autoimmune hepatitis

perinatal route. The severity of hepatitis B can range from mild to severe. Hepatitis C most commonly occurs in patients who received blood transfusion prior to routine screening for this agent in the blood supply.

The liver is sensitive to a variety of compounds that can produce hepatotoxic effects. Intrinsic hepatotoxins include direct hepatotoxins, like carbon tetrachloride, that directly damage liver cells. Indirect hepatotoxins, like acetaminophen, can damage the liver by disruption of hepatocyte metabolic pathways or secretory mechanisms. The effect of alcohol on the liver will be discussed later in more detail because of the relationship to alcohol dependence.

Cholestatic liver diseases produce primarily elevations in alkaline phosphatase and bilirubin. Primary biliary cirrhosis (PBC) is a progressive cholestatic liver disease of unknown cause that affects primarily middle-aged women. PBC commonly produces pruritis and can be associated with hyperpigmentation, gallstones, and osteoporosis. PBC can produce liver failure and is a common indication for liver transplant. Primary sclerosing cholangitis (PSC) is characterized by inflammation, fibrosis, and eventual obstruction of the bile ducts. PSC occurs more frequently in patients with inflammatory bowel disease like ulcerative colitis, and it is associated with cholangiocarcinoma. Granulomatous hepatitis can occur due to mycobacterial or fungal diseases of the liver or be associated with systemic granulomatous illnesses like sarcoidosis.

Metabolic diseases, such as Wilson's disease, produce liver damage. Primary liver cancer (hepatocellular carcinoma) strikes up to 15–20% of patients with hepatitis C. Metastatic liver cancer is common in colon cancer and other cancers. Vascular abnormalities of the liver include hepatic artery thrombosis (Budd-Chiari syndrome) and portal vein thrombosis. Abscess formation can occur in the liver due to bacterial agents or parasitic infections. Autoimmune chronic active hepatitis can be controlled with glucocorticoids, but it can become progressive and require liver transplantation.

Epidemiology of Alcoholic Cirrhosis

Chronic liver disease and cirrhosis is the ninth leading cause of death in the United States (2). In 1989 chronic liver disease was the underlying cause of death for 26,720 persons in the United States (3). In addition, chronic liver disease was a contributing cause of death for an additional 14,101 persons. Among deaths from chronic liver disease as an underlying cause, 46.1% were classified as attributable to alcohol. Alcohol-related liver deaths are coded alcoholic fatty liver, acute alcoholic hepatitis, alcoholic cirrhosis of the liver, and alcoholic liver damage—unspecified. Alcohol probably plays a significant role in many of the deaths coded as chronic liver disease with unspecified conditions (49.5% of liver disease deaths).

Alcoholic cirrhosis is associated with chronic heavy alcohol consumption (4–6). Despite this well-known link, only about 25% of heavy drinkers will develop significant cirrhosis. The risk of cirrhosis appears to be related to the duration of heavy drinking as well as the quantity of alcohol consumed. The severity of liver damage increases with increasing daily intake of alcohol exceeding 180 grams (approximately 14 drinks per day) (4). The duration of heavy drinking required for the development of cirrhosis usually ranges from 10 to 20 years. Women appear more likely to develop cirrhosis than men when quantity of alcohol is controlled (7–9). Once evidence of cirrhosis develops, patients become at risk for a significant number of medical complications.

Medical Complications of Alcoholic Cirrhosis

The process of liver damage and cirrhosis cause several pathophysiological changes that can result in a variety of medical complications (10) (Fig. 1). Liver cirrhosis produces an increase in portal venous pressure. This process can result in significant esophageal varices. Esophageal varices are prone to rupture, with gastrointestinal hemorrhage occasionally resulting in death from exsanguination. Portal hypertension is also associated with ascites—a process of abdominal fluid accumulation resulting in abdominal distention. Cirrhosis also increases the risk of spontaneous bacterial peritonitis, an abdominal cavity infectious disease that can also be life-threatening.

The loss of liver function associated with cirrhosis produces symptoms of liver

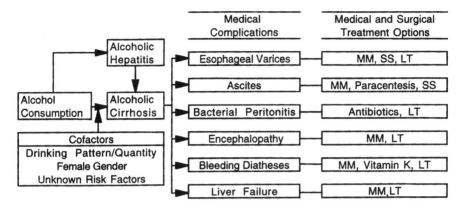

Figure 1 Medical complications and treatment options for cirrhosis. MM = Medical management specific to complication; SS = shunt surgery; LT = liver transplantation.

insufficiency. Because the liver is responsible for handling breakdown products, liver insufficiency can produce accumulation of central nervous system toxins such as ammonia. This waste accumulation can produce various degrees of encephalopathy from mild cognitive impairment to coma. Because the liver is essential in producing clotting factors, liver insufficiency can increase risk for hemorrhage due to bleeding diathesis. Finally cirrhosis can produce acute or chronic liver failure with life-threatening complications. Individual patients with cirrhosis may suffer from one or more of the complications of the disease.

The complications of cirrhosis can be treated with a variety of medical and surgical approaches, including endoscopic sclerotherapy and venous shunt surgery. Venous shunt therapy is aimed at minimizing the effect of portal hypertension. Paracentesis (draining of abdominal fluid) can temporarily relieve the distension associated with ascites. Bacterial peritonitis can be controlled with antibiotic therapy. Despite the availability of medical and surgical treatment, continued drinking after the onset of cirrhosis produces limited success in affecting the progression and dire outcome in alcoholic cirrhosis (11–14). Conversely, aggressive medical and surgical management linked with abstinence from alcohol can halt or slow the progression of the disease.

Liver transplantation is considered the only curative approach to the management of alcoholic cirrhosis. Indications for liver transplantation include presence of significant varices, ascites, spontaneous bacterial peritonitis, liver insufficiency, or encephalopathy.

THE ROLE OF LIVER TRANSPLANTATION IN TREATMENT OF ALCOHOLIC CIRRHOSIS

In 1983 the National Institutes of Health reported recommendations for liver transplantation in alcoholic cirrhosis. A Consensus Development Panel recommended that transplantation for cirrhosis should be considered in "only a small proportion of cases" (15). Two criteria were developed to select patients appropriate for transplantation. First the patient should have "established clinical indicators of fatal outcome" and second, the patient should be "judged likely to abstain from alcohol." This second selection criteria presents a significant clinical and research challenge. No commonly agreed indicators of alcoholism relapse risk for cirrhosis exist. Individual liver transplant centers have been left to develop their own criteria for assessing the indicators of good alcoholism prognosis in liver transplant candidates with a history of alcoholism (16–21).

Predictors of Relapse in Alcoholism Associated with Cirrhosis

The research tradition in seeking predictors of outcome in alcoholism is extensive (22–29). However, limited clinical research exists on the validity of predictors in cirrhotic patient populations. Candidate predictors that have been used clinically by liver transplantation centers include the duration of abstinence (17), psychosocial support (30), psychiatric comorbidity, and patient cooperation with alcoholism treatment recommendations (31), among others. Several scales combining several candidate predictors have been developed and have received some attention in clinical settings.

Predictors of Outcome in Alcoholism

The role of baseline factors in predicting alcohol-related readmission was evaluated in a study of male U.S. veterans admitted for treatment of alcoholism (32). This study examined drinking history, psychiatric illness, sociodemographic factors, and other substance abuse as candidate predictors of relapse and readmission for alcoholism treatment. Following an index treatment experience, computerized patient treatment file records were accessed for 15 months after discharge and compared to baseline characteristics. Several index variables were associated with relapse in the follow-up period (Table 3).

Using a Cox proportional hazards model, three variables entered an equation to define the risk for readmission controlling for all significant predictor variables. Duration of heavy drinking, daily alcohol intake, and history of alcoholism treatment independently contributed to risk of readmission. Using the proportional hazards model, we developed a high-risk alcoholism relapse scale from this study (33,34) (Table 4).

Using the Cox proportional hazards model and the ratings from the HRAR scale, a predictive relative risk equation for readmission in one year can be produced:

$$RR = e[(d * 0.3228) + (t * 0.5129) + (r * 0.6290)]$$

where:

d = duration of heavy drinking score
t = daily usual drink number score
r = treatment episode score

Table 3 Variables Examined for Effect on Readmission[a]

	Chi-square		Chi-square
Daily alcohol consumption	16.14[b]	Hamilton depression scale	0.40
Duration of heavy drinking	12.36[b]	Antisocial personality	0.44
Sum of DSM-III alcohol abuse		Stressful life events	3.38
dependence criteria	9.34[b]	Work adjustment	8.42[b]
Sum of DSM-III pathological		Financial difficulty	1.12
alcohol use criteria	16.35[b]	Living circumstances	4.75
Previous alcohol treatment	14.1[b]	Years of education	1.35
Sum of drinking behaviors	11.03[b]	Age	0.32
Days sober on interview	0.75	Length of stay in treatment	0.01
History of polydrug use	1.84		

[a] Log-rank tests for time to readmission.
[b] Statistically significant relationship to readmission.

Table 4 High-Risk Alcoholism Relapse Scale

Variable	Point value	
Years of heavy drinking:		
<11	0	
11–25	1	
>25	2	_____
Daily usual drink number		
<9	0	
9–17	1	
>17	2	_____
Number of prior alcohol- ism inpatient treat- ment episodes		
0	0	
1	1	
>1	2	_____
Total		_____

Low risk—Sum of three factors = 0, 1, or 2.
Moderate risk—Sum of three factors = 3 or 4.
High risk—Sum of three factors = 5 or 6.

This results in assigning a relative risk of 1 for a subject scoring 0 on all three criterion items from the HRAR rating scale. The relative risk estimate for the highest risk group (scoring the maximum of 6) using the equation is 18.7. This range of risk translated into a 3–5% readmission risk for the lowest score contrasted to a >60% readmission risk for the highest scoring group.

Although the predictive equation was developed without a specific theoretical model, the three variables in the model seem consistent with a model associating prognosis with severity of alcoholism. This severity model is similar to how severity for other psychiatric conditions and medical conditions are also categorized. Years of heavy drinking is an index of chronicity. Chronicity has been associated with poor prognosis in depression as well as in many medical conditions. Daily usual drink number can be considered a symptom frequency measure as well as a measure of physiological dependence on alcohol. Symptom frequency has been a predictor of outcome in bulimia and in coronary artery disease, where the target symptom is angina. Finally, history of relapse following previous treatment is an index of treatment refractoriness. Treatment refractoriness has been associated with poor prognosis in medical conditions such as cancer. We have therefore conceptualized the high risk for relapse model as a prognostic indicator using indices of illness chronicity, symptom frequency, and treatment responsiveness as separate measures of alcoholism severity.

PSYCHIATRIC ISSUES IN THE SELECTION OF LIVER TRANSPLANTATION CANDIDATES

At most U.S. institutions, patients with a medical indication for transplant undergo evaluation by a panel of specialists prior to listing for transplant. Patients must be able to survive the process of anesthesia for liver transplant, a procedure that might take 12–14 hours. Cardiac function and coronary artery status are routinely examined pre-transplant along with pulmonary function. Routine social work assessment is completed to evaluate the financial and interpersonal resources for potential candidates. Psychiatric pretransplant evaluation is also commonly done to evaluate for potential psychiatric contraindications to transplantation.

As the surgical and medical outcomes for liver transplantation have improved, psychiatric and behavioral issues play a larger role in contributing to an adverse outcome. This increases the importance of pretransplant psychiatric assessment and the importance of the availability of psychiatric services for the posttransplant population. There are several steps in the psychiatric pretransplant evaluation process. Table 5 outlines the criteria used by the University of Iowa Liver Transplant Service for psychiatric pretransplant screening (35).

For patients with alcohol-related liver transplant, estimating the prognosis for the patient's alcoholism is extremely important. As outlined earlier, there is no standard evaluation process for screening patients with alcoholic cirrhosis. To estimate prognosis,

Table 5 Transplant Guidelines for Patients with Cirrhosis Due to Alcoholic Liver Disease

	Risk category	
Criteria	Low	High
Favorable alcoholism prognosis[a]	Yes	No
Continued drinking after learning that alcohol had damaged their liver	No	Yes
Signed alcohol compliance agreement	Yes	No
Social support	Good	Poor
Psychiatric contraindication to transplant[b,c]	No	Yes

[a] HRAR score of three or less or >12 months documented sobriety.

[b] Relative psychiatric contraindication to transplant: polysubstance abuse, moderate personality disorder, major mood disorder.

[c] Absolute psychiatric contraindication to transplant: severe personality disorder, severe mental retardation, dementia, or chronic psychosis.

Acceptable candidates are generally ranked low risk in all five categories.

Occasional acceptance may be granted for candidates with a predominance of low-risk ratings.

rating of the patient's alcoholism severity using the High Risk Alcoholism Relapse scale can be done. At the University of Iowa, a patient is felt to have a favorable alcoholism prognosis when the HRAR score is 3 or less or when a patient with a higher score has a documented period of sobriety of at least 6 months. Patients who have continued drinking after being told the seriousness of their liver disease generally have a poor alcoholism prognosis.

Transplant candidates with alcoholism must acknowledge that alcohol is a problem for them and that they have accepted abstinence as a lifelong goal. A compliance agreement stating these issues is signed. Patients agree to undergo routine monitoring of their drinking status during the pretransplant period. Relapse to drinking during this time results in deactivation of the transplant status. Candidates are encouraged to continue some form of outpatient treatment during the assessment and waiting period. This treatment is expected to continue during the posttransplant period, as the stress of transplantation can serve as a significant contributor to the risk of relapse.

General social support appears to be important in alcoholism outcome as well as for liver transplantation outcome. The Psychosocial Assessment of Candidates for Transplantation (36) is a structured scale that assesses eight domains of psychosocial support and is appropriate for use in all types of transplantation. Patients with a stable occupational history and a job to return to after transplant are more likely to have a successful quality of life following transplant. Patients with geographic stability and a supportive spouse or significant other also appear to have better outcomes after successful transplantation.

Issues of psychiatric comorbidity are important to examine in the candidate-assessment process. This includes the potential role of drug abuse comorbidity as well as other axis I and axis II comorbidity (1). Active drug abuse at the time of transplant assessment is considered by most centers as an absolute contraindication for transplant. Routine pretransplant drug screening is important to detect potential drug use not endorsed by interview.

PHARMACOLOGIC ISSUES IN LIVER DISEASE AND TRANSPLANTATION

Most psychotropic agents are metabolized by the liver. This makes it necessary to carefully consider the pharmacokinetics of psychotropic drugs when treating patients with liver disease or those who have undergone transplantation. In hepatic and other gastrointestinal disease, all the essential steps in pharmacokinetics can be affected, including absorption, distribution, metabolism, and elimination.

Trzepacz and colleagues (37) reviewed the psychopharmacologic issues associated with organ transplantation. This reference can serve as a valuable resource for psychiatrists treating patients with liver disease. The issues associated with individual psychotropic drug agents will be reviewed.

Tricyclics

Tricyclic antidepressant drugs metabolize to a great extent on the first pass through the liver. This means that disruption of the normal blood flow from the gut to the liver will result in higher blood levels of tricyclic agents. In liver disease, portal hypertension produces significant shunting of the first pass of tricyclic agents around the liver and into the general circulation. Also the hypoalbuminemia associated with poor hepatic function can increase free tricyclic levels.

This does not mean that tricyclic agents are contraindicated in liver disease and transplantation. A reasonable rule would be to utilize approximate one half the dose of tricyclic as would be used in a patient without liver disease. Nortriptyline probably represents the best choice for tricyclic use in liver disease. A reasonable starting dose would be 25 mg increasing to 50 mg daily. After 5 days on 50 mg of nortriptyline, a serum blood level can be checked to determine if nortriptyline has reached the therapeutic range (50–150 ng/dl), and dosage adjustments can be made accordingly.

Nontricyclic Antidepressants

Fluoxetine, sertraline, paroxetine, bupropion, and venlafaxine provide clinicians with a wide choice of nontricyclic agents for the treatment of depression in liver disease. Fluoxetine and its metabolite have the longest half-lives of agents in this category (4 and 7 days, respectively). Studies of the half-life of fluoxetine and norfluoxetine in alcoholic cirrhosis documented approximately a doubling of the half-life for both compounds. This study suggests that a reasonable strategy for dosing patients with liver disease would be 10 mg of fluoxetine daily or even 20 mg every other day. There are limited studies of the effects of the other nontricyclic agents in liver disease. However, these agents have been used safely in a variety of medically ill patients.

Lithium

Lithium represents a psychotropic drug whose metabolism does not appear to be influenced by the presence of liver disease. However, liver disease can be accompanied by renal insufficiency, so it is important to document the renal status of patients prior to the institution of lithium. One potential lithium-drug interaction in liver transplantation deserves consideration. Cyclosporin appears to increase lithium levels and can induce lithium toxicity when it is added to patients receiving lithium. If cyclosporin is added to a patient receiving lithium, reduction by 50% of the lithium dose with close lithium therapeutic monitoring is indicated. Clinicians can also consider changing lithium to valproic acid for an antimanic agent. Valproic acid is hepatically metabolized and should be monitored closely for toxicity by clinical exam and serum blood levels.

Antipsychotics

Antipsychotics are indicated for liver transplant patients who develop delirium in the postoperative period. Delirium in this group of patients occurs more frequently when a history of alcohol dependence is present. Several of the low-potency antipsychotics have been associated with hepatic toxicity and cholestatic jaundice. Chlorpromazine can induce hepatotoxicity in patients with impaired sulfoxidation. Impaired sulfoxidation affects up to 80% of patients with primary biliary cirrhosis and so should be avoided in PBC patients. High-potency antipsychotic agents like haloperidol are the antipsychotics of choice in liver disease and liver transplantation. These agents produce fewer cardiovascular effects and less risk of hepatotoxicity.

Benzodiazepines

Benzodiazepines can be used safely in the majority of liver transplant patients. However, these agents should be used cautiously, if at all, for patients with cirrhosis. Encephalopathy associated with cirrhosis appears to be related to a gamma-aminobutyric acid (GABA) mechanism. Since benzodiazepines also work through a GABA channel, they can precipitate or worsen encephalopathy related to cirrhosis. Low-dose antipsychotics can be substituted for sedation in this population. Trazodone is another alternative, although risk for priapism in men needs to be considered.

ADVERSE PSYCHIATRIC EFFECTS ASSOCIATED WITH COMMONLY PRESCRIBED DRUGS FOR GASTROINTESTINAL CONDITIONS

Gastrointestinal prescription drugs comprise a significant percentage of all prescriptions. Several of these agents can produce psychiatric symptoms. Additionally, several of the gastrointestinal drugs can interact with common psychiatric prescription drugs.

Cimetidine has been available for over 20 years as a histamine receptor antagonist blocking gastric acid secretion. Cimetidine appears to have some anticholinergic effect and can produce delirium, especially in hospitalized patients with severe medical or surgical illness. The newer histamine receptor antagonists have fewer adverse central nervous system (CNS) effects and drug interaction problems with psychotropic drugs. Cimetidine has seen a resurgence in use in many hospitals in an effort to reduce hospital costs and as a preferred drug in some managed care settings. This change has resulted in a risk for more adverse CNS and drug interaction problems. Omeprazole is a blocker of acid secretion that works by inhibiting the proton pump in gastric cells. A possible drug interaction with omeprazole that increases carbamazepine levels has been described (40).

Gastrointestinal stimulants target delayed gastric emptying associated with diabetes and advanced age. Two drugs in this class include cisapride and metoclopramide. Metoclopramide appears to be able to induce a depressive state in some individuals. Metoclopramide also can occasionally cause adverse effects associated with the dopamine-blocking property of antipsychotics. Such parkinsonian symptoms noted with metoclopraminde include dystonic reactions, akathisia, and muscular rigidity.

Antipsychotic drugs reduce nausea and vomiting. Some common antipsychotic drugs like haloperidol and chlorpromazine are used in the medical setting for their antiemetic effect. The antipsychotic prochlorperzine can produce the adverse effects of other phenothiazines and potentiate the sedative effects of some psychotropics. Like other phenothiazines, concurrent tricyclic administration results in higher blood levels of the tricyclic agents. Two anti-infective agents used for gastrointestinal diseases deserve comment. Interferon therapy for hepatitis C, as previously noted, carries a risk of depression with reports of suicide attempts and completed suicide in several cases (38). Some centers recommend psychiatric consultation prior to the institution of interferon therapy. Flagyl is commonly prescribed for giardiasis and peptic ulcer due to *Helicobacter* infection. This agent may increase risk for nephrogenic toxicity associated with lithium and also can produce an Antabuse-like reaction when alcohol is consumed.

Irritable bowel syndrome can be treated with antispasmodic agents. These compounds often produce significant anticholinergic effects. It is important to monitor the potential for antidepressants and low-potency antipsychotics to produce an additive anticholinergic effect in patients receiving antispasmodics. Anticholinergic toxicity can produce delirium, especially in patients with preexisting cognitive impairment.

Psychiatrists and other physicians prescribing psychotropic agents need to consider these potential interactions when treating patients with gastrointestinal diseases.

Collaboration between psychiatrists and physicians treating gastrointestinal disorders is frequently necessary for patients with combined illnesses. This collaboration will often also be necessary for separating out gastrointestinal from psychiatric causes in the differential diagnosis of complex patients.

TREATMENT OF PSYCHIATRIC DISORDERS IN LIVER DISEASE

Evaluation of Liver Function

It is important to be aware of the individual patient's liver function when considering psychotropic treatment. A history of liver diseases should be noted. Liver function can be estimated by evaluating the serum transaminase levels, gamma-glutamyl transferase, alkaline phosphatase levels, serum bilirubin, serum albumin, and blood clotting parameters. If evidence of active liver disease is present, specific modifications of treatment regimens should be considered. Specific treatment recommendations for management of psychiatric problems in the liver-compromised patient is summarized in Table 6.

Alcohol Withdrawal

Alcohol withdrawal represents a serious medical emergency that can result in death. For patients with active liver disease, alcohol withdrawal presents a significant management challenge. Long-acting benzodiazepines may accumulate and the potential benefits of using a renal metabolized benzodiazepine like lorazepam should be considered. Gener-

Table 6   Treatment Recommendations for Psychiatric Syndromes in Patients with Active Liver Disease

Alcohol withdrawal	Lorazepam 2 mg q 4 h × 24 h, 2 mg q 6 h × 24 h, 1 mg q 4 h × 24 h, 1 mg q 6 h × 24 h Use only if objective withdrawal signs present, hold dose if sedated, ataxic
Alcoholic hallucinosis	Haloperidol 2–5 mg q 4 hr prn
Hepatic encephalopathy	Avoid benzodiazepines; use haloperidol 1–2 mg PO or IM q 4 hr prn for agitation
Agitated delirium posttransplant	Consider IV haloperidol 0.5 to 5 mg IV q hr alternating with IV lorazepam 0.5–2.0 mg q h (see Ref. 39 for more details)
Alcohol dependence	Both disulfiram and naltrexone can cause hepatotoxicity, avoid in active liver disease
Major depression	Reduce standard doses by one half, selective serotonin agents usually well tolerated
Anxiety disorders	Avoid benzodiazepines, consider antidepressants, buspirone, or short-term low-dose antipsychotics

ally 3–4 days of treatment is necessary. Benzodiazepine doses should be held during withdrawal if sedation, ataxia, or benzodiazepine-related nystagmus are present.

Alcoholic Hallucinosis

Hallucinosis can occur during alcohol withdrawal. Clinicians should search for evidence of alcohol withdrawal delirium such as cognitive impairment. Haloperidol can be used to target symptoms of hallucinosis or agitation. Haloperidol should not be substituted for lorazepam but be used in addition to the dose of lorazepam required to control withdrawal signs of tachycardia, elevated temperature and blood pressure, and withdrawal tremor.

Delirium Due to Hepatic Disease

Cirrhosis and fulminant liver failure produce cognitive impairment and clouding of consciousness. The clinical picture frequently includes various levels of sedation up to, and including, hepatic coma. The delirium associated with cirrhosis and liver failure is usually not associated with psychotic symptoms or agitation and may not require pharmacologic intervention. Benzodiazepines should be avoided. There is some evidence that benzodiazepine antagonists like flumazenil can temporarily reduce the signs of hepatic coma is some individuals.

Delirium in the Posttransplant Period

Delirium occurs in a significant number of patients following liver transplant. Impaired cognitive function prior to transplant and transplant for alcohol-related liver disease increases the risk of posttransplant delirium. Posttransplant delirium can be associated with psychotic symptoms and significant agitation. Haloperidol is frequently used in this setting, and intravenous haloperidol can be considered. Although haloperidol has not been approved for intravenous use, clinical studies suggest it can be safely considered especially when the patient receives cardiac monitoring. Haloperidol can be alternated with lorazepam until adequate sedation is achieved (39).

Alcohol Dependence

Pharmacologic strategies for alcohol dependence can provide adjunctive treatment to psychosocial treatments. Disulfiram and naltrexone appear to provide some long-term benefit for some individuals with alcohol dependence. Unfortunately, both disulfiram and naltrexone can produce hepatotoxicity. Clinicians should avoid these agents in severe active liver disease. For patients with milder illness, clinicians need to carefully consider the potential risks and benefits of trials with either disulfiram or naltrexone.

Mood and Anxiety Disorders

Mood and anxiety disorders are common in patients with liver disease. The use of individual antidepressants and antianxiety agents has been discussed in the section on pharmacology. In summary, it is best to avoid benzodiazepines for the treatment of mood and anxiety disorder in patients with liver disease. Selective serotonin agents appear to be well tolerated and effective. For sedation, clinicians can consider trazodone or low-dose antipsychotic use.

SUMMARY

Clinicians need to assess the potential of liver disease and its treatment to affect the diagnosis and management of psychiatric illnesses. Psychiatric treatment of mental illness in this population requires attention to several factors. First, how has the liver disease affected the psychiatric presentation? Have medical treatments contributed to the psychiatric symptoms experienced by the patient? Second, how will the liver disease affect the treatment options available? Which drugs can be used and which avoided? Careful consideration of these issues can avoid iatrogenic complications and increase the likelihood of successful management.

REFERENCES

1. American Psychiatric Association. Diagnostic and Statistical Manual. 4th ed. Washington, DC: American Psychiatric Press, 1994.
2. U.S. Bureau of the Census. Statistical Abstract of the United States (1992). 112th ed. Washington, DC, 1992.
3. Deaths and hospitalizations from chronic liver disease and cirrhosis: United States 1980–1989. MMWR 1993; 41:969–973.
4. Grant BF, Dufour MC, Harford TC. The epidemiology of alcoholic liver disease. Sem Liver Dis 1988; 8:12–25.
5. Batey RG, Burns T, Benson RJ, Byth K. Alcohol consumption and the risk of cirrhosis. Med J Aust 1992; 156:413–415.
6. Yates WR, Petty F, Brown K. Risk factors for alcohol hepatotoxicity among male alcoholics. Drug Alcohol Depend 1987; 20:155–162.
7. Hasin DS, Grant B, Harford TC. Male and female differences in liver cirrhosis mortality in the United States, 1981–1985. J Studies Alcohol 1990; 51:123–129.
8. Norton R, Bate R, Dwyer T, MacMahon S. Alcohol consumption and the risk of alcohol-related cirrhosis in women. Br Med J 1987; 295:80–82.
9. Loft S, Olesen KL, Dossing M. Increased susceptibility to liver disease in relation to alcohol consumption in women. Scand J Gastroenterol 1987; 22:1251–1256.
10. LaMont JT, Koff RS, Isselbacher KJ. Cirrhosis. In: Isselbacher KJ, Adams RD, Braunwald E, Petersdorf RG, Wilson JD, eds. Harrison's Principles of Internal Medicine. New York: McGraw-Hill, 1980:319–325.

11. Kawasaki S, Henderson JM, Hertzler G, Galloway JR. The role of continued drinking in loss of portal perfusion after distal splenorenal shunt. Gastroenterology 1991; 100:799–804.
12. Pugh S, Lewis S, Rees Smith P. Bleeding oesophageal varices in alcoholic cirrhosis: long-term follow-up of endoscopic sclerotherapy. Q J Med 1993; 86:241–245.
13. Borowsky SA, Strome A, Lott E. Continued heavy drinking and survival in alcoholic cirrhosis. Gastroenterology 1981; 80:1405–1409.
14. Spina GP, Santambrogio R, Opochner E, Pisani-Ceretti A, Ongari B, Rashidi B, Garancini P, Gallus G. Factors predicting chronic hepatic encephalopathy after distal splenorenal shunt: a multivariate analysis of clinical and hemodynamic variables. Surgery 1993; 114:519–526.
15. Liver Transplantation Consensus Conference (1983). JAMA 1983; 250:2961–2964.
16. Beresford TP, Turcotte JG, Merion R, Burtch G, Blow FC, Campbell D, Brower KJ, Coffman K, Lucey M. A rational approach to liver transplantation for the alcoholic patient. Psychosomatics 1990; 31:241–254.
17. Bird GLA, O'Grady JG, Harvey FAH, Calne RY, Williams R. Liver transplantation in patients with alcoholic cirrhosis: selection criteria and rates of survival and relapse. Br Med J 1990; 301:15–17.
18. Surman OS, Dienstag JL, Cosimi AB, Chauncey S, Russell PS. Liver transplantation: psychiatric considerations. Psychosomatics 1987; 28:615–621.
19. Kumar S, Stauber RE, Gavaler JS, Basista MH, Dindzans VJ, Schade RR, Rabinovitz M, Tarter RE, Gordon R, Starzl TE, Van Thiel DH. Orthotic liver transplantation for alcoholic liver disease. Hepatology 1990; 11:159–163.
20. Leventhal RI, Berman DH, Lasky S, Gavaler JS, Dindzans V, Urban E, Van Thiel DH. Liver transplantation: initial experience in the Veterans Administration. Dig Dis Sci 1990; 35:673–680.
21. Lucey MR, Merion RM, Henley KS, Campbell DA, Turcotte JG, Nostrant TT. Selection for and outcome of liver transplantation in alcoholic liver disease. Gastroenterology 1992; 102:1736–1741.
22. Edwards G, Brown D, Oppenheimer E, Sheehan M, Taylor C, Duckett A. Long term outcome for patients with drinking problems: the search for predictors. Br J Addict 1988; 83:917–927.
23. Elal-Lawrence G, Slade PD, Dewey ME. Predictors of outcome in treated problem drinkers. J Studies Alcohol 1986; 47:41–47.
24. Ellis D, McClure J. Inpatient treatment of alcohol problems: predicting and preventing relapse. Alcohol Alcoholism 1992; 27:449–456.
25. Gallant D. Common predictors of abstinence and relapse among alcoholic and other drug abusers. Alcoholism 1992; 16:837.
26. Glenn SW, Parsons OA. Prediction of resumption of drinking in posttreatment alcoholics. Int J Addict 1991; 26:237–254.
27. Sheeren M. The relationship between relapse and involvement in alcoholics anonymous. J Stud Alcohol 1988; 49:104–106.
28. Vaillant GE. The Natural History of Alcoholism. Cambridge, MA: Harvard University Press, 1983.
29. Vaillant GE: What can long-term follow-up teach us about relapse and prevention of relapse in addiction? Br J Addict 1988; 83:1147–1157.
30. Levenson JL, Olbrisch ME. Shortage of donor organs and long waits. Psychosomatics 1987; 28:399–403.

31. Gish RG, Lee AH, Keeffe EB, Rome H, Concepcion W, Esquivel CO. Liver transplantation for patients with alcoholism and end-stage liver disease. Am J Gastroenterol 1993; 88:1337–1342.

32. Booth BM, Yates WR, Petty F, Brown K. Patient factors predicting early alcohol-related readmissions for alcoholics: role of alcoholism severity and psychiatric comorbidity. J Stud Alcohol 1993; 52:37–43.

33. Yates WR, Booth BM, Reed D, Brown K, Masterson B. Descriptive and predictive validity of a high-risk alcoholism relapse typology. J Stud Alcohol 1993; 54:645–651.

34. Yates WR, Reed D, Booth B, Masterson B, Brown K. The prognostic validity of short-term abstinence in alcoholism. Alcoholism: Clin Exp Res 1994; 18:1–4.

35. Gerdes T, Yates W, Martin M, LaBrecque D. Transplantation of patients with alcoholic liver disease. Iowa Med 1994; 84:305–308.

36. Olbrisch ME, Levenson JL, Hamer R. The PACT: a rating scale for the study of clinical decision-making in psychosocial screening of organ transplant candidates. Clin Transplant 1989; 3:164–169.

37. Trzepacz PT, DiMartini A, Tringali RD. Psychopharmacologic issues in organ transplantation. Part 2. Psychopharmacologic medications. Psychosomatics 1993; 34:290–298.

38. Janssen HLA, Brouwer JT, van der Mast RC, Schalm SW. Suicide associated with alfa-interferon therapy for chronic viral hepatitis. J Hepatol 1994; 21:241–243.

39. Goldstein MG, Haltzman SD. Intensive care. In: Stoudemire A, Fogel BS, eds. Psychiatric Care of the Medical Patient. Oxford: Oxford University Press, 1993:241–266.

40. Dammann HG. Therapy with omeprazole and clarithromycin increases serum carbamazepine levels in patients with *H. pylori* gastritis. Dig Dis Sci 1996; 41:519–520.

8

Renal Failure, Dialysis, and Transplantation

Norman B. Levy
Coney Island Hospital and
State University of New York Health Science Center at Brooklyn
Brooklyn, New York

HISTORICAL BACKGROUND

End-stage diseases of vital organs always led to death until 1961. In that year an invention by a surgeon and nephrologist resulted in what was termed the Scribner shunt (1). To understand its background, one must know the following information. Kidney failure affects 150–250 people per 1,000,000 population per year, worldwide (2). Since kidneys are vital organs, in the past an individual with kidney failure died. This occurred despite the fact that artificial substitution for kidney function was possible. This was an osmotic process in which a patient's blood on one side of a semipermeable membrane and a fluid (dialysate) on the other achieved an osmotic flow in which wastes and fluid in the blood passed through the semipermeable membrane to the dialysate fluid on the other side (3).

The mechanical problem, however, was one of repeating the process, since it would have to be done a few times a week, every week in order to sustain the patient. The difficulty was in vascular access since multiple venipunctures, at least two for each run, one taking the blood out and the other bringing the blood back into the body, would eventually result in sclerosis of peripheral vasculature so that subsequent venipunctures would become impossible. The Scribner Group at the University of Washington in Seattle mentioned above perfected a very simple device in which the radial artery and the radial vein were isolated and joined together by a plastic tube, which was brought to the outside of the skin. This enabled the clamping off of artery and vein, disconnection of the tube, and direct delivery of blood from the radial artery into the dialysis equipment and return of the blood directly into the radial vein (1). This rather simple but remarkable invention thus enabled repeated access to the vascular system and heralded it in a new area of medicine, one in which for the first time the functions of a vital organ could be substituted over a long period of time by artificial means.

Keeping in mind the wide prevalence of renal failure, this presented every community with a major biomedical ethical problem. The cost of dialysis in terms of equipment and personnel even in the 1960s was roughly $20,000 per patient per year. Only wealthy countries could afford such an investment of opening opportunity for all to be dialyzed who needed it. In the United States in the early 1960s the National Institutes of Health funded several dialysis centers to perform these procedures and to educate medical professionals to perform them. In the New York City area the only center so funded was at Kings County Hospital in Brooklyn (4). Committees were set up by dialysis units to determine who should be accepted and who should be refused acceptance for dialysis treatment. Such committees essentially had the role of determining who should live and who should die. Probably the most famous and widely discussed committee existed in Seattle. That committee as well as others had to decide essentially on the value of human life. Should a married woman with two small children be given preference over a single woman of the same age? Should there be an age cutoff so that patients beyond 55 or 60 are refused treatment, thus enabling the younger to live longer? How do you measure the value of life of a 40-year-old sanitation worker compared with a 40-year-old physician or judge? These were among the issues presented to these committees.

One of the more remarkable aspects concerning the period of time between 1962 and 1973, the latter being the year in which dialysis essentially became available to all in the United States, was the paucity of applications to these units. One would think that, since renal failure occurs in roughly 30,000 people per year in a country of 150 million, these centers would be deluged with applicants. It is important to note that perhaps half of the 30,000 suffering with renal failure are individuals whose death would not be greatly delayed by dialysis because their renal failure is an aspect of a generalized medical disorder. Even eliminating from the remaining figure those with systemic diseases that would not be immediately fatal if they were dialyzed, such as lupus and diabetes, a considerable number of individuals remain who would be suitable for dialysis. The factor of importance in the early days (between 1962 and 1972) was the general lack of knowledge concerning dialysis and of dialysis centers by the patients and their physicians. Many physicians who knew about dialysis either did not believe in it or saw it as an extremely arduous treatment, perhaps not worth the effort, and did not fully know how to make application to such a unit.

At the Kings County Medical Center where I was a fellow, and later an attending physician on the Medical-Psychiatric Liaison Service under Dr. Franz Reichsman, our dialysis unit had the following criteria to even be considered. The prospective patient could neither be below the age of 18 or above the age of 55, and he or she could not be suffering from any generalized disorder. Acutely psychotic people and people with addictive disorders were excluded. Neither Dr. Reichsman nor I entered into the decision process, but rather supplied the two nephrologists and two urologists who constituted the selection committee at our center with psychosocial data enabling them to make their own determinations (5).

In 1972, chiefly through the action of the National Association of Patients on Dialysis and Transplantation, an organization founded at our Center, the U.S. Congress passed and the president signed a bill that extended Medicare enrollment to patients with kidney failure irrespective of their age. Together with Medicaid, this essentially made dialysis available to every individual domiciled in the United States. With a passing of time and an enlargement of centers, dialysis became available not only to people with systemic diseases, such as diabetes and lupus, but even to near-terminal people with Alzheimer's disease in nursing homes. With the rising cost of medical care, this has presented us with some interesting ethical issues concerning cost containment and arguments against the "overavailability" of dialysis treatment in this country.

Other modalities of treatment for renal failure emerged. Even before the availability of the Scribner shunt, the use of peritoneal dialysis was entertained. This essentially utilized the peritoneum as the semipermeable membrane and involved the infusion of dialysate fluid into the abdomen and, later, its removal. Early problems concerning this modality of treatment involved the rather high incidence of peritonitis, which essentially, aside from pain and other signs and symptoms of infection, compromised the peritoneal space, making the procedure a very time-limited one (6). Newer methods of treatment have subsequently enabled peritoneal dialysis to be a feasible alternate treatment. With a better understanding concerning methods of counteracting the immune mechanisms of the body, transplantation of kidneys from related compatible relatives as well as from cadaveric kidneys also emerged as a feasible and, in many ways, a more desirable method of treatment.

CASE HISTORY

A 42-year-old former policeman with chronic glomerulonephritis and preexisting untreated depression developed renal failure. He presented problems to the dialysis staff from the onset of his hemodialytic treatment in his attitude of hopelessness and disregard of dietary restrictions. I was initially consulted by telephone by the dialysis charge nurse late on a Friday afternoon because the patient had come in intoxicated with alcohol. Having seen him 6 months previously, just prior to the onset of his dialytic treatment, I knew his case relatively well and felt comfortable giving some advice over the telephone prior to seeing him at his next dialysis run. I suggested that he be told that he would be dialyzed that day subject to his having good behavior in the treatment unit and if his behavior was not acceptable that day that he be dismissed from the run and wait to be dialyzed at his next scheduled appointment. I also suggested to the charge nurse that, if the nephrologist in charge was in agreement with me, the patient be told that, should he appear again intoxicated, he will not be permitted to have that dialysis treatment. The nephrologist agreed, the patient presented no behavior problem at that time, and I saw him at his next treatment. He appeared severely depressed and expressed profound feelings of hopelessness, helplessness, and poor self-esteem. He had both a sleeping and an eating disorder with marked reduction in appetite. It was impossible to assess the significance of his weight loss because the initiation of dialysis resulted in a great diuresis of fluid. He related his despondency to the loss of his position as a police officer. He had been a lieutenant in the New York City Police Department with 22 years of service and had been in line for promotion to captain before the onset of his renal failure, which forced him to retire. In addition to helping him identify his several losses, which included position, esteem, money, and some diminution in sexual ability with a moderate problem with impotence, I recommended that he be started on a selective serotonin-uptake inhibitor (SSRI) antidepressant. The combination of behavioral limits set by the nurse and the effect of the antidepressant produced a marked lessening of his depression and change in his behavior. Although he did not change his eating habits, he restrained from alcohol, a problem that his father had and which the patient abhorred. He also was subsequently successful in being reemployed in a supervisory capacity as a Wells Fargo security guard.

PSYCHIATRIC PROBLEMS SEEN IN DIALYSIS PATIENTS

The above case illustrates at least four problems of psychiatric significance not uncommonly seen in patients with renal failure: depression, uncooperativeness, impairment of sexual function, and problems of dependency/independency. To understand these aspects better, one must understand the stressful aspects of kidney failure and its treatments. All patients with renal failure sustain many losses. During the period of uremia, while untreated and in the early phases of treatment, there is a marked loss of energy and a spectrum of physical symptoms including loss of appetite, nausea, itching, sleeplessness, and difficulty concentrating, which may be part of an early uremic delirium. Dialysis treatment, although it improves a patient's physical status, never produces the state of physical well-being that a patient has prior to renal failure. People with normal renal function have 24-hour, around-the-clock clearance of wastes and fluid from their bloodstream by their kidneys, whereas patients on dialysis have a three times weekly time-limited cleansing process. Between dialysis runs there is an accumulation of waste products resulting in relatively mild uremia.

Dependency-Independency Conflicts

The treatment process itself produces a very artificial state of unusual and abject dependency upon the procedure, which prevents the patient from having the degree of freedom that he or she experienced in the past (5). Several measures have lessened the degree of dependency, including home dialysis and an exchange of patients by dialysis centers so that they need not travel so far for treatment. Nevertheless, most patients do not travel, and even if they do they have constraints upon their freedom. Among patients whose premorbid personality was one of great independence, such a system of treatment can weigh very heavy and cause them a good deal of dissatisfaction over their lost freedom. Indeed this was the case for the former police officer in the above-mentioned case history. Most people on dialysis and many receiving renal transplants never return to the degree of outside work activity they had prior to the onset of renal failure. Although disability payments and insurance compensate many, it is very uncommon for a patient to receive the equivalent of the financial compensation from work that existed prior to kidney failure. Employment is also more than just a method of earning money; for many people it is very intimately attached to their sense of self-esteem and even their sense of gender identity. It has been estimated that two thirds of dialysis patients do not return to full-time work activity (7). Even the advent of Epogen, a substance that enables patients to virtually achieve the hematocrit that they had prior to renal failure, has not materially affected the rate of unemployment in these people (8,9). Most patients eventually experience a loss of sexual interest and ability, which will be discussed later. Needless to say, such losses may exacerbate a previous depression or precipitate a new one.

Depression

The prevalence of major depressive disorders in this group of patients is not fully known. However, it is the opinion of most people working in consultation liaison psychiatry that the most common psychological complication of medical or surgical illness is either depression or depression/anxiety, and renal failure is certainly no exception to this (10). Since depression can mean a number of different things, I have used the term here to imply a depressive syndrome, which is something more than a depressed mood, involving in addition feelings of low self-esteem, worthlessness, feelings of hopelessness and/or helplessness, and at times suicidal ideas and suicidal acts (11). The somatic concomitants of depression, which are more easily identified in a nonmedically sick group of people, include diminished sexual interest and eating and sleeping disorders. Since the latter set of symptoms may be part of the uremic syndrome, they may become difficult to identify as benchmarks of depression in these patients.

Delirium

Organic mental disorders, i.e., delirium and dementia, refer to mental illnesses connected with either destruction of brain tissue or interference with brain function due to metabolic, circulatory, or other toxic effects. The hallmark of this group of disorders is diminution in the cognitive (i.e., intellectual) functions. This may be manifested by loss of recent memory, diminished ability to concentrate, and diminished ability to perform other intellectual functions such as mental arithmetic and abstraction. In severe cases aphasia is seen as well as personality changes and, in some cases, florid psychosis.

Anxiety

Anxiety is a protective response of organisms to impending danger. This usually involves fight or flight, but in our species, for whom such an avenue of escape is not often opened, the individual may experience the somatic effects of a desire to escape without actually engaging in such behavior (13). This may produce a feeling of fright together with rapid heartbeat, perspiration, and even panic reaction. Anxiety is not uncommonly seen in patients actively receiving dialysis. This process involves the removal of blood from the body and its treatment in a piece of equipment, which then returns it to that individual. Virtually every patient on dialysis has experienced fellow patients having episodes of bleeding, coma, cardiac, and other emergencies, which may cause the patient anxiety when he or she receives this treatment.

Uncooperativeness

Uncooperative behavior, although not a category of a psychiatric illness, nevertheless is often determined by conflict and psychological symptoms. Its significance lies in the fact that it is one of the most vexing matters with which nephrology professionals must deal. With the "democratization" of dialysis in the United States, treatments for renal failure are available for the entire spectrum of the community. Renal disease, to a degree, favors the uncooperative patient and also the substance abuser. People who are unable or unwilling to adhere to their dietary restrictions and medical regimen, who are hypertensive and/or diabetic, are more prone to renal failure than those who follow their doctors' instructions. Therefore, the patient who is uncooperative with medical treatment stands a much better chance of developing renal failure and is more represented among those receiving dialysis. Furthermore, use of heroin and other addictive substances may lead to renal failure. Thus the population of people with kidney failure, although involving the entire spectrum of society, somewhat favors the substance abuser and uncooperative patient. In the days when the nephrologist could decide whom to accept as dialysis patients, those who caused difficulty for medical professionals were certainly less favored as patients. People who are depressed are not necessarily the easiest people to treat. Depression has been viewed as aggression expressed inwardly, but, some of the inward feeling of depressed people may express itself in the outward direction. Another factor is that gratitude among the medically ill is not common. Many sick people are very angry that they have been "chosen" to be sick and look with envy around them. Thus, a mother of two young children who is being dialyzed may look at an older, unmarried nurse and express feelings as to the unfairness that she has been "selected" for renal failure, while a person with fewer dependents remains healthy.

Suicide

Suicidal behavior is much more common among dialysis and transplant patients than among the general population. The studies measuring suicide, though not recent show that it is not an uncommon method of demise (14,15). Here I am referring to actual suicide rate and separating it from voluntary withdrawal from dialysis, which will be undertaken later in this chapter. The combination of depression, a difficult and compromised existence, and having a method of carrying through readily upon it make these patients much more prone to suicide. Populations that exhibit a greater incidence of suicide, such as policeman, physicians, dentists, and nurses, all have a common characteristic that they share with dialysis patients: they can more readily kill themselves than the general population. A dialysis patient may simply go on a potassium binge by eating some bananas or oranges and miss a couple of dialysis runs in order to guarantee his or her demise. Voluntary withdrawal from dialysis, although technically a suicide, is viewed somewhat differently (16–18). Provided one rules out a major depressive disorder with a suicide wish, voluntary withdrawal may be viewed as a realistic option in patients who face an extremely compromised quality of life (19).

Sexual Dysfunction

Sexual disorders are common in people receiving treatment for renal failure, by either dialysis or renal transplant (20,21). The observation was made many years ago that men on dialysis seem to have greater impotence problems than the general population or even other men with chronic medical illnesses. A number of epidemiological surveys of both men and women have been done that show that roughly one third of men on dialysis are totally impotent, another one third are partially impotent, and the remaining third have no significant problem in this area. In women, orgasm during intercourse as a measure of sexual pleasure has been used, and it has been found to be markedly diminished. When comparing the frequency of intercourse prior to either dialysis or renal transplantation, the data are rather striking, showing marked deterioration primarily in men on dialysis and least in transplanted women (21). Although psychological factors likely play a role (certainly a secondary one), most research points to an organic basis for these sexual dysfunctions, in particular impotence. Since men normally experience erections during phase I REM sleep, the failure to get an erection during sleep favors an organic explanation of this problem. Evaluations of nocturnal penile tumescence point in the direction of marked organic deterioration in men on dialysis (22,23). Psychological factors may also play a role. In both genders sexuality is very closely related to one's gender identity. In women on forms of dialysis, there tends to be a marked diminution in fertility and not infrequently a total cessation of menstruation. These factors may compromise a woman's gender identity, especially when her sense of femininity was somewhat compromised before becoming sick with kidney disease. Likewise, if a man's sense of masculinity is somewhat compromised to begin with, the impact of renal failure may significantly affect his sexual function. People with renal failure eventually get to a point in which they essentially stop urinating or urinate necessarily due to "bladder sweat." The effect upon men may be great here since the organ of urination is also the genital organ. By far the most common use of the penis in the course of a day is for the purpose of urination. The impact of this loss, especially in a man whose sense of masculinity is compromised, may also be felt as a loss of masculinity. Secondary sexual dysfunctions also play an important role here. In the case of sexual dysfunction of purely physical origin, the impact of compromise of this activity may have a profound psychological effect. For example, if a relatively young man with longstanding diabetes has a single episode of impotence on the basis of a peripheral neuropathy, it may have significant psychological importance. If he responds to this episode as evidence of a deterioration of his masculinity and withdraws from future sexual encounters, as is not uncommonly the case, he may have what is termed a secondary sexual dysfunction. Therefore, even organically caused sexual dysfunction may lead to the psychological difficulties that may further compound this problem (24,25).

RENAL TRANSPLANTATION

General Considerations

In the view of most nephrology professionals, a successful renal transplant offers the best opportunity to the patient to resume a life closest to that experienced prior to renal failure. However, there are major obstacles in attaining such a transplant. The resource of available kidneys is limited. In the case of cadaveric transplants, although throughout the United States driver's licenses permit individuals to state their preference for organ donation, the actual decision to donate belongs to the nearest relative of the deceased. Most relatives refuse such requests. This is also true of live related donations, since this involves major surgery and deprives the potential donors of an organ they often incorrectly assume may have present or future essential use. This is particularly true of African Americans, who have a much higher refusal rate than other groups. Additional limiting factors include the limited surgical resources. Last but not least, many people with renal failure are hesitant to undergo a surgical procedure that is potentially life-threatening and certainly results in a reasonably long period of postsurgical morbidity (26–28).

Psychological Problems

The psychological problems seen in renal transplant patients include the effect of immunosuppressant medications, especially prednisone and, to a lesser extent, cyclosporine. Patients receiving these medications may experience complications of anxiety, depression, and even emergence of psychosis. A dialysis patient may have a sense of feeling the sword of Damocles hanging over him or her, especially postoperatively when there is the greatest chance of rejection. The potential for rejection remains throughout the lifetime of the transplanted kidney. The successful use of denial as a coping mechanism can enable many if not most patients to push away their concern about rejection (26). Those who have difficulty in this area are usually anxious. Because of the action of immunosuppressive medication, people receiving renal transplants are much more prone to a wide variety of bacterial and fungal infections, including some very serious ones, as well as an increase in incidence of cancer. Needless to say, this can and often does take a significant psychological toll (27–29).

Treatment Options

Preventive Measures

Many treatment options are available to patients with renal failure. The selection of the modality of treatment should be made on the basis of psychosocial including family factors. As mentioned, one of the great stresses of dialysis is the feeling of abject dependence, which may place the very independent patient in a most uncomfortable and even untenable situation. Therefore, the personality style of the patient is a factor to consider. The very independent patient should be either transplanted or put into a form of dialytic treatment in which he or she can be active in the treatment process. Home dialysis offers one such opportunity. Another is that of continuous ambulatory peritoneal dialysis (CAPD). This is a treatment choice in which an individual perfuses his or her abdomen four to five times per day with dialysate fluid and slowly receives return dialysate in a plastic bag underneath the clothing. For individuals whose social support system is not great, the option of home dialysis is less available to them (29).

Patients should be informed about the psychological complications of their treatment so that, if they occur, they will understand it and more likely seek medical attention. For example, since the incidence of impotence is close to 70% in dialysis patients (21), every man should be told of this possibility. If this is done, it is more likely that a patient having the onset of impotence will see this as a complication of treatment and/or illness rather than something having to do with an innate defect in his body. He will also more likely call this to the attention of the medical staff, who may be able to help in its treatment. The issue of voluntary withdrawal should also be raised. Patients should be told that this option may arise in their minds, and if so it should be brought to the attention of nephrology and other professionals. This is an important point, because patients often hide these feelings and by the time they are known to the staff they have made firm commitments to their demise.

Patients should be interviewed by a psychologically trained person—social worker, nurse, psychologist, or psychiatrist—prior to onset of treatment so that individuals who are more prone to psychological complications may be identified early. People with a background of substance abuse, child abuse, and previous psychiatric illness are more vulnerable to psychological problems and should be identified as individuals who need to be more closely monitored for their emergence (30).

Talking Therapies

It is my experience as well as that of many others working in this area that patients on forms of treatment for renal failure tend to be most resistive to receiving any talking therapy for their psychological problems. They already feel "overdoctored" and also tend to see their problems as a result of their physical difficulties rather than having to do with emotional conflicts. However, among selected patients therapies may be conducted with or without the use of psychotropics, especially when they are done in the dialysis unit itself. The issue of confidentiality even in relatively close spaces seems to be of greater concern to the therapist than to the patient. Most individuals in a busy dialysis unit are so involved with themselves that they are not aware of the conversation occurring beyond the drawn curtains around the next dialysis chair.

Sexual Behavior Therapies

Behavior therapy holds great promise for the treatment of sexual dysfunction in dialysis patients. It permits them to regain sexual function by encouraging activity with their partners, not necessarily including sexual intercourse. A change of direction from avoidance to encounter is the therapeutic goal (31).

Exercise

A fair amount of research has shown that exercise not only may diminish blood pressure in dialysis patients but, also has a definite anxiolytic and antidepressant effect. Its use in patients with renal failure is encouraged.

Psychologically Active Medications

Several important factors need to be understood prior to the prescription of any medication to people with renal failure. Individuals without kidney function who are on dialysis or who have transplants that are not functioning well need to be monitored concerning the use of medications eliminated by the kidney (32,33). With some exceptions, no such medication should be prescribed for them. Such an exception is lithium, which will be discussed a bit later. Many factors influence the pharmacokinetics of medications in these patients. This includes their absorption, which may be compromised, as well as factors surrounding the issue of protein binding. Patients with renal failure have a diminished ability to protein-bind medications. Since many medicines and virtually all of the psychologically active ones are protein bound, this is a significant factor. It is the unbound form of the medication that is pharmacologically active and can cause side effects (34). Thus, an individual with an inability to protein bind will tend to have more medication available in a free form. Therefore, the general rule of thumb in patients with renal failure concerning the use of psychologically active medication is the following: one should use no more than two-thirds the maximum dose of medication that one would use on an individual with normal kidney function (33). An additional consideration concerning the medication of these patients is whether or not that medication is dialyzed. If it is, it may reach subtherapeutic levels during a dialysis run (34,35). Fortunately virtually all of the psychologically active medications (with exceptions to be mentioned) are fat soluble, pass the blood-brain barrier, are not removed by the kidney, but are detoxified by the liver and eliminated in bile in the feces. Exceptions to this include the barbiturates meprobamate and lithium.

Lithium

Lithium it is entirely removed by the kidney and is also completely dialyzed since it is a small molecule. Thus, patients who need to receive lithium who are on dialysis should get a single dose after each dialysis run. Since it is completely eliminated by the kidney, levels will be maintained between dialyses and the medication removed during the process of dialysis (36,37). Experience has shown that patients with bipolar disorder do not run into difficulties during the few-hour period during a dialysis run in which their lithium level is subtherapeutic.

Anxiolytic Agents

Anxiety can best be handled by the administration of short-acting benzodiazepines, such as lorazepam (Ativan) or alprazolam (Xanax) (38). Benzodiazepines that have pharmacologically active metabolites, such as librium and valium, should be avoided in dialysis patients because if they are given chronically, high blood levels can occur (39). Barbiturates should not be prescribed because they are less efficacious than benzodiazepines and some are only partially dialyzed.

Antidepressants

Antidepressants can play an important role in the treatment of depressant symptoms. It has been suggested that those that have been widely used in these patients should be favored since their track record is known. The tricyclic antidepressants have many disadvantages because of their side effects and because they can be used to commit suicide. The selective serotonin-reuptake inhibitors are preferable. Fluoxetine (Prozac) is very well tolerated, and there is published research showing its efficacy and that it is well tolerated in these patients (40–42).

Tranquilizers

Administration of haloperidol (Haldol) or similar agents is useful in controlling acute psychotic symptoms in patients with delirium or dementia. In general it is safer to use medications with a longer track record because their side effects are better known and because their safety in this group of patients has been clinically established.

CONCLUSION

The psychological treatment of people with renal failure is challenging. It requires some basic knowledge of the treatment modalities and the special considerations connected with this form of organ failure.

REFERENCES

1. Quinton W, Dillard D, Scribner BH. Cannulation of blood vessels for prolonged hemodialysis. Trans Am Soc Artif Organs 1960; 6:104–108.
2. Walser M. Conservative management of the uremic patient. In: Brenner BM, Rector FC Jr, eds. The Kidney. 2d ed. Philadelphia: Saunders, 1981:2383–2424.
3. Merrill JP, Smith S III, Calahan EJ III, Thorn GW. The use of an artificial kidney I. Technique. J Clin Invest 1950; 29:412–418.
4. Levy NB. Psychological studies at the Downstate Medical Center of patients on hemodialysis. Med Clin N Am 1977; 61:759–769.
5. Reichsman F, Levy NB. Problems in adaptation to hemodialysis: a four-year study of 25 patients. Arch Intern Med 1972; 130:850–865.
6. Majorca R, Cancarni G. Techniques, complications, and indications of peritoneal dialysis. In: Massry, SG, Glassock, RJ, eds. Textbooks of Nephrology. 3d ed. Baltimore: Williams & Wilkins, 1995:1563–1570.
7. Gutman RA. Stead WW. Robinson RR. Physical activity and employment status of patients on maintenance dialysis. N Engl J Med 1981; 304:309–313.
8. Antonoff A, Mallinger M. Vocational rehabilitation: limitations and resistance of renal patients. Dial Transplant 1991; 10:604–609.
9. Evans RW. Recombinant human erythropoietin and the qualtity of life of end-stage renal disease patients: a comparative analysis. Am J Dis 1991; 4:62–70.
10. Kaplan De Nour A. Social adjustment of chronic dialysis patients. Am J Psychiatry 1982; 139:97–100.
11. DSM IV: The Diagnostic and Statistical Manual of Mental Diseases. 4th ed. Washington, DC: American Psychiatric Association, 1994.
12. Lipowski ZJ. Delirium. Springfield, IL: Charles C. Thomas, 1980.
13. Colon EA, Popkin MK. Anxiety and panic. In: Rundell JR, Wise MG, eds. Textbook of Consultation-Liaison Psychiatry. Washington, DC: American Psychiatric Press, 1996:402–425.
14. Abram HS, Moore GC, Westervelt FB Jr. Suicidal behavior in chronic dialysis patients. Am J Psychiatry 1971; 127:1199–1204.
22. Karacan I. Assessment of nocturnal penile tumescence as an objective method for evaluating sexual functions in ESRD patients. Dial Transplant 1978; 7:872–876.
23. Procci WR, Goldstein DA, Adelstein J. Sexual dysfunction in the male uremic patient: a reappraisal. Kidney Int 1982; 19:317–323.
24. Levy NB. Psychological complications of disalysis: psychonephrology to the rescue. Bull Menninger Clin 1984; 48:237–250.
25. Levy NB. Coping with maintenance hemodialysis: psychological considerations in the care of patients. In: Messry SG, Sellers AL, eds. Clinical Aspects of Uremia and Dialysis. Springfield, IL: Charles C. Thomas, 1976:53–68.
26. Levy NB. Psychological aspects of renal transplantation. Psychosomatics 1994; 35:427–433.
27. Surman OS. Hemodialysis and transplantation. In: Cassem NH, ed. Handbook of General Hospital Psychiatry. 3d ed. St. Louis: Mosby Yearbook, 1991:401–430.
28. Wolcott DL. Organ transplant psychiatry: psychiatry's role in the second gift of life. Psychosomatics 1990; 31:91–97.

29. Fricchione GL. Psychiatric aspects of renal transplantation. Aust NZ J Psychiatry 1989; 23:407–417.
30. Friedman EA. Strategy in Renal Failure. New York: John Wiley, 1978.
31. McKevitt PM. Treating sexual dysfunction in dialysis and transplant patients. Health Soc Work 1976; 1:132–157.
32. Bennett WM, Aronoff GR, Golper A, Morrison G, Singer I, Brater DC. Drug Prescribing in Renal Failure: Dosing Guidelines for Adults. Philadelphia: American College of Physicians, 1987.
33. Brater DC. Drug Use in Kidney Disease. Sydney: AIDS Health Science Press, 1985.
34. Wagner JG. Fundamentals of Clinical Pharmacokinetics. Hamilton, IL: Drug Intelligence Publications, 1975.
35. Reidenberg MM. The biotransformation of drugs in renal failure. Am J Med 1977; 62: 882–485.
36. Port FK, Kroll PD, Rosenweig J. Lithium therapy during maintenance hemodialysis. Psychosomatics 1977; 20:130–132.
37. Levy NB. Use of psychotropics in patients with kidney failure. Psychosomatics 1985; 26: 699–709.
38. Greenblatt DJ, Divoll M, Abernathy R, Ochs HR, Shader RI. Clinical pharmacokinetics of the newer benzodiazepines. Clin Pharmacokinetics 1983; 8:223–252.
39. Levy NB. Psychopharmacology in patients with renal failure. Int J Psychiatr Med 1990; 20:325–334.
40. Bergstrom RF, Beasley CM Jr, Levy NB, Blumenfield M, Lemberger L. Fluoxetine pharmacokinetics after daily doses of 20 mg. of fluoxetine in patients with severly impaired renal function. Int Clin Psychopharmacol 1993; 8:261–266.
41. Levy NB, Blumenfield M, Beasley CM Jr, Dubey AK, Solomon RJ, Todd R. Fluoxetine in depressed subjects with renal failure and subjects with normal kidney function. Gen Hosp Psychiatry 1996; 18:8–13.
42. Blumenfield M, Levy NB, Spinowitz B, Charytan C, Beasley CM Jr, Dubey A, Solomon RJ, Todd R, Goodman A, Bergstrom RF. Fluoxetine in depressed patients on dialysis. Int J Psychiatr Med 1997; 27:71–80.

9

Endocrine Disorders

Caroline Carney
University of Iowa College of Medicine
Iowa City, Iowa

ILLUSTRATIVE CASE

KG is a 54-year-old, recently divorced man who had been evaluated and treated for type II diabetes mellitus 3 years prior to presentation. He presented with a 2-month history of complaints of fatigue, tremulousness, diaphoresis, vague abdominal pain (for which he requested narcotic analgesia), and intermittent brief losses of consciousness. Previous evaluation revealed normal metabolic indices except for intermittent plasma glucose values ranging from 50 to 60 mg/dl. Abdominal imaging studies and upper and lower endoscopy were unremarkable. No evidence for diabetes mellitus was found. He was admitted and placed on a 48-hour fast. He frequently requested pain medications. Approximately 4 hours into the fast, he developed diaphoresis and confusion. A plasma glucose was noted at 51 mg/dl. The patient's C-peptide level was not suppressed. A urine screen was remarkable for measurable levels of glyburide. The patient left the hospital against medical advice.

INTRODUCTION

An association between endocrine disease and psychiatric disorder has been noted over centuries of medical practice. Psychiatric manifestations of endocrine disease may appear so similar to a primary psychiatric process that even the most astute clinician may have difficulty considering an underlying medical diagnosis. Psychiatric disorders, conversely, may covertly influence the course and prognosis of primary endocrine disorders. In the extreme, medical treatments such as insulin may be the means of creating illness such as occurs in factitious disorders. The aims of this chapter are to provide an overview of the primary medical process, discuss the physical and mental presentation of the illness, provide a guide to the laboratory evaluation of a patient presenting with symptoms suggestive of an endocrine disorder, discuss the psychiatric morbidity associated with the endocrine disorder, and provide a brief synopsis of treatment issues.

DIABETES MELLITUS

Overview

The relationship between emotional factors and diabetes mellitus was referred to as early as 1679 by the English physician Thomas Willis (1). Diabetes mellitus is a disease of impaired glucose metabolism affecting children and adults, which has profound physical and psychological effects. The morbidity associated with the disease is extreme and includes renal failure, blindness, increased rates of vascular disease, and amputation. Given the substantial morbidity and the obligatory lifestyle modifications associated with adequate treatment, it is no surprise that psychiatric morbidity is common to the disease.

Diabetes mellitus is divided into three subclasses: Type I, or insulin-dependent diabetes mellitus (IDDM); Type II, or non–insulin-dependent mellitus (NIDDM); and diabetes mellitus attributable to another cause such as primary pancreatic disease (2). Additionally, gestational diabetes and impaired glucose tolerance are associated with the development of diabetes mellitus. This section will focus primarily on Type I and Type II diabetes mellitus.

Type I diabetes mellitus results from an autoimmune destruction of pancreatic beta-cells and subsequent loss of pancreatic insulin secretory capacity and secondary insulin resistance. Beta-cell destruction is likely mediated by T-cell–and macrophage-released cytokines or cytotoxic T cells. The disease is thought to be caused by an interplay of genetic, environmental, and autoimmune factors. The evidence for genetic factors is compelling given reported concordance rates ranging from 30 to 50% in identical twins. Class II HLA haplotype antigens DR3/x, DR4/x, and DR3/4 are linked to Type I diabetes mellitus. Environmental factors believed to contribute to the pathogenesis include viral illness such as rubella, coxsackievirus, and mumps. Finally, approximately 80% of newly diagnosed individuals express islet cell antibodies (2).

Type II diabetes mellitus is mediated by genetic and environmental causes that lead to impaired insulin secretion and tissue resistance to the action of insulin. Concordance rates in identical twins are nearly 100%, but a specific genetic defect has not yet been identified. Environmental factors are believed to modify the expression of the disorder. Upper body and abdominal obesity versus lower body or peripheral obesity is associated with insulin resistance (2). Reduced physical activity and increased caloric intake may contribute to the genesis of the disease in some population groups.

The prevalence of Type I diabetes mellitus in the United States is approximately 0.03%. Prevalence rates are variable among ethnic groups consistent with a genetic mechanism for the disease. The prevalence of Type II diabetes mellitus varies with the population assessed. The overall prevalence in the United States is estimated at 3–5%, but increases to 10–15% among individuals older than 50 years. Native Americans, African Americans, Mexican descendants, and Japanese immigrants to the United State have higher prevalence rates in the United States (2).

Patient Presentation

Type I diabetes mellitus may have a gradual or abrupt presentation. The disease most commonly presents in children and young adults. Classic symptoms include weight loss, polyuria, polydipsia, and polyphagia. Patients may complain of fatigue or an antecedent illness. Persons with advanced disease will have complaints consistent with end-organ involvement such as neuropathy. Type II diabetics tend to be obese persons older than 40 years of age. Although the symptoms may be the same as in Type I, they are mild in comparison, delaying the diagnosis.

Physical Examination

The physical examination may be unremarkable early in the course of the disease. Advanced disease is associated with physical findings including hypertension. Diminished visual acuity is noted with both Type I and Type II diabetes and is usually the result of proliferative retinopathy. Fundascopic examination reveals the presence of preproliferative microaneurysms, hemorrhages, and exudates ("cotton wool" patches). Proliferative changes occur with the initial growth of minute bunches of blood vessels and fibrous tissue on the retina or optic nerve head, which ultimately extend to the vitreous. The neurological examination may be remarkable for diminished, usually symmetrical sensory loss (thermal and vibratory discrimination), diminished reflexes, and muscle wasting of the hands and feet. Examination of the feet may reveal the skin surface to be warm and dry. Persons with advanced atherosclerotic disease may have diminished peripheral pulses and plantar ulcerations, which are frequently painless.

Mental Status Examination

The mental status examination may be entirely normal if no coexisting psychiatric syndrome is present. A depressed diabetic patient will present similarly to a nondiabetic patient with major depressive disorder (3). The presence of weight loss may not discriminate depressed from nondepressed diabetics; however, it may be an important discriminator in diabetics with an eating disorder (3). Cognitive functioning in insulin-dependent diabetic patients is generally well maintained, even at substantially elevated levels of blood glucose (4). Discrete hypoglycemic episodes, conversely, appear associated with impaired performance in simple reaction time, digit vigilance, trail-making part B, word recall, serial digit learning, and verbal fluency (4). A prospective 9-year study assessing the relationship between intensive insulin therapy, sometimes associated with frequent episodes of hypoglycemia, did not reveal impairment in neuropsychological performance (5).

Laboratory Evaluation

The diagnosis of diabetes mellitus is made if (1) a random fasting serum glucose ≥ 200 mg/dl or is noted in a patient with "classic" diabetic symptoms including polydipsia, polyuria, and weight loss, (2) glucose is >140 mg/dl on at least two occasions, (3) fasting glucose is <140, but following a 75-g glucose load, both the 2-hour sample and some other value between the fasting and 2-hour value are >200 mg/dl.

Role in Psychiatric Conditions

Diabetes mellitus has been commonly associated with two psychiatric conditions: affective disorders and eating disorders. Both types of condition are thought to begin early in the disease, complicate the course of the diabetes, and likely affect long-term prognosis of the medical condition.

Major Depressive Disorder

The existence of a biological association between depression and diabetes exists is supported by two theories: (1) both conditions have been associated with dysregulation of hypothalamic-pituitary-adrenocorticol activity, resulting in abnormal cortisol production, and (2) functional deficiencies in norepinephrine and serotonin are associated with both depression and animal models of diabetes (6–8).

The prevalence of major depressive disorder in diabetes mellitus is variable depending on the population studied. Confounding biases include age, sex, socioeconomic status, obesity, concomitant medical illness, severity of diabetes, time frame of depression, participation rate, ascertainment of subjects, and differences in diagnostic assessment (6). Gavard et al. conducted a systematic review of the literature, which revealed prevalence rates of depression in Type I (IDDM) and Type II (NIDDM) diabetes ranging from 8.5 to 27.3% in controlled studies and 11.0 to 19.9% in uncontrolled studies using different diagnostic instruments (6). An increased prevalence of major depressive disorder and depressive symptoms is suggested by the review, however, the authors conclude that future studies that assess biases and methodological issues need to be conducted.

The mean age of onset of depression in IDDM may be earlier than in the general population (22.1 years vs. 27–35 years), but not in NIDDM (28.6 years). Given that the onset of NIDDM generally occurs later in life, depression may antedate the onset of diabetic illness (9). Females are more commonly affected than males.

Diagnostic approaches using structured interviews and accepted psychiatric criteria are relatively sensitive in detecting depression in patients with diabetes (10). Depressed diabetics and depressed nonmedically ill persons score similarly when assessed by the Beck Depression Inventory. The only significant differences between the two groups were noted in the items assessing fatigue, health worries, decreased interest in sex, and decreased interest in other people (3). However, both depressed groups scored significantly different than nondepressed diabetics on all measures except weight loss. One may conclude that a diabetic patient with depression will present similarly to psychiatric depressed patients without diabetes (3).

Major depressive disorder affects youths with diabetes and may influence diabetic-related complications. Major depressive disorder has been noted in 27.5% of juveniles who were 8–13 years old at the time of onset of IDDM and were studied longitudinally from initial diagnosis for a median interval of 9 years (11). The highest incidence rates were noted in the first year after diagnosis. Conduct and generalized anxiety disorder were also noted in this population (11). Young women with diabetes are at nine times greater risk for recurrent depression than their male counterparts (12). Antecedent clinical depression has been shown to be a risk factor for retinopathy in young adults with IDDM (13). The literature reviewing the effects of depression on retinopathy, nephropathy, and neuropathy in adult diabetics is controversial and inconsistent, although depression may be associated with poorer glycemic control (10). Depression may also affect compliance with weight loss programs and have significant correlation with hyperglycemic and hypoglycemic symptoms (14,15).

Effective treatments for depressed diabetics include pharmacotherapy, psychotherapy, and electroconvulsive therapy (ECT). Goodnick et al. (16) reviewed the available literature on the pharmacological management of depressed diabetics. Given the potential for significant side effects with monoamine oxidase inhibitors and tricyclic antidepressants, the drugs of choice in the treatment of diabetic depression are the selective serotonin-reuptake inhibitors (SSRIs). Monoamine oxidase inhibitors in combination with insulin and sulfonylureas have been shown to exaggerate the hypoglycemic response and lead to a delayed recovery to normal glucose concentrations (16,17). Risks associated with the use of tricyclic antidepressants in diabetic patients are related to the well-known side effects of this class of medications. Diabetic complications, including neuropathy, may be worsened by the anticholinergic and orthostatic hypotensive effects of the tricyclics. Additionally, tricyclics are noted to increase carbohydrate craving, which has implications related to weight gain and glycemic control. The noradrenergic effects of tricyclics are associated with hyperglycemia when these agents are used in long-term administration (16). SSRIs do not appear to have an adverse effect on glycemic control (16). Preliminary results by Goodnick et al. reveal reductions in depression severity and improved dietary compliance with an SSRI (16).

ECT is a beneficial treatment for the depressed medically ill patient (18). Vigilant monitoring of the diabetic patient is a necessity during the course of ECT therapy. Oral hypoglycemic agents and insulin doses may need to be held or lowered by as much as one half on treatment days. Blood glucose monitoring should be performed prior to and following the procedure to avoid hypoglycemic complications.

Eating Disorders

The association between disordered eating symptoms and eating disorders with diabetes mellitus has been hypothesized to occur related to the following issues: (1) coincidence, (2) IDDM-affiliated food preoccupation leading to disordered eating habits, (3) IDDM-affiliated chronic dietary restraint leading to disordered eating habits, (4) insulin omission providing an easily accessible and covert weight loss method, (5) insulin-associated weight gain triggering body dissatisfaction, (6) IDDM leading to early disturbances in ego development, and (7) altered family dynamics secondary to the chronic disease increasing the risk for development of an eating disorder (19).

Similar to major depressive disorder, the ascertainment of prevalence between eating disorders and diabetes mellitus is confounded by methodological issues such as characteristics of the study population (e.g., clinical vs. community samples), the response rate of the sample, measures, methods, and diagnostic criteria used (19). Three controlled studies utilizing standardized research interviews to determine the prevalence of eating disorders in a sample of diabetics and nondiabetics drawn from the case register of a hospital outpatient clinic revealed no increased incidence of clinical eating disorders in young adults (17–25 years old), adolescents (11–18 years old), and adolescents and preadolescents (8–18 years old) (20–22).

What is common to these and other studies, however, are the findings that disordered eating habits adversely affect the course of the IDDM. Several studies and case reports now document the presence of intentional insulin withholding for weight control. Intentional insulin withholding may manifest as elevated hemoglobin Alc (HbAlc) levels, recurrent bouts of diabetic ketoacidosis, more negative attitudes toward diabetes, more diabetes-related hospitalizations, and higher rates of retinopathy and neuropathy.

The identification of an eating disorder in a diabetic seen in psychiatric consultation setting may be difficult (23). The physician should attempt to obtain a history from persons in addition to the primary source and use metabolic markers such as weight loss and potassium and HbAlc levels to assist in the diagnosis. Low potassium levels may indicate vomiting or diuretic abuse.

Treatment of patients with eating disorders and diabetes mellitus may be complex. A three-step plan has been proposed (24): (1) stabilization of the diabetes mellitus, followed by (2) formal treatment for the disordered eating behavior, and (3) long-term treatment to maintain proper glycemic control and control of eating-disordered symptoms. Treatment of eating and weight symptoms should be designated to a specialist. Additional benefit may be obtained with education about the risks of eating disorders, the use of insulin, family dynamics, and normal eating habits (25).

Treatment of Diabetes Mellitus

The key elements in the comprehensive management of the diabetic patient are to (1) avoid the short-term consequences of insulin insufficiency, including symptomatic hyperglycemia, diabetic ketoacidosis, and nonketotic hyperosmolar syndrome, and

(2) ameliorate the complications of longstanding disease such as nephropathy, retinopathy, neuropathy, and vascular disease (26). Glycemic control remains the cornerstone underlying these elements. Glycemic control is best achieved in IDDM with a combination of insulin, dietary modification, physical activity, and avoidance of alcohol. Regimens should vary according to patient need and compliance. Typical regimens include (1) conventional therapy, which warrants at least two daily injections of more than one insulin type to address both the basal and dietary insulin requirements, (2) multiple daily insulin injections (also known as intensive conventional therapy), which employs treatment of the basal insulin requirement with once or twice daily injections and treatment of the dietary insulin requirement with preprandial injections, and (3) treatment of the basal requirement with a continuous infusion of insulin delivered via a subcutaneously implanted pump and meeting dietary requirements with preprandial injections (26).

Treatment of Type II diabetes is quite variable. Some patients can be managed with a combination of diet and exercise alone, while others ultimately require insulin therapy. Pharmacotherapy is achieved with the use of sulfonylureas, biaguanides, or alpha-glucosidase inhibitors. The sulfonylureas most commonly used in the United States are glyburide and glipizide. These drugs are contraindicated in children, Type I diabetes mellitus, and pregnancy. Complications include hypoglycemia and toxic reactions.

The biaguanide metformin may be used for primary treatment of Type II diabetes mellitus, especially in obese, insulin-resistant patients. It acts by inhibiting hepatic gluconeogenisis and by enhancing glucose uptake in the peripheral tissues. Metformin has been shown to cause a reduction in triglycerides and low-density lipoprotein while increasing high-density lipoprotein. This medication is contraindicated in persons with severe renal or liver disease, heart failure, pulmonary insufficiency, pregnancy, or alcoholism. Metformin does not cause hypoglycemia. Complications include nausea, anorexia, diarrhea, metallic taste, and rarely lactic acidosis (26). Metformin has been reported to have caused panic attacks in one individual, presumably due to elevated lactic acid levels (27).

Alpha-glucosidase inhibitors such as acarbose function by competitively inhibiting intestinal disaccharidases, leading to postprandial reductions in glucose. They do not effect the fasting glucose. Given the local mechanism of action, complications of acarbose include abdominal pain, flatulence, and diarrhea. The drug is contraindicated in persons with liver disease, obstructive bowel disease, and inflammatory bowel disease.

HYPOGLYCEMIA

Overview

Hypoglycemia is a clinical condition characterized by intermittent episodes of low plasma glucose, commonly, but not absolutely, defined as a value below 50 mg/dl, with or without symptoms (28). The disorder has been classically described by Whipple as exhibiting three components: documented low blood sugar, characteristic signs and symptoms, and improvement of signs and symptoms with administration of glucose (29). A discussion of hypoglycemia is pertinent to medical psychiatry because of the neuropsychiatric manifestations of the documented condition and the comorbid psychiatric conditions of persons who may inappropriately bear the diagnosis.

The etiology of hypoglycemia can be divided into two major classifications: diabetes-related and spontaneous. The former is found in both Type I and Type II diabetics and occurs with (1) increase or overdose of medications (insulin, sulfonylureas, alcohol, beta-blockers), (2) dietary changes, and (3) increased physical activity. Spontaneous hypoglycemia has a broader differential diagnosis, which includes both fasting (>6 hours following last food ingestion) and postprandial (<5 hours from last food ingestion) elements. Fasting hypoglycemia may be secondary to liver disease, insulinoma, alcohol intoxication, adrenocortical insufficiency, hypothyroidism, growth hormone deficiency, and renal failure–related malnutrition. Postprandial hypoglycemia results from insulin secretion following meals in persons with partial gastrectomy or glucose-intolerant individuals (26). An important third cause of hypoglycemia is factitious hypoglycemia, which will be discussed later.

Patient Presentation

The presentation of symptoms in a patient with hypoglycemia is generally stable within the patient but may be vastly different between patients (28). Symptoms are classically divided into two categories: adrenergic and neuroglycopenic. The use of the term "adrenergic" may be incorrect as symptoms in this category are the result of both catecholamine and acetylcholine-mediated systems. Hypothalamic activation is responsible for the "adrenergic" symptoms. The parasympathetic, sympathetic, and cholinergic systems are also activated. Neuroglycopenic symptoms have been attributed to the effects of hypoglycemia on the cerebral cortex, followed by the cerebellum, basal ganglia, thalamus, hypothalamus, midbrain, brain stem, spinal cord, and peripheral nerves (28). The presentation of these symptoms can lead to difficulty in making the diagnosis, because patients may appear to have syndromes ranging from panic to stroke (Table 1). Hypoglycemic patients may initially be given an incorrect diagnosis because of the complexity of symptom presentation.

Physical Examination

During an episode of hypoglycemia, the vital signs may be remarkable for tachycardia and cardiac ectopy. The pulse pressure may become widened with increased systolic and decreased diastolic readings. Hypothermia and hyperthermia have been reported. The patient may appear diaphoretic and have excessive salivation. Localizing neurological deficits such as paresis, aphasia, and Babinski reflexes will resolve at the normalization of plasma glucose. The patient may seize. Visual reaction time may increase. Peripheral neuropathy may complicate repetitive episodes of hypoglycemia.

Table 1 Symptoms of Hypoglycemia

Neuroglycopenia	Adrenergic
Headache	Anxiety
Blurred vision	Nervousness
Paresthesias	Tremulousness
Weakness	Sweating
Amnesia	Hunger
Incoordination	Palpitations
Tiredness	Irritability
Confusion	Pallor
Dizziness	Nausea
Abnormal mentation	Flushing
Behavioral change	Angina
Feeling cold	
Difficulty waking in a.m.	
Senile dementia	
Organic personality syndrome	
Transient hemiplegia	
Transient aphasia	
Seizures	
Coma	

Mental Status Examination

The patient with acute hypoglycemia may appear anxious or distracted. He or she may complain of hunger. In the extreme, the patient may be obtunded and unable to communicate. Observers may note behavioral changes, memory loss, and personality change. Temper outbursts and psychotic behavior have been reported.

Laboratory Examination

Hypoglycemia may be the result of excess insulin, sulfonylureas, or a late effect of exercise in an individual with diabetes. The laboratory diagnosis of acute hypoglycemia in a symptomatic individual is made by determining the plasma glucose, insulin, and C-peptide levels. Symptoms should improve after administration of intravenous glucose. Care must given to ensure that patients with a history of alcohol abuse or dependence are treated with intravenous thiamine prior to glucose.

The diagnosis of insulinoma may be made based on history and documented plasma levels of glucose, insulin, and C-peptide. Insulinomas generally become symptomatic after 4 hours of fasting. Patients may present with complaints of symptoms occurring after they have been asleep for several hours and may eat regularly to avoid symptoms. Four diagnostic criteria must be met for evaluation of insulinoma: (1) documented plasma hypoglycemia, (2) neuroglycopenic symptoms occurring simultaneously with hypoglycemia, (3) inappropriately elevated plasma insulin ($>$5 μU/ml), and (4) inappropriately elevated C-peptide ($>$0.6 mg/dl). Monitored, controlled, inpatient 48- to 72-hour fasts may be necessary to determine the diagnosis. Baseline mental status and plasma glucose, insulin, and C-peptide levels are drawn. Labs and mental status are evaluated every 4 hours until the blood glucose has declined below 60 mg/dl, and hourly thereafter. Confirmation of two glucose levels below 40 mg/dl and evidence of neuroglycopenia should be accomplished before terminating the fast. Insulinoma is considered if the plasma and C-peptide levels do not decline with fasting plasma glucose below 40 mg/dl (30). Further work-up for insulinoma includes angiography and imaging studies.

An insulin-to-glucose ratio greater than 0.3 may be indicative of inappropriate insulin secretion. However, the test is confounded in conditions of obesity, and neuroglyopenic symptoms must be present with documented C-peptide levels. The tolbutamide stimulation test may be useful, but it must be done in centers with standardized protocols. Finally, the C-peptide suppression test may be useful in the diagnosis of insulinoma (30).

Role in Psychiatric Conditions

Three psychiatric syndromes have been described in affiliation with hypoglycemia: factitious hypoglycemia, "functional" hypoglycemia, and insulin as a vehicle for suicide. Factitious hypoglycemia describes the condition in which an individual or a caregiver administers insulin or sulfonylureas to the self or a proxy (Munchausen's syndrome by proxy). An individual with factitious insulin or sulfonylurea use is typified by several factors: (1) unconstrained access to insulin or sulfonylureas (diabetics, relatives of diabetics, or health care personnel), (2) prior history of multiple surgical procedures, hospitalizations, or bizarre physical complaints, and (3) female gender. The diagnosis of factitious hypoglycemia previously relied upon patient admission, patient observation, or the presence of anti-insulin antibodies. The diagnosis may best be made by documenting a simultaneous elevation of plasma insulin and suppression of C-peptide. Sulfonylurea levels must be measured in the serum or urine at the time of hypoglycemia. Each level must be measured individually. Outcomes for persons with factitious hypoglycemia are poor and similar to factitious disorder. Patients should be evaluated for the presence of other psychiatric syndromes such as major depressive disorder.

"Functional" or "reactive" hypoglycemia are terms designating persons who exhibit symptoms of hypoglycemia within 1–3 hours following meals and do not have clearly documented laboratory evidence for hypoglycemia. Frequently these persons have many poorly defined somatic complaints such as fatigue. These individuals have been previously described as "highly nervous," "intense, driving, and overly conscientious," and "thin, tense, neurotic individuals" (31). Formal Minnesota Multiphasic Personality Inventory testing has revealed a profile of the conversion-V triad of scales

HS, D, Hy, consistent with an emotional disturbance underlying somatic complaints (32).

Insulin injection has been reported as a means of suicide. Kaminer and Robbins reviewed insulin misuse and commented that although only 19 cases of suicide by insulin overdose had been documented, the numbers may actually be higher due to lack of information concerning adolescents and incomplete attempts (33). There are no gender differences in insulin-related suicide attempts. These authors propose that psychiatric evaluation must be considered in cases of inadequately explained hypoglycemia (33).

Differential Diagnosis

Diagnosis includes panic disorder, volume depletion, myocardial ischemia, gastritis, stroke, epilepsy, brain tumor, and medication side effects, in addition to the known causes of hypoglycemia.

Treatment

Treatment of hypoglycemia is directed at the underlying cause.

CUSHING'S SYNDROME

Overview

Cushing's syndrome is the condition resulting from either pituitary- or adrenal-mediated overproduction of cortisol. The most common cause (60–70%) of Cushing's syndrome is Cushing's disease, which is caused by an adrenocorticotropic hormone (ACTH) secreting adenoma of the pituitary (34). Cushing's disease is eight times more common in women than men. Other causes of Cushing's syndrome include adrenal causes such as primary adrenal tumors, ectopic production of ACTH by malignant neoplasms, chronic alcoholism, and physiologic states that result in overproduction of cortisol. The syndrome can be iatrogenic, induced by chronic administration of glucocorticoids.

Patient Presentation

Symptoms and signs are insidious in onset. Patients will present with complaints of increased weight and skin changes including hyperpigmentation, hirsutism, complexion changes including acne, and easy and excessive bruisability. Weakness may be reported, as well as diminished sexual drive, impotence and oligo- or amenorrhea. Back pain may be of concern. Persons with a pituitary tumor large enough to cause compression symptoms may complain of visual field loss and headache. Finally, patients may note depressed mood, fatigue, and emotional lability.

Physical Examination

The physical examination of a patient with Cushing's syndrome reveals several classic findings. Hypertension is observed. Patients may have a "buffalo hump" and centripetal obesity with thin extremities. A "moon facies" develops, as does a facial plethora, acne, and hirsuitism. Purple striae greater than 1 cm in width are found on the abdomen. The skin may be hyperpigmented, thin, and bruised. Gynecomastia and testicular atrophy are noted in men. The neurologic exam may reveal proximal muscular weakness and visual field loss.

Mental Status Examination

The patient will have the appearance described above. He or she may be uncooperative and display emotional lability. Psychomotor retardation may be observed. The mood may be depressed and the affect restricted. In severe cases, psychoses may be perceived.

Laboratory Examination

Random cortisol levels are not useful because of diurnal variation. Screening should begin with an overnight dexamethasone-suppression test. The false-negative rate of this test is less than 2%; therefore, a normal result virtually eliminates a diagnosis of Cushing's syndrome. False positives, or lack of suppression of plasma cortisol levels ($>5\mu g/$ dl), may result from improper timing of the test components; significant obesity; renal failure; elevated cortisol-binding globulin, such as occurs during pregnancy or with the use of oral contraceptives or estrogen; stress, inpatient hospitalization; alcoholism, major depressive disorder, and anorexia nervosa. False positives may also be caused by phenytoin, phenobarbital, carbamazepine, and rifampin. If a positive result is found, a 24-hour urine collection that shows a cortisol excretion rate of >100 μg is suggestive of Cushing's syndrome (35). If excess cortisol is present, low- and high-dose dexamethasone-suppression tests are conducted to determine the source of the excess cortisol or ACTH. Failure to suppress on the low-dose test confirms the diagnosis of Cushing's syndrome. Pituitary, but not ectopic, etiologies of Cushing's syndrome show suppression on the high-dose dexamethasone test. Adrenal causes will fail to suppress to both the high- and low-dose test, but will be distinguished by a low plasma ACTH level.

Other laboratory abnormalities in Cushing's syndrome include hypokalemia, metabolic alkalosis, hypercalciuria, glucosuria, granulocytosis, and lymphopenia. Imaging studies may reveal cerebral and cerebellar atrophy (36,37).

Clinical Variants

One important variant of cortisol excess is the iatrogenic production of physical and mental signs and symptoms as a result of supraphysiological doses of glucocorticoids. Unlike persons with Cushing's syndrome who primarily develop affective syndromes, persons receiving exogenous steroids may be at risk for developing symptoms of mild euphoria ranging to frank psychosis (38). Steroid psychosis is characterized by emotional lability, anxiety, distractibility, pressured speech, sensory flooding, insomnia, depression, perplexity, agitation, auditory and visual hallucinations, intermittent memory impairment, mutism, disturbances of body image, delusions, apathy, and hypomania (39). Patients receiving a daily dose of ≥40 mg or its equivalent are at greater risk (39). Symptoms usually occur in the first 5 days of treatment (39). Females may be at greater risk than males; other factors such as previous history of steroid psychosis do not appear to affect risk (39,40). Treatment is indicated with antipsychotics or electroconvulsive therapy. Tricyclic antidepressants may exacerbate symptoms (41). Symptoms usually improve when cortisol doses are lowered, but improvement may take weeks to months.

Role in Psychiatric Conditions

Psychiatric disorder has been reported in up to 50% of patients with Cushing's syndrome (42,43). Depression may precede the onset of the endocrine disorder, and emotional changes may be noted very early in the illness (44). Up to 86% of selected populations have mild to severe depression, characterized by mood lability, irritability, fatigue, diminished concentration and memory, paranoid features, and insomnia. There does not appear to be an association between serum cortisol levels and the severity of depression (44).

The psychoses associated with Cushing's syndrome are usually affective in nature, with paranoid delusions and hallucinations. Neuropsychological testing reveals deficits in verbal and nonverbal cognitive and memory functions and of somatosensory and motor functions (45). Deficits were generally more frequent and severe in nonverbal visual ideational and spatial-constructional abilities than in language and verbal reasoning (45).

Treatment

Treatment modality is directed at the underlying cause of Cushing's syndrome. Transphenoidal resection of pituitary microadenomas generally results in a 75–90% remission rate (34). Alternative forms of treatment include pituitary irradiation. Pharmacotherapy has its primary role in preparation for surgery or for control of hypercortisolism during the interval when radiation is taking effect (34). Surgical resection of an ectopic source of ACTH production is indicated. Unilateral adrenalectomy is appropriate for treating an adrenal adenoma (35).

Psychiatric symptoms usually resolve with treatment of the underlying cause of Cushing's syndrome. Depressive symptoms may begin to improve within days to weeks but may take up to a year to clear completely (44). Psychopharmacology may be indicated in cases of severe mental illness or persistence of symptoms despite normalization of cortisol levels.

ADDISON'S DISEASE

Overview

Primary adrenal insufficiency, or Addison's disease, occurs secondary to ACTH-independent and ACTH-dependent causes. At least 90% of the adrenal gland must be destroyed before failure occurs. ACTH-independent causes of destruction include autoimmune, infectious, metastatic, or hemorrhagic processes. Infectious causes include tuberculosis, sarcoidosis, histoplasmosis, and AIDS-related cytomegalovirus, mycobacterial, or fungal infections. Hemorrhage may occur in sepsis or due to anticoagulant therapy. Although malignancy-associated primary adrenal insufficiency is rare, amyloidosis can lead to this condition. Medication-induced failure has been noted with ketoconazole, rifampin, and anticonvulsants. ACTH-dependent causes affect the hypothalamic-pituitary system through mechanisms such as neoplasm, infection, head trauma, and sarcoidosis. ACTH and glucocorticoid therapy may also be responsible. The most common worldwide cause of primary adrenal insufficiency is tuberculosis. Autoimmune processes are the most common causes in the industrialized west (46).

Patient Presentation

Individuals may present with nonspecific complaints including weakness, fatigue, and anorexia. They may develop nausea, vomiting, and weight loss. An acute presentation may occur in a patient with impending adrenal failure who contracts an acute illness or injury or undergoes a surgical procedure. Additionally, abrupt discontinuation of longstanding glucocorticoid replacement may lead to acute failure. The adrenal or Addisonian crisis is manifested by hypovolemic shock with profound hypotension and impairment of vital organ function.

Physical Examination

The physical examination in an individual with Addison's disease will be in part dependent on the underlying process. Typical Addison's findings include orthostatic hypotension. Hyperpigmentation occurs in primary adrenal failure.

Mental Status Examination

Depression associated with primary adrenal failure was described originally by Addison and has since been described by other authors. Patients may present with symptoms of depressed mood, negativism, social withdrawal, nervousness, irritability, paranoid psychosis, anxiety, poverty of thought, and apathy (47). Patients may be seclusive.

Addisonian encephalopathy presents as a delirium characterized by memory deficit and clouding of consciousness progressing to stupor and coma (48). Psychiatric symptoms may antedate physical complaints.

Laboratory Examination

Hyponatremia is common to both primary and secondary adrenal failure, whereas hyperkalemia occurs in primary adrenal failure. The diagnosis of Addison's disease may be made by the cosyntropin stimulation test. Cosyntropin (250 µg) is administered, and plasma cortisol is measured 30 minutes later. A normal response is a stimulated plasma cortisol level of >20 µg/dl. Additionally, plasma ACTH may be used to discriminate primary from secondary adrenal failure. If secondary adrenal failure is found, further workup assessing for other pituitary hormone deficiencies should be performed.

Hyponatremia, hyperkalemia, hypoglycemia, and metabolic acidosis are noted in adrenal or Addisonian crisis.

Role in Psychiatric Conditions

Addison's disease may complicate the diagnosis of a major depressive disorder. Depressive symptoms may abate with treatment of Addison's disease and its underlying causes. If treatment of the underlying medical etiology and glucocorticoid and mineralocorticoid replacement does not improve the depressive symptoms, antidepressant therapy may be warranted.

Treatment

Adrenal crisis must be treated immediately with hydrocortisone and fluid replacement. If a diagnosis of Addison's disease has not been established, the critically ill patient should be given a single dose of dexamethasone and a cosyntropin test performed. Chronic treatment is directed at treating the underlying disorder and glucocorticoid and mineralocorticoid replacement. Typically, prednisone is used for replacement, adjusting the dose as needed for acute illness, injury, or surgery. Fludrocortisone therapy and liberal salt intake are used for management of mineralocorticoid deficiencies in persons with primary adrenal failure.

HYPERTHYROIDISM

Overview

Hyperthyroidism is the condition resulting from increased formation and release of thyroid hormone from the thyroid gland. Thyrotoxicosis describes the clinical syndrome that results from tissue exposure to excess amounts of thyroid hormone, resulting in metabolic changes and pathophysiological alterations in organ function (49). Thyrotoxicosis results from increased thyroid hormone production or stimulation, excess thyroid hormone administration, or autonomous hormone production. The most common conditions are those caused by increased production/stimulation, such as in Graves' disease, Hashitoxicosis, hydatidiform moles, choriocarcinoma or neoplasm including thyroid-stimulating hormone (TSH)-producing pituitary tumors, toxic adenomas, toxic multinodular goiter, or follicular cancer. Conditions resulting in increased thyroid hormone release such as subacute granulomatous thyroiditis and subacute lymphocytic thyroiditis also occur. One must also consider exogenous sources of thyroid hormone such as thyrotoxicosis factitia, improper slaughterhouse technique, and ectopic production of thyroid hormone (49).

Hyperthyroidism affects approximately 2% of women and is 10 times more common in women than in men (50). Women aged 20–40 years are at highest risk for the condition. The most common cause of hyperthyroidism is Graves' disease, accounting for 60–90% of all cases (49). Graves' disease is an autoimmune disorder in which thyroid-stimulating antibodies cause hyperthyroidism by stimulating the (TSH) receptor. The second most common cause is iatrogenic caused by the administration of excessive levels of thyroid hormone supplementation.

Patient Presentation

Signs and symptoms involve many organ systems. Patients may present with physical complaints including muscular weakness, hair loss, increased appetite with either weight gain or weight loss, fatigability, hyperdefecation, menstrual cycle abnormalities, heat intolerance, excessive perspiration, dyspnea, and palpitations. Cognitive complaints include feelings of irritability, anxiousness, restlessness, emotional lability, and changes in personality.

Physical Examination

The physical examination may reveal cardiovascular findings including sinus tachycardia, atrial fibrillation, elevated systolic blood pressure, widened pulse pressure, and systolic murmur. The skin may be warm, moist, and thin. Spider angiomas may be detected. The patient may have a fine hand tremor. Ophthalmic findings include stare, exophthalmos, lid lag, failure of pupillary accommodation, and periorbital edema. Depending on the etiology, the thyroid gland may be diffusely enlarged or a nodule(s) may be palpated. A vascular bruit may be present over the gland. The thyroid may be hard and tender to palpation in subacute thyroiditis. Fine and silky hair accompanied by shedding of the hair upon combing is noted. Other physical findings include pretibial myxedema, gynecomastia, hyperreflexia, proximal muscular weakness and atrophy, and lymphadenopathy and splenomegaly (49).

Mental Status Examination

The mental status examination may be remarkable for an anxious or apprehensive-appearing facies, rapid speech, psychomotor agitation noted by hyperkinesis, irritability, diminished concentration, short attention span, and emotional lability.

Laboratory Examination

Laboratory findings include high total thyroxine ($T_4 > 12.5$ µg/dl), high free thyroxine (free $T_4 > 2$ ng/dl), normal to high triiodothyronine ($T_3 > 220$ ng/dl), and low thyroid-stimulating hormone (TSH < 0.5 µU/ml). A suppressed TSH alone does not indicate hyperthyroidism and may reflect severe illness, pituitary disease, or be caused by drugs (glucocorticoids and dopamine). The 24-hour radioactive iodine (RAI) and radionuclide scans are used to differentiate causes of hyperthyroidism. A normal or high RAI indicates the presence of hot nodules, toxic multinodular goiters, Graves' disease, or TSH-induced hyperthyroidism. A low or zero uptake is caused by factitious thyroid hormone ingestion, silent or subacute thyroiditis, struma ovarii, or recent iodide exposure (35). Other laboratory anomalies are infrequent and may include low serum cholesterol, elevated alkaline phosphatase, increased direct bilirubin, mild anemia, lymphocytosis, moderate neutropenia, and hypokalemia.

Clinical Variants

Two important clinical variations of hyperthyroidism must be noted: apathetic or "masked" hyperthyroidism and thyroid storm. Apathetic hyperthyroidism is the clinical syndrome of hyperthyroidism with an atypical clinical presentation including complaints of confusion, fatigue, weakness, weight loss, cardiovascular complications including congestive heart failure, depression, and psychomotor retardation. The state was first described in elderly patients, but it may occur in patients of all ages, including children (51–53). Approximately 10% of elderly patients may present with apathetic hyperthyroidism (54). Thyroid storm is denoted by extreme manifestations of thyrotoxicosis coexistent with fever above 37.8°C reaching to 41°C, tachycardia out of proportion to the fever, decompensation in one or more organ systems, and acute changes in mental status. Mental status changes include confusion, delirium, stupor, obtundation, and psychosis. In most, but not all, cases of thyroid storm, a precipitating event can be identified. The most common precipitants are infection, sepsis, and both thyroidal and nonthyroidal surgery. The incidence is approximated at less than 10%, and mortality ranges from 20 to 30% if untreated (55,56).

Role in Psychiatric Conditions

The presence of psychiatric morbidity in hyperthyroidism was described in early descriptions of Graves' disease and included the presence of fatigue, anxiety, excitability, emotional lability punctuated by episodes or crying, irritability, and restlessness. The patient may have increased work activity complicated by poor concentration and a diminished ability to complete tasks. Cognitive deficits include difficulty with simple arithmetic and recent memory (57).

The prevalence of psychosis has been reported to range between 1 and 20% in variable populations (58). Psychotic presentations reported in the literature include paranoid, hebephrenic, and catatonic schizophrenia, psychotic depression, delirium, and psychosis resembling that observed in bipolar affective disorder (58). Psychotic symptoms include hallucinations, delusions, and paranoia. No clearly defined psychotic syndrome is unique to hyperthyroidism. Thyroid-induced psychotic symptoms should clear with proper treatment of the underlying disorder.

The psychiatric differential diagnosis for the constellation of symptoms bearing a similarity to hyperthyroidism includes anxiety disorders such as panic disorder, bipolar and unipolar affective disorders, substance abuse including the use psychostimulants and cocaine, anorexia nervosa, dementia, and schizophrenia. Importantly, thyrotoxicosis factitia is the deliberate ingestion of large quantities of thyroid hormone and is seen occasionally in medical and paramedical personnel (59). These patients show thyrotoxicosis in the presence of thyroid atrophy and hypofunction. Features that discriminate between a patient with a primary psychiatric disorder and primary hyperthyroidism embody the findings of constant rather than intermittent anxiety; cognitive impairment; resting tachycardia; warm and dry, not cold and clammy palmar surfaces; and fatigue accompanied by a desire to be active (60).

Treatment

Treatment of hyperthyroidism may be directed at the cause of the hyperthyroidism, the thyroid hypersecretion, or the clinical manifestations of the condition. Proper diagnosis of the etiology of the hyperthyroidism is paramount. Antithyroid drugs include methimazole, carbimazole, and propylthiouracil (PTU) and are used as first-line treatment for Graves' disease and for short-term therapy before radiation or surgery. These agents act to inhibit the synthesis of thyroid hormones. Common minor side effects include pruritis, arthralgia, fever, gastrointestinal distress, and abnormal sensation of taste. Serious rare side effects include agranulocytosis, an idiosyncratic reaction more common in persons over 40 years old. The onset is sudden and is characterized by fever and sore throat. Although recovery is likely, the side effect may be fatal. Other rare side effects include hepatitis and a lupus-like syndrome (61).

Beta-adrenergic antagonistic drugs are used as adjunctive therapy and provide symptomatic relief by ameliorating the action of thyroid hormone in the body tissues. They do not affect synthesis of thyroid hormone and should not be used for primary treatment (61).

Radioiodine (RAI) I[131] is safe and effective in the treatment of Graves' disease. It is used for primary treatment or for recurrences after treatment with antithyroid drug treatment. The therapy may not take immediate effect, and treatment with beta-blockers or antithyroid drugs may still be necessary. The primary side effect of RAI treatment is the development of hypothyroidism (61).

Subtotal surgical resection of the thyroid gland is appropriate treatment for those who refuse RAI therapy and for those with large goiters who have symptoms of compression or cosmetic concerns (61).

HYPOTHYROIDISM

Overview

Hypothyroidism is a clinical condition resulting from decreased secretion of thyroid hormone from the thyroid gland. The vast majority of cases (90–95%) are the consequence of failure of the thyroid gland (e.g., primary hypothyroidism). The remainder of cases are attributed to pituitary disease (secondary hypothyroidism) or hypothalamic disease (tertiary hypothyroidism) (49). The prevalence of hypothyroidism ranges from 1 to 10% depending on the population studied (62). Hypothyroidism occurs more frequently in iodine-poor geographic areas, among females, and among the elderly.

Etiology

Primary hypothyroidism occurs with processes related to the destruction of the thyroid gland. The most common cause of destruction is from an autoimmune process such as Hashimoto's thyroiditis or end-stage Graves' disease. Destruction of the thyroid gland can also occur secondary to an iatrogenic procedure such as external radiation or thryoidectomy performed for the treatment of another thyroid disease. Additionally, infiltrative processes such as lymphoma, scleroderma, or amyloidosis may destroy the gland. Congenital hypothyroidism is rare, affecting 0.003–0.02% of American neonates (49). Iodine deficiency or excess may interfere with thyroid hormone synthesis, leading to hypothyroidism.

Drug-induced hypothyroidism develops when biosynthesis of thyroid hormone is altered. It has been attributed to lithium and carbamazepine, but does not appear to be caused by antipsychotics, tricyclic antidepressants, or benzodiazepines (63). Lithium interferes with both the synthesis and release of thyroxine and may also inhibit the action of TSH. Lithium-induced hypothyroidism usually occurs within the first 2 years of initiation (64). Some authors recommend checking TSH levels every 2–3 months for the first 2 years, then biannually thereafter (64), although all authors are not in agreement on the frequency (63). Lithium-induced hypothyroidism usually fully reverses upon discontinuation of the drug. Carbamazepine's reduction of T_4 levels is dose-dependent. TSH levels usually remain normal, and patients remain clinically euthyroid. Other drugs thought to induce hypothyroidism include sulfonamides, interleukins, and thionamides (49).

Secondary forms of hypothyroidism result from pituitary gland failure secondary to conditions such as neoplasm or surgery. Hypothalamic failure occurs secondary to infiltrative and infectious processes (49).

Patient Presentation

As with hyperthyroidism, hypothyroidism affects many organ systems and can cause a myriad of symptoms and signs. The onset of symptoms is usually insidious and may go unnoticed by the patient or close relatives. Patients present with complaints including forgetfulness, low mood, fatigue, menorrhagia, impotence, headache, tinnitus, hearing loss, constipation, muscular stiffness and cramping, joint pain, intolerance to cold, dry or rough skin, weight gain despite diminished appetite, and paresthesias, commonly in the carpal tunnel region. Relatives may note social withdrawal, personality changes, snoring, or vocal hoarseness.

Physical Examination

The physical examination may reveal changes in the skin that include dry, rough skin with hyperkeratosis. The hair may be thinning and have a coarse, brittle texture. Non-pitting edematous skin changes may be found in the face, limbs, and supraclavicular fossa. The voice may be dysarthric, and an ataxic gait may be noted. A distal peripheral neuropathy may be detected. Deep tendon reflexes are slowed with a delayed relaxation phase. A pleural effusion may be present. Bradycardia and hypertension are detected on cardiovascular examination (49,58).

Mental Status Examination

Mental status examination may be remarkable for an irritable or anxious individual with a depressed, puffy, or stoic-appearing facies. Speech may be slow and toneless. Psychomotor retardation is noted. Memory may be diminished. Formal memory testing reveals deficits in all scales except mental control on the Wechsler Memory Scale (65). The affect may be depressed, with mood complaints including dysphoria, anhedonia, and suicidality. In severe cases, a thought disorder characterized by agitation, paranoid ideation, persecutory delusions, hallucinations, and disorientation may be observed.

Laboratory Examination

Laboratory abnormalities confirm the diagnosis. Grade I, or overt, primary hypothyroidism is characterized by an elevated TSH (>6 μU/ml), diminished free T_4 (< 0.9 ng/dl), and diminished total T_4 (<4.5 μg/dl). The T_3 usually remains normal early in the course, but later becomes diminished (<80 ng/dl) (49). A hypothyroid state induced by hypothalamic or pituitary disease will be distinguished by a normal or low TSH in spite of a decreased free or total T_4. The presence of antithyroid antibodies is compatible with Hashimoto's disease. Thyroid-releasing hormone (TRH) testing may be used to delineate the cause of secondary hypothyroidism. Other laboratory findings include hypercholesterolemia; normocytic/normochromic, hypochromic/microcytic, or macrocytic anemias; prolonged bleeding time; elevated serum lactate dehydrogenase, serum creatinine kinase of MM origin, and serum aspartate aminotransferase. Cerebral spinal fluid protein may also be elevated (62).

Role in Psychiatric Conditions

The psychiatric syndromes in hypothyroidism date to 1874, when Gull first described a "cretinoid state" in an adult woman. Within the next 15 years, the mental changes associated with advanced hypothyroidism were well documented and the term "myxedema" was coined. In 1949, Asher described 14 cases of "myxoedematous madness" in patients who were thought to suffer from a primary psychotic process (66). It is currently believed that 5–15% of myxedema patients have overt psychoses, although these figures may be lower as thyroid disease is now generally diagnosed earlier. Hypothyroidism may reduce central 5-hydroxytryptamine and result in depression (67). Other proposed mechanisms include reduced cerebral flow resulting in a relative cerebral hypoxia.

Psychiatric syndromes occurring with advanced hypothyroidism are variable and include psychotic depression, delirium, dementia, manic-like syndrome, and a schizophrenic-like syndrome. Patients may present with depressed mood, personality change with lability of mood, anxiety, emotional withdrawal, generalized agitation, mental slowing, persecutory delusions, paranoid ideation, and auditory hallucinations (58,62,63,66). Myxedema is an important cause of reversible psychiatric and dementia syndrome. Psychiatric symptoms usually respond to thyroid hormone replacement, but reversal may take days to months. A manic-like state can ensue if replacement is too rapid. During the initial treatment, psychotropic medications may be needed to control symptoms while the thyroid replacement is taking effect.

The literature evaluating the role of hypothyroidism in unipolar major depressive disorder, bipolar affective disorder, and dysthymia is mixed. The issue becomes further complicated when considering the influence of subclinical hypothyroidism on the affective state. Subclinical hypothyroidism (grades 2 and 3) denotes the circumstance in which free T_4 and total T_4 are normal but TSH is elevated. Typical symptoms of hypothyroidism are either absent or present to only a minimal degree (68).

Some studies suggest that clinical depression occurs in over 40% of hypothyroid patients (57,69) and at a rate of 12% in depressed inpatients (70). Antithyroid antibodies are found in 9–20% of those with unipolar depression (71,72). Patients over 65 years old who have subclinical hypothyroidism have a lifetime history of major depressive disorder (68). These findings must be interpreted with caution, however, because of small sample populations and/or lack of control groups (68). More recently, Haggerty and Prange (68) showed that 50% of a population of general medical patients with TSH values of >3.0 IU had been treated for depression compared with only 18% of those with TSH of <3.0 IU. Using structured psychiatric interviews, they further showed a higher lifetime prevalence of depression in a group of young and middle-aged women with grade 2 or 3 hypothyroidism than in women who were euthyroid (68).

Subclinical hypothyroidism has been associated with rapid cycling bipolar affective disorder in some, but not all, studies (73). Some findings suggest that subclinical hypothyroidism may be present in up to 40% and overt hypothyroidism in 25–50% of rapid-cycling bipolar patients (68). Antithyroid antibodies have been found in 33% of mixed episodes, but the frequency of subclinical hypothyroidism is no different between subjects with and without mixed states (68,73). The role of lithium-induced hypothyroidism complicates the interpretation of the role of thyroid hormone in bipolar affective disorder.

A review of comorbidity in dysthymia showed that a subgroup of patients with dysthymia are at risk for subclinical or overt hypothyroidism (74).

Treatment

Levothyroxine sodium remains the primary treatment for overt hypothyroidism and may be used for treatment of subclinical hypothyroidism and as adjuvant treatment for affective disorders. Most patients with primary hypothyroidism can be treated with levothyroxine at an average daily dose of about 1.6 μg/kg ideal body weight. Healthy, young adults (<65 years old) may be initiated at the full treatment dose, generally 100 μg daily, but those older than 65 years old or who have a history of cardiac disease should begin with 25 μg/day with increases at approximately 6- to 8-week intervals. The goal of therapy is to normalize TSH and improve symptoms. TSH levels should be checked 2–3 months after initiation of treatment, as they are unlikely to normalize until that time. Symptomatic improvement may be noted within 3–4 weeks of initiation of therapy. Therapy is usually lifelong, although dose adjustments may be needed over time (75). Laboratory evaluation should be conducted on an annual basis once the TSH has normalized. Complications of overreplacement include the development of hyperthyroidism, increasing the nocturnal heart rate, and increasing bone resorption leading to osteoporosis (76).

Treatment of subclinical hypothyroidism remains controversial (75,76). Levothyroxine replacement has been recommended for patients with TSH of >10 μU/ml and for those with TSH of >5 μU/ml when a goiter or antithyroid antibodies are present (75). Treatment may be particularly important in the elderly (>65 years). Elderly persons with an elevated TSH and antithyroid have an 80% chance of developing hypothyroidism in a 4-year period. Some authors recommend that the list of index symptoms for initiating treatment of subclinical hypothyroidism should be broadened to include depression, memory faults, and fatigue (68).

Adjuvant treatment with thyroid hormone may be beneficial in the treatment of both unipolar and bipolar affective disorders. Data regarding the usefulness of adjuvant therapy are limited by a paucity of large sample sizes and few double-blind crossover trials. Persons with depression refractory to antidepressant therapy, especially those with subclinical hypothyroidism, may benefit from triiodothyronine (T_3) or levothyroxine supplementation. Additionally, levothyroxine has been reported to benefit patients with bipolar affective disorder who are euthyroid or have subclinical hypothyroidism (73). Until larger, well-designed studies are done to address this issue of adjuvant treatment, clinical judgment remains the best alternative.

REFERENCES

1. Greyanus DE, Hofmann AD. Psychological factors in diabetes mellitus: a review of the literature with emphasis on adolescence. Am J Dis Child 1979; 133:1061–1066.
2. Sherwin RS. Diabetes mellitus. In: Bennett JC, Plum F, eds. Cecil Textook of Medicine. Philadelphia: WB Saunders, 1996:1258–1277.
3. Lustman PJ, Freedland KE, Carney RM, Hong BA, Clouse RE. Similarity of depression in diabetic and psychiatric patients. Psychosom Med 1992; 54:602–611.
4. Draelos MT, Jacobson AM, Weinger K, Widom B, Ryan CM, et al. Cognitive function in patients with insulin-dependent diabetes mellitus during hyperglycemia and hypoglycemia. Am J Med 1995; 98:135–144.
5. Diabetes Control and Complications Trial Research Group. Effects of intensive diabetes therapy on neuropsychological function in adults in the diabetes control and complications trial. Ann Intern Med 1996; 124:379–388.
6. Gavard JA, Lustman PJ, Clouse RE. Prevalence of depression in adults with diabetes. Diabetes Care 1993; 16:1167–1176.
7. Cameron OG, Kronfol Z, Greden JF, Carroll BJ. Hypothalamic pituitary adrenocorticol activity in patients with diabetes mellitus. Arch Gen Psychiatry 1984; 41:1090–1095.
8. MacKenzie R, Trulson M. Effects of insulin and streptozotocin-induced diabetes on brain tryptophan and serotonin metabolism in rats. J Neurochem 1978; 30:205–211.
9. Lustman PJ, Griffith LS, Clouse RE. Depression in adults with diabetes: Results of a 5-yr follow-up study. Diabetes Care 1988; 11:605–612.
10. Lustman PJ, Griffith LS, Gavard JA, Clouse RE. Depression in adults with diabetes. Diabetes Care 1992; 15:1631–1639.
11. Kovacs M, Goldston D, Obrosky DS, Bonar LK. Psychiatric disorders in youths with IDDM: rates and risk factors. Diabetes Care 1997; 20:36–44.
12. Kovacs M, Obrosky DS, Goldston D, Drash A. Major depressive disorder in youths with IDDM. Diabetes Care 1997; 20:45–51.
13. Kovacs M, Mukerju P, Drash A, Iyengar S. Biomedical and psychiatric risk factors for retinopathy among children with IDDM. Diabetes Care 1995; 18:1592–1599.
14. Marcus MD, Wing RR, Guare J, et al. Lifetime prevalence of major depression and its effect on treatment outcome in obese type II diabetic patients. Diabetes Care 1992; 15: 253–255.
15. Lustman PJ, Clouse RE, Carney RM. Depression and the reporting of diabetes symptoms. Int J Psychiatry Med 1988; 18:295–303.
16. Goodnick PJ, Henry JH, Buki MV. Treatment of depression in patients with diabetes mellitus. J Clin Psychiatry 1995; 56:128–138.
17. Cooper AJ, Ashcroft G. Potentiation of insulin hypoglycemia by MAOI antidepressant drugs. Lancet 1966; i:407–409.

18. Weiner RD, Coffey CE. Electroconvulsive therapy in the medical and neurologic patient. In: Stoudemire A, Fogel BS, eds. Psychiatric Care of the Medical Patient. New York: Oxford University Press, 1993:207–224.

19. Rodin GM, Daneman D. Eating disorders and IDDM: a problematic association. Diabetes Care 1992; 15:1402–1412.

20. Fairburn CG, Peveler RC, Davies B, Mann JI, Mayou R. Eating disorders in young adults with insulin dependent diabetes mellitus: a controlled study. Br Med J 1991; 303:17–20.

21. Peveler RC, Fairburn CG, Boller I, Dunger D. Eating disorders in adolescents with IDDM: a controlled study. Diabetes Care 1992; 15:1356–1359.

22. Striegel-Moore RH, Nicholson TJ, Tamborlane WV. Prevalence of eating disorder symptoms in preadolescent and adolescent girls with IDDM. Diabetes Care 1992; 15:1361–1368.

23. Carney CP, Yates WR. The evaluation of eating and weight symptoms in the general hospital consultation setting. Psychosomatics. 1998; 39:61–67.

24. Hillard JR, Hillard PJ: Bulimia, anorexia nervosa, and diabetes: deadly combinations. Psychiatr Clin North Am 1984; 7:367–379.

25. Jones JM, Rodin GM, Daneman D. Controlling eating disorders in young women with IDDM. Contemporary Intern Med 1997; 9:33–41.

26. Orland MJ. Diabetes mellitus. In: Weald GA, McKenzie CR, eds. Manual of Medical Therapeutics. Boston: Little, Brown, 1995:437–463.

27. Gin H, Viala R, Rigal F, Morlat P, Beauviewx JM, et al. Panic attack caused by biguanides. Rev Med Intern 1989; 10:361–363.

28. Field JB. Hypoglycemia: definition, clinical presentations, classification, and laboratory tests. Endocrinol Metab Clin North Am 1989; 18:27–43.

29. Whipple AO. The surgical therapy of hyperinsulinism. J Int Chir 1938; 3:237–276.

30. Comi RJ. Approach to acute hypoglycemia. Endocrinol Metab Clin North Am 1993; 22:247–261.

31. Leggett J, Favazza AR. Hypoglycemia: an overview. J Clin Psychiatry 1978; 39:51–57.

32. Johnson DD, Dorr KE, Swenson WM, et al. Reactive hypoglycemia. JAMA 1980; 243:1151–1155.

33. Kaminer Y, Robbins DR. Insulin misuse: a review of an overlooked psychiatric problem. Psychosomatics 1989; 30:19–24.

34. Jameson JL. Anterior pituitary. In: Bennett JC, Plum F, eds. Cecil Textook of Medicine. Philadelphia: WB Saunders, 1996:1205–1221.

35. Landsberg L. Endocrinology and metabolism. In: Lee Goldman, ed. Medical Knowledge Self-Assessment Program. Philadelphia: American College of Physicians, 1995:1062–1064.

36. Momose KJ, Kjellberg RN, Kliman B. High incidence of cortical atrophy of the cerebral and cerebellar hemispheres in Cushing's disease. Radiology 1971; 99:314–348.

37. Heinz ER, Martinez J, Haenggela A. Reversibility of cerbral atrophy in anorexia nervosa and Cushing's syndrome. J Comput Assist Tomogr 1977; 1:415–418.

38. Rome HP, Braceland FJ. Psychological response to corticotropin, cortisone, and related steroid substances. JAMA 1952; 148:27–30.

39. Hall RCW, Popkin MK, Stickney SK, Gardner ER. Presentation of steroid psychoses. J Nerv Ment Dis 1979; 167:229–236.

40. Ling MH, Perry PJ, Tsuang MT. Side effects of corticosteroid therapy: psychiatric aspects. Arch Gen Psychiatry 1981; 38:471–477.

41. Hall RCW, Popkin MK, Kirkpatrick B. Tricyclic exacerbation of steroid psychosis. J Nerv Ment Dis 1978; 166:738–742.
42. Starkman MN, Schteingart DE. Neuropsychiatric manifestations of patients with Cushing's syndrome. Arch Intern Med 1981; 141:215–219.
43. Michael RP, Gibbons JL. Interrelationships between the endocrine system and neuropsychiatry. Int Rev Neurobiol 1963; 5:243–302.
44. Cohen SI. Cushing's syndrome: a psychiatric study of 29 patients. Br Psychiatry 1980; 136:120–124.
45. Whelan TB, Schteingart DE, Starkman MN, Smith A. Neuropsychological deficits in Cushing's syndrome. J Nerv Ment Dis 1980; 168:753–757.
46. Loriaux DL. Adrenal cortex. In: Bennett JC, Plum F, eds. Cecil Textook of Medicine. Philadelphia: WB Saunders, 1996:1245–1252.
47. Smith KC, Barish J, Correa J, et al. Psychiatric disturbance in endocrinologic disease. Psychosom Med 1972; 34:69–86.
48. Ettigi PG, Brouwn GM. Brain disorders associated with endorine dysfunctin. Psychiatr Clin North Am 1978; 1:117–136.
49. Dillman WH. The thyroid. In: Bennett JC, Plum F, eds. Cecil Textook of Medicine. Philadelphia: WB Saunders, 1996:1227–1245.
50. Tunbridge WMG, Evered DC, Hall R, et al. The spectrum of thyroid disease in a community: the Whickham survey. Clin Endocrinol 1977; 7:481–493.
51. Lahey FH. Non-activated (apathetic) type of hyperthyroidism. N Engl J Med 1931; 204: 747–748.
52. McGee RR, Whittaker RL, Tullis IF. Apathetic thyroidism: review of the literature and report of four cases. Ann Intern Med 1959; 50:1418–1432.
53. Grossman A, Waldstein SS. Apathetic thyroid storm in a 10-year old child. Pediatrics 1961; 28:447–451.
54. Davis PJ, Davis FB. Hyperthyroidism in patients over the age of 60 years: cinical features in 85 patients. Medicine 1974; 53:161–181.
55. Tietgens ST, Leinung MC. Thyroid storm. Med Clin North Am 1995; 79:169–185.
56. Mackin JF, Canary JJ, Pittman CS. Thyroid storm and its management. N Engl J Med 1974; 291:1396–1398.
57. Whybrow PC, Prange AJ, Treadway CR. Mental changes accompanying thyroid gland dysfunction. Arch Gen Psychiatry 1969; 20:48–63.
58. Hall RCW. Psychiatric effects of thyroid hormone disturbance. Psychosomatics 1983; 24: 7–18.
59. Tonks CM. Psychiatric aspects of endocrine disorders. The Practitioner 1977; 218:526–531.
60. Popkin MK, Mackenzie TB. Psychiatric presentations of endocrine dysfunction. In: Hall RCW, ed. Psychiatric Presentations of Medical Illness. New York: Spectrum Books, 1980: 142–143.
61. Franklyn JA. The management of hyperthyroidism. N Engl J Med 1994; 330:1731–1738.
62. Lamb AS. Hypothyroidism: the varied manifestations of a common disorder. NC Med J 1994; 55:124–126.
63. Wison WH, Jefferson JW. Thyroid disease, behavior, and psychopharmacology. Psychosomatics 1985; 26:481–492.
64. Vincent A, Baruch P, Pierre V. Early onset of lithium-associated hypothyroidism. J Psychiatr Neurosci 1993; 18:74–77.

65. Manzani F, Del Guerra P, Caraccio N, Pruneti CA, Pucci E, et al. Subclinical hypothyroidism: neurobehavioral features and beneficial effect of L-thyroxine treatment. Clin Invest 1993; 71:367–371.
66. Ascher R. Myxedematous madness. Br Med J 1949; 2:555–562.
67. Cleare AJ, McGregor A, O'Keane V. Neuroendocrine evidence for an association between hypothyroidism, reduced central 5-HT activity and depression. Clin Endocrinol 1995; 43: 713–719.
68. Haggerty JJ, Prange AJ. Borderline hypothyroidism and depression. Annu Rev Med 1995; 46:37–46.
69. Jain VK. A psychiatric study of hypothyroidism. Psychiatr Clin North Am 1972; 5:121–130.
70. Gold MS, Pottash ALC, Extein I. Hypothyroidism and depression. JAMA 1981; 245: 1919–1922.
71. Gold MS, Pottash ALC, Extein I. "Symptomless" autoimmune thyroiditis in depression. Psychiatry Res 1982; 6:261–269.
72. Nemeroff CB, Simon JS, Haggerty JJ, Evans DL. Antithyroid antibodies in depressed patients. Am J Psychiatry 1985; 142:840–843.
73. Joffe RT, Young LT, Cooke RC, Robb J. The thyroid and mixed affective states. Acta Psychiatr Scand 1994; 90:131–132.
74. Howland RH: General health, health care utilization, and medical comorbidity in dysthymia. Int J Psychiatry Med 1993; 23:211–238.
75. Mandel SJ, Brent GA, Larsen PR. Levothyroxine therapy in patients with thyroid disease. Ann Intern Med 1993; 119:492–502.
76. Toft AD. Thyroxine therapy. N Engl J Med 1994; 331:174–180.
77. Swanson JW, Kelly JJ, McConahey WM. Neurologic aspects of thyroid dysfunction. Mayo Clin Proc 1981; 56:504–512.
78. Isley WL. Thyroid dysfunction in the severely ill and elderly: forget the classic signs and symptoms. Postgrad Med 1993; 94:111–128.

10

Treatment of Psychiatric Disorders in Patients Infected with HIV

**Glenn J. Treisman, Marc Fishman,
Joseph M. Schwartz, Constantine G. Lyketsos,
and Paul R. McHugh**
*Johns Hopkins University School of Medicine
Baltimore, Maryland*

INTRODUCTION

Psychiatric disorders are common in HIV-infected patients. Impulsive behavior, intoxication, cognitive impairment, hopelessness, and disorganization produced by psychiatric disorders may lead to risk for HIV infection. At the same time, HIV infection produces both psychosocial stressors and brain injury that may lead to psychopathology (see Fig. 1). This chapter describes the clinical characteristics, assessment, and treatment of disorders that commonly occur co-morbidly with HIV, emphasizing the ways in which HIV may influence clinical variables. Diagnosis and treatment in this population is complicated by multisystem medical illness, stigma, and psychosocial stress, but treatment has been shown to be associated with clinical improvement. We also speculate that aggressive treatment of psychiatric disorders may improve outcome and risk behaviors in HIV-infected patients.

The population at risk for HIV infection in developed countries has changed dramatically since the epidemic began. Descriptions of the routes of transmission, the etiological agent, the risk factors, and the characteristics of risk populations have resulted in reduction of risk behaviors in many patients. Patients with high-risk behaviors are now likely to have some appreciation of the risks they take but are unable to respond to efforts to curb risk behaviors. This impels us to look for factors that distinguish those who take precautions from those who do not.

We have proposed that psychiatric disorders play an important role in continued high-risk behavior despite public health measures. This hypothesis predicts increasingly

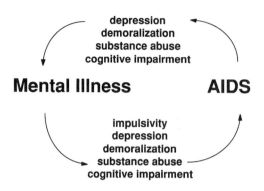

depression
demoralization
substance abuse
cognitive impairment

Mental Illness   AIDS

impulsivity
depression
demoralization
substance abuse
cognitive impairment

Figure 1   Hypothesized relationship between HIV-infection and psychiatric disorders.

high rates of psychiatric disorders in new cases of HIV as the epidemic progresses. We also believe that effective treatment of psychiatric disorders leads to better outcome and decreased spread of HIV. Wide variation in the rates of psychiatric disorders in populations at risk for HIV and HIV-infected persons has been reported, but differences in definition, methods of study, and population may partly explain this variation. We have reported very high rates of psychopathology in our study population, as have some others, but additional careful examinations of this issue will be useful in efforts to fight this epidemic.

Our discussion is organized around the perspectives proposed for understanding psychiatric disorders by McHugh and Slavney in their textbook *The Perspectives of Psychiatry* (1). We will first consider disorders that we believe to involve a lesion of brain, which are best viewed as diseases (schizophrenia, dementia, mania, major depression), then disorders related to character and temperament (personality traits and disorders), then disorders related to motivated behaviors (addictions, paraphilia), and finally those disorders that occur as psychological reactions to life circumstances and experiences (grief, demoralization, adjustment disorders).

AIDS DEMENTIA AND OTHER COGNITIVE DISORDERS

The AIDS dementia syndrome was one of the first clearly described neuropsychiatric consequences of AIDS. HIV infection is associated with a number of cognitive impairments. Early in the infection, patients may have a transient encephalitis with an accompanying delirium or mild difficulty with cognition. This is usually brief in duration with complete recovery. Later in the course of HIV with progressive decline in T-cell number, patients may develop variable isolated cognitive deficits that may be sustained or actually improve over time. These are the so-called minor cognitive features, and although they can be quite severe, they are usually limited in time, do not progress, and do not incapacitate patients. Psychiatrists are often called upon to evaluate such patients for "competence," and although patients have clearly demonstrable deficits in focal cognitive domains, it is rare at this stage for them to have any global intellectual impairment.

The AIDS dementia syndrome is a progressive disorder, affecting primarily subcortical brain areas and rapidly leading to complete disability for most patients. It usually occurs in advanced disease with <200 T cells. The syndrome is similar to other subcortical dementing illnesses such as Huntington's and Parkinson's diseases, and the disorder features the "subcortical triad" of motor dysfunction, mood dysfunction, and memory disturbance. Prominent are the deterioration of personality, with apathy, irritability, and the so-called coarsening of personality. Impairments in psychomotor speed, retrieval, and parallel cognitive processing are prominent features. Recognition recall is preserved compared with free recall, so a patient may name objects but have difficulty listing animals starting with a particular letter. Although impairment of cortical functions, such as aphasia and apraxia, are seen with advanced disease, these are not prominent early features as they are in Alzheimer's disease. For this reason screening tests that emphasize cortical tasks, such as the Mini-Mental State Exam, are not sensitive screens for AIDS dementia. Tests such as the Verbal Trials B, grooved pegboard, and digit-symbol substitution are more useful for identifying mild to moderate disease.

HIV dementia usually progresses to death. High-dose AZT provides some palliation in patients who can tolerate it (we often give a gram or more in divided doses each day). Because of the central nervous system (CNS) penetration of AZT, it has been maintained as part of the therapy even in previously exposed patients, but patients who cannot tolerate AZT may still respond to aggressive viral load reduction with other agents, and several trials to demonstrate the efficacy of non–CNS-penetrating regimens are underway. Dementia, particularly subcortical dementia, is often associated with mood disorder. Both major depression and mania have been associated with subcortical brain injury. We expect that ongoing research will confirm that AIDS dementia follows this pattern. Mania associated with AIDS dementia has been described by our group as well as others. (This manic syndrome is discussed below.)

Like other subcortical dementias, AIDS dementia can also produce disinhibition or an apathy syndrome in which motivation, energy, emotional range, and hedonic interests are all markedly diminished. Although sometimes difficult to distinguish from major depression, it is characterized by prominent affective blunting rather than strong negative affective states such as sadness. In its most severe forms, it may include abulia and akinesia and lead to such colloquial descriptions as "lights on, but nobody home." The apathy responds in some cases to antidepressants but more often to direct dopaminergic stimulation. We use stimulants for apathy, such as methylphenidate, pemoline, and amphetamines. These agents can give improvements in energy, activity, and mental speed, but side effects such as appetite suppression must be monitored. Depression, which may have associated apathy, may show initial improvement with stimulants as well, but in our experience antidepressants give a better and more sustained response, and sometimes depressed patients with dementia do best on both.

Many HIV patients have cognitive impairment, either from lifelong cognitive subnormality or from acquired cognitive deficits including AIDS dementia, head trauma, chronic substance use, or CNS infection. Our group at Hopkins found an 18% prevalence of cognitive impairment on intake to a medical HIV clinic (2). Many of the patients in this series had cognitive impairment prior to HIV infection by history. This suggests that cognitive impairment may be a risk factor for HIV risk behaviors and serotransmission. This would not be surprising, as cognitive deficits are associated with limitations in coping strategies in many domains as well as narrowed and maladaptive behavioral repertoires. Furthermore, people with cognitive deficits generally have difficulty modifying established behavior patterns and therefore can be expected to respond poorly to risk-behavior modification and education.

Once infected, patients with cognitive limitations have great difficulty understanding and adhering to complicated treatment plans, especially the polypharmaceutical regimens that are typical in the HIV clinic. Careful history is needed to ascertain the diagnosis of AIDS dementia as opposed to other cognitive disorders, and complicating diagnoses include CNS opportunistic infections, tumors, neurosyphilis, and intoxication. Additionally, patients must be evaluated prior to other psychiatric treatment for their cognitive capacity.

MOOD DISORDERS

The identification and impact of psychiatric disorders, including mood disorders, in persons with HIV infection has increased substantially over the course of the epidemic. This reflects the changing profile of the epidemic in several ways. First, HIV infection is increasingly being identified earlier in its course as public knowledge, concern, and screening become more widespread. Patients who are identified soon after seroconversion are now living with HIV much longer. This allows a longer period for psychiatric symptoms to manifest themselves and come to medical attention, primarily prior to AIDS. It also provides a longer period in which psychiatric diagnosis and treatment can potentially make a difference in quality of life, function, course of HIV infection, and ongoing risk behaviors. Second, with advancing treatments patients are living longer after AIDS develops. This prolongs the period during which neuropsychiatric sequelae of symptomatic HIV infection can develop. Third, as risk-behavior intervention programs become more common, those who can easily modify their risk behaviors do so. This means that risk groups are increasingly enriched with those who are less responsive to risk-behavior modification efforts. Presumably many of these persons will turn out to have one or more of a variety of psychiatric disorders. Finally, with increasing recognition of the impact of psychiatric disorders on HIV patients, there has been increasing emphasis on the need for a psychiatric presence in HIV care settings. With more frequent and careful assessment, there is better identification of psychiatric disorders, and affective disorders in particular.

Bipolar Disorders (Including Manic-Depressive Disorder)

Bipolar disorder (manic-depressive disorder) has been associated with increased rates of substance abuse and impulsive behavior, and there has been speculation that bipolar disorder may be a risk factor for HIV infection. Although a manic syndrome has been described in late-stage AIDS at increased rates, no study has been able to show increased bipolar disorder in a general population of HIV-infected patients (3). We found a trend toward increased rates of bipolar disorder in a population of HIV-positive clinic patients, but the effect was small and not statistically significant (unpublished data). Part of what complicates this issue is the changing nosology and improving diagnostic clarity of the psychiatric literature. The clearer description of bipolar type II, in which the mania is of lower grade and is often missed, may clarify whether bipolar disorder increases the risk for HIV infection.

Mania can occur either early or late in the course of HIV infection and stratifies clearly into two groups: preexisting bipolar disorder and secondary mania as a consequence of HIV brain involvement. In general, manic syndromes in HIV patients occur with higher frequency after the onset of AIDS (3,4). Furthermore, AIDS patients develop mania at rates substantially greater than the general population—in our series 8% of all AIDS patients seen at the HIV clinic over 17 months (more than 10 times the 6-month general population prevalence) (3). We categorized grouped mania patients into those whose first manic episode came late in their HIV course with CD4 count <200 and those whose episode came early with CD4 count >200. The late-onset patients were less likely to have a personal or a family history of mania or any mood disorder, which presumably means they were less likely to have bipolar disorder or a genetic predisposition to mania. They were also more likely to have dementia or other cognitive impairment indicating brain damage. Our group's preliminary findings from ongoing MRI studies have so far not demonstrated any focal injury.

We use the term AIDS mania to refer to late-stage onset of a *first* lifetime episode of mania without family history. Patients with preexisting bipolar disorder can develop mania at any time in the course of HIV infection, early or late. AIDS mania seems to have a somewhat different clinical profile than bipolar mania. Patients tend to have cognitive slowing or dementia. Although without a previous dementia diagnosis this may be difficult to ascertain on exam in the midst of an acute manic episode, the history will usually reveal progressive cognitive decline prior to onset of mania. Irritable mood is more common than euphoria. Sometimes prominent psychomotor slowing accompanying the cognitive slowing of AIDS dementia will replace the expected hyperactivity of mania, which complicates the differential diagnosis.

Our clinical experience suggests that AIDS mania is usually quite severe in its presentation and malignant in its course. In our series, late-onset patients had a greater total number of manic symptoms than early-onset patients. They were also more commonly irritable and less commonly hypertalkative (5). AIDS mania seems to be more characteristically chronic than episodic, has infrequent spontaneous remission, and usually relapses with cessation of treatment. Because of their cognitive deficits, patients have little functional reserve to begin with. They are also less able to pursue treatment independently or consistently.

One relatively common pathoplastic presentation of mania, either early or late, is the expression of grandiosity by a delusional belief of having discovered a cure for HIV or having been cured. When euphoria is a prominent symptom in otherwise debilitated late-stage patients, caregivers may wistfully question the humaneness of robbing patients of the illusion of happiness. It is the clearly impairing, often devastating effects of the other symptoms of mania that tip the balance of the risk/benefit equation towards treatment.

The treatment of mania in early-stage HIV infection is not substantially different from the standard treatment of bipolar disorder. However, as the infection advances, with lower CD4 counts, more medical illnesses, more CNS involvement, and greater overall physiological vulnerability, treatment strategies are somewhat different. First, single-agent therapy becomes an important goal because of the cumulative burdens of polypharmacy. AIDS mania patients in particular seem to respond well to treatment with a neuroleptic alone. We have had the best success with high-potency agents such as haloperidol and fluphenazine. In general, late-stage patients are far more sensitive to the therapeutic effects, but even more so to the toxic side effects, of neuroleptics. Therefore, doses much lower than customarily used in mania in other settings are sufficient. We usually begin with 1–2 mg/day, then titrate upward, but rarely above 15 mg/day. The more advanced the patients' HIV and/or dementia, the more sensitive they are to dosage changes that might otherwise seem trivial. We have sometimes seen patients overly sedated on 8 mg, but floridly manic on 6 mg. Some patients develop extrapyramidal symptoms but will also prove very sensitive to the side effects, especially delirium, of anticholinergic agents. We usually avoid them when possible, and when necessary start at low doses, e.g., benztropine ½ mg b.i.d. Additionally, we have used atypical agents such as respiridone, olanzapine, and quetiapine. Some patients have a good response to the agents and tolerate them better, but some require traditional neuroleptics.

We have also had success with mood-stabilizing agents in selected patients. Lithium use has been problematic for several reasons, including high rates of associated delirium and other toxicity, and because levels often fluctuate with constant dosing even in the hospital with wide changes in blood level and dramatic intoxication. We have used valproic acid with success, titrating to the usual therapeutic serum levels. This is sometimes limited by side effects, especially hepatotoxicity in the setting of chronic viral hepatitis. Monitoring of liver function tests has been essential, but in many cases we have not found hepatic toxicity to be a problem. In cases of severe hepatic mycobacterium avium complex (MAC) infiltration, e.g., with portal hypertension, we have avoided valproic acid, but this and related considerations have not been formally studied. Carbamazepine is also effective but more poorly tolerated because of sedation and because of the presumed potential for synergistic bone marrow suppression in combination with antiviral medications and HIV itself. We have little experience with calcium channel blockers or the newer anticonvulsants such as gabapentin and lamotrigene, but these agents are promising.

Major Depression

Except for substance abuse, major depression is the most frequent psychiatric disorder we encounter in either new patients or referred patients in the HIV clinic. We have suggested that major depression is increased in HIV-infected patients, and that depression may be a risk factor for infection. We have not been able to demonstrate the latter but have shown that as patients enter what Justin MacArthur refers to as the "neurologically vulnerable period" of advanced HIV infection, rates of major depression are increased (see below).

Widely varying estimates of the prevalence of major depression in HIV-infected patients have been reported, ranging from 4 to 20% (6). The differences arise from the use of varying definitions and assessment techniques, diverse clinical samples (including differences in risk factors and stage of infection), and other aspects of study design. We reported a 20% cross-sectional prevalence of current major depression among outpatients at initial intake into the HIV medical clinic (2). Although this is higher than rates reported by other investigators, most studies have found that major depression is more common among clinical samples of HIV patients than in the general population (6,7). The rates in HIV patients are also substantially higher than those found in general medical patients of similar age, including those with progressive and fatal diseases such as end-stage renal disease and cancer (8), but are similar to those reported in older patients with other chronic medical illnesses (9).

Patients with major depression also comprise a large portion of referrals to HIV psychiatric treatment settings. Of 252 referred patients evaluated by our group in an HIV psychiatry clinic over 2 years, 56% had a diagnosis of major depression (10). In a series of 40 medical hospital inpatients referred to our HIV psychiatric consultation service, 28% had a diagnosis of major depression (11). Other groups have reported comparably large proportions of adjustment disorders but low rates of major depression in referred populations (12–14). This may reflect differences in the patient populations examined or differences in diagnostic definitions used in assessment of patients with depressive symptoms.

Some authors have proposed that HIV patients with affective disorders be considered in two broad and overlapping groups: those with affective disorders that precede their HIV and those whose affective disorders emerge as a consequence of HIV. High rates of mood disorders would be expected to be associated with both groups. The first group, those presumed to have previous histories of affective disorder, should be expected to roughly reflect the background rates of affective disorders among the major HIV risk groups. Both homosexual men and drug users have high rates of depression compared to the general population. Several surveys have compared asymptomatic or early stage HIV-positive patients to HIV-negative controls from similar high risk groups and found high rates of major depression in both, but without significant increase with seropositivity (15–22). Additionally, patients with addictive disorders are known to have high rates of major depression (23). For many patients, mood disorders themselves are likely to have been significant risk factors for the contraction of HIV, although this has not yet been demonstrated.

The second group is presumed to have mood disorders provoked by HIV. This has been attributed to the systemic effects of viral infection, in particular brain involvement. This should not be surprising, given a neurotropic virus known to affect subcortical brain areas. By analogy with other pathological processes causing subcortical brain damage—such as Parkinson's disease, Huntington's disease, and stroke—AIDS would be expected to cause high rates of mood disorders along with the other deficits of the "subcortical triad" (dementia, depression, dyskinesis) (24). These cases of affective disorder would be expected to occur late in the course of HIV, around the time of other clinical manifestations of AIDS. In fact, longitudinal examination of a large cohort of HIV-infected men showed that rates of depressive symptoms and presumably index cases of depression (as measured by threshold scores on the CES-D mood scale) increase dramatically around 6–18 months preceding clinical AIDS, from about 10% to 25%. This increase occurs independent of both somatic symptoms and knowledge of progression and suggests symptoms produced directly by a pathological brain process (25).

For both groups of patients it has also been suggested that the chronic stresses associated with HIV infection may be a provocative or exacerbating factor in mood disorders. Activation of the hypothalamic-pituitary-adrenal axis and other physiological stress responses have been suggested as potential mechanisms. The known association between stressors and mood disorder in vulnerable individuals makes this an intriguing possibility.

The most frequent complaints in HIV patients presenting for psychiatric evaluation are depressive symptoms. Such symptoms may accompany any of a number of disorders (see Table 1), each requiring different treatment strategies. Probably the most frequently, though often erroneously, invoked explanation for depressive symptoms is understandable demoralization over having HIV infection. Patients with a progressively disabling fatal illness that provokes stigma and isolation do encounter life circumstances that produce disruption and sadness. Demoralization, or adjustment disorders, should

Table 1 Differential Diagnosis of Depressive Symptoms in HIV Infection

Major depression
Demoralization
Dementia
Delirium
Drugs

always be on the differential in the evaluation of depressive symptoms. Many persons do go through a transient period of demoralization and sadness on learning of their HIV diagnosis.

As with other severe chronic illnesses, though, most patients gradually recover and readjust as life goes on. In fact, most patients with HIV do not have high rates of depressive symptoms. If they arise, however, depressive symptoms should not be dismissed as understandable and "normal" but rather should be considered as possible evidence of an impairing disorder and cause for careful workup.

Major depression may have different features in the outpatient clinic, hospital, or nursing home settings. In the outpatient clinic setting, spontaneous complaints of low mood are the most frequent presentation for major depression. Many patients also present to primary care providers with complaints about sleep, appetite, anxiety, vague pain, general malaise, as well as specific medical problems with no clear "organic" cause. Patients complaining of insomnia may have been treated with hypnotics and may be dependent on them, complicating both diagnosis and treatment. Early morning awakening may suggest underlying mood disorder. Many patients will present with nonspecific feelings of anxiety or "nerves" and may have been treated with anxiolytics (especially benzodiazepines), which often worsen their depressions. Exaggerated fears regarding medical symptoms and preoccupying catastrophic worries about health are frequent. Some patients will express diminished self-attitude by concerns or suspicions of being stigmatized or rejected out of proportion to their actual circumstances or in some cases even when no one else knows about their serostatus. Sustained despair or hopelessness over the very fact of HIV positivity as a kind of "death sentence" may reflect enduring aspects of temperament in some patients, but in many may be an episodic symptom of major depression. Longitudinal assessments are helpful in sorting out confusing presentations or difficult differential diagnoses.

We have found it useful to screen routinely for psychiatric distress in HIV clinic patients rather than wait for progressive severity to warrant urgent referral. The combination of two brief self-administered questionnaires, the Beck Depression Inventory (BDI) and the General Health Questionnaire (GHQ), is a simple and efficient screening tool. A score of >14 on the BDI or >6 on the GHQ prospectively predicted a DSM-III-R axis I diagnosis (other than substance abuse) as made by a psychiatrist's evaluation, with a sensitivity of 81%, specificity of 61%, and a positive predictive value of 71% (5). Because of this we have instituted the policy of incorporating this screen into the standard HIV medical clinic intake evaluation. All patients who score above the screening thresholds are automatically referred to psychiatry for further evaluation.

Such screens identify psychiatric symptoms and the likelihood of a psychiatric disorder but cannot make a diagnosis or distinguish various disorders from each other. This is the role of psychiatric history and examination. The diagnosis of major depression requires careful clinical evaluation in the HIV-infected patient, who often has comorbid substance abuse, personality vulnerabilities, and severe psychosocial stressors.

The inpatient medical hospital setting, in which psychiatric diagnoses are typically made by a consultation service, presents a different set of difficulties. The overall severity of multisystem symptoms and the urgency generated by this setting may lead care providers to jump prematurely from a presentation of acute distress to a presumption of major depression. Additionally, delirium is very frequent in the hospital setting and can present with a bewildering array of symptoms, including emotional ones, often confused with mood disorders (both mania and depression). Because of the shifting symptoms of acutely medically ill patients, cross-sectional mental status examination is relatively unreliable in making a diagnosis. Because of the relatively brief duration of hospital stays, extended or longitudinal assessment is often impossible. Therefore, past history and reports from outside informants take on greater importance.

It is usually best to be conservative in making a *new* diagnosis of major depression, postponing it until the medical condition has stabilized, often after the patient is back in the outpatient setting. A lower threshold for diagnosis is appropriate for patients with known histories of mood disorder, although we believe it usually inappropriate to diagnose major depression or reinitiate treatment while patients are delirious, even if there is an underlying mood disorder.

The nursing home setting is notable for the fragility of advanced-stage AIDS patients with multiple medical illnesses. The majority of patients we see in this setting have dementia of varying severity. Depressive syndromes will often present with small or subtle changes. These debilitated or demented patients may not be able to clearly describe classic subjective symptoms of depression. Serial observations by caregivers are more useful. Fortunately, in this setting, patients will have well-known baselines, and longitudinal assessment should be the rule. Presentations will include dysphoria (either sadness or irritability), moping, apathy, decreased social interaction, negativism, sleep disturbances, and anorexia. Many patients with dementia develop behavioral disturbances, which may occur as catastrophic responses to unmanageable (even if minor) environmental provocations. Sometimes, however, when behavioral disturbances are accompanied by a prominent and persistent mood disturbance, a diagnosis of major depression may be warranted. Because these patients are very susceptible to frequent delirium, it is crucial to distinguish that syndrome from affective disorder.

The key to making the diagnosis of affective disorder in HIV patients is to follow standard psychiatric diagnostic practice, without overly discounting signs and symptoms either because of putative severity of stressors on the one hand or putative "organic" factors on the other. When depressive symptoms cluster together in the familiar syndromal pattern, the diagnosis of major depression should be made. In fact, patients themselves will often misinterpret depressive symptoms and attribute low mood to the burden of having HIV, in essence making a layman's diagnosis of adjustment disorder. On further inquiry, the patient's struggle with HIV may be long-standing and unchanged, while the depressive symptoms are new and atypical of the person's usual adaptive style.

Other frequently seen features include preoccupation with illness and fears of imminent death out of proportion to actual severity of medical condition. Patients with depression often feel that they are dying, when in fact they have virtually no symptoms of their infection. Accompanying features such as change in self-attitude (e.g., excessive guilt about having failed family by getting sick), change in vital sense, vegetative disturbance, or diurnal variation may help to confirm the diagnosis of affective disorder. In particular we have found anhedonia to be one of the most useful symptoms in difficult diagnoses. The diagnosis may remain counterintuitive to the patient, who insists that it is "understandable" to feel bad when you have HIV. The discontinuity of symptoms and lack of temporal correlation with stressors can help both the clinician and the patient differentiate major depression from demoralization.

Major depression can overlap with symptoms that accompany other HIV-related illnesses. Fatigue, sleep and appetite disturbance, general malaise, and feelings of illness are all such potentially overlapping symptoms. This is especially problematic because these nonspecific symptoms might occur in early-stage patients who are otherwise relatively healthy. However, these symptoms are less prominently related to HIV than many have supposed. Perkins et al. found no difference in fatigue, insomnia, or neurocognitive symptoms between early-stage HIV-infected homosexual men (average CD4 = 340) and noninfected homosexual controls (26). When these symptoms do occur in early-stage HIV infection, they are more likely to suggest mood disturbance than HIV disease progression. In evaluating early-stage homosexual HIV-infected men, fatigue and insomnia were highly correlated with both depressive symptoms and diagnosis of major depression but not with CD4 count (26). Additionally, worsening of fatigue and insomnia at 6-month follow-up was highly correlated with worsening depression but not CD4 count, change in CD4 count, or disease progression by CDC category. Others have also found that these symptoms are more closely associated with depression than with HIV disease progression (27).

These findings support the notion that somatic symptoms generally suggestive of depression should be cause for a full psychiatric evaluation and not explained away as resulting from HIV in its earlier stages. This is less applicable in later stage infection when a variety of illnesses are common. Somatic symptoms should always be evaluated carefully and considered in the context of the company they keep, i.e., either with other indicators or progression of HIV disease or with other indicators of depression. If somatic symptoms are misinterpreted, the diagnosis of major depression may be made too readily. In our experience, it is under- rather than overdiagnosis of major depression that has been a problem, but overdiagnosis could become a problem if the differential diagnosis is not fully considered.

Some HIV-related medical conditions and medications can cause depressive symptoms. These include the full range of CNS disorders such as toxoplasmosis, cryptococcus, lymphoma, syphilis, and many others (see Table 2). Some investigators have found significant rates of depressive symptoms among male HIV patients with hypotestosteronemia. Drugs such as AZT and other antiviral agents, metoclopramide, clonidine, propranolol, disulfiram, sulfonamides, anabolic and corticosteroids, muscle relaxants, cocaine, opioids, benzodiazepines, and many others have all been reported to produce major depression or similar syndromes. In these situations depressive symptoms

Table 2 Differential Diagnosis of Dementia in HIV-Infected Patients

AIDS dementia complex/HIV dementia
   Traumatic brain injury
   Organic brain injury (anoxia, toxic, metabolic, congenital)
   Mental retardation
   Poststroke dementia
Depression (pseudodementia)
Delirium
   Intoxication
     Prescribed medication
     Psychomotor stimulants, opiates, alcohol, sedative hypnotics (including
       alcohol)
   Withdrawal
     Sedative hynotics, opiates, others
   Anoxia/hypoxia
CNS infection (usually presenting as delirium, but may present with depression,
     dementia, or malaise)
   Toxoplasmosis
     Other parasites
   CMV encephalitis
   Herpes (zoster and simplex)
   JC virus—PML (progressive multifocal leukoencephalopathy)
     Other virus
Cryptococcal meningitis
     Other fungi
   Tuberculosis
   Other mycobacteria
   Syphilis
   Other bacteria
Stroke
CNS vasculitis
CNS tumors

and syndromes often respond to primary treatment for the underlying medical disorder or withdrawal of the offending drug. When they do not, they should be treated as secondary major depression with antidepressant medication.

Treatment of Depression

Several small preliminary open-label uncontrolled trials of antidepressants for major depression in HIV-infected patients, almost exclusively in homosexual men in early stages of infection, have shown both good tolerance and very good efficacy (28–33). Rabkin et al. (33) found imipramine significantly more effective than placebo in a double-blind controlled trial in depressed HIV patients, including many with AIDS. Of particular note was that the response rate (74%) was the same as those commonly seen in medically healthy patients with major depression. Further, patients' stage of HIV illness as indicated by CD4 count had no influence on response rate.

In our clinical experience, all of the antidepressants are effective against major depression in HIV-infected patients. This applies through the entire continuum of HIV, from asymptomatic to end-stage AIDS. To date, no study has demonstrated any effectiveness advantage of any individual agent or class of agents. We have used all of the available agents with good outcome, with side effect profile generally dictating our choice of drug. Although we have avoided bupropion in AIDS-defined patients because of the risk of seizures, this is generally an underused treatment option.

Although many patients do not have significant side effects, few patients have no side effects. Further, HIV patients as a group have increased difficulty with medications of all kinds. Therefore we have developed an approach to medication selection that emphasizes prescription based on consideration of potential side effects, using them deliberately when possible. Examples include adjunctive treatment for weight loss or diarrhea with tricyclics or for fatigue with selective serotonin-reuptake inhibitors (SSRIs) (see Fig. 2).

Not surprisingly, there are more severe side effects in medically symptomatic patients (32). This follows a progressive trend as patients advance in their HIV stage, with greater numbers of illnesses and greater overall organ system vulnerability. Considerations in drug choice and dosing must include decreased hepatic and/or renal clearance and increased susceptibility to bone marrow suppression. With progression, patients also tend to accumulate increasingly complicated polypharmaceutical regimens, which can affect antidepressant tolerance in unpredictable ways. In late-stage patients, medication trials should begin at low doses, and titrations should proceed more gradually than usual. Where relevant, serum drug levels should be checked earlier and more often than in standard circumstances. For example, it is not uncommon to see 25 mg/day (or even 10 mg) of nortriptyline produce a full therapeutic level. In general, the usual therapeutic levels apply, though the lower end of a given therapeutic range may often be preferable in late-stage patients because of side effect:benefit ratio.

Patients are especially sensitive to medications when they develop CNS sequelae including dementia. Although this tends to amplify susceptibility and severity for all potential side effects, delirium is the most significant. Because of this, tricyclics, which tend to provoke more delirium, should be used much more cautiously, with other agents such as SSRIs generally preferred in patients with advanced dementia or CNS infection.

Psychotherapy is also a critical component of the treatment of mood disorders in HIV patients. Patients often need guidance in traversing the potential pitfalls of life under the altered circumstances of HIV infection. They often need guidance in managing their complicated medical treatments. They certainly need guidance in strategies for coping with the world while afflicted with major depression. Randomized trials of time-limited psychotherapy have shown improvements in distress and depressive

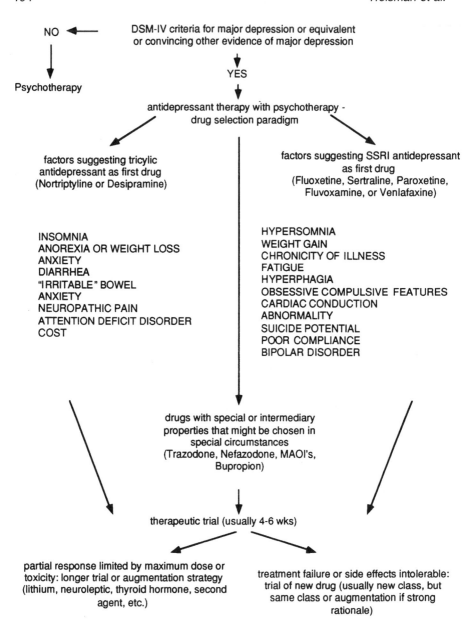

Figure 2   Algorithm for the antidepressant treatment of depression in HIV-infected patients.

symptoms in HIV patients. Preliminary observations suggest an advantage of an interpersonal approach focused on HIV-specific topics over a less direct supportive approach (34,35).

Many HIV patients with mood disorders are difficult to diagnose and treat because their course is complicated by other co-morbid psychiatric disorders. Because of these and other potentially complicating issues, assessment and treatment are often difficult. It is essential to formulate and frequently refine an explicit treatment plan and to review that plan with the patient. Furthermore, the success of the mood disorder treatment depends on the success of simultaneously treating any co-morbid condition.

PERSONALITY DISORDERS

Efforts to define personality disorder have been hampered by many conflicting ideas about etiology. Efforts to use operationalized criteria as in DSM-IV are unsatisfactory because of the dimensional nature of personality and the difficulty in distinguishing where to draw the line between traits and disorder. Additionally, many of the terms of personality disorder carry a psychodynamic interpretation while others are pejorative. We consider personality in a dimensional manner, and at the risk of oversimplification, we will discuss two prominent elements that underlie personality, extroversion versus introversion and stability versus instability (see Fig. 3). Although these dimensions do not correspond directly to DSM-IV personality disorders, they are prominent features of identified personality disorders (cluster A introversion, cluster B extroversion, and instability).

Extroverts find the present and its rewards very salient and have mercurial emotions. Introverts find the future and past salient and are consequence avoidant rather than reward seeking. Instability describes the magnitude of emotional excursion in response stimuli and the maximal excursion of emotion. Superimposition of these curves gives one the four quadrants shown in Figure 3. The patients in the choleric quadrant exhibit the borderline, histrionic, narcissistic, and antisocial traits (or cluster B traits). These patients tend to be impulsive, changeable, labile, driven by their feelings, and reward seeking. Patients with these vulnerabilities of temperament are not easily affected by negative consequences, and this makes them less likely to consider their consequences of high-risk behaviors and more vulnerable to intoxication that may lead to infection. Additionally, they may have difficulty in adapting to the persistent demands and slow frustrating pace of HIV, or any chronic medical treatment.

Rates of comorbid personality disorders are increased in HIV-infected patients (35,37–39). Features of personality disorders such as impulsivity are associated with high-risk sexual behaviors (40–42). Brooner et al. (43) showed an association between antisocial personality disorder and needle-sharing behavior among intravenous drug users. Uncontrolled studies have shown greater rates of personality disorder in HIV-positive persons than in the general population (38,39). Even more common has been the finding of increased rates of DSM-IV cluster B personality traits, such as impulsivity,

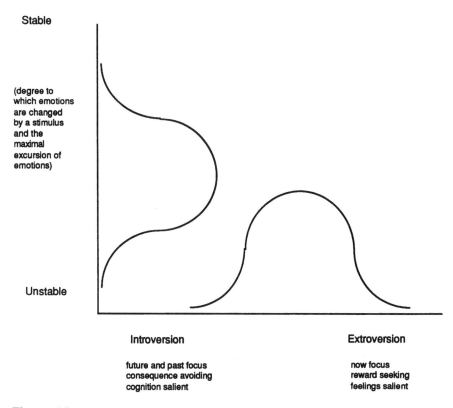

Stable

(degree to which emotions are changed by a stimulus and the maximal excursion of emotions)

Unstable

Introversion   Extroversion

future and past focus   now focus
consequence avoiding   reward seeking
cognition salient   feelings salient

Figure 3A   Our conceptualization of two independent axes of personality distributed in a dimensional manner. Each curve shows a hypothetical population distribution of people with the traits described on that axis.

emotional lability, instability of interpersonal relationships, etc., which can be component features of a personality disorder. In a study of 220 HIV testing volunteers, cluster B traits were correlated with an increased likelihood of a positive HIV test (36). Other semicontrolled studies have shown increased rates of personality disorders in groups of gay men (37) and intravenous drug users (44). One found a 19% rate of personality disorders in persons presenting for HIV testing, and although there was no difference between groups with positive and negative results, this very high rate again implies that personality disorders may be overrepresented in HIV risk groups in general.

Because we believe that these traits are distributed continuously, exacting definitions of who is afflicted by a full personality disorder and who merely has partial features has plagued research in this area. Nevertheless, clinicians agree these patients present a considerable challenge in treatment. The type of therapeutic approach we use has

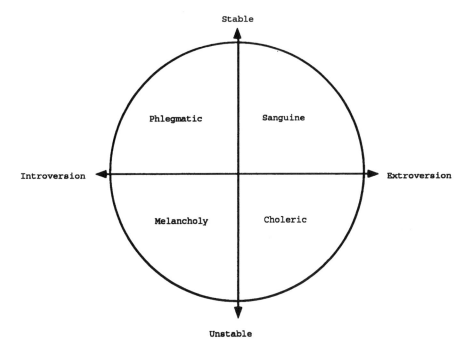

Figure 3B   The four types of personality as they derive from the humors described by the Hippocratic school of ancient Greece. They are shown as they correspond to the combination of the traits shown in Figure 3A.

usually been referred to as cognitive-behavioral therapy. These patients require additional encouragement, firm limits, and directive psychotherapy that emphasizes the rewards of treatment success.

Most descriptions of treatment methods emphasize three common practical components, despite widely varying theoretical underpinnings. These are (1) a clear set of goals for treatment, sometimes in the form of a contract, (2) a primary emphasis on behaviors and behavioral expectations, with the understanding that a patient may express their feelings but must not act on them, and (3) a clear description of the behavioral limits of treatment with a strategy for managing problem behaviors. Although perhaps counterintuitive, it is the principle that positive behavioral change will produce positive emotional change (and *not* vice versa) that provides these patients with a means for improvement.

We have recommended that patients with personality difficulties have a description of the treatment plan in the primary chart. All treating physicians must confer and agree on the plan to minimize splitting and staff frustration. Outrageous behavior is often the reason for psychiatric consultation, and a treatment contract that emphasizes rewards rather than punishments and is consistent around the clock will often help the staff as well as save the patient from destructive behavior patterns.

A final caveat is that personality influences the symptoms of other psychiatric disorders. Depression, mania, and dementia may be masked by chaotic behavior, conflict over treatment agendas, and substance abuse. It is therefore even more critical with the most challenging patients to clearly assess the needs for treatment of co-morbid substance use and affective disorders and to communicate the issues of the overall treatment plan to the patient and the treatment team.

DISORDERS OF MOTIVATED BEHAVIOR (ADDICTION)

Motivated behavior has been defined by McHugh and Slavney (1) as behavior provoked by internal changes such as visceral or endocrine phenomena or changes in responsiveness to behavior provoking external stimuli. Thus, addictions lead to motivated behavior because both external (availability of substance) and internal (withdrawal or craving) stimuli lead to an increase in the frequency of the addictive behavior.

Behavioral disorders (or addictions) are common in HIV-infected persons. The association between drug use disorders and HIV is well known. For those whose HIV risk factor is injection drug use (IDU), the etiological role of addiction is obvious. The proportion of AIDS patients in the United States who are IDUs increased from 17% during 1981–87 to 33% during 1993–1995 (45). Substance abuse plays a much broader role in HIV transmission than that. Heterosexual partners of injection drug users (mostly women) are one of the fastest growing groups of new seroconverters. In fact, in Maryland, 75% of all newly identified cases of HIV are IDUs or heterosexual partners of IDUs. Substance abuse, whether involving the injection route or not, is associated with other risk behaviors (46). This is not surprising given the chaotic relationships and behaviors frequent in drug abusers. Disinhibition and poor judgment often accompany intoxication and probably increase risk behaviors even in so-called recreational drug users. Drug use, independent of injection use, has been linked to sexual risk behaviors and high rates of various sexually transmitted diseases in both adults and adolescents. This presumably extends also to HIV transmission (47). The close link between crack cocaine use and high-risk sexual behaviors, such as prostitution and trading sex for drugs, has been well described (48). Among homosexual men estimates of substance use disorders are as high as 75% (20). Furthermore, drug use has been shown to correlate with high-risk sexual behaviors and seroconversion in homosexual men (49).

Ongoing addiction is common among HIV patients, and the overlap with other psychiatric disorders is very high as well. We found that 44% of HIV-infected new medical clinic intakes suffered from current substance use disorders (2). Further, 24% of patients had both current substance abuse and an additional non–substance abuse axis I diagnosis. This trend has continued, with about a quarter of all patients in our

HIV medical clinic having so-called "triple diagnoses"—HIV, addiction, and another psychiatric disorder. These patterns apply equally to patients whose risk factor was other than injection drug use. The use of intoxicants confounds treatment of mood disorders because they can provoke, exacerbate, and sustain affective symptoms. Illicit drugs and alcohol can have many potentially dangerous interactions with medicines. And the chaotic cycle of addiction often disrupts a patient's ability to pursue medical and psychiatric treatment (50,51). For these reasons, identification and treatment of drug disorders is an essential part of the overall treatment of HIV patients.

Another behavioral disorder associated with HIV, though less well studied, is paraphilia. Some patients report histories of unusually strong sexual drives or compulsive patterns of high-risk sexual behaviors that contributed to their contraction of HIV. Sexual risk behaviors often continue despite full understanding of risk and so-called safer sex practices. High frequency of "casual" sexual activity has been shown to correlate with both risk behaviors and actual seroconversion (49).

In our clinical experience, it is the patients who have active behavioral disorders who report the highest rates of ongoing risk behaviors despite full knowledge of the endangerment of others. Much controversy has arisen over the use of so-called harm-reduction strategies. Some of these strategies, such as needle exchange programs, bleach sterilization education, condom distribution to prostitutes, etc., have been quite effective (52). Although practical in their aims, implicit in these strategies is the idea that certain conditions are hopeless. This should be contrasted with rehabilitative strategies, which emphasize treatment and the hopeful prospect of recovery from behavioral disorders. Much encouraging work is ongoing in this field (53). Batki et al. (53) have shown the benefit of combined pharmacological and psychotherapeutic interventions in cocaine addicts. Our group has successfully combined addiction and paraphilia rehabilitation in the outpatient clinic with a full spectrum of medical and psychiatric treatments (see below under outcome).

LIFE CIRCUMSTANCES

Finally, while we must not "explain away" all suffering as understandable, demoralization is real. HIV patients can sustain numerous personal losses, many of them catastrophic. The stigma attached to HIV and AIDS is still enormous despite public education. Misconceptions about transmission sometimes lead to HIV-infected persons being treated as outcasts. They may be rejected by family and friends. Some keep their serostatus secret, even from their most intimate partners. Persons with HIV also may have frequent losses, when friends, acquaintances, and loved ones die from AIDS. Bereavement and reaction to loss are more likely to take on the form of grief and posttraumatic response than of a depressive disorder (54).

The event of new seroconversion can often lead to severe acute reactions. As with any devastating news, shock and/or denial may give way to sadness, anger, and hopelessness. Rates of suicidal thoughts and even actual suicide are increased temporarily during this acute response (55). Feelings of self-pity, guilt, victimization, imminent mortality, and being overwhelmed are also common. Eventually, feelings that life is over usually give way to feelings that life can continue, though under altered circumstances; acceptance seems to be the rule rather than the exception.

Later in the course of infection, with the development of HIV-related symptoms and eventually AIDS, additional life stressors accumulate. As their illness advances patients often struggle with pain and inability to care for themselves. Loss of employment and other features of independence are common, as are impoverishment and social disenfranchisement, understandably leading to varying degrees of demoralization. Patients tend to focus on and even overreact to small changes in laboratory indicators such as CD4 counts. Some will have an acute crisis response to the news of AIDS definition, even if they are clinically asymptomatic. Although demoralization is to some extent inevitable, as in any progressively disabling and debilitating condition, levels of social support, and more importantly *perceived* social support, can be protective against psychological distress. Counseling, support groups, family groups, family education programs, drop-in centers, and advocacy programs are all useful in countering demoralization. Treatment by compassionate physicians can very much improve feelings of hope and quality of life for these patients. Particularly, the ability to plan for changes in medical condition, a discussion of the options for treatment, and a sense of therapeutic optimism are essential to these patients and often perceived as a "lifeline" by them. If life stressors are exaggerated by affective disorder, especially depression, they are all the more burdensome, and can be helped by aggressive antidepressant treatment.

OUTCOME

There are few data on outcomes using multiple treatment modalities in "usual care" clinical settings. A retrospective chart review in our clinic at Johns Hopkins University examined treatment outcome in 110 patients treated for major depression (10). These were a heterogeneous group of patients with mixed risk factors; mixed stage of HIV infection; mixed demographic characteristics; mixed comorbidity (including active addiction and personality disorder); mixed duration of, and compliance with, treatment. Retrospective rating of severity of depressive symptoms at last observation revealed 85% of all patients were at least somewhat improved, including 51% who were very much improved. Confounding variables such as poor compliance or additional co-morbidity were associated with lower rates of full remission, but not lower rates of partial improvement.

In a later prospective study, we followed a cohort of 126 HIV-infected patients referred for psychiatric evaluation and treatment (5). The group was composed of mixed psychiatric diagnoses, including 62% with major depression. Otherwise they had a similar heterogeneous mix of characteristics as in our previous group. Treatment, including pharmacology and psychotherapy, was delivered according to individualized treatment plans.

All patients had at least one follow-up visit following evaluation, with an average follow-up period of 14 months (range 1–36). Using a global outcome measure including symptoms, overall function, and HIV risk behavior, 50% of patients were improved including 20% who were nearly well. Patients were abstinent from alcohol and illicit drugs 50% of the time. These results were similar regardless of non–substance abuse psychiatric diagnosis. The most powerful predictor of outcome was compliance with treatment, rated independently, with a vigorous dose-responsive effect. Of patients with "poor" compliance, 85% had outcomes of not improved or worse and achieved abstinence 32% of the time. Of patients with "good" compliance, 95% were at least somewhat improved, including 46% who were nearly well. These patients also achieved abstinence 68% of the time.

Although success rates vary depending upon the co-morbid diagnosis, type of addictive substance used, level of social and economic support available, and other factors, our follow-up data suggest that HIV-infected patients' psychiatric problems can be helped with both psychological and pharmacological treatment.

CONCLUSION

We believe that psychiatric disorders increase risk behaviors for HIV infection (Fig. 1). We also feel that HIV causes a variety of psychiatric disorders through both disenfranchisement and social deconstruction as well as by direct subcortical injury. Psychiatric disorders, including affective disorders (both major depression and mania), dementia, addiction, personality disorders, and demoralization are common and severely impairing in patients with HIV infection. These disorders have tremendous impact on subjective well-being, self-care, a level of overall function, compliance with medical treatment, and continuation of risk behaviors with implications for further HIV transmission.

While many caregivers have noted the burdens and deficits suffered by HIV patients because of their depression and despair, we would caution that compassion for the suffering of HIV patients may divert attention from potentially treatable psychiatric conditions such as affective disorders. Empathic understanding can become a kind of clinical nihilism in which all psychological distress is interpreted as deserving of comfort measures such as support, sedatives, and narcotics. Diagnosis of mood disorders in HIV patients, in particular discrimination of major depression from demoralization, can be difficult. Treatment of affective and other psychiatric disorders, however, leads to improved outcomes.

Mood disorders in HIV patients respond well to treatment, even in patients with advanced AIDS, dementia, or co-morbid conditions such as addiction and personality disorder. Substance abuse responds to treatment, and even though permanent abstinence is less common, intermittent sustained abstinence with progressive decrease in relapse frequency is common. Personality disorders, though chronic, can be managed so that life can proceed less chaotically and treatment more fruitfully. In our experience, patients who respond to treatment for their psychiatric disorders do better in a variety of domains. We expect that further research will reveal that effective treatment of major depression, mania, and other psychiatric disorders in HIV patients prolongs health and perhaps life. Furthermore, as psychiatric symptoms become more prominent among patients with HIV infection and perhaps contribute to HIV-transmission risk behaviors, we hope to show that aggressive treatment of psychiatric disorders will play a role in slowing the spread of HIV.

ACKNOWLEDGMENT

We thank Ms. Claire Mooney for help in preparing the manuscript.

REFERENCES

1. McHugh PR, Slavney PR. The Perspectives of Psychiatry. 2nd ed. Baltimore: Johns Hopkins University Press, 1998.
2. Lyketsos CG, Hanson AL, Fishman M, et al. Screening for psychiatric morbidity in a medical outpatient clinic for HIV infection: the need for a psychiatric presence. Int J Psychiatry Med 1994; 24:103–113.
3. Lyketsos CG, Hanson AL, Fishman M, et al. Manic episode early and late in the course of HIV. Am J Psychiatry 1993; 150:326–327.
4. Kieburtz K, Zettelmaier AE, Ketonen L, et al. Manic syndrome in AIDS. Am J Psychiatry 1991; 148:1068–1470.
5. Lyketsos CG, Schwartz J, Fishman M, Treisman G. AIDS mania. J Neuropsychiatry Clin Neurosci 1997; 9:277–279.
6. Lyketsos CG, Treisman GJ. Psychiatric disorders in HIV-infected patients: epidemiology and issues in drug treatment. CNS Drugs 1995; 4:195–206.
7. Regier DA, Boyd JH, Burke JD, et al. One-month prevalence of mental disorders in the United States. Arch Gen Psychiatry 1988; 5:977–986.
8. Chochinov HM, Wilson KG, Ennis M, et al. Desire for death in the terminally ill. Am J Psychiatry 1995; 152:1185–1191.
9. Derogatis LR, Morrow GR, Fetting J, et al. The prevalence of psychiatric disorders among cancer patients. JAMA 1983; 249:751–757.
10. Treisman G, Fishman M, Lyketsos C, McHugh PR. Evaluation and treatment of psychiatric disorders associated with HIV infection. In: Price RW, Perry SW, eds. HIV, AIDS and the Brain. New York: Raven Press, 1994:239–250.
11. Fishman M, Treisman G. Institute on Psychiatric Services [abstr]. Chicago, July 1996.
12. O'Dowd MA, et al. Characteristics of patients attending an HIV related psychiatric clinic. Hosp Commun Psychiatry 1991; 42:615–619.
13. O'Dowd MA, McKegney FP. AIDS patients compared with others seen in psychiatric consultation. Gen Hosp Psychiatry 1990; 12:50–55.

14. Dilley JW, Ochtill HN, Perl M, et al. Findings in psychiatric consultations with patients with acquired immune deficiency syndrome. Am J Psychiatry 1985; 142:82–86.

15. Maj M, Janssen R, Starace F, et al. WHO neuropsychiatric AIDS study, cross-sectional phase I: study design and psychiatric findings. Arch Gen Psychiatry 1994; 51:39–49.

16. Perkins DO, Stern RA, Golden RN, Murphy C, Naftolowitz D, Evans DL. Mood disorders in HIV infection: prevalence and risk factors in a nonepicenter of the AIDS epidemic. Am J Psychiatry 1994; 151(2):233–236.

17. Atkinson JH, Grant I, Kennedy CJ, et al. Prevalence of psychiatric disorders among men infected with human immunodeficiency virus: a controlled study. Arch Gen Psychiatry 1988; 45:859–864.

18. Gala C. Pergami A, Catalan J, et al. The psychosocial impact of HIV infection in gay men, drug users, and heterosexuals: controlled investigation. Br J Psychiatry 1993; 163:651–659.

19. Brown GR, Rundell JR, McManis SE, et al. Prevalence of psychiatric disorders in early stages of HIV infection. Psychosom Med 1992; 54:588–601.

20. Rosenberger PH, Bornstein RA, Nasrallah HA, et al. Psychopathology in HIV infection: lifetime and current assessment. Compr Psychiatry 1993; 34:150–158.

21. Williams JB, Rabkin J, Remien RH, et al. Multi-disciplinary baseline assessment of homosexual men with and without human immunodeficiency virus infection. II. Standardized assessment of current and lifetime psychopathology. Arch Gen Psychiatry 1991; 480:124–130.

22. Perry S, Jacobsberg LB, Fishman B. Psychiatric diagnosis before serological testing for the human immunodeficiency virus. Am J Psychiatry 1990; 147:89–93.

23. Regier DA, Farmer ME. Comorbidity of mental disorders with alcohol and other drug abuse. JAMA 1990; 264(19):2511–2518.

24. McHugh PR. The neuropsychiatry of basal ganglia disorder: a triadic syndrome and its explanation. Neuropsychiatry Neuropsychol Behav Neurol 1989; 2:239–247.

25. Lyketsos CG, Hoover DR, Guccione M, et al. Changes in depressive symptoms as AIDS develops. Am J Psychiatry 1996; 153:1430–1437.

26. Perkins DO, Leserman J, Stern RA, et al. Somatic symptoms and HIV infection: relationship to depressive symptoms and indicators of HIV disease. Am J Psychiatry 1995; 155(12):1776–1781.

27. Pugh K, Riccio M, Jadresic D, et al. A longitudinal study of the neuropsychiatric consequences of HIV-1 infection in gay men. II. Psychological and health status at baseline and at 12-month follow-up. Psycholog Med 1994; 24:897–904.

28. Rabkin JJ, Rabkin R, Wagner G. Effects of fluoxetine on mood and immune status in depressed patients with HIV illness. J Clin Psychiatry 1994; 55:92–97.

29. Rabkin JG, Harrison WM. Effect of imipramine on depression and immune status in a sample of men with HIV infection. Am J Psychiatry 1990; 147(4):495–497.

30. Fernandez F, Levy JK, Mansell PW. Response to antidepressant therapy in depressed persons with advanced HIV infection [abstr]. International Conference on AIDS, Montreal, 1989.

31. Lyketsos CG, Fishman M, Hutton H, et al. The effectiveness of psychiatric treatment for HIV-infected patients. Psychosomatics 1997; 38:423–432.

32. Hintz S, Kuck J, Peterkin JJ, et al. Depression in the context of human immunodeficiency virus infection: implications for treatment. J Clin Psychiatry 1990; 51:497–501.

33. Rabkin JG, Rabkin R, Harrison W, Wagner G. Effect of imipramine on mood and enumer-

ative measures of immune status in depressed patients with HIV illness. Am J Psychiatry 1994; 151(4):516–523.

34. Markowitz JC, Klerman GL, Clougherty KF, et al. Individual psychotherapies for depressed HIV-positive patients. Am J Psychiatry 1995; 152:1504–1905.

35. Kelly JA, Murphy DA, Bahr GR, et al. Outcome of cognitive-behavioral and support group therapies for depressed, HIV-infected persons. Am J Psychiatry 1993; 150(11):1679–1686.

36. Jacobsberg L, Frances A, Perry S. Axis II diagnoses among volunteers for HIV testing and counseling. Am J Psychiatry 1995; 152(8):1222–1224.

37. Perkins DO, Davidson JD, Leserman J, Liao D, Evans D. Personality disorder in patients infected with HIV: a controlled study with implications for clinical care. Am J Psychiatry 1993; 150(2):309–315.

38. Pace J, Brown GR, Rundell JR, Paolucci S, McManis DK. Prevalence of psychiatric disorders in a mandatory screening program for infection with human immunodeficiency virus: a pilot study. Military Med 1990; 155(2):76–80.

39. James ME, Rubin CP, Willis SE. Drug abuse and psychiatric findings in HIV seropositive pregnant patients. Gen Hosp Psychiatry 1991; 13(1):4–8.

40. McCusker J, Stoddard AM, Zapka JG, et al. Predictors of AIDS-preventive behavior among homosexually active men: a longitudinal study. AIDS 1989; 3:443–448.

41. Seal DW, Agostinelli G. Individual differences associated with high-risk sexual behavior: implications for intervention programmes. AIDS Care 1994; 6:393–397.

42. Perkins DO, Leserman J, Murphy C, Evans DL. Psychosocial predictors of high-risk sexual behavior among HIV-negative homosexual men. AIDS Educ Prev 1993; 5:141–152.

43. Brooner RK, Bigelow GE, Strain E, Schmidt CW. Intravenous drug abusers with antisocial personality disorder: increased HIV risk behavior. Drug Alcohol Depend 1990; 26:39–44.

44. Ellis D, Collis I, King M. A controlled comparison of HIV and general medical referrals to a liaison psychiatry service. AIDS Care 1994; 6:69–76.

45. Centers for Disease Control and Prevention. First 500,000 AIDS cases—United States, 1995. MMWR 1995; 46:849–853.

46. Centers for Disease Control and Prevention. Continued sexual risk behavior among HIV-seropositive, drug-using men—Atlanta; Washington, D.C.; and San Juan, Puerto Rico. MMWR 1996; 45:151–152.

47. Booth RE, Watters JK, Chitwood DD. HIV risk-related sex behaviors among injection drug users, crack smokers, and injection drug users who smoke crack. Am J Public Health 1993; 83:1144–1148.

48. Edlin BR, Irwin KL, Faruque S, et al. Intersecting epidemics: crack cocaine use and HIV infection among inner-city young adults. N Engl J Med 1994; 331:1422–1427.

49. Doll LS, Ostrow DG. Homosexual and bisexual behavior and HIV prevention. In: Holmes KK, Sparling PF, Mardh PA, Lemon SM, Stamm WF, Piot P, Wasserheit JN, eds. Sexually Transmitted Diseases. 3d ed. New York: McGraw-Hill, 1996.

50. Broers B, Morabia A, Hirschel B. A cohort study of drug users' compliance with zidovudine treatment. Arch Intern Med 1994; 154:1121–1127.

51. Wall TL, Sorensen JL, Batki SL, Delucchi KL, London JA, Chesney MA. Adherence to zidovudine (AZT) among HIV-infected methadone patients: a pilot study of supervised therapy and dispensing compared to usual care. Drug Alcohol Depend 1995; 37:261–269.

52. Des Jarlais DC, Hagan H, Friedman SR, et al. Maintaining low HIV seroprevalence in populations of injecting drug users. JAMA 1995; 274(15):1226–1231.

53. Batki SL, Manfredi LB, Jacob P III, Delucci K, Murphy J, Washburn A, Goldberger L, Jones RT. Double-blind fluoxetine treatment of cocaine dependence in methadone maintenance treatment (MMT) patients—Interim analysis. In: Harris LS, ed. Problems of Drug Dependence 1992: Proceedings of the 54th Annual Scientific Meeting of the College on the Problems of Drug Dependence. National Institutes of Health, 1993:102.
54. Goodkin K, Blaney N, Tuttle R, et al. Bereavement and HIV infection. Int Rev Psychiatry 1996; 8:267–276.
55. Perry SW, Jacobsberg L, Fishman B. Suicidal ideation and HIV testing. JAMA 1990; 263: 679–682.
56. Lyketsos CG, Fishman M, Treisman G, et al. Effectiveness of psychiatric treatment for HIV-infected patients [abstr]. 6th Annual Meeting of the American Neuropsychiatric Association, 1995.

11

Pulmonary Disease and Lung Transplantation

Catherine L. Woodman and Joel N. Kline

University of Iowa College of Medicine
Iowa City, Iowa

BACKGROUND

Respiratory disorders are a major medical and social problem. They are the cause of substantial morbidity and mortality, and are considered to be the largest single cause of absence from work (1). There is considerable comorbidity between pulmonary disorders and psychiatric disorders, with depression and anxiety disorders co-occurring most frequently. The psychiatric illness may be secondary to the pulmonary illness, either because the respiratory disorder is a severe and chronic illness or as a result of the physiological changes that occur with the respiratory disease. Alternatively, there may be a genetic basis linking a predisposition to respiratory and psychiatric disorders. Therefore, any discussion of the epidemiology, course, and treatment of lung disease should also include a discussion of the concomitant psychological and behavioral issues.

Anatomically, there is some limited evidence to connect pulmonary disease with psychiatric illness. The respiratory centers are positioned in the brainstem and are connected via the hippocampal formation to the parahippocampal region. The parahippocampal region has been hypothesized to be affected in patients with panic disorder. Using positron emission tomography to study patients with lactate-induced panic disorder, Reiman and associates (2) noted an abnormal hemispheric asymmetry of parahippocampal blood flow, blood volume, and oxygen metabolism, as well as abnormally high brain metabolism overall and increased susceptibility to hyperventilation. The hyperventilation may lead to abnormal parahippocampal activity in subjects with pulmonary disorders, and make these subjects more vulnerable to panic attacks. If hyperventilation and panic are then misconstrued as indicating worsening of the patient's respiratory disorder, then dosages of medications may be inappropriately increased.

Many of these medications increase anxiety, and may lead to worsening of the psychiatric disorder.

The behavior of the individual is an important component of the development and management of many respiratory diseases. Smoking is the behavior that is of greatest importance in pulmonary disorders. It is the primary cause of chronic obstructive pulmonary disease (COPD), and COPD is the most prevalent of all lung diseases, accounting for half of all mortality due to pulmonary causes. Smoking also plays a role in the development and exacerbation of other respiratory conditions, such as asthma and occupational lung disease. In addition, once the disease process has begun, the patient's behavior may affect management of the disease. In many conditions, the patient must take some action to control the disease, by taking medication, avoiding allergens, stopping smoking, or exercising regularly. The motivation of the patient to make and maintain the necessary changes over a long period of time is a major challenge. Figure 1 summarizes the biopsychosocial model of how psychological factors and the environment contribute to the manifestation and course of pulmonary disorders. This chapter reviews the influence of psychiatric illness on pulmonary disorders and the effect of pulmonary disorders on the management and course of psychiatric disorders.

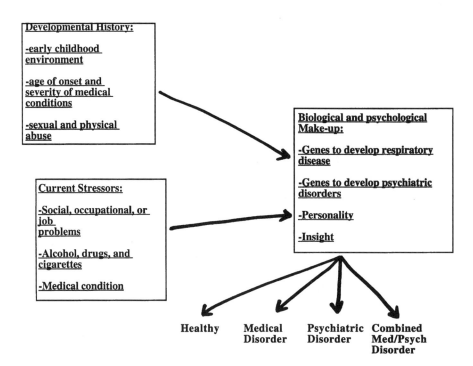

Figure 1   Biopsychosocial model of interaction between respiratory and psychiatric disorders.

CASE HISTORIES

Case 1: Panic Disorder and Asthma

Ms. A. is a 29-year-old nurse with moderate persistent to severe persistent asthma since early childhood. Her asthma is characterized by both atopic (allergic) and nonatopic triggers. It is further complicated by chronic sinusitis, which has necessitated multiple surgical procedures and continues to cause the patient substantial pain on a daily basis. Control of her asthma has required repeated bursts of prednisone, averaging six bursts per year since childhood; additional medications include inhaled steroids, oral and inhaled beta-agonists, and theophylline, as well as self-administered terbutaline or epinephrine injections for severe acute attacks. Ms. A.'s acute asthma exacerbations are characterized by chest tightness, wheezing, tachypnea, tachycardia, and severe dyspnea; she has been hospitalized for asthma exacerbations at least twice yearly for the past decade. Ms. A was diagnosed with panic disorder at age 27. At the time of her diagnosis she had a number of recent life stressors, the importance of which she minimized. The patient was experiencing marital difficulties and caring for a mildly mentally retarded child at the time that she was diagnosed with panic disorder. Her panic attacks mimicked her asthma exacerbations in all ways except for the lack of bronchospasm. Prior to the diagnosis of panic disorder, the treatment for her attacks of dyspnea centered on sympathomimetic agents that exacerbated her anxiety and panic. The patient required a combination of an antidepressant and a benzodiazepine to control episodes of panic. Her asthma was not substantially changed by treatment for panic disorder, but her emergency room visits diminished substantially.

Case 2: Asthma, Prednisone, and Disorders of Thought and Mood

Dr. B. is a 63-year-old male biochemist with a 15-year history of severe persistent asthma, which has resulted in permanent medical disability. His FEV_1 is 1.54 L (48% predicted) at baseline. Although steroid bursts have been used to treat exacerbations, use of corticosteroids has resulted in severe mood and thought disturbances with symptoms of sleeplessness, irritability, pressured speech, flight of ideas, and occasional visual hallucinations. In addition, his course has been complicated by major depressive episodes associated with the deaths of two sons. Medications include paroxetine, inhaled short- and long-acting beta-agonists, antihistamines, and inhaled steroids. Because of worsening control of his asthma, requiring several hospitalizations, the patient was referred for a second opinion. To maximize his anti-inflammatory therapy without resorting to systemic steroids, the patient was started on high-dose inhaled fluticasone (Flovent 220; four puffs b.i.d.), the most potent inhaled steroid currently available in the United States. One week after institution of this therapy, the patient's wife called to report that he was sleeping only 2–3 hours nightly and was "acting weird." This behavior improved when his dose was reduced, and then disappeared completely when fluticasone was discontinued and a less potent inhaled steroid was used.

These cases represent two situations in which psychiatric illness impacts on the management of a common pulmonary disorder, asthma. In the first case, the treatment of the patient's medical condition impacts significantly on the expression of her psychiatric disorder; sympathomimetic medications such as beta-agonists, anticholinergics, and theophylline are mainstays of the treatment of asthma and other pulmonary disorders; and these agents can cause or exacerbate anxiety and panic attacks. Careful attention to the relationship between the patient's symptoms and physiological parameters allowed differentiation between asthma and panic attacks. Treatment of her panic disorder focused on anxiolytic medication as well as on diminishing the use of sympathomimetic agents as much as possible. In the second case, hypomania and psychosis secondary to corticosteroids impact on and limit their use in a disabled patient who could otherwise benefit from them. Although altered mental status is not uncommon secondary to high-dose corticosteroids, it is rarely induced by inhaled corticosteroids. Patients with this side effect can be successfully treated with thymoleptic medications, such as lithium or valproate, but these medications necessitate additional monitoring. As higher-potency steroid agents are being used with increased frequency, psychiatric side effects may become more common.

CLINICAL ATTRIBUTES OF PULMONARY DISORDERS

Dyspnea

Dyspnea, an uncomfortable increased awareness of breathing, is a cardinal symptom of many pulmonary disorders, and may also be caused by abnormalities of cardiac, endocrine, or other organ systems. In many cases, relief of dyspnea is the primary goal of the treating physician, especially when the symptom is out of proportion to physiological parameters such as hypoxemia, hypercarbia, or pulmonary functions. In addition, dyspnea can be a symptom of anxiety or depression in the absence of nonpsychiatric disease. Differentiating between pulmonary and psychiatric causes of dyspnea can be challenging for the practitioner, but it is vital since the treatment of dyspnea will significantly depend on its cause (Table 1).

The two main physiological correlates to the sensation of dyspnea are increased respiratory effort and "length-tension inappropriateness." As the efficiency of breathing decreases or ventilatory demand increases, progressive increases in respiratory effort are required. At some point, which varies between individuals, the increased work of breathing is noted as dyspnea. Respiratory drive is affected by oxygen (PaO_2) and carbon dioxide ($PaCO_2$) levels in the blood, pH, thyroid hormones, and level of sympathetic activation, among other factors. There is a considerable range in sensitivity to these factors, both in health and in lung disease. For example, in COPD with equivalent impairment in lung function, a "pink puffer" generally has a low or normal $PaCO_2$ and normoxemia, and notes dyspnea even at rest, whereas a "blue bloater" is relatively dyspnea-free, but may have an increased $PaCO_2$ and hypoxemia. These expressions of obstructive lung disease are not dependent on its etiology or absolute severity, and they

Table 1 Etiologies of Dyspnea

Pulmonary
  Obstructive physiology
    Asthma
    Emphysema
    Chronic bronchitis
    Bronchiectasis
    Intrathoracic bronchial obstruction (polypoid tumor, tracheomalacia)
  Restrictive physiology—pulmonary
    Idiopathic pulmonary fibrosis
  Secondary pulmonary fibrosis (collagen-vascular disease, pneumoconioses, postinfectious, etc.)
  Pulmonary edema (congestive heart failure, neurogenic, adult respiratory distress syndrome, capillary leak syndromes)
  Restrictive physiology—extrapulmonary
    Thoracic cage (kyphoscoliosis, flail chest)
    Obesity and abdominal mass (tumor, ascites, pregnancy)
    Pleural disease (thickening, mesothelioma, pleural effusion, pneumothorax)
Vascular
  Pulmonary emboli
  Pulmonary hemorrhage
  Vasculitis (pulmonary)
  Pulmonary hypertension
Neurological
  Neuromuscular (diaphragmatic weakness)
    Polio and post-polio syndrome
    Demyelinating disorders (Guillain-Barré, chronic inflammatory demyelinating polyneuropathy)
    Posttraumatic (cervical spinal injury)
    Toxins (botulism, hyperthyroidism)
  Central (increased respiratory drive)
    Acidosis
      Metabolic
      Respiratory
    Hypoxemia
    Increased metabolic drive
      Hyperthyroidism
      Stimulants (theophylline, amphetamines, cocaine)
  Peripheral/Sensory
    Irritant receptors
    Stretch receptors (air trapping in COPD, asthma)
    Pulmonary hypertension
Psychiatric
  Anxiety
  Depression
  Somatization
  Factitious

may be genetically determined. Of interest, sensitivity to CO_2 is also important in the evaluation of panic attacks.

Length-tension inappropriateness is a description for the perception that diaphragm and accessory muscle activation has not led to sufficient muscle contraction (ventilation). This may be due to increased airway resistance (as in obstructive lung disease) or elastic recoil of the lungs (as in pulmonary fibrosis) or to dysfunction of the chest wall (as in kyphoscoliosis) or respiratory muscle (as in neuromuscular disease). The ability to sense alterations in length-tension relationships depends on innervation of respiratory muscles (patients with high cervical spinal cord injuries lack this sensation).

Assessment of dyspnea is subjective, but a number of scales have been devised for its quantification. Some of these include the Borg Scale, the American Thoracic Society Shortness of Breath Scale, and the Visual Analog Scale for Dyspnea. These scales, although imprecise, allow for determination of improvement or worsening in individuals; they have been shown to be reproducible and they are easy to use.

Treatment of dyspnea depends on its etiology. If respiratory drive is increased due to hypoxemia or hypercarbia, specific therapies may include oxygen, and measures designed to improve pulmonary function such as bronchodilators and anti-inflammatory agents. Failing that, sedation and opiates can directly reduce ventilatory drive; surgical interventions such as carotid body excision and vagal nerve sectioning are rarely indicated. Pulmonary rehabilitation, with components of education and physical training, may lead to enhancement of respiratory muscle efficiency. Muscle rest, through invasive or noninvasive mechanical ventilation, can also lead to subsequent improved respiratory muscle strength. Psychiatric interventions include anxiolytic and sedative medication, the safety of which has not been well studied, as well as psychotherapy.

Asthma

Asthma is a chronic disorder of the airways characterized by inflammation, bronchial hyperreactivity to various stimuli, and bronchospasm, or reversible airflow obstruction. Its presenting symptoms are variable and may include wheezing, chest tightness, dyspnea, and cough. Diagnosis is made through an appropriate clinical history; spirometry during an acute attack reveals airflow obstruction (decreased FEV_1) that is significantly reversible using bronchodilators. Although wheezing is often considered a characteristic symptom of asthma, it can also occur in other lung diseases, in congestive heart failure, in vocal cord dysfunction, and in malingering or factitious disorder.

Asthma may develop at any age. Childhood-onset asthma develops before age 5, and is diagnosed twice as often in boys as in girls. In adult asthma, with onset usually after the age of 25, there is no gender predilection. Age of onset of asthma does not appear to predict its course, but severity of asthma at presentation does. Although many asthmatics are atopic, atopy can develop without asthma and asthma often occurs without an atopic component. Despite advances in therapy, asthma prevalence and mortality may be increasing, particularly among youths in low socioeconomic classes.

Asthma attacks may be triggered by a variety of factors. Airway infection, allergic stimuli, irritant inhalations, smoke, dust, pollens and exercise are common triggers. Emotional stressors can also trigger attacks in some individuals. Treatment of asthma relies on control of airway inflammation (with corticosteroids, cromolyn or nedocromil, or leukotriene pathway inhibitors) and relief of bronchoconstriction (with beta-agonists and/or theophylline, most commonly).

Chronic Obstructive Pulmonary Disease

COPD most commonly refers to emphysema and chronic bronchitis. These disorders are overwhelmingly caused by cigarette smoking, although genetic factors, such as $alpha_1$-antitrypsin deficiency, clearly play a central role in rare individuals. In emphysema, an imbalance of proteolytic and antiproteolytic enzymes results in destruction of alveolar walls, leading to enlargement of the airspace distal to the terminal bronchiole. This leads to expiratory airway collapse due to loss of tethering of the bronchi, which leads to air-trapping and hyperinflation. Loss of alveolar capillary units may be measured by decreased single-breath carbon monoxide diffusion capacity (DLCO); this correlates with the development of hypoxemia and lack of pulmonary reserve. Chronic bronchitis often overlaps with emphysema. It is defined as a productive cough on most days for 3 months in at least 2 consecutive years.

Treatment of COPD is often supportive. The only medication shown to prolong life in advanced COPD is oxygen, which should be prescribed for patients whose PO_2 is less than 55 mm Hg, or is between 55 and 60 when polycythemia or cor pulmonale (right-sided heart failure) are present, or if desaturation (O_2 saturation, usually measured by pulse oximetry) below 88% develops at rest, while exercising, or while sleeping. Although bronchodilators and anti-inflammatory agents are often used, not all patients have a reversible component to their disease. Ipratropium bromide may be the bronchodilator of choice for COPD patients. In advanced emphysema, lung-reduction surgery holds some promise for temporary improvement in pulmonary mechanics. Lung transplantation is a final resort for some otherwise healthy patients with end-stage lung disease (see below).

Since therapeutic options are relatively limited in this disorder, prevention is of great importance. Cigarette smoking is the single greatest preventable cause of pulmonary morbidity and mortality in the United States. Smoking cessation is a multibillion-dollar industry that includes proponents of behavioral (such as hypnotism and group therapy) and pharmacological (e.g., nicotine patches and gums) intervention. Although experts differ on the benefits of "cold turkey" abrupt cessation compared with gradual tapering amounts of cigarettes, there is general agreement that external stimuli, including physicians' advice and peer and family support, enhance the success of smoking cessation with or without other interventions. Regardless of the methods used, most studies show a 12-month success rate for smoking cessation of no higher than 20%.

Cystic Fibrosis

Cystic fibrosis is the most common lethal genetic disorder in Caucasians, with an incidence of 1 in 2000 live births, and a carrier rate of approximately 5%. It is caused by an autosomal recessive genetic defect, which is responsible for abnormal production of a protein called the cystic fibrosis transmembrane conductance regulator (CFTR). A single genetic mutation, known as ΔF508, which causes the deletion of a single phenylalanine at position 508, is responsible for approximately 70% of cystic fibrosis cases. Patients with cystic fibrosis are unable to transport chloride normally across epithelial cell membranes. This abnormal ion transport leads to accumulation of thick secretions in many organ systems. The most important pathophysiological abnormalities develop in the pancreas and lung.

Pulmonary disease is the most significant cause of morbidity and mortality in patients with cystic fibrosis. These patients develop clogged bronchi and suffer chronic infections due to a reduced ability to clear and eliminate organisms. Although some genetic variations are less severe, most patients with cystic fibrosis begin to develop pulmonary dysfunction in childhood. Recurrent infections, especially with *S. aureus* and mucoid strains of *P. aeruginosa* lead to the development of bronchiectasis, or the abnormal permanent dilation of airways due to destruction of their walls, which leads to an even greater susceptibility to infection.

Formerly almost universally fatal in the pediatric patients, the median age of survival is now more than 30 years. Although some of the long-term survivors have milder forms of the disease, others have been chronically ill since childhood. This is a significant stressor on the family as well as the child, and significantly affects the patient's psychological health.

Although gene transfer may lead to a cure for this disease in the future, therapy now focuses on treatment of infections. Measures designed to improve clearance of secretions from the lungs (e.g., chest physiotherapy and postural drainage) and aggressive use of antibiotics remain the state-of-the-art treatment. As with emphysema, lung transplantation remains an option for patients with end-stage lung disease.

Lung Transplantation

Lung transplantation is a therapeutic option for a limited number of patients with end-stage lung disease and no other significant medical condition. Despite early successes with solid-organ transplantation, lung transplantation lagged significantly behind because of the difficulty in balancing the prevention of rejection with the risk of infection. The lungs are active immune organs; thus, rejection is a common problem. In addition, during respiration they are exposed to the outside environment, and are thus at increased risk of infection. With the development of cyclosporine in 1980, successful lung transplantation became possible. Although the first long-term success was a combined heart–lung transplantation in 1982, single-lung transplantation is now the most common procedure. This allows the greatest number of recipients to benefit from a single donor, and in most cases has the best outcome.

With increased experience in the procedure, the indications for transplantation have broadened. Lung transplantation is currently performed for end-stage patients with a wide range of diseases, including pulmonary hypertension, obstructive lung disease, pulmonary fibrosis, and even cystic fibrosis, despite the universal bacterial colonization of these patients. Exclusion criteria vary from center to center, and include the presence of concurrent disease (e.g., coronary artery disease, malignancy, or renal failure), previous chest surgery or trauma, nutritional state, functional status, and psychosocial issues. Although psychosocial contraindications to transplantation are difficult to quantify, active problems with cigarette, alcohol, or illegal drug use are felt to portend poor compliance with posttransplant regimens and worsen the likelihood of successful transplantation; there are few data on the impact of psychiatric diagnoses on transplant outcomes.

IMPACT OF PSYCHIATRIC ILLNESS ON PULMONARY DISEASE

There appears to be a higher than predicted comorbidity of anxiety disorders, particularly panic disorder, with pulmonary disease (3). In one study of psychiatric outpatients, the lifetime prevalence of respiratory disorders was 47% in patients with panic disorder compared with 13% in patients with obsessive-compulsive disorder. Conversely, the prevalence of anxiety disorders among pulmonary patients appears to be disproportionately high. Pollack et al. (4) found the prevalence of panic disorder among patients referred for pulmonary-function testing at a large urban medical center to be 11%, compared with 2–4% in the general population.

Psychological stressors can modulate the interactions between the central nervous system (CNS) and the immune system. It is generally accepted that hormones and neuropeptides are part of the control system(s) through which the CNS interacts with the immune system. These interactions could operate at the receptor level and at the gene level, affecting the production of cytokines and other messenger molecules used by subpopulations of mononuclear cells to interact with one another. Stress may also alter susceptibility to infectious illness, particularly respiratory illness, as well as morbidity and mortality following infection.

The association between anxiety and pulmonary disease is not surprising given that the sensation of dyspnea and impending suffocation occurs in many patients with pulmonary disease. Pulmonary dysfunction, with its associated symptoms, can trigger fear of death and panic in anxiety-prone individuals. Alternatively, pulmonary disease could unmask panic in predisposed patients because of recurrent episodes of hypercarbia and acidosis that trigger the suffocation alarm system.

Asthma

Asthma is a leading cause of chronic medical illness in childhood, and the illness is widely acknowledged to be associated with psychiatric illness. There is an increased lifetime prevalence of anxiety disorders as well as depression in adult asthmatics who seek treatment for their pulmonary condition (5). During periods of breathing difficulty, asthmatics often describe feeling frightened, panicked, or afraid of dying, so it is not surprising that the anxiety disorder with which asthma is most frequently associated is panic disorder. Approximately 6–30% of patients with asthma meet criteria for panic disorder and/or agoraphobia (6–8), with higher rates in clinical populations and lower rates in community studies.

In 1941, French and Alexander (9) proposed that the asthmatic patient is subject to an underlying conflict between dependence on the mother and other emotional conflicts that are incompatible with the dependency. Although there is no convincing evidence that this is true, or that asthma can be caused by psychological disturbances, psychological factors clearly play a role in asthma exacerbations and their management. Emotional factors can trigger an attack in some asthmatics. Purcell and associates (10) showed that the severity of asthma in children whose asthma was triggered by emotions such as depression, anger, or anxiety was improved by a 2-week separation from the parents. Children whose asthma was not precipitated by emotional stimuli displayed no improvement with separation.

A patient's reaction to the onset of an asthmatic attack governs his experience of symptoms. Typically, an asthmatic must take precautions against precipitating an asthma attack and take appropriate action when an attack develops. Regardless of what precipitates the attack, the individual's reaction to the symptoms of asthma may inhibit proper management. Patients who overreact to symptoms may have a greater severity and variety of symptoms of asthma. This personality trait has been called the panic-fear reaction, and the scale to measure it is derived from the Minnesota Multiphasic Personality Inventory (MMPI). Kinsman et al. (11) found that 42% of 100 inpatient asthmatic subjects described panic-fear during asthma attacks. Persons with panic-fear are more fearful, emotionally labile, and rejection-sensitive, and less able to cope in the face of stress. Dirks and associates (12) found that patients who scored high on the panic-fear scale had more hospitalizations and longer hospital stays, as well as more medication overuse. High levels of panic-fear and anxiety were associated with higher use of steroid regimens. Whether the panic-fear reaction increases the severity of asthma symptoms, causes the physician to increase the level of asthma therapy, or is induced by more severe asthma has not been clearly established.

Subjects with anxiety and asthma are more sensitive to the experience of dyspnea than subjects without respiratory disease, and the fear of dyspnea may actually trigger episodes of panic in some people (13). They may develop a cycle of excessive fear and avoidance of activities, with resulting diminution in quality of life. Studies that have reported the prevalence of panic disorder in asthmatics have not reported the prevalence of agoraphobia, but asthmatics appear to have risk factors for this type of panic disorder.

Chronic Obstructive Lung Disease

Anxiety is associated with impaired quality of life in patients with COPD, and higher levels of anxiety have been associated with greater intensity of breathlessness in these patients. Estimates of the prevalence of anxiety and other psychiatric disorders in patients with COPD are well above the prevalence of psychiatric illness seen in the general population (see Table 2). Patients' fear of breathlessness may lead to avoidance of otherwise achievable physical activity and cause further deconditioning. Anxious patients with COPD often fear emotionally charged situations because of their concern that their emotional arousal will trigger an episode of breathlessness. As a result, they may severely restrict not only their activities but the quality and number of their interpersonal relationships. In a study of 50 consecutive patients with chronic obstructive airway disease admitted to a respiratory-disease unit, 34% met criteria for an anxiety disorder and 24% met criteria for panic disorder. Neither pulmonary function testing nor response to bronchodilators differentiated those who had an anxiety disorder from those who did not.

It is known that there is relatively poor correlation ($r = 0.60$) between the exercise tolerance of a patient and any measure of his pulmonary function (14). This indicates that less than 40% of the variance in exercise tolerance can be explained by the level of pulmonary function. Light and associates (15) provided support for the hypothesis that the psychological status of the patient is an important determinant of the functional capacity of a given patient. They found that changes in the functional capacity of their patients, as assessed by the distance walked in 12 minutes, were more closely correlated with changes in depression and anxiety symptoms than they were with changes in results of pulmonary-function tests.

The degree of dyspnea experienced by patients with COPD appears to be related more to their sensitivity to carbon dioxide rather than to the degree of airway obstruction. Klein (16) has hypothesized that "blue bloaters," usually patients with chronic bronchitis who retain carbon dioxide, who experience relatively little dyspnea despite chronic hypercarbia, have a blunted suffocation-alarm sensitivity. On the other hand,

Table 2 Lifetime Prevalence (%) of Psychiatric Disorders in Patients with Chronic Obstructive Pulmonary Disease

	Depressive disorders	Anxiety disorders	Substance abuse	Any psychiatric disorder	No psychiatric disorder
Karajgi et al., 1988 (54)	18	16	—	42	58
Wells et al., 1989 (55)	19.4	21	36	—	—
Light et al., 1985 (56)	42	2	—	50	50
McSweeney et al., 1982 (57)	42	12	—	66	33
Agle and Baum, 1977 (58)	70	96	20	96	4

"pink puffers," usually patients with emphysema who maintain relatively normal carbon dioxide levels by increasing ventilation (number of respirations per minute) maintain their responsiveness to carbon monoxide and experience marked dyspnea. When dyspnea increases, there is a concomitant increase in distress and anxiety. There has been one open-label trial using benzodiazepines in "pink puffers" (17). Four patients with severe dyspnea were treated with a flexible dose of diazepam until dyspnea was reduced (dosage range: 15–40 mg per day). All patients had striking relief of dyspnea. The patients had an increased tolerance of carbon dioxide during rebreathing while on diazepam, which suggests that the inhibition of various drives to the medullary respiratory center may be the mechanism of the improvement. Alternatively, the relief of anxiety that three of the four patients experienced may also have contributed to the improvement. Further study of the use of benzodiazepines in COPD is warranted.

Patients with chronic medical illness and depressed mood are reported to be more disabled than patients without psychiatric illness, but data related to the benefits and risks of treating depression in this patient population are limited. Borson et al. (18) examined multiple outcome indicators in patients with disabling COPD and comorbid depression. They reported that nortriptyline was clearly better than placebo for the treatment of depression in these patients. They found that the nortriptyline-treated group also had significant improvement in respiratory symptoms and day-to-day function, although physiological measures were unchanged. The study highlights the detrimental effect of psychiatric illness related to COPD, and suggests that the diagnosis and treatment of the comorbid disorder improve not only the psychiatric disorder but the patient's quality of life and ability to function.

Smoking and Nicotine Dependence

Cigarette smoking is the largest preventable cause of respiratory illness in the United States. The percentage of the American population that report smoking has decreased since the Surgeon General's Report in 1964 describing the association between smoking and pulmonary disease. In 1965, 52.1% of men stated that they smoked. By the mid-1980s that number was reduced to 34.8% and has remained at about a third. For females, the 1965 smoking rate was 34.8%, a figure that fell to 29.5% by 1983. However, the proportion of the population that smokes more than 25 cigarettes per day and is therefore more likely to be nicotine-dependent has increased since 1965. In 1965, 24.1% of men smoked a pack or more a day, which rose over the next two decades to 33.6%. Of women, 13.0% reported smoking 25 cigarettes a day, increasing to 20.6% by the mid-1980s. So, while fewer people are smoking, more of them are nicotine-dependent.

Breslau (19) reported on an epidemiological study of young adults aged 21–34 in an urban area. He found that nicotine dependence was 20%. Higher rates were reported in Caucasians, persons with lower levels of education, and persons who were separated or divorced. Among smokers, lifetime prevalence of major depression and all anxiety disorders, as well as of substance abuse, was significantly higher than in nonsmokers. Major depression was specifically associated with nicotine dependence, and the association was partly explained by the personality trait of increased neuroticism. Nicotine dependence is hypothesized to have an antidepressant effect, rather than causing the depressive disorder, but the relationship is not clear.

Cystic Fibrosis

There have been a number of studies of the prevalence of psychiatric illness in children with cystic fibrosis. Thompson et al. (20) found that 58% of children with cystic fibrosis had a DSM-III-R diagnosis, as compared with 23% of control children and 77% of psychiatrically referred children. The children with cystic fibrosis had high levels of anxiety and worry, and were comparable to the psychiatrically referred children on those illness variables.

There have been few psychological and psychiatric studies of adults with cystic fibrosis. Strauss and Wellisch (21) found that patients over 23 years old had increased somatization and social isolation compared to younger patients, but no increase in depression or other anxiety symptoms with age. These additional problems in adults with cystic fibrosis could adversely affect overall adjustment with the increasing lifespan seen with cystic fibrosis patients. Stern and associates (22) evaluated psychoactive drug use in adults with cystic fibrosis and found that 11% regularly smoked tobacco, 20% used marijuana, and 60% used alcohol. All psychoactive substance use was associated with some adverse effects on the patient's cystic fibrosis and, with an aging cystic fibrosis population, is an issue that warrants further evaluation. Strauss et al. (23) reported that a time-limited psychosocial support group helped to reduce resentment and doubt in adults with cystic fibrosis. This is the only treatment-outcome study in the literature, and it did not include structured psychiatric diagnosis or stringent outcome evaluation and criteria.

Lung Transplantation

Psychiatric disorders are common in patients with end-stage lung disease who are candidates for lung transplant. Craven (24) found that 50% of applicants for lung transplant had a lifetime history of psychiatric illness. Lack of hope for the future, poor energy, poor sleep, and poor concentration are common in patients with end-stage lung disease. Optimizing the emotional health of candidates prior to transplant is an important role for the consult-liaison psychiatrist. Woodman et al. (25) studied 34 patients who underwent either single or bilateral lung transplant, and found that psychiatric disorders were common. All patients were followed psychiatrically preoperatively as well as postoperatively. To find predictors of survival, patients who survived for more than 12 months were compared to patients who did not survive 12 months. There were no significant differences between the two groups related to age, gender, education, or smoking history. The 1-year survivors had significantly more psychiatric illness (56% vs. 18%; $p < 0.001$) and use of prednisone in the month prior to transplant (62.5% vs. 31%;

$p < 0.01$). All patients with psychiatric illness were treated pretransplant, and the presence of a psychiatric illness did not adversely affect outcome. Patients with significant noncompliance with the treatment program were excluded from eligibility for transplantation. The finding that preoperative prednisone use is associated with increased 1-year survival is consistent with the hypothesis that immunosuppression pretransplant may decrease rejection posttransplant.

EFFECT OF PULMONARY DISORDER ON THE MANIFESTATIONS AND COURSE OF PSYCHIATRIC DISORDERS

The diagnosis of a psychiatric illness in conjunction with a medical illness was first formally included in psychiatric diagnostic criteria in Feighner's criteria in 1972 (26) and refers to a psychiatric syndrome that follows in time and parallels the medical illness. Since then, each edition of the *Diagnostic and Statistical Manual of Mental Disorders* has included a similar diagnostic concept. The incidence and prevalence of psychiatric illness in conjunction with one or more chronic illnesses were evaluated using data from the National Institute of Mental Health (NIMH) Environmental Catchment Area study in Los Angeles ($n = 2554$), and found that medical illness was associated with a 41% higher adjusted prevalence rate of recent psychiatric illness and a 28% higher prevalence of lifetime psychiatric disorder (27). Psychiatric illness that occurs in conjunction with medical illness has been associated with higher utilization of health care services (28) and a worse outcome for medical illness (29).

Medications used to treat respiratory diseases can be anxiogenic, including glucocorticoids, beta-adrenergic agonists, methylxanthines, and anticholinergics (see "Frequently Used Pulmonary Medications" below). Thus, pulmonary disease may be a risk factor for the development of anxiety disorders and panic disorder specifically. In a retrospective, case-control study of 150 consecutive anxiety patients, 42.7% of those with panic disorder had a history of respiratory disease that predated their anxiety disorder, compared with only 16.2% of patients with other anxiety disorders (30).

Asthma

The frequent co-occurrence of asthma with psychiatric disorders can complicate the correct identification of which disorder is in need of treatment. In patients who have panic disorder as well as asthma, it can be particularly difficult to separate these diagnoses. As noted above, the treatment for asthma involves anxiogenic medications that inherently complicate the panic disorder and may increase the difficulty in controlling both disorders simultaneously.

The problem of noncompliance with medication is associated with personality and behavior. It is a major reason for the high rate of emergency-room use in asthmatics. Hulka et al. (31) found that 75.5% of emergency-room visits by 50 asthmatic children were due to medication noncompliance and the remaining 24.5% to treatment with inappropriate medications, such as antihistamines and decongestants, or to prescription of inadequate doses of bronchodilators. Avery and associates (32) studied 157 adult asthmatics and found that 66% had no bronchodilator medication at home and 24% used the bronchodilator ineffectively. In addition, 44% did not contact their physician when they had a serious asthma attack. Bosley et al. (33) studied psychological factors associated with poor compliance with the treatment for asthma in 102 asthmatic outpatients. They defined noncompliance as taking less than 70% of the prescribed dose of medications each week, and found that these patients with depression were more likely to be noncompliant with treatment. They found that asthmatics who have comorbid depression were less compliant with their medications. Noncompliance with treatment has been associated with increased health care utilization, and increased mortality and morbidity in asthmatics. There has not been a prospective treatment study of asthmatics with comorbid depression to determine if treatment of the depression is associated with a decrease in complications secondary to asthma. There was a trend toward anxiety being associated with noncompliance, but it did not reach significance.

Chronic Obstructive Pulmonary Disease

It has been hypothesized that COPD predisposes to the development of anxiety and depressive disorders by means of classic conditioning (34). A related hypothesis, more consistent with the cognitive model of panic, is that COPD patients who have experienced anxiety-provoking somatic sensations during acute episodes of respiratory deregulation are more prone to panic or to developing an anxiety disorder because they have learned to interpret the arousal symptoms as catastrophic (35). Spinhoven and associates (36) studied 100 panic disorder patients, 100 major depressive disorder patients, and 100 patients without an axis I or axis II diagnosis from an outpatient psychiatric clinic population. They found that 16% of the panic disorder patients had a lifetime prevalence of respiratory disorders, compared with 9% of patients with major depressive disorder and 5% of controls ($p < 0.05$). They confirmed the observations of Kinsman et al. (37) that anxiety is more closely related to intermittent respiratory disorders, such as asthma, whereas depression is associated with continuous pulmonary obstruction, such as chronic bronchitis. It is possible that disturbed respiratory function may have a different effect, depending on the nature of the disorder and the interpretation of symptoms by the patient. Intermittent attacks of severe respiratory dysfunction that is life-threatening may be more anxiety-inducing, whereas more continuous forms of airway obstruction, which are associated with loss of physical function and mobility, may predispose to depressive episodes.

Smoking and Nicotine Dependence

Smoking and nicotine dependence are comorbid with psychiatric disorders more frequently than reported in the general population, with up to 90% of patients with schizophrenia having a current or past diagnosis of nicotine dependence. Smokers are more likely than nonsmokers to have a history of major depression (38,39).

Breslau et al. (40) described the epidemiology of nicotine dependence and its association with psychiatric disorders. Lifetime prevalence of nicotine dependence was 20% in an urban population. Males and females with nicotine dependence had increased odds for alcohol and drug dependence, major depression, and anxiety disorders when compared with nonsmokers and non-dependent smokers. Major depression and all anxiety disorders were specifically associated with nicotine dependence.

It has been hypothesized that nicotine may act as an antidepressant in some smokers (41,42). The development of a depressed affect or frank depression after smoking cessation has been associated with relapse (43,44). Therefore, antidepressants may have a role in smoking-cessation treatment plans. However, results of clinical trials using antidepressants for smoking cessation have been mixed. The initial experience was promising, but no large trials have been reported (45). There have been a number of reports about the safety and efficacy of sustained-release bupropion for smoking cessation (46–48). Hurt et al. (46) followed 615 nondepressed smokers for 1 year and reported that sustained-release bupropion at 150 mg and 300 mg was significantly more effective for smoking cessation than placebo. Probands on bupropion had minimal side effects and gained less weight than on placebo.

Further investigation of the psychopharmacology of nicotine may explain the relationship between psychiatric disorders and pulmonary disorders caused or exacerbated by smoking.

Cystic Fibrosis

Cystic fibrosis has been shown to be associated with psychiatric illness at the same rate as other chronic, severe illnesses with a childhood onset. Canning et al. (49) found that 41% of chronically ill patients, which included children with cystic fibrosis, diabetes, inflammatory bowel disease, and cancer, met criteria for a psychiatric diagnosis. Burke and associates (50) found an increase in obsessional symptoms in children with cystic fibrosis, as has been reported with other pediatric chronic illness. Steinhausen and Schindler (51) evaluated cystic fibrosis patients and healthy controls and found that psychiatric illness was significantly more common in the cystic fibrosis group. They found moderate correlations between impaired psychiatric function and increased psychopathology, and the data suggest that children with cystic fibrosis require psychiatric help. They hypothesized that this need would increase as the disease progresses.

In contrast to these studies, Bennett (52) carried out a meta-analysis of depression in children with chronic illness, and did not find a higher incidence among children with cystic fibrosis. This analysis did not include all psychiatric disorders, and studies that have suggested an increase in psychiatric illness have noted that no single psychiatric diagnosis is associated with cystic fibrosis. The author also noted the lack of information about adults with cystic fibrosis, and hypothesized that as the children reach adulthood, the incidence of depression will rise, as the literature on childhood cancer has shown.

It has been hypothesized that the stress of having a chronic illness is responsible for the increased prevalence of psychiatric illness. The physiological effect of the illness and the treatment the illness entails may contribute to the expression of psychiatric disorders, but the comparable rates of comorbid psychiatric illness across chronic childhood illnesses supports the hypothesis of a shared underlying etiology.

Lung Transplantation

The respiratory disorders that lead to lung transplantation are discussed above. Although patients who are candidates for transplant are in the end stage of their respiratory disorder, they are not a different group of patients at that point. The limited literature available on the prevalence of psychiatric illness in the population of patients who are evaluated or listed for lung transplantation shows higher rates of lifetime psychiatric illness compared with control populations, but similar rates to those in end-stage disease populations.

Posttransplant patients may or may not have their pretransplant disorder, but they all become immunocompromised and at risk for episodes of rejection. Such episodes are difficult to distinguish from infectious episodes based on symptoms alone, and both can be confused with the symptoms of either minor or major depression. The medications used for immunosuppression can cause psychiatric symptoms as well. Because the patient is not able to choose whether to continue the immunosuppression, any depressive or anxious symptoms that do not clear with a reduction or change in medication need to be treated. Psychiatric symptoms that occur secondary to medications respond to conventional treatment regimens at dosages similar to those used for primary psychiatric disorders.

Psychiatric illness pretransplant does not adversely affect 1-year survival (25), but may affect the ability to return to work posttransplant. This has not been well studied in patients with lung transplants. In a study of 250 patients who had undergone heart transplantation, Paris and associates (53) found that patients' self-perception pretransplant influenced their return to work, as well as the length of medical disability pretransplant and the loss of health insurance and/or disability income. Patients' self-perception could be influenced by psychiatric disorders. The quality of life after lung transplantation has not been studied, and is another area where untreated psychiatric illness could affect the success of the transplant.

FREQUENTLY USED PULMONARY MEDICATIONS

Medications commonly used in patients with pulmonary disorders can be divided into several categories. Bronchodilators include inhaled and systemic agents that directly relieve bronchospasm. These include beta$_2$-agonists, anticholinergics, and theophylline. Anti-inflammatory agents include corticosteroids (systemic and inhaled), cromolyn sodium and related compounds, and the newly available leukotriene-pathway blockers.

Antihistamines, decongestants, and antibiotics are common therapeutic agents in patients with pulmonary disorders, but are not covered in this chapter. Although each of the pharmacological classes discussed below may be used in a wide variety of pulmonary diseases, where appropriate we have indicated the "niche" in which the drug is most often used.

Beta-agonists are sympathomimetic agents with specificity for the beta$_2$-receptor that cause bronchodilation. They are available in systemic and inhaled dosage forms; in general, the inhaled forms are preferable because of greater specificity of effect, more rapid onset of action, and fewer systemic side effects. Some patients, however, prefer the oral agents because of their activating properties. Systemic (i.m./i.v.) agents are used for the emergent treatment of acute asthma episodes only. Side effects of all beta-agonists include restlessness, anxiety, tremor, and tachycardia. At higher doses they can lead to seizures and cardiac arrhythmias. Technique is important to maximize benefits from metered-dose inhalers, but the use of spacers and some new delivery forms (e.g., the Maxair Autohaler™) can be used to treat patients who have difficulties coordinating inhaler actuation and inhalation. Inhaled beta-agonists are first-line therapy for mild asthmatics with occasional bronchospasm; all patients for whom bronchospasm is a component of the illness may utilize these agents to prevent and acutely treat bronchoconstriction.

Ipratropium bromide (Atrovent™) is the anticholinergic agent most commonly used for bronchospasm. Because of its quaternary structure, it is less absorbable and has fewer side effects than atropine sulfate. Anticholinergic agents act through blockade of cholinergic receptors, which cause large-airway bronchoconstriction. Adverse effects of anticholinergic agents include delerium, urinary retention, and decreased gastrointestinal motility. Although anticholinergic agents are less effective bronchodilators than beta-agonists in asthmatics, they appear to be at least as effective in patients with chronic obstructive lung disease, and are therefore often used for bronchodilation in emphysema and chronic bronchitis.

Theophylline, a member of the methylxanthine family, has multiple beneficial effects on airway physiology. Although its mechanism of action remains unknown, it acts as a bronchodilator, and it has been shown to improve right ventricular function as well as diaphragmatic strength. In addition, it may also have anti-inflammatory effects. Unfortunately, the toxic-therapeutic ratio may be low in some patients, and side effects are not uncommon, especially at the upper end of the "therapeutic" range. Adverse reactions may include insomnia, anxiety, agitation, gastrointestinal disturbances, cardiac arrhythmias, and seizures. Theophylline metabolism is significantly affected by a number of agents (including phenobarbital, erythromycin, oral contraceptive agents, cimetidine, and ethanol) and conditions (including congestive heart failure, liver disease, and viral infections), so monitoring of drug levels is particularly important in acutely ill patients. Theophylline is now rarely used as monotherapy for pulmonary disorders, but may be of value in providing "background" bronchodilation in COPD and asthma patients, especially in cases of nocturnal bronchospasm.

Corticosteroids remain the cornerstone of anti-inflammatory therapy for pulmonary disorders. They are available in oral, parenteral, and inhaled forms. Enteral and parenteral doses are used to treat acute inflammation and exacerbations of asthma and COPD. The inhaled forms are used to prevent airway inflammation, and they have significantly fewer systemic side effects than systemic corticosteroids do. Increasingly potent inhaled corticosteroids have recently become available, and they have allowed a number of steroid-dependent patients to be tapered off oral steroids. Acute adverse effects of high-dose corticosteroids include neuropsychiatric problems such as mood lability, mania, and psychosis. Long-term usage may cause bone demineralization, adrenal suppression, hypertension, weight gain, and a host of other effects. Both inhaled and systemic corticosteroids are used to treat airway and parenchymal inflammation; to varying degrees, inflammation is an important aspect of many pulmonary disorders.

Other anti-inflammatory agents used to treat airway inflammation include sodium cromoglycate and nedocromil sodium. These inhaled agents prevent triggering of bronchospasm through mast-cell-membrane stabilization and prevention of release of inflammatory mediators from mast cells. Zyleuton and zafirleukast are members of a new class of agents, inhibitors of the leukotriene pathway. These agents appear to be moderately effective in preventing triggered bronchospasm in asthma; both are well tolerated, although the use of zyleuton has been associated with some reversible liver-enzyme abnormalities.

FUTURE RESEARCH AND CONCLUSIONS

This chapter raises many interesting questions about the relationship between pulmonary disorders and psychiatric disorders. Why are chronic lung conditions so strongly associated with psychiatric disorders? How is the prevalence of psychiatric disorders affected by the presence of one or more pulmonary disorders? How does the course of the psychiatric disorder over time co-vary with the course of the pulmonary disorder? Data related to these questions would help unravel the complicated causal relationships among medical and psychiatric disorders.

Genetic, developmental, and social investigations should identify whether a predisposition toward psychiatric disorders causes an increased vulnerability to pulmonary disorders. These studies could confirm that knowing the personal and family history of patients with psychiatric disorders is helpful in managing their pulmonary disorder.

Psychobiological methods should be used to better understand the relationship between pulmonary and psychiatric disorders. For example, a therapeutic trial of an antidepressant in patients with panic disorder and asthma could lead to both a functional and an objective improvement in their medical status, as well as an improvement in their panic disorder as compared with an anxious control group.

There is reason to believe that pulmonary disease is a risk factor for the development of a psychiatric disorder. The risk is probably related to repeated experiences with dyspnea, as well as life-threatening exacerbations or pulmonary dysfunction, hypercapnia, hyperventilation, the use of anxiogenic medications, and the stress of coping with a chronic disease.

REFERENCES

1. Williams SJ. Chronic respiratory illness and disability: a critical review of the psychosocial literature. Soc Sci Med 1989; 28:791–803.
2. Reiman EM, Raichle ME, Robins E. The application of positron emission tomography to the study of panic disorder. Am J Psychiatry 1986; 143:469–477.
3. Smoller JW, Pollack MH, Otto MW, Rosenbaum JF, Kradin RL. Panic anxiety, dyspnea, respiratory disease. Am J Respir Crit Care Med 1996; 154:6–17.
4. Pollack MH, Otto MW, Sabatino S, Majcher D, Worthington JJ, McArdle ET, Rosenbaum JF. Relationship of childhood anxiety to adult panic disorder: correlates and influence on course. Am J Psychiatry 1996; 153(3):376–381.
5. Yellowlees PM, Kalucy RS. Psychobiological aspects of asthma and the consequent research implications. Chest 1990; 97:628–634.
6. Yellowlees PM, Haynes S, Potts N, Rurrin RE. Psychiatric morbidity in patients with life-threatening asthma: initial report of a controlled study. Med J Aust 1988; 149:246–249.
7. Shavitt RG, Gentil V, Mandetta R. The association of panic/agoraphobia and asthma: contributing factors and clinical implications. Gen Hosp Psychiatry 1992; 14:420–423.
8. Carr RE, Lehrer PM, Rausch LL, Hochron SM. Anxiety sensitivity and panic attacks in an asthmatic population. Behav Res Ther 1994; 32:411–418.
9. French TM, Alexander F. Psychogenic factors in bronchial asthma. Psychosom Med Monogr 1941; 4:2–94.
10. Purcell K, Brady K, Chai H, Muser J, Molk L, Gordon N, Means J. The effect of asthma in children of experimental separation from the family. Psychosom Med 1969; 31:144–164.
11. Kinsman RA, Luparello T, O'Banion K, Spector S. Multidimensional analysis of the subjective symptomatology of asthma. Psychosom Med 1973; 35:250–267.
12. Dirk JF, Horton DJ, Kinsman RA, Fross KH, Jones NF. Patient and physician characteristics influencing medical decisions in asthma. J Asthma Res 1978; 15:171–178.
13. Carr RE, Lehrer PM, Hochron SM. Panic symptoms in asthma and panic disorder: a preliminary test of the dyspnea–fear theory. Behav Resp Ther 1992; 30:251–261.
14. Light RW. Exercise, exercise testing, and disability evaluation. In: George RB, Light RW, Matthay RA, eds. Chest Medicine. New York: Churchill Livingstone, 1983.
15. Light RW, Merrill EJ, Despars J, Gordon GH, Mutalipassi LR. Doxepin treatment of depressed patients with chronic obstructive pulmonary disease. Arch Intern Med 1986; 146:1377–1380.
16. Klein DF. False suffocation alarms, spontaneous panics, and related conditions: an integrated hypothesis. Arch Gen Psychiatry 1993; 50:306–317.
17. Mitchell-Heggs P, Murphy K, Minty K, Guz A, Patterson SC, Minty PSB, Rosser RM. Diazepam in the treatment of dyspnoea in the "pink puffer" syndrome. Quarterly J Med 1980; 193:9–20.
18. Borson S, McDonald GJ, Gayle T, Deffebach M, Lakshminarayan S, Van Tuinen C. Improvement in mood, physical symptoms, and function with nortriptyline for depression

in patients with chronic obstructive pulmonary disease. Psychosomatics 1992; 33:190–201.

19. Breslau N. Psychiatric comorbidity of smoking and nictoine dependence. Behav Genet 1995; 25:95–101.
20. Thompson RJ, Hodges K, Hamlett KW. A matched comparison of adjustment in children with cystic fibrosis and psychiatrically referred and nonreferred children. J Pediatr Psychol 1990; 15:745–759.
21. Strauss GD, Wellisch DK. Psychological assessment of adults with cystic fibrosis. Int J Psychiatry Med 1980–1981; 10:265–272.
22. Stern RC, Byard PJ, Tomashefski JF, Doershuk CF. Recreational use of psychoactive drugs by patients with cystic fibrosis. J Pediatrics 1987; 111:293–299.
23. Strauss GD, Pedersen S, Dudovitz D. Psychosocial support for adults with cystic fibrosis: a group approach. Am J Dis Child 1979; 133(3):301–305.
24. Craven J and the Toronto Lung Transplant Group. Psychiatric aspects of lung transplant. Can J Psychiatry 1990; 35:759–764.
25. Woodman CL, Geist L, Vance S, Laxson C, Kline JN. Predictors of survival in lung transplant: the Iowa experience. Psychosomatics 1997; 38:192.
26. Feighner JP, Robins E, Guze SB, Woodruff RA, Winokur G, Munoz R. Diagnostic criteria for use in psychiatric research. Arch Gen Psychiatry 1972;26:57–63.
27. Wells KB, Golding JM, Burnam MA. Psychiatric disorder and limitations in physical functioning in a general population. Am J Psychiatry 1988; 145:712–717.
28. Noyes R, Woodman C, Garvey M, Cook B, Clancy J, Anderson DJ. Generalized anxiety disorder versus panic disorder: is the distinction valid? J Nerv Ment Disord 1992; 180:369–379.
29. Cassem E. Depression and anxiety secondary to medical illness. Psychiatr Clin N Amer 1990; 13:597–612.
30. Verburg K, Griez E, Meijer J, Pols H. Respiratory disorder as a possible predisposing factor for panic disorder. J Affect Disord 1995; 33:129–134.
31. Hulka BS. Patient-clinician interactions and compliance. In: Haynes RB, Taylor DW, Sackett DL, eds. Compliance in Health Care. Baltimore: Johns Hopkins University Press, 1981.
32. Avery CH, March J, Brook RH. An assessment of the adequacy of self care in adult asthmatics. J Commun Health 1980; 5:167–180.
33. Bosley CM, Fosbury JA, Cochrane GM. The psychological factors associated with poor compliance in asthma. Eur Resp J 1995; 8:899–905.
34. Zandbergen J, Bright M, Pols H, Fernandez I, deLoof C, Griez EJL. Higher lifetime prevalence of respiratory diseases in panic disorder? Am J Psychiatry 1991; 148:1583–1585.
35. Clark NM, Feldman CH, Evans D, Levinson MJ, Waselewski Y, Mellins RB. The impact of health education on frequency and cost of health care by low income children with asthma. J Allergy Clin Immunol 1986; 78:108–115.
36. Spinhoven P, Ros M, Westgeest A, Van der Does AJW. The prevalence of respiratory disorders in panic disorder, major depression, and V-code patients. Behav Res Ther 1993; 647–649.
37. Kinsman RA, Fernandez E, Schocket M, Dirks JF, Covino NA. Multidimensional analysis of the symptoms of chronic bronchitis and emphysema. J Behav Med 1983; 6:339–357.
38. Glassman AH, Helzer JE, Covey LS. Smoking, smoking cessation, and major depression. JAMA 1990; 264:1546–1549.

39. Hall SM, Munoz R, Reus V. Smoking cessation, depression, and dysphoria. NIDA Res Monogr 1991; 105:312–313.
40. Breslau N, Kilbey MM, Andreski P. DSM-III-R nicotine dependence in young adults: prevalence, correlates, and associated psychiatric disorders. Addiction 1994; 89:743–754.
41. Hughes JR. Dependence potential and abuse liability of nicotine replacement therapies. In: Pomperleau O, Pomperleau C, eds. Progress in Clinical Evaluation. New York: Alan R Liss, 1988:261–277.
42. Glass RM. Blue mood, blackened lungs: depression and smoking. JAMA 1990; 264:1583–1584.
43. Covey LS, Glassman AH, Sterner F. Depression and depressive symptoms in smoking cessation. Comprehen Psychiatry 1990; 31:350–354.
44. Hall SM, Munoz RF, Reus V. Cognitive-behavioral intervention increases abstinence rates for depressive-history smokers. J Consult Clin Psychol 1994; 62:141–146.
45. Edwards NB, Murphy JK, Downs AD, Ackerman BJ, Rosenthal TL. Am J Psychiatry 1989; 146:373–376.
46. Hurt RD, Sachs DPL, Glover ED, Offord KP, Johnston JA, Dale LC, Khayrallah MA, Schroeder DR, Glover PN, Sullivan CR, Croghan IT, Sullivan PM. A comparison of sustained-release bupropion and placebo for smoking cessation. N Engl J Med 1997; 337:1195–1202.
47. Bupropion (Zyban) for smoking cessation. Medical Letter Drug Ther 1997; 39:77–78.
48. Leif HI. Bupropion treatment of depression to assist smoking cessation. Am J Psychiatry 1996; 153:442.
49. Canning EH, Hanser SB, Shade KA, Boyce WT. Mental disorders in chronically ill children: parent-child discrepancy and physician identification. Pediatrics 1992; 90:692–696.
50. Burke P, Meyer V, Kocoshis S, Orenstein DM, Chandra R, Nord DJ, Sauer J, Cohen E. Depression and anxiety in pediatric inflammatory bowel disease and cystic fibrosis. J Am Acad Child Adolesc Psych 28:948–951, 1989.
51. Steinhausen HC, Schindler HP. Psychological adaptation in children and adolescents with cystic fibrosis. J Dev Behav Pediatrics 1981; 2:74–77.
52. Bennett DS. Depression among children with chronic medical problems: a meta-analysis. J Pediatr Psychol 1994; 19:149–169.
53. Paris W, Woodbury A, Thompson S, Levick M, Nothegger S, Hutkin-Slade L, Arbuckle P, Cooper DKC. Social rehabilitation and return to work after cardiac transplantation. Transplantation 1992; 53:433–438.
54. Karajgi B, Rifkin A, Doddi S, Kolli R. The prevalence of anxiety disorders in patients with chronic obstructive pulmonary disease. Am J Psychiatr 1990; 147:200–201.
55. Wells KB, Golding JM, Burman MA. Affective, substance abuse, and anxiety disorders in persons with arthritis, diabetes, heart disease, high blood pressure, or chronic lung conditions. Gen Hosp Psychiatry 1989; 11:320–327.
56. Light RW, Merrill EJ, Despars JA, Gordon GH, Mutalipassi LR. Prevalence of depression and anxiety in patients with COPD. Chest 1985; 87:35–38.
57. McSweeney AJ, Grant I, Adams KM, Timms RM. Life quality of patients with chronic obstructive pulmonary disease. Arch Med 1982; 142:473–478.
58. Agle DP, Baum GL. Psychological aspects of chronic obstructive pulmonary disease. Med Clinics N Am 1977; 61:749–758.

12

Cancer

Simon Wein*

Memorial Sloan-Kettering Cancer Center
New York, New York

Cancer is a word, not a sentence.

—W. F. Moon, M.D.

INTRODUCTION

Psychiatry has a crucial role to play in the management of the cancer patient. Oncology and psychiatry share the common experience of having to overcome a taboo. For its part, psychiatry has had to contend with "spirits" and other such invisible forces, whereas oncology has been portentously linked with death. To a large extent, both specialties have been normalized, but the legacy of those prejudiced taboos lingers and is one of the challenges facing psycho-oncology.

The purview of psycho-oncology is broad, as it encompasses the two main psychological dimensions of cancer. The first, the psychosocial aspect, refers to the psychological response of patients, families, and caregivers to cancer in all its stages. The second, the psychobiological aspect, covers the psychological, behavioral, and social factors that influence risk, detection, and survival (1). Hence, psycho-oncology, in its clinical and research arenas, encompasses quality-of-life issues; epidemiology; cancer control and prevention; bioethics, including euthanasia and physician-assisted suicide; psychiatric care; psychoneuroimmunology, looking at links between brain, immune, and endocrine systems; pain control and palliative care; and more recently genetic counseling. The breadth of psycho-oncology means that practitioners from many and varied fields are brought under its rubric, providing a necessary critical mass not only to

---

* Current affiliation: Shaare Zedek Medical Center, Jerusalem, Israel.

treat the individual patient as a whole, but to address the broader societal issues that arise.

HISTORICAL PERSPECTIVE

The word cancer has been unmentionable for centuries because of its association with death, pain, and suffering. Intercalated with these fears were ignorance, superstition, and religious symbolism equating suffering with purification (2). Together, these factors contributed to the dictum that patients should not be told the truth about their cancer, and death became a taboo. Only recently, initially with the discovery in the nineteenth century of anesthesia, antisepsis, and surgery and then the introduction of radiation therapy and chemotherapy in this century, has the treatment of cancer been successful. Of equal importance, our knowledge about the causes and treatments of cancer increased greatly. These advances implied the need for public education about the early signs of cancer. No longer would we have to be passive and hopeless in the face of cancer.

In parallel with these breakthroughs, the hospice movement evolved in Europe and the United States in the 1950s, reflecting both societal changes and medical advances (3,4). The Nuremberg trials following World War II emphasized the importance of patient consent, autonomy, and rights and arguably have a significant legacy in medical ethics (5). Similarly, the post–Vietnam war era, when authority and paternalism were challenged, influenced society, including medical practice. Medical advances that not only offered patients new therapeutic options also required their informed consent and active participation in often life-threatening procedures. Patients lived longer both with their disease and with posttreatment complications, such as second malignancies, deformities, infertility, and more recently a genetic legacy. Epidemiological research revealed potentially preventable lifestyle habits, particularly obesity and the use of tobacco and alcohol. In recent years, bioethical issues with obvious psychological overtones have been a new and fertile area of discussion and research (physician-assisted suicide, euthanasia, and advanced directives, to name but a few). Paradoxically, as oncology and radiation therapy became scientific disciplines emphasizing curative and life-prolonging outcomes, the gap vis-a-vis quality-of-life issues widened. All these factors in the 1970s and 1980s proved a tremendous impetus to treat, describe, and then investigate these "new" psychological and behavioral aspects of cancer. Psycho-oncology, as a new subspecialty of oncology, emerged from this need to deal with the human dimension of cancer not merely as an "art of care" but also as a scientific discipline.

CASE HISTORY

Mr. T., a 71-year-old retired dairy farmer, was being treated for acute leukemia. Following induction chemotherapy he had been admitted with febrile neutropenia. Restaging investigations did not show disease progression, hence his withdrawn, uncooperative, and unmotivated state was thought to be contributing to a decline in medical status. Psychiatry was consulted to assess possible depression. Mr. T., who appeared older than his years, was cachectic and disheveled. He pointed to a bedside photograph of himself taken only 2 months earlier, dancing at his wedding to his second wife. He had had no significant medical illnesses except for an episode of major depression some 30 years prior, related to a fatal road accident in which he killed a motorcyclist. There was no psychiatric family history. He drank little alcohol and did not smoke or use other drugs. He spoke at length about the disappointment of becoming sick so soon after remarrying with plans of retiring to Florida.

His wife and daughter described him as a positive, optimistic man who loved life. His mood and affect were flat and restricted, but given the extent of other physical symptoms it was difficult to assess the severity of the depressive syndrome. The Mini-Mental State Examination was at the lower limit of normal, and other than an altered sleep-wake cycle, staff had not reported hallucinations or inappropriate behavior. His medication included broad-spectrum antibiotics and low-dose opiates.

We tentatively diagnosed an adjustment disorder with depressed mood but emphasized the need to rule out delirium and suggested low-dose pemoline to improve his well-being. Over the next few days, medical and nursing staff became increasingly frustrated by his persistent withdrawal, refusal to cooperate, and apparent loss of will to live. He became progressively unable to given a coherent account of events and was disorientated in time and place with increasing somnolence. We indicated that psychostimulants alone were contraindicated and a trial of haloperidol should be instituted as our diagnosis was now hypoactive delirium due to multiple medical problems. The medical staff nevertheless commenced an antidepressant, paroxetine, hoping to bolster his mood. Friction between the medical and psychiatric staff increased over the diagnostic and therapeutic approach. His condition worsened and investigations confirmed disease recurrence. He died shortly thereafter. A sense of resignation had pervaded the case with, in the end, blame being apportioned equally to the disease and the patient's "loss of will to live."

This vignette demonstrates a number of important clinical points:

1. The difficulties in diagnosing an affective disorder in the presence of a delirium.
2. The importance of actively diagnosing delirium and looking for a medical (or "organic") cause.
3. The importance of not allowing psychiatry to be the "dumping ground" for diagnoses of exclusion. Just as a myocardial infarction has positive and minimum criteria for diagnosis, so too have depression, anxiety, and delirium.
4. The importance of liaison psychiatry to recognize the dynamic issues at play in medical oncologists who deal with critically ill patients.
5. The importance of serving as liaison between staff, family and patient to expedite acceptance of an unwanted but painful reality.

The common psychiatric disorders have traditionally been poorly defined in the cancer population and hence underdiagnosed and undertreated; however, today many more and complex treatments are available. Patients live longer with their cancers, allowing old problems to be magnified and new ones to come to light. This chapter outlines the clinical presentation and management of the common problems and seeks to give a flavor of the unique variations and nuances created by the cancer setting.

PSYCHOLOGICAL RESPONSE TO CANCER

The diagnosis of cancer, or news that it has relapsed, is a major life stressor. Psychological reactions range from appropriate adaptation to disabling psychiatric disorders. A given cancer might not have worse health implications than other serious illnesses, however, the meaning and significance of cancer, like tuberculosis of old, adds a dimension of stress. Fear of death is primary, which incorporates the fears of pain, disfigurement, dependence, and loss. Cancer interrupts the assumptions, the "forward life trajectory," even the meaningfulness of a person's life. Hope, essential to a sense of well-being, is prematurely dashed (6).

The spectrum and prevalence of psychiatric reactions and disorders was studied by the Psychosocial Collaborative Oncology Group in 215 randomly selected cancer patients in a cross-sectional study. Using the criteria of the third edition of the *Diagnostic and Statistical Manual of Mental Disorders* (as listed in Ref. 7), about one half (53%) of the patients had adjusted normally to the stresses of cancer. However, the remainder (47%) had clinically apparent psychiatric disorders at the time of interview. Of these 47%, adjustment disorder with depressed or anxious mood was the most common (68%), followed by major depression (13%), organic mental disorder (mainly delirium) (8%), and prior psychiatric disorders (mainly personality and anxiety) comprising 11% (Fig. 1).

It is important to note that many psychiatric symptoms and diagnoses are comorbid and tend to fluctuate in concert with the disease progression.

NORMAL ADAPTATION TO CANCER

Although individual variation is great, a characteristic pattern of normal responses is seen (8) (Table 1). The initial phase is one of disbelief and denial at the diagnosis ("they must have mixed up the slides"). Some patients feel "numb" and appear not to understand. Less commonly, despair is present at the outset. Phase II follows once the initial information has been acknowledged. Emotional distress with dysphoria, anxiety, panic, and depression characterize this difficult time. Sleep, appetite, and the ability function day-to-day are often disturbed. Phase III represents progressively more sophisticated levels of adaptation. Treatment plans, therapeutic alliances, and mobilization of social resources help in the adjustment to a different set of expectations. This sequence of disbelief, dysphoria, and adaptation may reappear with each new medical

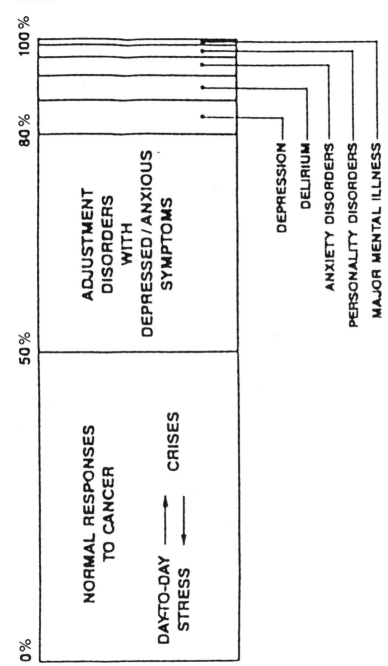

Figure 1 Prevalence of psychiatric disorders in 215 adult cancer patients indicated that slightly more than half were adjusting normally to the crisis of illness. Adjustment disorder with depressed and/or anxious mood was the most common psychiatric disorder diagnosed. (From Ref. 7, and derived from PSYCOG Prevalence Data.)

Table 1 Initial Response to Diagnosis of Cancer

Phase	Symptoms	Time interval
I: Initial response	Disbelief or denial or despair ("I knew it all along")	Usually less than 1 week
II: Dysphoria	Anxiety, depressed mood, anorexia, insomnia, poor concentration, inability to function	Usually 1–2 weeks, but variable
III: Adaptation	Accepts validity of information and begins dealing with the options available Finds reasons for optimism and resumes usual activities	Usually by 2 weeks, but adaptation continues over months; may or may not be successful

Source: Ref. 9.

crisis. Psychological defenses characteristic for that individual are tapped and, where adaptive, should be encouraged. However, as the disease progresses and loss of function accumulates, the overall level of adaptation may change, for better or for worse (1).

While the three-phase model of acute response to catastrophic news is generally applicable, the infinite individual variation is influenced by three interacting factors: societal attitudes, patient-related factors, and medical factors (Table 2).

Societal attitudes are dynamic. In America today it is more accepted to tell the truth and give the patient the option and autonomy of decision making. The ready access of information on the Internet enables and encourages patients and their families to take control. However, the burden of decision making does not sit well on some individuals' shoulders, and they may feel isolated or pressured.

Patient-related factors are crucial and self-evident. In particular, personality style, maturity, concurrent life stresses, and flexibility are strong influences.

Medical factors are important beyond immediate prognosis. For an elderly woman, a mastectomy might be relatively uneventful, whereas for a young mother it would be a catastrophe. Summarized differently, Table 3 provides a practical list of factors that predict poor coping with cancer (9). Overall, cancer patients as a group represent a psychologically healthy population adapting to uncommon stress. When adaptation fails, or becomes maladaptive, the patterns of normal adjustment are likely to evolve into psychiatric disorders. The task of the psychiatrist is to diagnose and treat these patients, to facilitate their strengths and adaptive capacities, and to help engage external resources (10).

Table 2 Factors Influencing Psychological Adaptation to Cancer

Societal
Paternalistic and secretive; or autonomous and open
Taboos, stigmata, myths, e.g., stress causes cancer
Health care system, e.g., if uninsured
Patient
Coping ability, emotional maturity, "hardiness"
Premorbid psychiatric illness
Philosophical, spiritual, religious beliefs
Development of life's goals and meaning of loss, e.g., marriage, children
Support of spouse, family, friends
Medical
Tumor: site, stage, prognosis
Treatment: severity and complications
Symptom accumulation, disability, disfigurement
Psychosocial attentiveness of staff

Source: Ref. 9.

Table 3 Predictors of Poor Coping with Cancer

Social isolation
Low socioeconomic status
Alcohol or drug abuse
Prior psychiatric history
Prior experience with cancer (e.g., family member)
Recent losses/bereavement
Flexibility and rigidity of coping
Pessimistic philosophy of life
Absence of belief/value system
Multiple obligations

Source: Ref. 39.

PSYCHIATRIC DISORDERS IN CANCER

Anxiety and depression are the most common psychiatric disorders seen in cancer patients, and they often appear as comorbid states. In the absence of a premorbid diagnosis, each can be seen as ranging on a continuum from normal fears through to generalized anxiety and panic disorder, from sadness to major depression. Throughout the illness these emotions will shift back and forth along the spectrum (Table 4).

Advanced disease and pain, two interrelated factors, are associated with higher prevalence of depression and delirium. Approximately 25% of all cancer patients experience severe depressive symptoms, with the prevalence increasing to 77% in advanced illness (11). Similarly delirium ranges from 25% to a high of 85% during terminal phases of illness (12). In the Psychosocial Collaborative Oncology Group study (8), 39% of patients with a psychiatric diagnosis experienced significant pain, whereas only 19% of patients without a psychiatric diagnosis had significant pain. Adjustment disorder with depressed or anxious mood and major depression constituted the majority of

Table 4 Common Psychiatric Disorders in Cancer

Illness-related
  Adjustment disorder—anxiety, depression, mixed
  Major depression
  Delirium
Preexisting disorders, exacerbated
  Personality disorders—histrionic, narcissistic,
    borderline, paranoid, schizotypal
  Bipolar
  Schizophrenia
  Anxiety disorder—phobia, panic, generalized

diagnoses and were seen more frequently in patients with pain. Clinical experience and data support a causal relationship between uncontrolled pain and psychiatric symptoms (13). Pain must be controlled before a psychiatric diagnosis can firmly be made.

Anxiety, depression, and delirium, the most common psychiatric disorders in cancer, should be viewed as symptoms which, like fever, may have many different etiologies. Empiric treatment is initially directed at relieving the symptoms, but the causes must be investigated in order to direct management.

ANXIETY

Some degree of anxiety is universal in cancer patients. Recognition of anxiety can be difficult as patients often present with physical symptoms overshadowing psychiatric or cognitive ones. Patients may not be aware that their complaints are due to anxiety. A high index of suspicion on the part of the clinician is helpful. It is important to ask about breathing difficulties, concentration, jitteriness, restlessness, appetite, feeling overwhelmed, ruminating, and problems making decisions and following instructions. Speaking with family members is important in order to corroborate or add information.

Anxiety as a symptom is seen in adjustment disorder, generalized anxiety disorder, phobia, agitated depression, and delirium and secondary to physical illnesses and medications (14) (Table 5). The course of cancer is punctuated with situations that exacerbate anxiety, such as at diagnosis or relapse, awaiting a test result, a new pain, fear of recurrence, a frightening procedure, or termination of treatment. Underpinning these apprehensions is the gnawing existential fear of death. Poorly controlled pain, hypoxia, hypoglycemia, sepsis, pulmonary emboli, bleeding, delirium, hyperthyroidism, and, less commonly, paraneoplastic endocrine tumors such as pheochromocytoma and carcinoid can all cause anxiety (15). Adverse drug reactions or side effects of corticosteroids, antiemetics, neuroleptics, and certain chemotherapeutic agents as well as withdrawal states from alcohol, opiates, and benzodiazepines are examples of medication-related anxiety syndromes.

Personality styles and preexisting anxiety disorders, including claustrophobia or fear of needles and hospitals contribute to difficulties adjusting to a new reality. Past traumatic experiences with death, either in war or of loved ones, especially if related to cancer, bring painful associations. In deciding whether to treat the anxiety, the patient's subjective level of distress and presence of problematic behavior, such as noncompliance, disruption of interpersonal relationships, and inability to perform daily functions, help guide the physician.

Treatment is both nonpharmacological and pharmacological. Supportive psychotherapy and behavioral interventions, alone or in combination, deal with situational anxiety and existential issues. Supportive activities include clarifying treatment options and teaching patients to recognize anxiety and its causes (psychoeducation); offering emotional support (such as being with patients for procedures or for critical interviews with internists); providing relaxation tapes; teaching hypnosis, progressive muscle relax-

Table 5   Causes of Anxiety in Patients with Cancer

Situational
    Diagnosis, prognosis
    Conflicts with family, staff
    Test result pending
    Fear of recurrence
Disease
    Pain, poorly controlled
    Hypoxia, other metabolic problems
    Hormone-secreting tumors and paraneoplastic
    Delirium
Exacerbation of preexisting anxiety disorder
    Phobias
    Panic or generalized anxiety disorder
    Posttraumatic stress disorder (e.g., Holocaust,
        Vietnam, death of a loved one with cancer)
Treatment
    Procedures (MRI, injections, debridement)
    Anxiety-producing drugs
    Withdrawal states (opiates, alcohol, benzodiazepines)
    Conditioned vomiting (cyclic chemotherapy)

Source: Ref. 1.

ation, and guided imagery; serving as liaison to other treating doctors and mobilizing ancillary help. All play a role.

It is important to include family members or loved ones in discussions (16). The fear of death often manifests as a fear of loneliness and separation. Encouraging patients to verbalize these fears by gentle and appropriate questioning is in itself therapeutic. It is not easy to ask personal and intrusive questions; we are concerned they will upset the patient. We must overcome our own fears, embarrassment, and denial. It is useful to enlist the help of pastoral care when appropriate.

Another common scenario is that patients who have just received bad news assume incorrectly that they are about to die. Specific reassurances are helpful. Similarly, when fear of pain is at issue, reassurances, explanations, and referral to a pain specialist are effective interventions. For more complex problems, such as anticipatory vomiting following chemotherapy or claustrophobia during radiation therapy, cognitive-behavioral techniques are used, supplemented with anxiolytics (17).

Pharmacotherapy of anxiety in oncology involves the use of benzodiazepines, neuroleptics, antihistamines, antidepressants, and opioid analgesics (Table 6). Anxiety is seen in cancer patients from the day of diagnosis to the final stages of palliative care. Hence, a wide range of medications is required to deal with the physiological and psychological symptoms of anxiety.

Table 6 Anxiolytic Medications Used in Cancer

Generic name	Approximate daily dosage range (mg)	Route
Benzodiazepines		
Very short-acting		
Midazolam	10–60 per 24 h	IV, SC
Short-acting		
Alprazolam	0.25–2.0 tid-qid	PO, SL
Oxazepam	10–15 tid-qid	PO
Lorazepam	0.5–2.0 tid-qid	PO, SL, IV, IM
Intermediate-acting		
Chlordiazepoxide	10–50 tid-qid	PO, IM
Long-acting		
Diazepam	5–10 bid-qid	PO, IV, PR
Clorazepate	7.5–15 bid-qid	PO
Clonazepam	.05–2 bid-qid	PO
Nonbenzodiazepines		
Buspirone	10–30 bid	PO
Neuroleptics		
Haloperidol	0.5–5 q2–12 h	PO, IV, SC, IM
Methotrimeprazine	10–20 q4–8 h	SC, PO, IM
Thioridazine	10–75 tid-qid	PO
Chlorpromazine	12.5–50 q4–12 h	PO, IM, IV
Antihistamine		
Hydroxyzine	25–50 q4–6 h	PO, IV, SC
Tricyclic antidepressants		
Imipramine	12.5–150 hs	PO, IM
Clomipramine	10–150 hs	PO

PO, Peroral; IM, intramuscular; PR, per rectum; IV, intravenous; SC, subcutaneous; SL, sublingual; bid, two times a day; tid, three times a day; qid, four times a day; q4–8 h, every 4–8 hours; hs, at bedtime. Parenteral doses are generally twice as potent as oral doses; intravenous bolus injections or infusions should be administered slowly.

Benzodiazepines are the most helpful class of medication. In physically well patients, the longer-acting drugs, such as clonazepam and diazepam, have the advantages of avoiding breakthrough anxiety, end-of-dose failure, and a withdrawal syndrome. Addiction, even with chronic anxiety, is usually not a problem in cancer patients.

Alprazolam is preferred for acute anxiety or panic attacks related to planned procedures or known precipitants. As patients become sicker, the shorter-acting anxiolytics, namely oxazepam, aprazolam, and lorazepam, are preferred as they are less likely to accumulate, have a mild euphoric effect, and prove less of a problem interacting adversely with opiates in terms of central nervous system and respiratory depression. Lorazepam is important because it is commonly used to help control the nausea and vomiting of chemotherapy and, if anxiety is a comorbid disorder, the "double effect" can be utilized. Lorazepam is safely administered parenterally. Midazolam is effective as a continuous subcutaneous infusion for anxiety and agitation in the terminally ill (18). Diazepam can be administered rectally in doses equivalent to oral regimes if other routes are unavailable in the dying patient.

Buspirone is an effective, nonbenzodiazepine anxiolytic. It is more useful in chronic anxiety because it takes 5–10 days to be effective. Buspirone is non–cross-tolerant with benzodiazepines and will not prevent withdrawal when stopping a benzodiazepine. Buspirone is less sedating than benzodiazepine and is helpful when respiratory depression is an issue. Some experience has been gained using maximal doses of buspirone (30 mg twice daily) to achieve rapid anxiolysis within a few days. The dose can then be tapered as guided by side effects. Buspirone has no significant abuse potential.

Selective serotonin-reuptake inhibitors (SSRIs) as a class have been shown to have an important role in the long-term control of panic disorders. We have found combining an SSRI of choice with a long-acting benzodiazepine to be effective in treating the continuous panic-like state that occurs with some patients as they experience loss of control in the face of disease progression.

Neuroleptics are useful when benzodiazepines are ineffective, when respiratory depression is a concern, and when delirium, with psychotic symptoms, is driving or accompanying the anxiety. Haloperidol is safe either orally or parenterally and is not significantly sedating. Thioridazine, a low-potency neuroleptic, is more sedating and is helpful when insomnia, agitation, and anger are prominent. The main side effects of the low-potency agents are anticholinergic symptoms and hypotension.

Hydroxyzine, an antihistamine with sedating, anxiolytic, and analgesic properties, is effective in hospitalized patients either in combination or when benzodiazepines are contraindicated; 100 mg parenterally is equivalent to 8 mg of morphine and potentiates the analgesia of opiates (19). Tricyclic antidepressants are effective for anxiety and insomnia in the setting of depression and/or neuropathic pain. Opioid medications have a limited but important role in treating anxiety when it presents due to dyspnea or pain; however, they should not be used alone in the treatment of anxiety that is occurring on a psychological basis.

DEPRESSION

The incidence of depression (major, 5–8%; adjustment disorder, 20%) increases with advanced illness, greater disability, and uncontrolled pain (1). It is incorrect to think that significant depression is "understandable" in a patient with cancer and therefore there is no need to treat. Depression should be and is successfully treated. Risk factors for developing depression that are helpful in the diagnostic assessment are: personal or family history of depression, alcoholism, or substance abuse, recent loss, poor social support, previous suicide attempt, medications (corticosteroids, amphotericin, vinca alkaloids, asparaginase, tamoxifen, interferon, interleukin), and various paraneoplastic, endocrine, and metabolic illnesses that affect the central nervous system.

The medically ill can have physical symptoms that are the same as the diagnostic criteria for depression (20). Thus, the neurovegetative symptoms of anorexia, fatigue, insomnia, and weight loss are unreliable because they lack specificity. The diagnosis of depression in the physically ill relies more on psychiatric and cognitive symptoms such as worthlessness, hopelessness, guilt (in being a burden to the family), inability to concentrate, suicidal ideation, and an unrelenting awareness of the diagnosis. Each of these symptoms must be analyzed in detail and evaluated against the stage and state of the illness. For example, a patient with terminal cancer might be hopeless about cure but hopeful about symptom control. If, however, the hopelessness pervades all thoughts and is associated with despairing ruminations, then it is more likely part of a depressive syndrome.

Suicide is more common in cancer patients than in the general population but not as high as is often assumed (21). Table 7 lists factors known to be associated with an increased risk of suicide (22). Studies have shown that loss of hope is a better predictor for suicide than depression (23). It is likely that drug overdose at home during the terminal stage of cancer is underdiagnosed and underreported. It is important to evaluate suicidal ideation at every consultation, bearing in mind that asking about it does not create the thought nor precipitate the action and that it is more often a relief to express it. Thinking about suicide is, in a paradoxical way, a form of comforting oneself with hope and maintaining a sense of control. The act of saying "If things get too bad, I can kill myself" creates a breathing space and functions as a coping mechanism by implying that the situation is not as bad as it could be.

Management of depression involves supportive psychotherapy, cognitive-behavioral techniques, and antidepressant medications. Electroconvulsive therapy is rarely needed, although it may be indicated in an agitated, psychotic elderly patient who is refractory to medications. The mainstay for treatment of major depression in cancer

Table 7   Risk Factors for Suicide in Cancer

Pain, suffering, fatigue
Advanced illness and poor prognosis
Depression and hopelessness
Loss of control and helplessness
Preexisting psychopathology
Substance/Alcohol abuse
Suicide history (family and personal)
Delirium with disinhibition
Social isolation

Source: Ref. 21.

patients is antidepressants, including in patients whose depression is due to a medical mechanism (e.g., brain tumor) or treatment side effects (e.g., corticosteroids). The choice of antidepressant in the individual patient depends on target symptoms and knowledge of side effects, which are avoided as necessary but utilized where appropriate (Table 8).

The SSRIs have been dramatically successful in treating depression in the medically ill because of their relatively benign side-effect profile vis-a-vis the tricyclics (24). The SSRIs have little or no anticholinergic properties and are not cardiotoxic. The most common side effects are nausea, headaches, somnolence (long-term), and impaired sexual function. The SSRIs can cause drowsiness, activation, or insomnia, but by changing the dosing from morning to evening the problem can be overcome. Less commonly, extrapyramidal symptoms including akathisia and dyskinesia are seen. Rarely, hyponatremia and platelet dysfunction have been reported. Renal impairment does not alter pharmacokinetics, but liver disease prolongs the half-life.

The major cause for concern in the medically ill are the drug interactions with SSRIs via the cytochrome P_{450} enzymes. Fluoxetine is reported to increase serum levels of tricyclics, haloperidol, diazepam, alprazolam, and valproate. Fluoxetine has no effect on warfarin levels or prothrombin time. Cimetidine can increase paroxetine levels by up to 50%, and sertaline and paroxetine significantly increase tricyclic blood levels (25). If the SSRIs are started in low doses, some of the milder side effects can be accommodated. However, if sexual dysfunction develops, it can be ameliorated by providing a "drug holiday," adding a psychostimulant, lowering the dose, or changing to another medication such as bupropion, mirtazapine, or nefazadone.

In cancer patients who are significantly ill, lower doses of antidepressants have been shown to be equally effective. This may or may not translate into fewer side effects. With tricyclics, which are especially useful in depressed patients who have insomnia, anorexia, and/or neuropathic pain, it is often sufficient to start at doses of 10–25 mg at night and build up to a maximum of 150 mg per day. Drug levels are available (except for doxepin) and should be used particularly in the medically ill and elderly.

Bupropion, with sympathomimetic activating properties, is effective in treating depression in the physically ill, especially in individuals with neurovegetative symptoms. However, it should not be used if there is a history of seizure or if a risk of seizure exists. Tremor, insomnia, and nausea are early side effects. Mirtazapine, an antidepressant that targets serotonin and norepinephrine receptors, has the curious characteristic of being very sedating at low doses (15 mg/day) but not at higher doses (45 mg/day). Mirtazapine does not have the anticholinergic properties of tricyclics but has the potentially beneficial property—in cancer patients, at least—of increasing appetite and weight.

Tricyclics and SSRIs take at least 1–2 weeks to start working. In the medically ill, when a more rapid response is needed, psychostimulants prove useful. Psychostimulants have been shown to improve attention and concentration in neuropsychological testing in the medically ill (26). They are effective within a day in depressed patients with psychomotor slowing and fatigue and anergia due to the cancer or its treatment. At low doses, psychostimulants increase appetite, lift depression, and improve a sense

Table 8 Antidepressant Use in Cancer Patients

Medication	Start/Daily dose	Primary side effects/ Comments
Tricyclics (TCAs)		All TCAs can cause cardiac arrhythmias; blood levels are available for all but doxepin; get baseline EKG
Amitriptyline (Elavil)	10–15/50–100	Sedation; anticholinergic; orthostasis
Imipramine (Tofranil)	10–25/50–150	Intermediate sedation; anticholinergic; orthostasis
Desipramine (Norpramin)	25/75–150	Little sedation or orthostasis; moderate anticholinergic
Nortriptyline (Pamelor)	10–25/75–150	Little anticholinergic or orthostasis; intermediate sedation; therapeutic window
Doxepin (Sinequan)	25/75–150	Very sedating; orthostatic hypotension; intermediate anticholinergic effects; potent antihistamine
Second Generation		
Buproprion (Wellbutrin)	75/200–450	May cause seizures in those with low seizure threshold/brain tumors; intially activating
Trazodone (Desyrel)	50/150–200	Sedating; not anticholinergic; risk of priapism
Selective-serotonin reuptake inhibitors (SSRIs)		Serotonin-reuptake inhibitors have few anticholinergic or cardiovascular side effects; sexual dysfunction including anorgasmia
Fluoxetine (Prozac)	10/20–40	Headache; nausea; anxiety; insomnia; has a very long half-life; may be even longer in debilitated patient
Sertraline (Zoloft)	25/50–150	Nausea; insomnia
Paroxetine (Paxil)	10/20–50	Nausea; somnolence; asthenia; no active metabolites
Psychostimulants		
D-Amphetamine (Dexedrin)	2.5/5–30	All psychostimulants may cause insomnia, nightmares, psychosis, anorexia, agitation, and restlessness
Methylphenidate (Ritalin)	2.5/5–30	Possible cardiac complications; should be given in two divided doses at 8 a.m. and noon; can be used as analgesic adjuvant and to counter sedation of opiates

Table 8   Continued

Medication	Start/Daily dose	Primary side effects/ Comments
Pemoline (Cylert)	18.75/37.5–150	Follow liver tests
Other		
Venlafaxine (Effexor)	75/225–375	Inhibits reuptake of both serotonin and norepinephrine; achieves steady state in 3 days; may increase blood pressure
Nefazodone (Serzone)	100/200–500	Affects serotonin 5HT$_2$, and norepinephrine; sedating; decreased cardiotoxicity; less reported sexual dysfunction than SSRIs
Mirtazapine (Remeron)	15/30–45	Sedating at low dose; increase weight; less sexual dysfunction; reduced clearance in elderly and liver/renal impairment

Source: Ref. 40.

of well-being. Pemoline, which is unrelated to amphetamines, is as effective in cancer patients. It has little abuse potential and can be chewed and absorbed through the buccal mucosa. However, since pemoline can cause liver impairment, it must be monitored. Amphetamines can be used for many months without risk of abuse in this population, although tolerance does develop and doses must be adjusted. The other important use of psychostimulants is to counteract sedation secondary to opiates, while at the same time potentiating their analgesia. Side effects include anxiety, insomnia, and paranoia. Typically, the psychostimulants are prescribed in divided doses at 8 a.m. and 12 noon and slowly increased over several days, with monitoring of desired benefit against side effect.

Lithium carbonate should be used cautiously and monitored closely in the sick oncology patient in whom fluid and electrolyte abnormalities are common and risk of lithium toxicity is significant. This is particularly true with cisplatinum, where the potential for nephrotoxicity is high. Nonetheless, if a patient has been previously stable on lithium it should be continued. Monoamine oxidase inhibitors (MAOIs) are rarely used in cancer patients. The dietary restrictions are unacceptable and unreasonable in this population, and the risk of adverse drug interaction in a polypharmacy setting are high. Tricyclics and SSRIs are preferable alternatives.

Insomnia is a frequent and distressing problem in oncology. It is seen both with psychiatric and medical conditions. The underlying cause, be it pain, hypoxia, or anxiety, must be corrected, while at the same time treating, if necessary, the insomnia with hypnotics. Zolpidem (5–20 mg), trazadone (50–150 mg), diphenhydramine (25–50 mg), chloral hydrate (25–100 mg), benzodiazepines, and tricyclic antidepressants, given at bedtime, are effective agents. Behavioral techniques have also been shown to successfully treat secondary insomnia in cancer patients. One study using progressive muscle relaxation showed a marked reduction in mean sleep onset latency (27).

DELIRIUM

Delirium is common in cancer. It is frequently underrecognized, misdiagnosed, and improperly treated. The two hallmark features are a disturbance of level of consciousness in association with global impairment of cognitive functions. As a consequence, abnormalities of mood (depression or anxiety), perception (hallucinations), and altered sleep-wake cycle are frequent psychiatric symptoms (28). Other critical features are the relatively abrupt onset of symptoms in a medical setting and the waxing and waning of symptoms over a period of several hours. Delirium is a syndrome due to global cerebral dysfunction without a clear neurophysiological mechanism. The typical causes of delirium in a cancer setting are listed in Table 9. The most common scenario is that multiple factors interact to precipitate a delirium.

Medications are a common cause of delirium, especially when organ failure is present. Benzodiazepines and any opioid analgesics are frequently implicated. Chemo-

Table 9 Causes of Delirium in Cancer

Direct CNS causes
    Primary brain tumor
    Seizures
    Metastatic spread to CNS
Indirect causes
    Metabolic encephalopathy due to organ failure
    Electrolyte imbalance
    Treatment side effects
        chemotherapy
        corticosteroids
        radiation to brain
        opioids
        anticholinergics
        antiemetics
        antibiotics
    Infection
    Hematological abnormalities
    Nutritional deficiencies
    Paraneoplastic syndromes

Source: Refs. 9, 41.

therapeutic drugs known to cause delirium include ifosfamide, intrathecal methotrexate, fluouracil, vinca alkaloids, asparaginase, cytosine arabinoside, procarbazine, bleomycin, cisplatinum, interferon, and the corticosteroids. The spectrum of mental disturbances related to corticosteroids includes minor mood lability, affective disorders (mania, agitation, depression), cognitive impairment, and delirium ("steroid psychosis"). Doses causing delirium are usually higher than the equivalent of 40 mg of prednisolone per day. The timing and nature of the neuropsychiatric complications are poorly predictable from one course of corticosteroids to the next and prior psychiatric illness is not a significant risk factor.

Delirium is more likely to occur in the elderly and in those with preexisting brain damage, especially dementia, cerebrovascular disease, and alcoholism (29). Delirium is reversible except in the presence of irreversible organ failure, typically in terminal disease. Whatever the etiology, delirium is a bad prognostic sign in terms of morbidity and mortality and thus is important to diagnose. The Delirium Rating Scale and the Mini-Mental State Examination (MMSE) are two bedside tools that help in the diagnostic process (30). The MMSE screens for cognitive failure but does not distinguish between delirium and dementia. There is no pathognomonic test to diagnose delirium, which is often misdiagnosed because behavioral changes are attributed to "understandable" psychiatric reactions. Early symptoms of delirium can present as affective disorders with anxiety, anger, depression, and paranoia. It is therefore important to check for the presence of impaired cognition and fluctuating levels of consciousness.

Delirium presents as a clinical spectrum from hypoactive to hyperactive. Hypoactive patients are lethargic and withdrawn and are typically seen in metabolic derangements such as liver failure. This group of patients can be misdiagnosed as depressed. The hyperactive delirium presents with agitation, delusions, and hyperarousal and can be misdiagnosed as anxious or hysterical behavior. Finally, it is not uncommon for delirium itself to be the presenting symptom of the underlying medical illness.

The principles of management of delirium are straightforward. They include ensuring the physical safety of patient, family, and staff; pharmacotherapy to control symptoms of delirium; and searching for and reversing the underlying etiology. If the patient is violently agitated, physical restraints with one-on-one nursing care may be necessary initially. In less disturbed patients a quiet, well-lit room with familiar objects such as calendars and photographs and the presence of a supportive relative or friend help reduce disorientation and anxiety. Controlling the situation and reassuring the family reduces their stress while liaison is initiated with medical staff to coordinate investigations and treat any reversible causes. In the terminally ill, the cause of delirium was found in less than 50% of the cases in one study. Depending upon the extent of the disease, extensive search for an etiology may be inappropriate because no further treatment is possible and intrusive tests are inappropriate (31).

Neuroleptics alone or combined with benzodiazepines are the medications of choice in treatment of delirium (Table 10). Haloperidol is the drug of choice in treating delirium in the medically ill. It controls agitation, clears sensorium, and improves cognitive function with minimal hypotensive and anticholinergic properties. Low doses (0.5–

Table 10 Medications Useful in Managing Delirium in Cancer Patients

Generic name	Approximate daily dosage range (mg)	Route
Neuroleptics		
Haloperidol	0.5–5.0 q2–12 h	PO, IV, SC, IM
Thioridazine	10–75 q4–8 h	PO
Chlorpromazine	12.5–50.0 q4–12 h	PO, IV, IM
Methotrimeprazine	12.5–50.0 q4–8 h	IV, SC, PO
Benzodiazepines		
Lorazepam	0.5–2.0 q1–4 h	PO, IV, IM
Midazolam	30–100 per 24 h	IV, SC

IM injections should be avoided if repeated use becomes necessary; SC infusions are generally accepted modes of drug administration in the terminally ill; parenteral doses are generally twice as potent as oral doses; IV infusions or bolus injections should be administered slowly.

3 mg) are started, with repeat doses every 45–60 minutes titrated against symptoms. Oral administration is often adequate; however, the intravenous route—especially in agitated paranoid patients—is safe and rapidly effective. Parenteral doses are twice as potent as oral doses. Extrapyramidal problems (especially in combination with neuroleptic antiemetics) are a concern, however, anecdotally, parenteral haloperidol is said not to be strongly associated with extrapyramidal side effects. Tardive dyskinesia and neuroleptic malignant syndrome are rarely seen, in part because treatment courses are short and doses required are low. After 24 hours, the total dose of haloperidol is calculated and then, if the clinical situation has stabilized, it is given in two or three divided doses for the next 24-hour period.

Because haloperidol tends not to be very sedating, lorazepam (0.5–2 mg) orally or intravenously can be given every 1–2 hours with the haloperidol to achieve rapid sedation. It is a common error to treat with benzodiazepines alone, which might give transient control but does nothing to improve sensorium or cognition. The only randomized double-blinded study comparing haloperidol, chlorpromazine, and lorazepam showed that lorazepam alone worsened delirium and cognitive function (31).

In terminally ill cancer patients, the goals of care are different. Delirium is often irreversible, especially in the last few days of life, and sedation may be the only effective way to control symptoms (32). Midazolam given as an intravenous or a continuous subcutaneous infusion is an example in which benzodiazepines are appropriately used alone in delirium. Methotrimeprazine has unique analgesic properties (being equipotent with morphine without the constipating effect) and is effective in terminal cancer patients with pain, anxiety, and delirium. Its major dose-limiting drawback is hypotension and sedation (33).

STAFF SUPPORT

A number of studies (34) have looked at the stressors experienced by the oncology staff. The doctor still carries much of the burden of decision making despite increasing patient autonomy and erosion of medical authority (8). To an extent, doctors are a self-selected group of individuals who tolerate stress, have a strong work ethic, see life as a challenge, not a burden, and are "hardy." However, within these characteristics there is often a characteristic of rigidity that predisposes to chronic stress (35). Physicians have difficulty saying no, taking vacation, forgoing responsibility, being able to divulge feelings—in short, they develop a "superman syndrome." Nowhere is this more apparent than in oncology, where they face the desperation of young families, patients' feelings of helplessness, anxiety, and panic, the repeated deaths of parents and children, the low efficacy and painful nature of many cancer treatments, the difficulties of decision making in end-of-life issues, the unpleasantness of giving bad news, and bearing the brunt of patients' and families' projected anger and unrealistic expectations (36).

Among oncologists and psycho-oncologists, two countertransference issues in particular are common (34). The first is the need to "save" the patient. Feelings of helplessness and futility at the progression of the disease, coupled with low self-esteem and depression, may lead doctors to become overinvolved or to encourage excessive and inappropriate therapies. Alternatively, the feelings of helplessness, impotence, and futility may build resentment or anger towards the patient and cause the doctor to avoid or prematurely give up the case. These issues typically arise at crises in the course of the disease, particularly in the transition from active treatment to palliative care.

The second common countertransference reaction is the need to "protect" the patient. Personal fears of the doctor prevent discussing important issues with the patient such as feelings and thoughts about death, loss, suffering, a will, and financial arrangements. We rationalize the patient's avoidance and denial by claiming that these issues will be too painful. But for whom? Being conscious of countertransference issues goes a long way to preventing problems. Physicians with emotional fatigue or burnout might not recognize their own symptoms. Loss of enthusiasm, exhaustion, irritability, depression, detachment from family and friends, and the use of alcohol to relax are some of the signs of accumulating stress (37) (Table 11).

Psychiatry has a role in educating about work stress. An effective forum is in the multidisciplinary team meeting in which the psychiatrist is an active member and the focus is initially on the psychosocial needs of the patients. As members become more familiar and comfortable with each other they feel safer and more able to express their emotions and private thoughts without feeling ashamed or inadequate. In particular, insight into personal views and fears of death and losses are useful. The psychiatrist can facilitate these discussions. At the same time tactics on how to survive can be shared. Methods include use of gallows humor, recognition of personal and medical limitations, controlling overtime, varying work by allocating time to writing or attending conferences, and using social events to increase camaraderie. Regularly discussing and ad-

Table 11 Symptoms of Burnout in Medical Staff

Physical
  Headaches
  Intestinal disorders
  Chronic fatigue
  Sleep disorders
  "Cancer phobia"
Emotional
  Depression
  Detachment
  Guilt
  Hopelessness
  Powerlessness
Maladaptive coping mechanisms
  Altered work patterns (absenteeism, arriving late,
    leaving early, clock watching)
  Excessive death watch
  Negativism, cynicism ("I hate medicine")
  Withdrawal from patients and coworkers
  Overinvolvement ("I must do everything")
  Uncontrollable crying
  Family and relationship conflicts
  Substance abuse (alcohol, nicotine, caffeine, other
    drugs)

Source: Ref. 37.

justing the goals of care of each patient helps the physician retain an objective perspective from which realistic hope and appropriate care can be delivered. At the end of the day, the work will retain its meaningfulness and burnout can be avoided.

CONCLUSION

Psycho-oncology has three roles. The first is to treat the psychiatric disorders complicating medical care with psychopharmacology, psychotherapy, and behavioral therapy. The second is to identify research questions among the many topics that come under its umbrella. The third is to become involved in disseminating this knowledge to colleagues, which is in many ways the most difficult but potentially the most rewarding.

It is difficult to work with sick and dying cancer patients. It is more difficult to be suffering oneself or losing a loved one. Maintaining a perspective does not always protect the health professional from the sadness and suffering of a cancer ward. Achieving a high level of medical competence is important and rewarding, but too often patients' and families' psychosocial needs are not met. Psycho-oncolgy has an important clinical role, developed and designed to help the patient, the family, and the staff.

REFERENCES

1. Holland JC. Principles of psycho-oncology. In: Holland J, Frei E III, Bast RC, Kufe DW, Morton DL, Weichselbaum RR, eds. Cancer Medicine. 4th ed. Baltimore: Williams & Wilkins, 1997:1327–1343.
2. Aries P. Western Attitudes Towards Death from the Middle Ages to the Present. London: Open Forum Series, Marion Boyars, 1976.
3. Saunders CMS. In: Doyle D, Hanks GWC, MacDonald N, eds. Oxford Textbook of Palliative Medicine. New York: Oxford University Press, 1993:v–viii.
4. Twyross RG. Hospice care: redressing the balance in medicine. J Roy Soc Med 1980; 73: 475–481.
5. Burt RA. The suppressed legacy of Nuremberg. Hastings Center Report 1996; 5:30–33.
6. Fawzy FI, Natterson B. Psychological care of the cancer patient. In: Cameron R, ed. Clinical Oncology: A Lange Clinical Manual. San Mateo, CA: Simon and Schuster Higher Education Group, 1994:40–44.
7. Derogatis LR, Morrow GR, Fetting J, et al. The prevalence of psychiatric disorders among cancer patients. JAMA 1983; 249:751–757.
8. Massie MJ, Spiegel L, Lederberg MS, Holland JC. Psychiatric complications in cancer patients. In: Murphy GP, Lawrence W, Jr, Lenhard RE, Jr, eds. American Cancer Society Textbook of Clinical Oncology. Atlanta: American Cancer Society, 1995:685–698.
9. Holland JC, Rowland JH, eds. Handbook of Psycho-Oncology: Psychological Care of the Patient with Cancer. New York: Oxford University Press, 1989.
10. Breitbart W. Identifying patients at risk for, and treatment of, major psychiatric complications of cancer. Support Care Cancer 1995; 3:45–60.
11. Bukberg J, Penman D, Holland JC. Depression in hospitalized cancer patients. Psychosom Med 1984; 43:199–212.
12. Massie MJ, Holland JC, Glass E. Delirium in terminally ill cancer patients. Am J Psychiatry 1983; 140:1048–1050.
13. Ahles TA, Blanchard EB, Ruckdeschel JC. The multidimensional nature of cancer related pain. Pain 1983; 17:277–288.
14. Breitbart W, Passik SD. Psychiatric aspects of palliative care. In: Doyle D, Hanks GWC, MacDonald N, eds. Oxford Textbook of Palliative Medicine. Oxford: Oxford University Press, 1993:609–626.
15. Strain JJ, Liebowitz MR, Klein DF. Anxiety and panic attacks in the medically ill. Psychiatr Clin North Am 1981; 4:333–348.
16. Fawzy FI, Fawzy NW, Pasnau RO. Critical review of psychosocial interventions in cancer care. Arch Gen Psychiatry 1995; 52:100–113.
17. Jacobsen PB, Bovbjerg DH, Schwartz H, Hudis CA, Gilewski TA, Norton L. Conditioned emotional distress in women receiving chemotherapy for breast cancer. J Consult Clin Psychol 1995; 63:108–114.
18. Bottomley DM, Hanks GW. Subcutaneous midazolam infusion in palliative care. J Pain Symptom Manage 1990; 5:259–261.

19. Hollister LE. Pharmacotherapeutic considerations in anxiety disorders. J Clin Psychiatry 1986; 47:33–36.

20. McDaniel JS, Musselman DL, Porter MR. Depression in patient with cancer diagnosis, biology and treatment. Arch Gen Psychiatry 1995; 52:89–99.

21. Breitbart W. Cancer pain and suicide. Adv Pain Res Ther 1990; 16:399–412.

22. Bolund C. Suicide and cancer. II. Medical and care factors in suicide by cancer patients in Sweden 1973–1976. J Psychosoc Oncol 1985; 3:17–30.

23. Beck AT, Kovacs M, Weissman A. Hopelessness and suicidal behavior: an overview. JAMA 1975; 234:1146–1149.

24. Stoudemire A. New antidepressant drugs and the treatment of depression in the medically ill patient. Psychiatr Clin North Am 1996; 19:495–514.

25. Nemeroff CB, DeVane CL, Pollock BG. Newer antidepressants and the cytochronic P450 system. Am J Psychiatry 1996; 153:311–320.

26. Fernandez F. Cognitive impairment due to AIDS related complex and its response to psychostimulants. Psychosomatics 1988; 29:38–46.

27. Cannici J, Malcolm R, Peck LA. Treatment of insomnia in cancer patients using muscle relaxant training. J Behav Ther Exp Psychiatry 1983; 14:251–256.

28. Lipowski ZJ. Update on delirium. Psychiatr Clin North Am 1992; 15:335–344.

29. Beresin E. Delirium in the elderly. J Geriatr Psychiatry Neurol 1988; 1:127.

30. Folstein MF, Folstein SE, McHugh PR. Mini-mental state. Psychiatric Res 1975; 12:189–198.

31. Breitbart W, Marotta R, Platt M, et al. A double-blind trial of haloperidol, chlorpromazine and lorazepam in the treatment of delirium in hospitalized AIDS patients. Am J Psychiatry 1996; 153:231–237.

32. Bruera E, Miller L, McCalion S. Cognitive failure in patients with terminal cancer: a prospective longitudinal study. Psychosoc Aspects Cancer 1990; 9:308–310.

33. Adams F, Fernandez F, Andersson BS. Emergency pharmacotherapy of delirium in the critically ill cancer patient. Psychosomatics 1986; 27:33–37.

34. Kash KM, Breitbart. The stress of caring for cancer patients. In: Breitbart W, Holland JC, eds. Psychiatric Aspects of Symptom Management in Cancer Patients. New York: American Psychiatric Press, 1993:243–260.

35. Kobasa CS, Pucceti MD. Personality and social resources in stress-resistance. J Pers Soc Psychol 1983; 45:839–850.

36. Mount BM. Dealing with our losses. J Clin Oncol 1986; 4:1127–1134.

37. Fawzy FI, Greenberg DB. Oncology. In: Rundell JR, Wise MG, eds. Textbook of Consultation-Liaison Psychiatry. Washington, DC: American Psychiatric Press, 1996:672–694.

38. Bolund C. Loss, mourning and growth in the process of dying. Palliative Med 1993; 7(suppl 1):17–25.

39. Weisman AD. Coping with Cancer. New York: McGraw-Hill, 1979.

40. Roth AJ, Breitbart W. Psychiatric emergencies in terminally ill cancer patients. Haematol/Oncol Clin North Am 1996; 10(1):235–259.

41. Posner JB. Neurologic complications of cancer. Disease-a-Month 1978; 25:1–60.

13

Pregnancy and Postpartum

Michael W. O'Hara and Scott Stuart

University of Iowa
Iowa City, Iowa

INTRODUCTION

Pregnancy and the postpartum are sometimes complicated by psychiatric illness. Women with schizophrenia, bipolar illness, recurrent depression, and severe anxiety disorders may represent difficult management problems during pregnancy because of the physician's concern about the possible teratogenicity of the patient's psychotropic medications and because the patient's prenatal care may be compromised by her inability to take proper care of herself and her fetus. Of perhaps greater notoriety are the acute psychoses, known as postpartum psychosis, which may develop within the first few weeks after childbirth. These illnesses, which are often affective in their presentation, usually require immediate hospitalization and are of great concern to the patient's physician and her family. Although severe psychopathology will prove the greatest challenge for the primary care physician, the relatively common occurrence of nonpsychotic depression and anxiety disorders among pregnant and postpartum women makes them an important source of concern as well.

HISTORICAL BACKGROUND

Hippocrates, it is generally acknowledged, was the first physician to describe postpartum mental illness. In the fourth century B.C. in the Third Book of the Epidemics he described the clinical course of a woman who gave birth to twins and experienced severe insomnia and restlessness on the sixth day postpartum (1). Hippocrates attributed these illnesses to lochial discharge carried to the head resulting in agitation, delirium, and attacks of mania (1). Tortula of Salerno, an eleventh-century gynecologist, described the postpartum blues as follows: "if the womb is too moist the brain is filled with water, and the moisture running over to the eyes compels them involuntarily to shed tears" (2). In more recent times, two psychiatrists, Esquirol (3) and Marce (4), described a large series of cases of psychiatric illness arising during pregnancy and in the postpartum period, which they encountered at the same mental hospital at Ivry-sur-Seine in France. They described cases of postpartum mania, melancholia, and other "mixed" disorders. In sum, by the middle of the nineteenth century, severe mental illness associated with childbearing had been well characterized. Very little attention, however, was given to nonpsychotic depressive and anxiety disorders until the 1950s, even though in his 1845 book Esquirol indicated that many cases of mild to moderate psychiatric illness were cared for at home and never recorded (1). It has only been with the clinical work on prevention by the Gordons (5,6) and the epidemiological research by Ryle (7), Tod (8), and Pitt (9) that postpartum depression has come into clear focus as a serious and treatable psychiatric illness.

There are several enduring controversies about the nature of psychiatric disorders observed during pregnancy and the postpartum period. First, there is disagreement about whether postpartum psychoses are distinct illnesses that should have their own place in our diagnostic nomenclature. The current wisdom embodied in the DSM-IV (10) is that the symptomatology of postpartum major depressive, manic, or mixed episodes does not differ from the symptomatology of nonpostpartum mood episodes and may include psychotic features. If these disorders emerge in the first 4 weeks after childbirth, they are given the specifier "with postpartum onset." This view is not universally accepted, and Brockington et al. (11), Hamilton (1), and others have argued that psychoses emerging early in the postpartum period are unique disorders that should be classified and studied as such.

The second enduring controversy is whether the postpartum period is a high-risk time for psychiatric illness. As we will discuss later, there is no question that psychotic illness is much more common in the first 90 days after childbirth than at any other time in a woman's life (12). However, the case for nonpsychotic depression is much more equivocal (13). Although there has been a general presumption that women are at increased risk for depression after childbirth, controlled studies published since 1990 have called that assumption into question. Although rates of depression in the postpartum period range from 10 to 15% when minor depressions are included, nonchildbearing women experience major and minor depressions at similar rates (14). The high rate of depression and anxiety disorders in women of childbearing age (15) should alert the primary care physician to consider these disorders in the routine care of young and middle-aged women.

DESCRIPTION AND PREVALENCE

Traditionally, postpartum psychiatric disorders have been divided into three categories reflecting increasing degrees of severity: postpartum blues, postpartum depression, and

Table 1 Symptoms of the Postpartum Blues

1.	Tearful	15.	Emotionally numb
2.	Mentally tense	16.	Depressed
3.	Able to concentrate	17.	Overemotional
4.	Low spirited	18.	Happy
5.	Elated	19.	Confident
6.	Helpless	20.	Changeable in your spirits
7.	Difficulty showing feelings	21.	Tired
8.	Alert	22.	Irritable
9.	Forgetful, muddled	23.	Crying without being able to stop
10.	Anxious	24.	Lively
11.	Wishing you were alone	25.	Oversensitive
12.	Mentally relaxed	26.	Up and down in your mood
13.	Brooding on things	27.	Restless
14.	Feeling sorry for yourself	28.	Calm, tranquil

For the positive symptoms (e.g., 5, 8, 12, etc.), it is their absence that reflects a symptom of the blues. These symptoms are included in a measure of the postpartum blues.
Source: Adapted from Ref. 16.

postpartum psychosis. Although these are the most frequently encountered problems, any psychiatric disorder may be manifest during the postpartum or during pregnancy.

Postpartum Blues

It is important for the primary care physician to recognize the postpartum blues and distinguish it from depression even though the postpartum blues typically do not require treatment. Within the first week of childbirth many women experience periods of tearfulness and crying, mood lability, anxious or sad mood, sleep and appetite disturbance, and irritability (16,17). One or more of these symptoms occurring together is often called the postpartum blues. Depending upon the criteria used, the prevalence of the blues ranges from 26 to 85% (17). Although these symptoms are usually mild in their intensity and brief in their duration, they are often experienced as unpleasant and may be atypically severe or persistent (17) (Table 1). The symptoms of blues often peak between the fifth and seventh day postpartum (18,19). This pattern distinguishes the blues from the psychological consequences of other stressful medical events such as surgery. Several studies have demonstrated that postsurgical symptoms are high immediately after surgery and diminish over time (20). Finally, there is little evidence that there are significant negative sequelae of the blues. However, there is evidence that the blues may serve as a risk factor for later depression (19).

Depression and Anxiety

Mood and anxiety disorders may emerge at any time during pregnancy or the postpartum, or they may they represent preexisting conditions. Depression, particularly depression that emerges in the postpartum period (postpartum depression), has received the bulk of the attention in the research literature. Figure 1 illustrates the varieties of onset and duration of depression that may afflict women during pregnancy and the postpartum. It should be clear that there is no particular time when these depressive episodes are most likely to occur. Moreover, these depressive episodes can be quite persistent and should not be regarded as transitory phenomena.

In the research literature postpartum depression has been defined in various ways; however, in recent years most studies have used diagnostic criteria such as the RDC (21) and the DSM-III-R (22). If minor depressions are included, the prevalence of

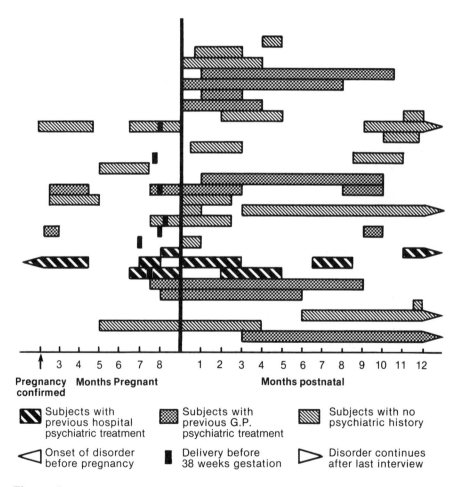

Figure 1 Varieties of onset and duration of depression that may afflict women during pregnancy and the postpartum.

postpartum depression is in the range of 10–15% (23). Including only depressions that meet criteria for major depressive disorder results in a prevalence rate of 5–8%. Although there has been a great deal of debate on this issue, the presentation of postpartum depression does not seem to differ significantly from depressions that occur at other times for women (24).

Although there have been numerous studies of the prevalence of depression in the postpartum and the factors that put women at increased risk for depression after delivery, there has been very little similar work with anxiety disorders. Much of the work that has been done has concerned the course of panic and obsessive-compulsive disorders during pregnancy and the postpartum (25,26). These conditions will be discussed in more detail in the section on treatment.

Risk Factors

Many hormonal theories have been offered as explanations for postpartum mood disturbance (27). Because levels of the estrogens and progesterone increase greatly during pregnancy (> 100-fold change) and drop rapidly after delivery, it has been suggested that the blues and depression may result from the abrupt withdrawal of these hormones. Only modest evidence, at best, supports this hypothesis (19,27). Thyroid dysfunction during pregnancy or after delivery has also been related to postpartum depression (27). Here the case is somewhat stronger, and it has been estimated that there may be a prevalence rate of postpartum depression of 4% due specifically to thyroid dysfunction (27). Although replacement estradiol and progesterone have been prescribed as treatments for postpartum depression (27), norms for thyroid levels are much better established and indications for treatment are much clearer.

A recent meta-analysis identified a number of social risk factors for postpartum depression (23). Women who experience postpartum depression are more likely to have lower incomes and come from lower social classes. These women will also be more likely to have experienced significant life-stressors during pregnancy and will have had a more difficult than normal pregnancy and delivery. With respect to social support, women at risk for postpartum depression are more likely to have a poor marital relationship and perceive others in their social networks as not particularly supportive. Finally, these women will often have a history of depression or dysthymia and show evidence of being at least mildly depressed or anxious during pregnancy.

Mood and anxiety disorders may develop during pregnancy or, in fact, predate pregnancy. Prevalence studies of depression during pregnancy have found that levels of depressive symptomatology are often higher than during the postpartum period; rates of syndromal depression tend to be lower, but not significantly so (13,28). Figure 1 nicely illustrates this phenomenon. Risk factors for depression during pregnancy are similar to those for postpartum depression and include past history of psychopathology (both syndromal and symptomatic), lack of support from partner, social disadvantage, and the occurrence of stressful life events (13,29).

Psychosis/Severe Psychopathology

Although pregnancy is a relatively low-risk time for the emergence of severe psychopathology, the early postpartum period is the time in a woman's life when she is at greatest risk for being hospitalized for a psychotic disorder (12). Figure 2 illustrates this phenomenon graphically. Kendell et al. (12) linked obstetric and psychiatric records for more than 50,000 women over a 20-year period in Edinburgh, Scotland. They plotted the number of psychiatric admissions for psychosis for a period spanning 2 years prior to delivery to 2 years subsequent to delivery (a total span of 4 years) for every subject and found that the vast majority of psychiatric admissions for psychosis occurred in the first 90 days after delivery. For example, they determined that the risk of hospitalization for psychosis within 30 days of delivery was 22 times greater than the risk of being hospitalized for psychosis during a 30-day nonchildbearing period. These findings make clear that the postpartum period is a high-risk time for psychosis in childbearing women. However, the actual prevalence of postpartum psychosis is approximately 0.1–0.4%, suggesting that the risk of a postpartum psychosis for the average woman is not high.

Postpartum psychosis usually develops early in the postpartum period, often within the first 2 weeks of childbirth (30). Although some episodes resemble schizophrenia, postpartum psychosis is usually considered to be an affective disorder or a variant of an affective disorder (11,12). As a consequence, symptoms of depression and mania are most common in postpartum psychosis. Also, these women often display symptoms related to cognitive impairment and bizarre behavior compared to nonchildbearing women experiencing an affective psychosis (31). Unusual psychotic symptoms such as

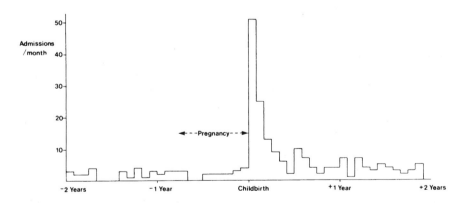

Figure 2 Number of psychiatric admissions for psychosis over a 4-year period (from 2 years before to 2 years after delivery) in a study of more than 50,000 women over 20 years in Edinburgh, Scotland. The vast majority of psychiatric admissions for psychosis occurred in the first 90 days after delivery. (From Ref. 12.)

tactile, olfactory, and visual hallucinations are also frequently observed in postpartum psychosis (31). It has been hypothesized that factors such as sleep deprivation during labor and the care demands of the newborn may lead to the development of disorganized mood states in vulnerable women (31).

Risk Factors

Several psychosocial and clinical risk factors for postpartum psychosis have been identified in the research literature. Primiparous women have a risk level twice that of multiparous women (12,32). Unmarried women and women who have had a cesarean section also are at increased risk for postpartum psychosis (33). However, none of these features elevates the risk of postpartum psychosis to a level that would require special clinical surveillance. Women who have previously experienced a postpartum or nonpostpartum psychosis have rates of recurrent psychotic episodes following delivery as high as 50%. The risk of postpartum psychosis associated with having a first-degree relative with a history of psychosis is on the order of 3%, well above the base rate of 0.1–0.2% (32). In sum, women who have a history of postpartum or nonpostpartum psychosis should be carefully followed throughout pregnancy and the postpartum period. Women with a family history of psychosis should be alerted to their risk of postpartum illness and should be counseled to contact their physician at the first sign of problems.

As illustrated in Figure 2, the risk of being hospitalized for a psychotic disorder during pregnancy is low, less than the risk before pregnancy and about 1/25 the risk during the first 30 days after delivery (12). Although new onset psychotic episodes are rare during pregnancy, women with severe mental illness do become pregnant and there is little question that prenatal care may be compromised by their mental illness (34). Problems include the following: refusal of prenatal care, poor nutrition, attempts at premature self-delivery, fetal abuse or neonaticide, and precipitous delivery (34). These risks to the mother and fetus suggest that prenatal care must be closely coordinated between the obstetrician and the woman's psychiatrist.

MANAGEMENT ISSUES

Screening for current or past mental illness should occur during the first prenatal visit (35). This recommendation may seem obvious, but it rarely appeared in basic textbooks of obstetrics before *Williams Obstetrics* (20th edition) (35). In fact, careful screening of psychiatric illness does not routinely occur during prenatal visits despite the commonness of psychiatric illness in childbearing-aged women and the potential serious consequences of psychiatric illness during pregnancy or the postpartum period for the mother, fetus, and child. A three-stage process that includes screening, monitoring, and treatment or referral will suffice in the prenatal care of most women (17).

Screening involves a brief assessment of past and current psychopathology, particularly mood and anxiety disorders. Women who are currently ill can be referred for treatment if they are not already receiving it. Women with a past history of depression, anxiety, or serious psychopathology (e.g., schizophrenia or bipolar disorder) can be followed more or less intensively by obstetrical staff or by mental health professionals.

Monitoring can be accomplished in several ways. For example, the Edinburgh Postnatal Depression Scale (36) (EPDS) (see Appendix) was designed to identify women with postpartum depression. It is also useful for identifying depression during pregnancy. It is easy and quick to administer and score. The EPDS can be completed by women while they wait for a prenatal visit, and for women determined to be at risk, it can be completed at home and returned by mail to the woman's physician.

TREATMENT OF PSYCHIATRIC DISORDERS DURING PREGNANCY

Despite concerns about the effects of the use of psychoactive drugs during pregnancy, approximately 35% of expectant women are given prescriptions for at least one psychotropic medication during their pregnancy (37). The FDA assigns medications used during pregnancy to one of four categories: category A (no evidence of teratogenicity or embryogenicity in controlled human studies); category B (no evidence of fetal risk based on animal studies, but for which there are no human studies available); category C (evidence exists for fetal risk based on animal studies, or there are no studies of either humans or animals regarding risks); or category D (positive evidence of human fetal risk). In general, the use of psychotropic medication during pregnancy should involve cautious clinical judgment, and a careful assessment of the benefits of the medication and the risks to the developing child should be undertaken. Risk assessment must include not only evaluation of teratogenic effects, but perinatal effects and postnatal neurodevelopmental effects as well. In addition to the risks to the newborn, there are substantial risks associated with the avoidance or discontinuation of psychotropic medication during pregnancy. Relapse or exacerbation of the patient's psychiatric illness may occur, with a concomitant increase in the risk of suicidal behavior or inability of the woman to care for herself and her unborn child.

Depression

The tricyclic antidepressants (TCAs), because of their long history of use, are the medications for which there is the most evidence of safety. Several prospective studies evaluating the use of these medications during the first trimester have shown no association between the use of TCAs and increased rates of congenital malformations (38,39). Altshuler et al. (40) analyzed the findings of 14 studies examining the teratogenic effects of TCAs and concluded that they do not pose an increased risk for major malformations.

There are reports, however, that newborns exposed to TCAs late in pregnancy may develop perinatal withdrawal syndromes. Newborns so exposed typically exhibit symptoms such as irritability and jitteriness; convulsions, bowel obstruction, and urinary retention have also been reported. The long-term effects on development following fetal exposure to TCAs appear to be minimal. Misri (41) followed children up to age 3 and noted no abnormalities in behavior or motor skills, and a study by Nulman et al. (38) did not find developmental differences when children exposed to TCAs in utero were compared to controls at age 18–68 months.

The selective serotonin-reuptake inhibitors (SSRIs) have not been as extensively studied as the TCAs. Data collected to date indicate that fluoxetine is relatively safe, while published data regarding the use of other SSRIs are limited. Pastuszak et al. (39) found no increases in the rates of major malformations when children exposed in utero to fluoxetine, tricyclic antidepressants, and nonexposed controls were compared. A prospective study by Chambers et al. (42) demonstrated that there were no significant increase in the rates of major malformations in children exposed in utero to fluoxetine compared to nonexposed controls, a finding replicated by Nulman et al. (38), who prospectively compared infants exposed to TCAs or fluoxetine to nonexposed infants. A single study examining 63 infants with first-trimester exposure to paroxetine did not show an increased incidence of malformations (43). There have been no controlled studies regarding the use of any of the other SSRIs during pregnancy.

The incidence of SSRI withdrawal syndromes are unknown. Chambers et al. (42) did find an increased rate of perinatal complications in women treated with fluoxetine during the third trimester of pregnancy compared to nonexposed controls and women who had taken fluoxetine only during the first two trimesters. These complications included higher rates of premature delivery, lower birth weight, and higher risk for perinatal admission to special care nurseries, as well as respiratory difficulty, cyanosis on feeding, and jitteriness.

The long-term effects of the SSRIs on child development have been examined only for fluoxetine. Nulman et al. (38) reported no differences in cognitive, language, and behavioral development in children assessed between 16 and 86 months when children exposed in utero to TCAs, those exposed to fluoxetine, and unexposed controls were compared. This finding held whether children were exposed only in the first trimester of pregnancy or throughout the entire pregnancy.

In contrast to the TCAs and SSRIs, the use of monamine oxidase inhibitors (MAOIs) has been associated with a higher-than-normal rate of congenital malformations, and the use of MAOIs is contraindicated during pregnancy. The safety of amphetamines during pregnancy is unclear; while there have been numerous studies demonstrating deleterious effects on newborns of mothers who abused amphetamines, none has examined the effects of children whose mothers were using antidepressant dosages. Reported effects of amphetamine abuse include fetal growth retardation and premature delivery.

Little information is available regarding the use of the atypical antidepressants. Two case reports regarding the use of buproprion reported no teratogenicity; however, one of the exposed infants (whose mother was also taking lithium) experienced some increased irritability and tremors following delivery (45). Trazodone, venlafaxine, nefazodone, and mirtazapine are all categorized as class C drugs for use during pregnancy, and there are no reports available regarding their effects in utero, perinatally, or on infant development.

In cases of severe depression, the use of electroconvulsive therapy (ECT) in the treatment of depression may be warranted. ECT appears to be safe during pregnancy (46), and reports of long-term follow-up have failed to show any developmental abnormalities in children exposed to ECT in utero.

Rational clinical management of antenatal depression suggests that antidepressant medication be avoided unless the benefits of its use clearly outweigh the potential risks. Thus usage of medication during the first trimester should be avoided if at all possible, and use during the second and third trimester should be reserved for patients with moderate to severe depression. Patients with mild to moderate antenatal depression may benefit from psychotherapeutic treatment including interpersonal psychotherapy (47) and cognitive behavior therapy (48).

For women with moderate to severe depression, or for those who do not respond to psychotherapy, the use of TCAs or fluoxetine is reasonable. In order to minimize side effects and potential withdrawal syndromes, TCAs with lower anticholinergic activity, such as nortriptyline or desipramine, should be used. For those women with recurrent depression, or those who are being treated pharmacologically for depression at the time of pregnancy, attempts should be made to wean the patient off the medication if possible during the first trimester. Treatment should be resumed if symptoms recur or if suicidal ideation develops during the first trimester, and can be restarted with a relative degree of safety during the second trimester if needed.

Bipolar Disorder

The treatment of bipolar disorder during pregnancy has been much more controversial than the treatment of depression primarily because of concerns regarding the use of lithium, one of the first-line treatments for the disorder. Early studies demonstrated an increased risk of congenital malformations, particularly of the cardiovascular system, for newborns exposed to lithium during the first trimester. More recent reports, however, have revised the risk of exposure. These reports indicate a relative risk of 10–20 for the development of Ebstein's anomaly in children exposed to lithium during the first trimester, but go on to note that the disorder occurs at a baseline rate of about 1:20,000 births (49). Thus, the clinical significance of the risk (about 1:1000) of developing the anomaly must be considered when the risks and benefits of using the medication are considered. Moreover, the only prospective study examining the use of lithium during the first trimester did not show any difference in the rates of malformations, spontaneous abortions, prematurity, or stillbirth when exposed children were compared to controls (50). The small sample size (148 women) precludes any firm conclusions but does suggest that the risk may less than that reported in earlier retrospective studies.

With respect to perinatal effects, there have been reports of neurotoxicity associated with late exposure to lithium: the so-called floppy baby syndrome of hypotonicity and cyanosis (51). Only one report has been published regarding the long-term effects of in utero exposure to lithium. Parents of children exposed during the second and third trimester of pregnancy did not report any behavioral differences in their exposed children as compared to their nonexposed siblings (62).

The use of anticonvulsants for treatment of bipolar affective disorder during pregnancy is also associated with an elevated risk of congenital malformation. Though no studies have been conducted specifically assessing the use of these medications in the treatment of antenatal mania, there are data regarding the use of anticonvulsants for seizure disorders during pregnancy. Both carbamazepine and valproic acid have been associated with an increased risk of spina bifida. Both have also been associated with an increased risk of minor malformations, particularly craniofacial abnormalities (53,54). There have been no published reports regarding the perinatal effects of the medications. The research regarding long-term developmental effects is sketchy, but seems to suggest that there are no adverse neurobehavioral outcomes associated with in utero exposure to carbamazepine (55). Tegretol is categorized as a class C medication during pregnancy, whereas valproic acid is categorized as class D and is not recommended for use during pregnancy.

Given the risks associated with the use of antimanic agents during the first trimester, prudent clinical management dictates that neither anticonvulsants nor lithium be used during the first trimester unless the risks of the untreated illness clearly outweigh the known increased risk of teratogenicity. If possible, these medications should be avoided during the entire pregnancy. Ideally, patients with bipolar illness should plan their pregnancy, with attempts at conception preceded by a slow taper of the antimanic medication.

If relapse occurs, however, the risk of untreated mania should be weighed carefully against the risks of teratogenicity. In general, clinical wisdom is that the mania should be treated, as the illness and its associated impulsive behavior are far greater risks to the woman and her child than is the medication. This is certainly true during the second and third trimester, as there is less compelling evidence that the medications cause malformations when used later in pregnancy. Alternatively, other treatments such as ECT or high potency neuroleptics could be utilized rather than the antimanic agents.

Anxiety Disorders

The most frequently used medications for the treatment of anxiety disorders are the benzodiazepines. The effects of benzodiazepines on fetal development are controversial and not well studied. Adding to the confusion is the fact that the use of benzodiazepines is often associated with abuse of alcohol and other illicit or prescription drugs. The current majority opinion is that use of benzodiazepines during the first trimester is associated with a two- to threefold increase in the risk of development of cleft lip and cleft palate. However, given the low base rate of the malformation (approximately 0.06%), it is unclear whether this represents a significant clinical risk. Several studies examining first trimester exposure to alprazolam have not revealed any increase in malformations or spontaneous abortions (56,57).

There are several case reports regarding perinatal syndromes in children who were exposed to benzodiazepines late in pregnancy, with symptoms including muscular hypotonicity and apnea. There are no controlled studies examining the perinatal effects of the use benzodiazepines, however. Animal studies have demonstrated that long-term behavioral effects result from the use of benzodiazepines, and there is some evidence that supports an association with developmental delays in humans exposed in utero to these medications (58,59), although no definitive conclusions can be drawn from the data that do exist.

Given the possible association between benzodiazepine use and increased risk for cleft lip and palate, a reasonable strategy for the management of prenatal anxiety disorders is to advise women to taper all benzodiazepines prior to attempting conception. The patient should be maintained off medication through the first trimester if possible. Cognitive-behavioral therapy, particularly for panic disorder, can be considered as an alternative treatment during this time and throughout the pregnancy (60). After the first trimester, once the highest period of risk for malformations has passed, benzodiazepines can be used if needed, but should be tapered if possible prior to delivery. An alternative strategy is to use TCAs which have also been shown to be efficacious in the treatment of anxiety disorders. Fluoxetine is a reasonable second-line treatment for patients who require antianxiety medication during the first trimester.

Psychotic Disorders

Psychotic disorders during pregnancy are medical emergencies that require immediate treatment. Pregnant schizophrenic women have been found to attend fewer prenatal medical appointments than normal controls despite having a higher frequency of physical problems, and they have a higher risk for delivery complications, shorter gestation periods, and lower birth weight babies (61). Schizophrenic women have also been shown to be less likely than controls to detect labor, and their infants are at higher risk for perinatal death (62). Although there is some controversy about the teratogenicity of the antipsychotic medications, it appears that the presence of a psychotic illness and the factors associated with it (such as substance abuse and lack of adequate prenatal medical care) are much more significant risk factors for adverse pregnancy outcome than is use of antipsychotic medication.

The data regarding the use of low-potency neuroleptics during pregnancy come primarily from studies examining women who were treated with these medications for hyperemesis gravidarum. Phenothiazines in particular appear to be problematic and are associated with a nonspecific increase in congenital malformations in comparison to the nonphenothiazine antipsychotics (63). The risk appears to be highest at approximately weeks 10–16.

Less is known about the effects of exposure to high-potency neuroleptics, and less still regarding exposure to the newer antipsychotic agents such as clozapine and risperidone. Two small retrospective studies investigating the teratogenic effects of haloperidol (used to treat hyperemeses gravidarum) found no associations between the use of the medication and congenital abnormalities (64,65). Information regarding clozapine consists of a single case report describing an uncomplicated pregnancy (66). Clozapine is a category B medication for use during pregnancy, while olanzepine is category C. There is no category rating for risperidone, but prescribing information states that risperidone should not be used during pregnancy.

One case series regarding perinatal syndromes in children whose mothers were using neuroleptics has been reported (67). The symptoms noted, particularly with the phenothiazines, include motor restlessness, tremor, and hypertonicity and are essentially analogous to the extrapyramidal symptoms observed in adults treated with the medications. Children exposed to neuroleptics in utero have not been shown to have neurobehavioral development problems when compared to nonexposed children, but there is some evidence from animal studies suggesting that long-term developmental effects may occur (68).

There are also risks attendant with the use of medications used to treat the side effects of the antipsychotics. The use of anticholinergic agents (benztropine, trihexyphenidyl) during pregnancy has been associated with increased rates of minor congenital malformations (69). An anticholinergic withdrawal effect has also been reported in newborns whose mothers were taking these agents. There have been reported associations between the use of diphenhydramine and congenital anomalies, and withdrawal symptoms have also been reported with this medication (69). Amantidine has been associated with a high risk for organ dysgenesis in animals, and a case describing cardiovascular malformations in a human infant exposed to amantidine in utero has been reported (70).

Given the high risks associated with untreated psychotic illness, women with chronic psychotic disorders should be maintained on doses of neuroleptic medication that are adequate to control their psychoses. Women with acute onset disorders should also be treated immediately with therapeutic doses, though the medication can be tapered over time as clinically indicated. In addition, though there is some evidence that neonatal withdrawal syndromes can occur, the risk of decompensation if medication were to be withdrawn and the risk for postpartum psychosis dictates that the medication be continued through the last stages of pregnancy and delivery, as well as in the postpartum period. Antiparkinsonian medications to counter the side effects of neuroleptics should be avoided during the first trimester as well as for the remainder of the pregnancy if possible.

TREATMENT OF PSYCHIATRIC DISORDERS DURING THE POSTPARTUM PERIOD

Psychotropic medications that may be used during the postpartum are, like those used during pregnancy, classified into four categories according to their potential for adverse affects on the newborn. Potential concerns during breastfeeding include both short-term neurologic and physiologic effects on infants, as well as long-term neurobehavioral effects. As is the case with use of psychotropic medication during pregnancy, a careful risk-benefit analysis must be conducted before initiating treatment. Particularly important to consider are the serious adverse effects of untreated maternal psychopathology on the development of the child. Additionally, though many women strongly desire to breastfeed and there appear to be benefits to infants who are breastfed, bottle-feeding or supplementing breastfeeding with bottle-feedings are obvious alternatives to exposing newborns to potential harm from medication. In many cases, drug levels in both breast-milk and in the neonate can be measured to aid in decision making about the use of medication.

Postpartum Depression

There are several antidepressant medications that are not associated with adverse effects in the breastfed newborn. None of the tricyclics has been associated with an increase in adverse effects on the newborn. Further, there was no evidence of accumulation of TCAs in breastfed newborns. A study evaluating the neurobehavioral development of breastfed children whose mothers were receiving TCAs did not note any abnormalities at follow-up at 9–36 months of age (41).

Information regarding the effects of SSRIs on breastfed newborns is limited. Case reports suggest that fluoxetine may accumulate at significant levels in breastfed newborns, though the effects of this accumulation are not clear. Sertraline, because of its shorter half-life, appears less likely to accumulate in newborn sera than fluoxetine (71). Current product labeling for fluoxetine recommends that it not be used for women who are breastfeeding.

The newer antidepressant medications have not been adequately studied. Prescribing information for trazodone, venlafaxine, nefazodone, and mirtazapine advise caution in use when treated women are breastfeeding. There are no studies regarding the use of MAOI antidepressants during breastfeeding, and their use is not recommended.

In general, the data suggest that use of tricyclics is not associated with high serum levels in newborns and is relatively safe. Further, Wisner et al. (72) suggest that the use of TCAs in infants more than 10 weeks of age is relatively safe due to the increased metabolic activity of newborns beyond this age. Because of the extensive data documenting the adverse effects that maternal depression has on children, the clinician should be sensitive to the risks posed by untreated depression. Fluoxetine should be avoided if possible when breastfeeding. It is possible that the SSRIs with shorter half-lives, such as fluvoxamine and sertraline, are safer than fluoxetine and should be used with women requiring this type of medication.

Psychotherapy may be an appropriate treatment for postpartum depression instead of pharmacotherapy. There is good evidence that interpersonal psychotherapy (47) is an effective short-term treatment for depression (73) and an effective treatment for postpartum depression in particular (74). Health care professionals who work with pregnant and postpartum women are well advised to develop relationships with mental health professionals who are experienced in working with this population.

Postpartum Bipolar Disorder

As is the case with the use of lithium during pregnancy, the significance of the effects of maternal usage of lithium on breastfeeding newborns is controversial. There is a developing consensus that women with bipolar disorder are at very high risk for postpartum relapse and that they should be treated prophylactically with lithium or another mood stabilizer (75). However, the adverse effects of these medications on newborns exposed to them during breastfeeding have not been well studied.

It is known that lithium does pass to the infant in breastmilk, usually resulting in infant serum concentrations of one-tenth to one-half those in the mother's serum. The product information for lithium strongly suggests avoidance of the medication in breastfeeding women, and the American Academy of Pediatrics recommends that lithium be considered contraindicated during breastfeeding (76).

It has been suggested that because of its rapid metabolism, carbamazepine may be a safer medication than lithium to use during breastfeeding; this conclusion, however, is not based on any prospective data. Both carbamazepine and valproic acid are considered by the American Academy of Pediatrics to be compatible with breastfeeding (76), although prescribing information for carbamazepine advises against its use during breastfeeding. It has been recommended by some authors that because of the risk of hepatotoxicity, valproic acid should not be used when nursing, though this conclusion is not supported by data. The long-term effects of exposure to the mood-stabilizing medications are not known.

Postpartum Anxiety Disorders

Benzodiazepines are secreted in breastmilk and appear to have some adverse effects in newborns. Diazepam, for example, has been reported to cause EEG changes, lethargy, and loss of weight in neonates (77), and it has been recommended that diazepam not be used when breastfeeding, particularly because it may accumulate in breastfed infants. Zolpidem has been studied in five lactating women and was measured in excreted milk at 0.004–0.019% of the administered dose 3 hours after ingestion (78). No detectable levels were found after this time, implying that zolpidem may be safe to use during breastfeeding. Other benzodiazepines have not been studied in detail.

Reasonable clinical practice suggests the use of short-acting benzodiazepines such as lorazepam and oxazepam when benzodiazepines are required during breastfeeding. Additionally, because of the immature excretory mechanisms in newborns, benzodiazepines should be used with particular caution perinatally. Alternate treatments for panic disorder include the TCAs, which are associated with less risk to the breastfeeding infant.

Postpartum Psychotic Disorders

The effects of nursing while using neuroleptics has not been well studied. Haloperidol was found in breastfed infants at very low levels, and no adverse effects in exposed children have been noted (79). The American Academy of Pediatrics recommends caution when using low-potency neuroleptics such as chlorpromazine and notes that drowsiness and lethargy have been observed in breastfed infants exposed to these medications (76). Pons et al. (78) have shown that chlorpromazine concentrations can actually be higher in milk than in maternal serum and recommend that chlorpromazine not be used because it can cause drowsiness in infants exposed to the doses found in breastmilk. Though no studies have been conducted with humans examining the neurobehavioral effects of newborns exposed to neuroleptics, animal studies have demonstrated adverse behavioral effects even at doses within the therapeutic range.

Prescribing information regarding clozapine strongly recommends that it not be used when breastfeeding, as does information regarding risperidone and olanzepine. No information is available regarding the anticholinergic medications used to treat the side effects of the neuroleptics.

Given the potential risks associated with the use of low-potency neuroleptics, reasonable clinical practice is to treat women requiring medication with haloperidol or other high-dose neuroleptics. Risperidone and olanzepine should be avoided; clozapine should likewise be avoided unless it is required to adequately treat the psychotic disorder.

CASE HISTORY

A 26-year-old woman was seen for initial obstetrical evaluation at 6 weeks gestation. During the evaluation, she revealed that she had experienced two previous episodes of depression, both of which were successfully treated with the SSRI antidepressant medication sertraline. She had been off the medication for about a year, following resolution of her most recent episode of depression. Her history was otherwise unremarkable, and no prenatal problems were noted. Her score on the Beck Depression Inventory (BDI) (80) used to screen for depression was 3.

She contacted her obstetrician 2 weeks later complaining of frequent unexplained crying spells, poor sleep, lack of energy, and lack of motivation. On exam, her obstetrician noted that she had continued to gain weight normally and also noted that she did not have any suicidal ideation. Her BDI score was 13. The patient expressed concern about using medication while pregnant. Both the patient and her obstetrician agreed on a diagnosis of mild depression and agreed to an immediate referral for cognitive-behavioral therapy (48).

The patient did fairly well for several weeks, but by week 12, her BDI score had increased to 25, and she had failed to gain weight since her last appointment. The patient and her obstetrician agreed to treat this more severe depression with medication. Rather than use sertraline, they opted for treatment with fluoxetine, which has much more evidence supporting safe use during pregnancy. The patient voiced less concern about medication use as she was near the end of her first trimester.

Her depression resolved after several weeks, and she continued to be symptom-free on fluoxetine until the delivery of a healthy infant at term. As the patient desired to breastfeed, she consulted with her obstetrician about continuing medication usage. Both agreed that given the high risk for relapse during the postpartum period, she should continue on antidepressant medication while nursing. Her obstetrician recommended a switch back to sertraline because of data suggesting that the shorter half-life of sertraline made it less likely to accumulate in her newborn. The patient stopped fluoxetine and resumed sertraline, which she continued to use for the next year.

CONCLUSION

Psychiatric disorders during pregnancy and the postpartum are common and are associated with a great degree of morbidity and dysfunction. Not only is the patient affected by psychiatric illness, but her child may be affected as well. Lack of psychiatric treatment during pregnancy can affect the woman's ability to obtain appropriate prenatal care, and disorders during the puerperium can dramatically affect the newborn's ability to regulate itself emotionally and to form stable attachments.

Clinicians must be sensitive to these problems, and we recommend that systematic screening of women during both prenatal visits and postpartum visits be conducted. Perinatologists should also be aware of postpartum psychiatric disorders, as it is not unusual that pediatricians identify maternal psychopathology at well-baby visits. Close monitoring of patients with identified disorders should also be part of a comprehensive treatment plan and should include routine assessment of depressive symptoms as well as suicidal ideation.

The decision to use (or to refrain from using) psychotropic medications should be carefully considered. The apparent risks of medication usage during pregnancy and the postpartum should be weighed against the less obvious but very significant risks of nontreatment, particularly with the more severe psychotic illnesses. Guidelines to medication usage and relative safety can be found in Tables 2 and 3. It is essential that physicians discuss treatment options fully with the patient and the patient's family and explicitly document the basis for their treatment decisions. Optimal outcomes can be

Table 2 Recommendations for Treatment of Antenatal Psychiatric Disorders

I. Depression	
Mild-moderate	Interpersonal psychotherapy, cognitive behavioral therapy (A)
Moderate-severe	Nortriptyline, desipramine (B)
	Fluoxetine (B)
	ECT (B)
II. Bipolar disorder	Lithium (C)
	Haloperidol (C)
III. Anxiety disorders	Cognitive-behavioral therapy (A)
	Nortriptyline, desipramine (B)
	Fluoxetine (B)
	Benzodiazepines (C)
IV. Psychotic disorders	Haloperidol (C)
	ECT (B)

The risks of medication usage are reduced after the first trimester. In each case, the risk of not treating the illness must be weighed against the risks of medication usage.
Estimated risk: A = none; B = minimal; C = moderate; D = high.

Table 3 Recommendations for Treatment of Postpartum Psychiatric Disorders

I. Depression	
Mild-moderate	Interpersonal psychotherapy (A)
Moderate-severe	Nortriptyline, desipramine (B)
	Sertraline (B)
	ECT (B)
II. Bipolar disorder	Valproic acid (C)
	Carbamazepine (C)
	Haloperidol (C)
III. Anxiety disorders	Cognitive-behavioral therapy (A)
	Nortriptyline, desipramine (B)
	Sertraline (B)
	Zolpidem (B)
IV. Psychotic disorders	Haloperidol (B)
	ECT (B)

The risks of medication usage are reduced as infant age increases. In each case, the risk of not treating the illness must be weighed against the risks of medication usage.
Estimated risk: A = none; B = minimal; C = moderate; D = high.

achieved as physicians work flexibly and collaboratively with their patients during these important phases of life.

APPENDIX: THE EDINBURGH POSTNATAL DEPRESSION SCALE (EPDS)

As you have recently had a baby, we would like to know how you are feeling. Please *circle* the number next to the answer which comes closest to how you have felt *in the past 7 days*, not just how you feel today.

Here is an example, already completed.

I have felt happy:

0 Yes, all the time.
1 Yes, most of the time.
2 No, not very often.
3 No, not at all.

In the past 7 days:

1. I have been able to laugh and see the funny side of things.

    0 As much as I always could.
    1 Not quite so much now.
    2 Definitely not so much now.
    3 Not at all.

2. I have looked forward with enjoyment to things.

    0 As much as I ever did.
    1 Rather less than I used to.
    2 Definitely less than I used to.
    3 Hardly at all.

3. I have blamed myself unnecessarily when things went wrong.

    0 Yes, most of the time.
    1 Yes, some of the time.
    2 Not very often.
    3 No, never.

4. I have been anxious or worried for no good reason.

    0 No, not at all.
    1 Hardly ever.

2   Yes, sometimes.
3   Yes, very often.

5. I have felt scared or panicky for no very good reason.

    0   Yes, quite a lot.
    1   Yes, sometimes.
    2   No, not much.
    3   No, not at all.

6. Things have been getting on top of me.

    0   Yes, most of the time I haven't been able to cope at all.
    1   Yes, sometimes I haven't been coping as well as usual.
    2   No, most of the time I have coped quite well.
    3   No, I have been coping as well as ever.

7. I have been so unhappy that I have had difficulty sleeping.

    0   Yes, most of the time.
    1   Yes, sometimes.
    2   Not very often.
    3   No, not at all.

8. I have felt sad or miserable.

    0   Yes, most of the time.
    1   Yes, quite often.
    2   Not very often.
    3   No, not at all.

9. I have been so unhappy that I have been crying.

    0   Yes, most of the time.
    1   Yes, quite often.
    2   Only occasionally.
    3   No, never.

10. The thought of harming myself has occurred to me.

    0   Yes, quite often.
    1   Sometimes.
    2   Hardly ever.
    3   Never.

Scoring and Other Information

Response categories are scored 0, 1, 2, and 3 according to increased severity of the symptom. Items 3 and 5–10 are reverse-scored (i.e., 3, 2, 1, and 0). The total score is calculated by adding together the scores for each of the ten items. Users may reproduce the scale without further permission providing they respect copyright (which remains with the *British Journal of Psychiatry*), quoting the names of the authors, the title, and the source of the paper in all reproduced copies.

The Edinburgh Postnatal Depression Scale (EPDS) has been developed to assist primary care health professionals to detect mothers suffering from postnatal depression, a distressing disorder more prolonged than the "blues" (which occur in the first week after delivery) but less severe than puerperal psychosis.

Previous studies have shown that postnatal depression affects at least 10% of women and that many depressed mothers remain untreated. These mothers may cope with their baby and with household tasks, but their enjoyment of life is seriously affected and it is possible that there are long-term effects on the family.

The EPDS was developed at health centres in Livingston and Edinburgh. It consists of ten short statements. The mother underlines which of the four possible responses is closest to how she has been feeling during the past week. Most mothers complete the scale without difficulty in less than 5 minutes.

The validation study showed that mothers who scored above a threshold 12/13 were likely to be suffering from a depressive illness of varying severity. Nevertheless, the EPDS score should *not* override clinical judgement. A careful clinical assessment should be carried out to confirm the diagnosis. The scale indicates how the mother has felt *during the previous week*, and in doubtful cases it may be usefully repeated after 2 weeks. The scale will not detect mothers with anxiety neuroses, phobias, or personality disorders.

Instructions for Users

1. The mother is asked to underline the response which comes closest to how she has been feeling in the previous 7 days.
2. All ten items must be completed.
3. Care should be taken to avoid the possibility of the mother's discussing her answers with others.
4. The mother should complete the scale herself, unless she has limited English or has difficulty with reading.
5. The EPDS may be used at 6–8 weeks to screen postnatal women. The child health clinic, postnatal check-up, or a home visit may provide suitable opportunities for its completion.

Source: Ref. 36. Cox JL, Holden JM, Sagovsky R. Detection of postnatal depression: development of the 10-item Edinburgh Postnatal Depression Scale. Br J Psychiatry 1987; 150:782–786.

REFERENCES

1. Hamilton JA. Postpartum Psychiatric Disorders. St. Louis: CV Mosby, 1962.
2. Steiner M. Postpartum psychiatric disorders. Can J Psychiatry 1990; 35:89–95.
3. Esquirol E. Mental maladies: a treatise on insanity. Philadelphia: Lea and Blanchard, 1845.
4. Marcé LV. Traitee de la Folie des Femmes Enceintes, des Nouvelles Accouchees et des Nourrices. Paris: Bailliere, 1858.

5. Gordon RE, Gordon KK. Social factors in the prediction and treatment of emotional disorders of pregnancy. Am J Obstet Gynecol 1959; 77:1074–1083.
6. Gordon RE, Gordon KK. Social factors in the prevention of postpartum emotional problems. Obstet Gynecol 1960; 15:433–438.
7. Ryle A. The psychological disturbances associated with 345 pregnancies in 137 women. J Mental Sci 1961; 107:279–286.
8. Tod EDM. Puerperal depression: a prospective epidemiological study. Lancet 1964; 2:1264–1266.
9. Pitt B. "Atypical" depression following childbirth. Br J Psychiatry 1968; 114:1325–1335.
10. American Psychiatric Association. Diagnostic and Statistical Manual of Mental Disorders. 4th ed. Washington, DC: American Psychiatric Press, 1994.
11. Brockington IF, Cernik KF, Schofield EM, Downing AR, Francis AF, Keelan C. Puerperal psychosis: phenomena and diagnosis. Arch Gen Psychiatry 1981; 38:929–933.
12. Kendell RE, Chalmers JC, Platz C. Epidemiology of puerperal psychoses. Br J Psychiatry 1987; 150:662–673.
13. O'Hara MW. Postpartum Depression: Causes and Consequences. New York: Springer-Verlag, 1994.
14. O'Hara MW, Zekoski EM, Phillips LH, Wright EJ. A controlled prospective study of postpartum mood disorders: comparison of childbearing and nonchildbearing women. J Abnorm Psychol 1990; 99:3–15.
15. Myers JK, Weissman MM, Tischler GL, et al. Six-month prevalence of psychiatric disorders in three communities. Arch Gen Psychiatry 1984; 41:959–967.
16. Kennerley H, Gath D. Maternity blues I. Detection and measurement by questionnaire. Br J Psychiatry 1989; 155:356–362.
17. O'Hara MW. Childbearing. In: O'Hara MW, Reiter R, Johnson S, Milburn S, Engeldinger J, eds. Psychological Aspects of Women's Reproductive Health. New York: Springer, 1995.
18. Kendell RE, Rennie D, Clarke JA, Dean C. The social and obstetric correlates of psychiatric admission in the puerperium. Psychol Med 1981; 11:341–350.
19. O'Hara MW, Schlechte JA, Lewis DA, Wright EJ. Prospective study of postpartum blues. Arch Gen Psychiatry 1991; 48:801–806.
20. Iles S, Gath D, Kennerely H. Maternity blues II. A comparison between post-operative women and post-natal women. Br J Psychiatry 1989; 155:363–366.
21. Spitzer RL, Endicott J, Robins E. Research diagnostic criteria: rationale and reliability. Arch Gen Psychiatry 1978; 35:773–782.
22. American Psychiatric Association. Diagnostic and Statistical Manual of Mental Disorders. 3rd ed revised. Washington, DC: American Psychiatric Press, 1987.
23. O'Hara MW, Swain AM. Rates and risk of postpartum depression: a meta-analysis. Int Rev Psychiatry 1996; 8:37–54.
24. Whiffen VE, Gotlib IH. Comparison of postpartum and nonpostpartum depression: clinical presentation, psychiatric history, and psychosocial functioning. J Consult Clin Psychol 1993; 61:485–494.
25. Cohen LS, Sichel DA, Faraone SV, Robertson LM, Dimmock JA, Rosenbaum JF. Course of panic disorder during pregnancy and the puerperium: a preliminary study. Biol Psychiatry 1995; 37.
26. Sichel DA, Cohen LS, Dimmock JA, Rosenbaum JF. Postpartum obsessive compulsive disorder: a case series. J Clin Psychiatry 1993; 54:156–159.
27. Harris B. Hormonal aspects of postnatal depression. Int Rev Psychiatry 1996; 8:27–36.

28. O'Hara MW, Zekoski EM. Postpartum depression: a comprehensive review. In: Kumar R, Brockington IF, eds. Motherhood and Mental Illness: Causes and Consequences. London: Wright, 1988:17–63.

29. Kitamura T, Shima S, Sugawara M, Toda MA. Clinical and psychosocial correlates of antenatal depression: a review. Psychother Psychosom 1996; 65:117–123.

30. Brockington IF, Cox-Roper A. In: Kumar R, Brockington IF, eds. Motherhood and Mental Illness: Causes and Consequences. London: Wright, 1988.

31. Wisner KL, Peindl K, Hanusa BH. Symptomatology of affective and psychotic illnesses related to childbearing. J Affective Disord 1994; 30:77–87.

32. O'Hara MW. Postpartum mental disorders. In: Sciarra JJ, ed. Gynecology and Obstetrics. Vol. 6. Philadelphia: Harper & Row, 1991:1–17.

33. Kendell RE. Emotional and physical factors in the genesis of puerperal mental disorders. J Psychosom Res 1985; 29:3–11.

34. Miller LJ. Psychiatric disorders during pregnancy. In: Stewart DE, Stotland NL, eds. Psychological Aspects of Women's Health Care. Washington, DC: American Psychiatric Association Press, 1993:55–70.

35. Cunningham FG, MacDonald PC, Gant NF, et al. Neurological and psychiatric disorders. In: Cunningham FG, MacDonald PC, Gant NF, eds. Williams Obstetrics. 20th ed. Stamford, CT: Appleton & Lange, 1997.

36. Cox JL, Holden JM, Sagovsky R. Detection of postnatal depression: development of the 10-item Edinburgh Postnatal Depression Scale. Br J Psychiatry 1987; 150:782–786.

37. Lewis P. Drug usage in pregnancy. In: Lewis P, ed. Clinical Pharmacology in Obstetrics. Boston: Wright-PSG, 1983.

38. Nulman I, Rovet J, Stewart DE, et al. Neurodevelopment of children exposed in utero to antidepressant drugs. N Engl J Med 1997; 336:258–262.

39. Pastuszak A, Schick-Boschetto B, Zuber C, et al. Pregnancy outcome following first-trimester exposure to fluoxetine (Prozac). JAMA 1993; 269:2246–2248.

40. Altshuler LL, Cohen L, Szuba MP, Burt VK, Gitlin M, Mintz J. Pharmacologic management of psychiatric illness during pregnancy: dilemmas and guidelines. Am J Psychiatry 1996; 153:592–606.

41. Misri S, Sivertz K. Tricyclic drugs in pregnancy and lactation: a preliminary report. Int J Psychiatry Med 1991; 21:157–171.

42. Chambers CD, Johnson KA, Dick LM, Felix RJ, Jones KL. Birth outcomes in pregnant women taking fluoxetine. N Engl J Med 1996; 335:1010–1015.

43. Inman W, Kubotu K, Pearce G. Prescription event monitoring of paroxetine. Prescription Event Monitoring Reports 1993; 1–44.

44. Reference deleted in proof.

45. Goldberg HL, Nissim R. Psychotropic drugs in pregnancy and lactation. Int J Psychiatry Med 1994; 24:129–149.

46. Miller LJ. Use of electroconvulsive therapy during pregnancy. Hosp Commun Psychiatry 1994; 45:444–450.

47. Klerman GL, Weissman MM, Rounsaville BJ, Chevron ES. Interpersonal Psychotherapy of Depression. New York: Basic Books, 1984.

48. Beck AT, Rush AJ, Shaw BF, Emery G. Cognitive Therapy of Depression. New York: Guilford Press, 1979.

49. Cohen LS, Friedman JM, Jefferson JW, Johnson EM, Weiner ML. A reevaluation of risk of in utero exposure to lithium. JAMA 1994; 271:146–150.

50. Jacobson SJ, Jones K, Johnson K, et al. Prospective multicentre study of pregnancy outcome after lithium exposure during first trimester. Lancet 1992; 339:530–533.

51. Woody JN, London WL, Wilbanks GD. Lithium toxicity in a newborn. Pediatrics 1971; 47:94–96.

52. Schou M. What ever happened to the lithium babies? A follow-up study of children born without malformations. Acta Psychiatr Scand 1976; 54:193–197.

53. Shaw GM, Wasserman CR, O'Malley CD, Lammer EJ, Finnell RH. Orofacial clefts and maternal anticonvulsant use. Reproductive Toxicol 1995; 1:97–98.

54. Jones KL, Lacro RV, Johnson KA, Adams J. Patterns of malformations in the children of women treated with carbamazepine during pregnancy. N Engl J Med 1989; 320:1661–1666.

55. Scolnik D, Nulman I, Rovet J, et al. Neurodevelopment of children exposed in utero to phenytoin and carbamazepine monotherapy. JAMA 1994; 271:767–770.

56. St. Clair SM, Schirmer RG. First-trimester exposure to alprazolam. Obstet Gynecol 1992; 80:843–846.

57. Schick-Boschetto B, Zuber C. Alprazolam exposure during early human pregnancy. Teratology 1992; 45:460.

58. Laegreid L, Olegard R, Conradi N, Hagberg G, Wahlstrom J, Abrahamsson L. Congenital malformations and maternal consumption of benzodiazepines: a case-control study. Child Neurol 1990; 32:432–441.

59. Viggedal G, Hagberg BS, Laegreid L, Aronsson M. Mental development in late infancy after prenatal exposure to benzodiazepines: a prospective study. J Child Psychol Psychiatry 1993; 34:295–305.

60. Robinson L, Walker JR, Anderson D. Cognitive-behavioral treatment of panic disorder during pregnancy and lactation. Can J Psychiatry 1992; 37:623–626.

61. Wrede G, Mednick SA, Huttunen MO, Nilsson CG. Pregnancy and delivery complications in the births of an unselected series of Finnish children with schizophrenic mothers. Acta Psychiat Scand 1980; 62:369–381.

62. Spielvogel A, Wile J. Treatment and outcomes of psychotic patients during pregnancy and childbirth. Birth 1992, 19:131–137.

63. Rumeau-Rouquette C, Goujard J, Huel G. Possible teratogenic effects of phenothiazines in humans. Teratology 1977; 15:57–64.

64. Hanson JW, Oakley GP. Haloperidol and limb deformity. JAMA 1975; 231:26.

65. Van Waes A, Van de Velde E. Safety evaluation of haloperidol in the treatment of hyperemesis gravidum. J Clin Pharmacol 1969; 9:224–237.

66. Waldman MD, Safferman AZ. Pregnancy and clozapine. Am J Psychiatry 1993; 150:168–169.

67. Auerbach JG, Hans SL, Marcus J, Maeir S. Maternal psychotropic medication and neonatal behavior. Neurotoxicol Teratol 1992; 14:399–406.

68. Cagiano R, Barfield RJ, White NR, Pleim ET, Weinstein M, Cuomo V. Subtle behavioral changes produced in rat pups exposed in utero to haloperidol. Eur J Psychopharmacol 1988; 157:45–50.

69. Heinonen OP, Slone D, Shapiro S. Birth Defects and Drugs in Pregnancy. Littleton, MA: Publishing Services Group, 1977.

70. Nora JJ, Nora AH, Way GL. Cardiovascular maldevelopment associated with maternal exposure to amantidine. Lancet 1975; ii:607.

71. Mammen OK, Perel JM, Rudolph G, Foglia JP, Wheeler SB. Sertraline and norsertraline levels in three breastfed infants. J Clin Psychiatry 1997; 58:100–103.

72. Wisner KL, Perel JM, Findling RL. Antidepressant treatment during breast-feeding. Am J Psychiatry 1996; 153:1132–1137.

73. Elkin I, Shea MT, Watkins JT, et al. National Institute of Mental Health Treatment of Depression Collaborative Research Program: general effectiveness of treatments. Arch Gen Psychiatry 1989; 46:971–982.

74. Stuart S, O'Hara MW. Treatment of postpartum depression with interpersonal psychotherapy. Arch Gen Psychiatry 1995; 52:75–76.

75. Cohen LS, Sichel DA, Robertson LM, Heckscher E, Rosenbaum JF. Postpartum prophylaxis for women with bipolar disorder. Am J Psychiatry 1995; 152:1641–1645.

76. American Academy of Pediatrics Committee on Drugs. The transfer of drugs and other chemical into human breast milk. Pediatrics 1994; 93:137–150.

77. Patrick MJ, Tistone WJ, Reavey P. Diazepam and breastfeeding. Lancet 1973; 1:542–543.

78. Pons G, Francoual C, Guillet PH. Zolpidem excretion in breast milk. Eur J Clin Pharmacol 1989; 37:245–248.

79. Stewart RB, Karas B, Springer PK. Haloperidol excretion in human milk. Am J Psychiatry 1980; 137:849–850.

80. Beck AT, Ward CH, Mendelson M, Mock J, Erbaugh J. An inventory for measuring depression. Arch Gen Psychiatry 1961; 4:561–571.

14

Menstrual Cycle–Associated Syndromes

Susan R. Johnson

University of Iowa College of Medicine
Iowa City, Iowa

INTRODUCTION

Mood symptoms are commonly ascribed to various aspects of menstrual functioning including the premenstrual phase, menses itself, and the cessation of menses, or menopause. This chapter will discuss situations in which women may experience adverse mood symptoms linked to a specific part of her menstrual life. For each condition, basic information is presented regarding epidemiology, pathophysiology, clinical presentation, and differential diagnosis, although the major emphasis is placed on a suggested method of evaluation and management.

MENSTRUAL CYCLE–ASSOCIATED MOOD SYMPTOMS

Description of the Menstrual Cycle

At least a cursory knowledge of the normal characteristics of the menstrual cycle is necessary to understand menstrual cycle–associated mood problems. The onset of menses (menarche) occurs on average at age 12, with a normal age range of 9–16. Regular ovulatory cycles may not begin immediately, with the result that girls may have irregular bleeding for several months after menarche. After that, most women have ovulatory cycles until they are in their fifth decade. The average age of menopause (marked by the occurrence of the last menstrual period) is age 51.

The relevant features of the menstrual cycle are shown in Figure 1. The average cycle length, defined as the interval from the first day of bleeding in one cycle to the first day of bleeding in the next cycle, is 28 days. This 28-day cycle can be divided

279

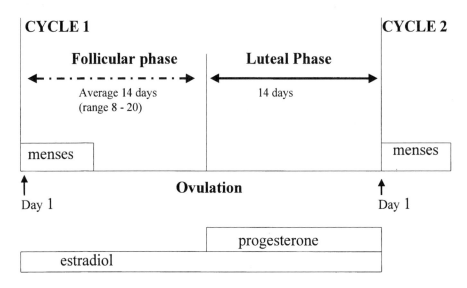

Figure 1 Menstrual cycle characteristics.

into two discrete phases: the follicular and luteal phases. The follicular phase, by defini-tion, begins with the first day of menstrual flow, and ends on the day of ovulation. The average duration of this phase is 14 days, but the length varies between women from about 8 days to 20 or more. During the follicular phase, the ovary is stimulated by follicle-stimulating hormone (FSH) to secrete estradiol.

A luteinizing hormone (LH) surge at the end of the follicular phase triggers ovula-tion. The follicle that contained the ovum that was released at ovulation, under the continued influence of LH, is transformed into the corpus luteum. The function of the corpus luteum is to secrete progesterone throughout the luteal phase. The luteal phase is of similar length in all women, lasting 14 days. At the end of the luteal phase, the corpus luteum disintegrates, and the resulting rapid drop in progesterone levels precipitates changes in the endometrium that lead to endometrial shedding, or menses.

The hallmark of ovulatory cycles is predictability. Even though the range of nor-mal for various parts of the menstrual cycle between women is wide, the pattern for each individual woman tends to be the same from cycle to cycle. For this reason, the "diagnosis" of ovulation can be made with a high degree of certainty in a woman who gives a history of longstanding predictable menstrual cycle events.

Premenstrual Syndrome and Premenstrual Dysphoric Disorder

Case Study

A 35-year-old woman married woman with two children seeks care for a 3-year history of intermittent mood symptoms. She describes the onset of this problem as gradual, and it has been serious enough for the past year to interfere with her marriage and her ability to work efficiently at her job as a supervisor. Her primary symptoms are irritability, unprovoked crying spells, and angry outbursts. Additionally, she describes bloating, appetite cravings, difficulty concentrating, fatigue, and insomnia. She says that her symptoms begin about 2 weeks before her menstrual period and start to go away almost immediately with the onset of bleeding. She feels like her "old self" during the 2 weeks after her period begins. She has no other medical problems and had a single episode of major depressive disorder treated several years ago with a tricyclic antidepressant. She has been off this medication for over 4 years.

Nomenclature

A luteal phase syndrome has been described in the medical literature since the early twentieth century, beginning with Frank's description in 1932 (1). Understanding of the phenomenology and appropriate classification of this problem first called "premenstrual tension" and later "premenstrual syndrome" has evolved over that same time period.

The modern era in the understanding of this problem is often dated from 1983, when the National Institutes of Mental Health held a consensus conference that resulted in agreement about basic elements of acceptable diagnostic criteria for use in research (2). Since then, although many sets of diagnostic criteria have been developed by individual investigators, the essential elements of requiring a measurable significant increase in symptoms in the luteal phase and the prospective timing of symptoms are usually included.

The most recent changes in nomenclature are the terms introduced by the American Psychiatric Association in its Diagnostic and Statistical Manual (DSM). In recognition that the most severe form of this problem is almost invariably associated with a presenting complaint of dysphoric mood, primarily irritability, a set of diagnostic criteria with the name "late luteal phase dysphoric disorder" was included on a trial basis in the appendix of the DSM-IIIR (3). These criteria were subsequently revised for the DSM-IV, and the name changed to "premenstrual dysphoric disorder (PDD)," a more appropriate name since symptoms typically begin early, not "late" in the luteal phase (4). In this scheme, premenstrual syndrome (PMS) is reserved for the description of women who have a luteal phase condition in which physical symptoms are prominent (5). Alternatively, PMS can be described as "severe" to refer to women otherwise classified as PMDD and "moderate" for all others. Both of these systems are used in the current medical literature. In this chapter, the acronym PMS will be used to refer to the clinical situation referred to by the terms PMDD and severe PMS.

Epidemiology

Based on surveys in which symptoms were assessed retrospectively, approximately 5% of menstruating women experience luteal phase symptoms severe enough to be categorized as PMDD or severe PMS. Another 15–20% experience moderate symptoms, and the remainder have either mild symptoms or none at all (6).

The natural history of PMS is not well understood. The most common age for symptomatic women to seek help for PMS is in the mid-thirties, even though symptoms may have been present for several years. Clinical experience suggests that many women experience monthly symptoms until menopause, although others may experience spontaneous remissions.

The only proven risk factors for PMS are female sex and ovulatory cycles. PMS has been reported among women in diverse geographical locations, cultural and ethnic groups, and historical periods. Racial, socioeconomic, or marital status differences have not been identified. Women with a prior history of a depressive disorder, including postpartum depression, or with a family history of PMS may represent high-risk groups.

Clinical experience suggests that one of the major sequela of PMS for most women is difficult family relationships. Whether the rate of divorce or child abuse is increased has not been demonstrated. Women with severe symptoms may perceive that they work less efficiently, but changes in cognitive function have not been demonstrated, and objective effects on job performance, such as absenteeism, and loss of employment have not been proven (6,7). Other adverse consequences attributed to PMS include substance abuse, violence, crime, work absenteeism, legal difficulties, and suicide, but none of these has been proven.

The relationship between depressive disorders and PMS has not yet been fully elucidated. Women with PMS appear to have a higher risk for psychiatric disorders, especially affective disorders (8–10). This observation, in addition to the similarity in symptoms between PMS and affective disorder, has led to an ongoing debate as to whether PMS is a variant of depression or is a unique, independent disorder (11–13).

There is evidence that the premenstrual affective state experienced by women with rigorously defined PMS differs from that experienced by women with PMDD (14,15). However, to make the situation even more difficult to sort out, there may be more than one distinct syndrome characterized by premenstrual affective change (16). For example, "pure" PMS may differ from a vulnerability to depression in which depressive symptoms are precipitated by the menstrual cycle (17).

Diagnostic Criteria

Although there is still no agreed-upon single set of diagnostic criteria for all luteal phase syndromes, all adequate criteria must address three fundamental elements: characteristic symptoms, adversity, and timing. Most women with PMS report six or more symptoms, usually distributed across the categories of emotional, somatic, and cognitive (18). Emotional symptoms are the most common reason for seeking help, and the hallmark symptom is irritability (19). Others include easily precipitated crying spells, low self-esteem, anxiety, and depression. The full range of depressive symptoms including low mood, sleep disturbance, and abnormal eating can be encountered. Two features help distinguish PMS from the depressive disorders: in PMS, the symptoms are restricted to the premenstrual phase, and depression is less prominent than irritability.

The somatic, or physical, symptoms of PMS include breast tenderness, bloating,

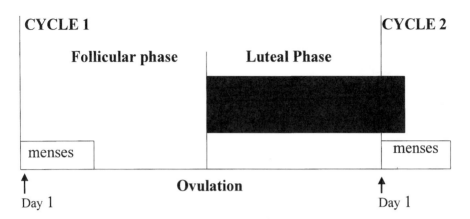

Figure 2 Timing of PMS/PMDD symptoms.

appetite increase and food cravings, insomnia, fatigue, hot flushes, headaches, and musculoskeletal discomfort. Finally, cognitive problems, although less frequently reported, can have a significant impact, particularly on a woman's work efficiency. These symptoms include short-term memory problems, difficulty concentrating, and "fuzzy" thinking.

Assessment of the level of adversity caused by the symptoms is critical. The majority of menstruating women experience symptoms that are qualitatively similar to those associated with PMS. The difference between these normal symptoms, also referred to as "molimina," and PMS is quantitative. Moliminal symptoms are typically present for a few days prior to the onset of menses and do not interfere with daily functioning. PMS, in contrast, begins 2 weeks or so before menses and results in problems with daily functioning. Although most women clearly fall into one of these two groups, there is a spectrum of experience in between.

The distinctive feature of PMS is the timing of symptoms during the menstrual cycle. Only women who ovulate are at risk for PMS, and the symptoms are confined to the luteal phase, which begins about 14 days before the onset of menses. The timing of symptoms is shown graphically in Figure 2. Symptom timing must be assessed prospectively, because reliance on the retrospective history will lead to inaccurate diagnoses (20). This is particularly important in perimenopausal women because of irregularities in the menstrual cycle, which can lead to the appearance of an inconsistent symptom pattern.

Differential Diagnosis

The most common condition that must be distinguished from PMS is menstrual magnification of another disorder, typically a mood disorder. Figure 3 graphically illustrates

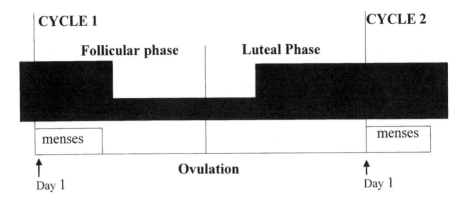

CYCLE 1   CYCLE 2

Follicular phase   Luteal Phase

menses   menses

↑   Ovulation   ↑
Day 1   Day 1

Figure 3   Timing of menstrual-magnification symptoms.

the type of symptom pattern in this situation. Briefly, the woman will experience symptoms characteristic of the underlying disorder in both phases of the cycle, but the symptoms will be more severe in the late luteal phase, and severe symptoms often persist into the early follicular phase.

Some women experience mood symptoms in association with dysmenorrhea (21), a severe form of menstrual cramps, which is caused by excessive effect of prostaglandins produced at the end of the luteal phase. Dysmenorrhea symptoms may begin a day or two prior to the onset of bleeding, rarely sooner, and usually spontaneously remit on the second or third day of bleeding. The cardinal symptom is lower mid-abdominal cramping pain, sometimes in association with diarrhea, nausea, headache, and fatigue.

Diagnosis

The evaluation of women suspected of having PMS can usually be completed in two office visits, with two menstrual cycles in between during which the woman prospectively records her symptoms ("charting") (20,22). Because it is not unusual for a woman to experience both depression and PMS simultaneously, the diagnostic challenge is to sort out those with PMS only, another diagnosis only, or both diagnoses concurrently.

First visit: The history should focus on: (1) establishing the presence of ovulation; (2) obtaining a description of the symptoms; (3) reviewing prior psychiatric diagnosis and treatments and any other medical problems. Ovulation can be presumed if a woman does not take exogenous hormones, and if she has menstrual periods characterized by regular intermenstrual interval, consistent flow, and menstrual cramps. Sophisticated testing (basal body temperature, mid–luteal phase progesterone level, urinary LH determination) is reserved for cases that are not clear. There are no characteristic physical examination findings associated with PMS. "Hormone tests," by which the patient usually means estrogen and progesterone levels, are of no value other than for the

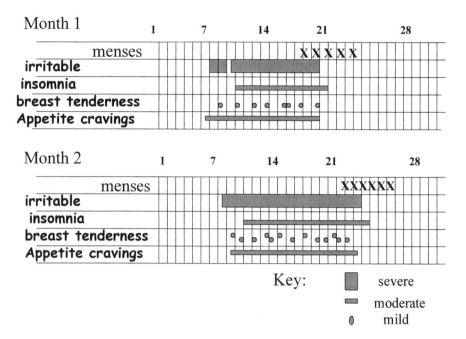

Figure 4   Sample 2-month menstrual calendar.

assessment of other suspected conditions. The physical examination and laboratory testing should be aimed at identifying other disorders suspected in the individual case.

Charting: For clinical purposes, a simple method of charting can be used. Figure 4 illustrates one such method, a grid on which to record the presence and severity of up to four symptoms each day, as well as the days of menstrual bleeding (22). The woman should be instructed to complete the chart each evening for a minimum of two cycles (20).

Second visit: The symptom charts should be evaluated and their interpretation integrated into the remainder of the clinical picture. Symptoms associated with PMS typically begin abruptly at or shortly after ovulation and resolve promptly with the onset of menstrual bleeding. Sometimes the onset is more gradual, although still occurring no sooner than ovulation, and the "offset" may involve a tapering over 2 or 3 days after the period begins.

Management

Many diverse etiologies have been proposed for PMS. While no single hypothesis adequately accounts for the entire clinical picture of PMS, there is now convincing evidence that the primary basis is biological. Considerable evidence suggests a role for altered serotonergic function in the pathogenesis of PMS (5,23,24). For example, normal women experience an increase in serotonin receptors in the luteal phase, perhaps induced by the increasing levels of estradiol from the late follicular phase. This "up-regulation" of receptors appears not to occur in women with PMS. As a result, there is an increase in serotonin reuptake and a lower level of active serotonin, which may result in adverse effects on mood. The clinical trials (described in a subsequent section) that have found a beneficial effect of selective serotonin-reuptake inhibitors (SSRIs) on PMS provide indirect support for this hypothesis.

Self-Help Therapies

For most women with mild to moderate luteal phase symptoms and as many as 20% of women with severe symptoms, self-help interventions, including dietary alterations, exercise, and nutritional supplements should be recommended as initial therapy. Dietary alterations include reductions in caffeine, salt, alcohol, and sugar intake; avoidance of prolonged fasting; and increased intake of complex carbohydrates. Two controlled clinical trials have demonstrated that increasing complex carbohydrate intake leads to a reduction in luteal phase symptoms among women with PMS (25,26).

Epidemiological evidence suggests that women who engage in regular exercise experience fewer premenstrual phase symptoms than sedentary women (27,28). The biological basis for this finding may be linked to exercise-induced modulation of central β-endorphin levels. Although there has been no controlled trial of exercise in women with PMS, a regimen of moderate, regular aerobic exercise (e.g., walking 1–2 miles briskly five times a week) has been shown to reduce premenstrual symptoms (29).

Finally, calcium and magnesium supplements have each been shown in controlled clinical trails to reduce both the physical and the emotional symptoms of PMS. Calcium is given daily as 1000 mg elemental Ca^{2+} (30,31). Magnesium may be given during the luteal phase only at a dose of 400 mg daily (32).

Pharmacological Therapies

If self-help interventions are ineffective after two to four menstrual cycles, pharmacological therapy should be considered. For most patients, use of a SSRI is the treatment of choice. Fluoxetine, the most extensively studied of this class for PMS, has been found to significantly reduce the symptoms of PMS compared to placebo in several clinical trials (33–39). The starting dose is 20 mg daily. Higher doses are not usually required, and some women respond to as little as 10 mg daily.

Other SSRIs shown to be effective in the treatment of PMS include clomipramine, up to 75 mg daily (40), paroxetine, 20 mg daily (41), and sertraline, between 50 and 150 mg daily (42). The effectiveness of SSRIs is not due to a nonspecific antidepressant effect. In comparative trials, SSRIs were superior in the treatment of PMS symptoms to bupropion (43), desipramine (44), and the noradrenaline reuptake inhibitor maprotiline (45).

The SSRIs may be administered during the luteal phase only (i.e., during the symptomatic phase) (46,47). The proportion of women who will respond to this less frequent dosing is not known, but in one study the response rate was 73% (47). This regimen can be effective even with the long half-life drug fluoxetine. This luteal-phase-only regimen has the advantages of lowered cost and the potential for fewer side effects.

The anxiolytics alprazolam and buspirone have also been shown in placebo-controlled trials to reduce PMS symptoms (48,49), although the effect has not been consistently demonstrated (50). The anxiolytics are associated with a higher rate of undesirable side effects, such as sedation, and in the case of alprazolam, at least, can be abused more easily.

Nortriptyline and perhaps other tricyclic antidepressants may help reduce the emotional symptoms, but are not helpful in reducing the physical symptoms of PMS (50). The patients who may benefit the most from this class of drugs are either women with severe insomnia or those with combined depression and PMS who do not respond to SSRIs.

Finally, progesterone in its "natural" form (in contrast to the synthetics such as medroxyprogesterone) has been widely touted in the past as an effective therapy (51). Multiple controlled trials of progesterone administered as a vaginal suppository, however, have failed to establish a beneficial effect of this regimen. The ineffectiveness of oral micronized progesterone was recently demonstrated in a large randomized trial in which 1200 mg daily during the luteal phase was no better than placebo (48).

Ovulation Inhibition

Ovulation inhibition was first suggested as a treatment for PMS in 1979, when Day reported on a small series of women treated with continuous danazol therapy. Although the high rate of side effects led to the conclusion that this was not an ideal primary therapy, the author felt that further study was warranted (53). In 1984, Muse et al. found, in a placebo-controlled crossover trial, that gonadotropin-releasing hormone agonist (GnRH) therapy reduced luteal phase symptoms to normal, follicular phase levels (54). Since then, controlled trials of ovulation-suppressive doses of GnRH, danazol, and estradiol have confirmed the finding that interruption of ovulation is beneficial (55–57).

GnRH agonist therapy is probably the most effective regimen. The agonists available in the United States are leuprolide acetate and nafarelin. Leuprolide is most easily administered in the depot formulation and is given in a dose of either 3.75 mg intramuscularly on a monthly basis or 11.25 mg every 3 months. Nafarelin is administered as a nasal spray, 200 μg twice daily, making this route somewhat inconvenient for long-term use. The practical effect of the GnRH agonists is to render the woman temporarily menopausal, and standard postmenopausal hormone-replacement therapy must be given concomitantly to avoid the adverse long-term effects of estrogen deficiency (58,59). The major drawback of GnRH is expense; the typical monthly cost for the agonist is between $400 and $500.

Danazol is a synthetic androgen-like hormone that has been used primarily to treat endometriosis. The most effective doses are 200 or 400 mg daily, given orally, usually in a divided dose (56,60). Danazol is not as predictably effective as the GnRH agonists and has a variety of effects that make it a poor choice for long-term therapy.

Among the "minor" side effects are weight gain, facial hair growth, and exacerbation of acne. Of more concern is the potential for long-term cardiovascular effects, due to known metabolic alternations such as depression of high-density lipoprotein (HDL) (61). If it is to be used beyond the recommended FDA limit of 9 months, lipids must be monitored.

Estradiol, given in a sufficiently high dose to inhibit ovulation, has been shown to be superior to placebo as well (57). This regimen is relatively inexpensive compared to GnRH agonists or danazol. The estrogen should be given by the transdermal route in a dose of at least 0.1 mg daily. In order to prevent endometrial hyperplasia and neoplasia, cyclic progestin must be given concomitantly. The effectiveness of this regimen is probably lower than for GnRH, with only approximately 50% of subjects rating the therapy as acceptable after 8 months (57).

Oral contraceptives also have the effect of inhibiting ovulation, but unfortunately have not been shown to have a beneficial effect on the emotional symptoms associated with PMS. This choice may be appropriate for women who have physical symptoms as their primary complaint (62).

One practical alternative to these more expensive and side effect–producing regimens is medroxyprogesterone acetate, either given orally as 20–30 mg per day or as depo-medroxyprogesterone acetate, 150 mg every 3 months. Only one small, short-term clinical trial has been conducted testing this regimen, but the results were encouraging (63). This regimen is inexpensive and has few long-term side effects.

In summary, none of the regimens shown to be effective is ideal for long-term therapy. Ovulation inhibition should therefore be reserved for situations in which other therapy has been unsuccessful, immediate control of severe symptoms is desirable, or the diagnosis is unclear.

Surgical

Oophorectomy (usually accompanied by a hysterectomy) appears to be effective in women with rigorously diagnosed PMS (64,65). However, this approach is costly, associated with risk of acute morbidity and mortality, and can lead to adverse long-term consequences, including cardiovascular disease and osteoporosis. With the increasing availability of effective pharmacological therapy, the need for surgical treatment should be rare. It is a particularly problematic choice for the perimenopausal women who have only a few months or years of menstrual functioning. In general, oophorectomy should be reserved for the woman who has disabling symptoms that do not respond to serotonin-reuptake inhibitor therapy and that are *only* eliminated by either GnRH agonist therapy for a minimum of four to six cycles.

Premenstrual Magnification

Case Study

A 24-year-old woman with a diagnosis of major depressive disorder complains of recurrent intermittent severe depression at the time of her period each month. On three occasions in the last year, she has been admitted to a local psychiatric hospital for suicidal ideation, and on each occasion her menstrual period began the day after admission. She is currently treated with a combination of three drugs, and has not noted an improvement in these episodes.

Clinical Presentation and Epidemiology

The term premenstrual magnification (PMM) is now commonly used to describe the situation in which a woman with an affective disorder experiences an exacerbation in her symptoms perimenstrually (66,67). An example of a typical pattern of symptoms is shown in Figure 3. Yonkers and White also provide empirical evidence based on intensive study of five women that this category may be further subdivided into one group with PMM only and a group that has PMS in addition to the affective disorder (68).

The pathophysiology of this phenomenon has not been determined. Some demographic differences between PMM and PMS have been found. In a community-based investigation of menstrual cycle–associated symptom patterns, the women with menstrual magnification tended to be younger than women with premenstrual symptoms, had less education, and reported more stress than the PMS group (67).

Although the prevalence of PMM among the population of women with affective disorders is not known, it is a common diagnosis among women who seek care for possible PMS. For example, in one university-based premenstrual syndrome clinic, 24 of the first 100 women evaluated were diagnosed with menstrual magnification (66).

The clinical presentation of PMM is usually in one of two circumstances. The first is among women who seek evaluation for possible PMS, and the risk is higher in women with a past history of affective disorder (69). The second setting is a woman who is being treated for an identified affective disorder, but who has recurrent "breakthough" symptoms each month in association with her menses.

Evaluation and Management

The diagnostic approach is identical to that for PMS. Briefly, a careful history is taken, the woman asked to chart her symptoms (see Fig. 4) for at least two menstrual cycles, after which an assessment can usually be made. Ovulation suppression is appropriate as a diagnostic test if the diagnostic picture remains unclear. A GnRH agonist such as leuprolide acetate is ideal for this purpose, because this drug effectively eliminates PMS symptoms without adding mood side effects of its own. If the symptoms do not improve after 3 months with this therapy, a menstrual cycle effect is an unlikely explanation for the recurring symptoms.

The cornerstone of management is adequate therapy directed at the underlying mood disorder. The aim should be to find therapeutic agents that will adequately control the mood symptoms during the nonperimenstrual part of the cycle. Then, if significant symptoms persist, hormonal suppression of ovulation should be added. The choices for ovulation suppression are the same as those described previously for PMS.

In our clinical experience, suppression with medroxyprogesterone acetate is often effective and provides the safest, most inexpensive alternative. Ovulation suppression may need to be continued until menopause.

MENOPAUSE-ASSOCIATED MOOD SYMPTOMS

Many women who develop emotional symptoms during the perimenopause assume these symptoms are caused by "hormone changes." For this reason, physicians who provide psychiatric or gynecological care to women in this age group must be aware of the appropriate differential diagnosis of these symptoms. The use of a methodical approach to diagnosis will allow most women to be accurately categorized and to be offered an effective treatment plan.

Case Study

A 49-year-old woman seeks treatment for mood symptoms. She reports that this problem began several months ago and has worsened in recent weeks. The major symptoms are irritability, depression, fatigue, and headaches. She has no history of depressive illness and has not experienced a similar episode in the past. She denies suicidal ideation and is able to continue working. Her appetite is unchanged, and she has neither gained nor lost weight. She has frequent insomnia, described as awakening in the middle of the night. She is certain that her hormones are the cause of her symptoms. Her menstrual periods have become less frequent over the past 8 months, and she has hot flashes that have been increasing in frequency.

Menopause and Its Transition Described

Figure 5 graphically illustrates the stages of the average women's menstrual life, from menarche through the postmenopause. "Perimenopause" has typically been used to describe the symptomatic months or years before and after the menopause. The term "menopause transition" has more recently been used to describe the time from when a woman begins to experience changes reflective of decreasing ovarian function to the last menstrual period, or menopause itself (69). This transition lasts on average 4 years, and is typically accompanied by alterations in menstrual pattern and flow and/or the beginning of vasomotor symptoms. After the last period, even more women experience vasomotor symptoms, and some go on to develop other symptoms associated with estrogen deficiency such as vaginal atrophy. In one large longitudinal study, the number of women who reported vasomotor symptoms increased from 10% during the pretransition years to 50% during that time (69). The rate rose to over 80% after menopause and did not begin to wane significantly until after 5 years.

The average age of menopause is 51 years, so that the typical transition begins in the mid- to late forties. However, because menopause can normally occur at a much

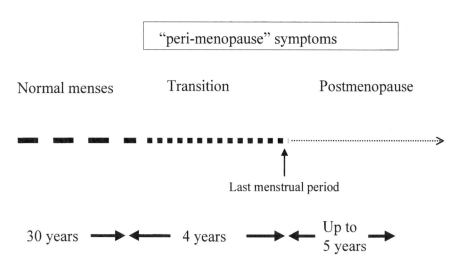

Figure 5   Time course of menopause.

younger age, the transition should be suspected even in women in their late thirties who have appropriate symptoms.

Menopause and Mood Symptoms

The nature of emotional symptoms at the time of menopause has been the subject of considerable controversy. Clinicians believed for many years that the menopause represented a time of increased risk for depressive illness. More recently, carefully designed epidemiological research has demonstrated that there is not an increased risk for major depressive disorder at this time (70).

Minor depressive symptomatology, however, is another matter. The few longitudinal cohort studies have found that vasomotor symptoms are directly related to menopause, whereas depressive symptoms and other physical symptoms are not clearly independently related (71–74). Vasomotor symptoms are important to this discussion because of their association with psychological symptoms. Hammar et al. showed that women who experienced the most severe hot flashes were also most at risk for severe depressive symptoms (75).

The mechanistic explanation for this association is not completely explained. However, a partial explanation may be related to sleep disturbance. Vasomotor symptoms tend to be more pronounced at night and have been shown to interfere with REM sleep. This sleep disturbance, in turn, can result in the phenomenon (well known to sleep-deprived physicians!) of irritability, fatigue, and depressive feelings.

Transition-Associated Symptoms

Women in the menopause transition commonly seek help from primary care physicians and gynecologists for emotional symptoms that they attribute to impending menopause. The approach to these women depends on an understanding of both luteal phase syndromes and menopause-related symptoms, and so this section is presented out of order to take advantage of the discussions of these two topics.

The primary differential diagnosis of the most common complex of emotional symptoms such as depression, irritability, and anxiety includes the depressive disorders, "perimenopause"-associated symptoms, and, in the woman who is still menstruating, premenstrual syndrome. Substance abuse, domestic violence, and other more uncommon causes of these emotional symptoms must also be considered when appropriate. "Perimenopause-associated emotional symptoms" is used in this chapter to refer to those emotional (and physical) symptoms that are best explained by the hormone fluctuations of the perimenopause. Until recently, there has been little interest in this stage of menstrual life, and we have much to learn about the epidemiology, risk factors, and etiology of these symptoms.

Diagnosis

The diagnosis of perimenopause-associated emotional symptoms is one of exclusion and should be suspected in the woman who develops irritability, dysphoric mood, and fatigue following the onset of vasomotor symptoms. A change in menstrual pattern, including amenorrhea, further supports the diagnosis of "perimenopause."

Hormone testing is of limited value. Follicle-stimulating hormone (FSH) can fluctuate during the transition years, so that a single value does not predict future symptoms or menstrual pattern. However, an elevated value (>20 mIu/ml) supports the diagnosis of the transition.

Management

A trial of hormone therapy is the most direct test of the diagnosis. Unless there is a medical contraindication, estrogen should be given for a minimum of 4–6 weeks. The initial dose should be selected to maximize the likelihood of effectiveness, and in many cases a higher-than-usual dose is appropriate, such as the equivalent of conjugated equine estrogens 0.9 or 1.25 mg. Progestin can be added initially or after the initial few weeks, when it is established that the symptoms are improved. Delay in adding progestin is sometimes advisable in this group of patients because they may have depressive side effects from the medication that may confuse the clinical picture.

Overall Evaluation

The first step is to determine the woman's menstrual status. If the woman is still menstruating, premenstrual syndrome must be considered. The woman should be asked if her emotional symptoms are linked temporally to the menstrual cycle. For PMS, the symptoms should be confined to the luteal phase (Fig. 2), a length of time that does not usually exceed 2 weeks. If PMS is a consideration at this point, the woman should be asked to record her menstrual periods and symptoms for at least two cycles and return for reevaluation. However, if the emotional symptoms are severe, evaluation and appropriate treatment of any other suspected disorders, particularly depression, should proceed during these 2 months.

A history of symptoms occurring on a daily basis suggests a diagnosis other than PMS. The next step is to determine whether or not the woman is perimenopausal. To do this, information is needed about menstrual cycle pattern changes and vasomotor symptoms (hot flashes and night sweats in particular). If menses are abnormal (irregular pattern or amenorrhea), consider other causes of the menstrual disturbance, especially in young women who have no vasomotor symptoms.

If the woman seems to be in the perimenopausal stage, an assessment of vasomotor symptoms is critical. The woman should be asked about hot flashes, night sweats, and sleep disturbance and the extent to which these are a problem. If vasomotor symptoms are present, determine if the emotional symptoms began prior to, coincident with, or after any transition period symptoms. Next, the woman should be asked about the temporal relationship between the onset of the emotional symptoms and the onset of the vasomotor symptoms. If the depressive symptoms came first, perimenopause is an unlikely cause.

If the onset of the emotional symptoms accompanied or started within a few months of the vasomotor symptoms, a trial of estrogen should be considered. The dose should be individualized. If the vasomotor symptoms are severe, a relatively high dose should be used, such as the equivalent of either 0.9 or 1.25 mg conjugated equine estrogens. If the vasomotor symptoms resolve within a few weeks but the emotional symptoms do not, depression should be considered.

If PMS and perimenopause-associated etiologies are unlikely, depression is the most likely explanation. However, other etiologies for the emotional symptoms should be considered as well, including domestic violence, substance abuse, or other psychiatric conditions.

If depression remains the most likely diagnosis, the severity and nature of the depression should be assessed. In addition to determining the type of depression according to the usual criteria, the need for consultation should be determined. The need for consultation will depend on the training and experience of the physician. Consultation should be considered in particular for the woman who might be psychotic (suggested by delusions or hallucinations), the woman who may have bipolar disorder, the woman who is actively suicidal, and the woman with recurrent depressive episodes or a history of past noncompliance.

A FINAL NOTE REGARDING PRIMARY MOOD DISORDERS

Because primary mood disorders (especially major depressive disorder and dysphoric disorder) are so common, the clinician must maintain a high index of suspicion any time a woman attributes her symptoms to the menstrual cycle. These historical features should increase suspicion: (1) history of prior major depressive episode in that a single episode predicts a 50% recurrence risk, and three episodes a 90% risk; (2) a mood disorder in first-degree relatives; and (3) a history of suicide attempts.

The primary method of diagnosing depressive illness is the clinical interview. In addition to determining the presence and duration of the symptoms consistent with the diagnostic criteria for each disorder, a complete medical and psychiatric history should be obtained. Some clinicians screen women at risk with a screening inventory, such as the Beck Depression Inventory. This type of survey is very sensitive, in that virtually all cases of depression will be identified, but it has many false positives. Importantly, an elevated score in the luteal phase of the menstrual cycle does *not* help distinguish between a primary mood disorder and one of the menstrual-related conditions described in this chapter. Therefore, a positive screening test should always be followed by a clinical evaluation.

Features that help in distinguishing depression from symptoms associated with the menopause transition include an absence of significant hot flashes, lack of response to a trial of exogenous estrogen, and severe vegetative symptoms or significant suicidality.

SUMMARY

The evaluation of women with mood symptoms can present a challenge. Specialized health care providers must deal with a differential diagnosis that includes disorders outside their training experience. History alone may not lead to a characterization of the clinical situation. Finally, women often have firm, but potentially inaccurate, ideas about the role that hormones play in their own situation.

However, these challenges can be met. This chapter includes an overview of the diagnostic territory with which the practitioner should be familiar. Mastery of this content, or the use of appropriate consultation, will lead to consideration of the appropriate diagnoses. The use of prospective symptom assessment, when indicated, will result in a markedly improved level of diagnostic accuracy in the menstruating woman. Finally, most women will respond favorably to an approach that involves the methodical approach described in this chapter, because it both allows a logical assessment of the role of hormones and a high likelihood of a successful treatment outcome.

REFERENCES

1. Frank RT. The hormonal basis of premenstrual tension. Arch Neurol Psychiatry 1931; 26:1053–1057.
2. Workshop on Premenstrual Syndrome. Cosponsored by the Center for Studies of Affective Disorders and the Psychobiological Processes and Behavioral Medicine Section, Clinical

Research Branch, National Institutes of Mental Health, Rockville, MD, Apr 14–15, 1983. Cited in Roy-Byrne PP, Hoban MC, Rubinow DR. The relationship of menstrually related mood disorders to psychiatric disorders. Clin Obstet Gynecol 1987; 30:386–395.

3. American Psychiatric Association. Diagnostic and Statistical Manual of Mental Disorders. 3d ed. Washington, DC: American Psychiatric Press, 1987.

4. American Psychiatric Association. Diagnostic and Statistical Manual of Mental Disorders. 4th ed. Washington, DC: American Psychiatric Press, 1994.

5. Steiner M. Premenstrual syndromes. Ann Rev Med 1997; 48:447–455.

6. Johnson, SR. The epidemiology and social impact of premenstrual symptoms. Clin Obstet Gynecol 1987; 30:367–376.

7. Morgan M, Rapkin AJ, D'Elia L, Reading A, Goldman L. Cognitive functioning in premenstrual syndrome. Obstet Gynecol 1996; 88:961–966.

8. Pearlstein TB, Frank E, Rivera-Tovar A, Thoft JS, Jacobs E, Mieczkowski TA. Prevalence of axis I and axis II disorders in women with late luteal phase dysphoric disorder. J Affect Disord 1990; 20:129–134.

9. MacKenzie TB, Wilcox K, Baron H. Lifetime prevalence of psychiatric disorders in women with perimenstrual difficulties. J Affect Disord 1986; 10:15–19.

10. Stout AL, Steege JF, Blazer DG, George LK. Comparison of lifetime diagnosis in premenstrual syndrome clinic and community samples. J Nerv Ment Dis 1986; 174:517–521.

11. Halbreich U. Premenstrual dysphoric disorders: a diversified cluster of vulnerability traits to depression. Acta Psychiatr Scand 1997; 95:169–176.

12. Rubinow DR, Schmidt PJ. Models for the development and expression of symptoms in premenstrual syndrome. Psychiatr Clin North Am 1989; 12:53–68.

13. Mortola JF. Issues in the diagnosis and research of premenstrual syndrome. Clin Obstet Gynecol 1992; 35:587–598.

14. Mortola JF, Girton L, Yen SS. Depressive episodes in premenstrual syndrome. Am J Obstet Gynecol 1984; 161:1682–1687.

15. Rapkin AJ, Chang LC, Reading AE. Mood and cognitive style in premenstrual syndrome. Obstet Gynecol 1989; 74:644–649.

16. Endicott J, Nee J, Cohen J, Halbreich U. Premenstrual changes: patterns and correlates of daily ratings. J Affect Disord 1986; 10:127–135.

17. Endicott J. The menstrual cycle and mood disorders. J Affect Disord 1993; 29:193–200.

18. Hurt SW, Schnurr PP, Severino SK, Freeman EW, Gise LH, Rivera-Tovar A, Steege JF. Late luteal phase dysphoric disorder in 670 women evaluated for premenstrual complaints. Am J Psychiatry 1992; 149:525–530.

19. Bloch M, Schmidt PJ, Rubinow DR. Premenstrual syndrome: evidence for symptom stability across cycles. Am J Psychiatry 1997; 154:1741–1746.

20. Mortola JF, Girton L, Beck L, Yen SSC. Diagnosis of premenstrual syndrome by a single, prospective and reliable instrument: the calendar of premenstrual experiences. Obstet Gynecol 1990; 76:302–307.

21. Johnson, SR. Dysmenorrhea and premenstrual syndrome. In: Moore TR, Reiter RC, Rebar RW, Baker VV, eds. Gynecology and Obstetrics: A Longitudinal Approach. New York: Churchill-Livingstone, 1993:773–787.

22. Johnson SR. Clinician's approach to the diagnosis and management of premenstrual syndrome. Clin Obstet Gynecol 1992; 35:637–657.

23. Dinan TG, O'Keane V. The premenstrual syndrome: a psychoneuroendocrine perspective. Baillieres Clin Endocrinol Metab 1991; 5:143–165.

24. Su TP, Schmidt PJ, Danaceau M, Murphy DL, Rubinow DR. Effect of menstrual cycle phase on neuroendocrine and behavioral responses to the serotonin agonist m-chlorophenylpiperazine in women with premenstrual syndrome and controls. J Clin Endocrinol Metab 1997; 82:1220–1228.

25. Wurtman JJ, Brzezinske A, Wurtman RJ, Laferrere B. Effect of nutrient intake on premenstrual depression. Am J Obstet Gynecol 1989; 161:1228–1234.

26. Sayegh R, Schiff I, Wurtman J, Spiers P, McDermott J, Wurtman R. The effect of a carbohydrate-rich beverage on mood, appetite, and cognitive function in women with premenstrual syndrome. Obstet Gynecol 1995; 86:520–528.

27. Aganoff JA, Boyle GJ. Aerobic exercise, mood states and menstrual cycle symptoms. J Psychosom Res 1994; 38:183–192.

28. Prior JC, Vigna Y, Sciarretta D, Alojado N, Schulzer M. Conditioning exercise decreases premenstrual symptoms: a prospective, controlled 6-month trial. Fertil Steril 1987; 47:402–408.

29. Steege JF, Blumenthal JA. The effects of aerobic exercise on premenstrual symptoms in middle-aged women: a preliminary study. J Psychosom Res 1993; 37:127–133.

30. Thys-Jacobs S, Ceccarelli S, Bierman A, Weisman H, Cohen MA, Alvir J. Calcium supplementation in premenstrual syndrome: a randomized crossover trial. J Gen Intern Med 1989; 4:183–189.

31. Penland JG, Johnson PE. Dietary calcium and manganese effects on menstrual cycle symptoms. Am J Obstet Gynecol 1993; 168:1417–1423.

32. Facchinetti F, Borella P, Sances G, Fioroni L, Nappi RE, Genazzani AR. Oral magnesium successfully relieves premenstrual mood changes. Obstet Gynecol 1991; 78:177–181.

33. Steiner M, Steinberg S, Stewart D, Carter D, Berger C, Reid R, Grover D, Streiner D. Fluoxetine in the treatment of premenstrual dysphoria. N Engl J Med 1995; 332:1529–1534.

34. Pearlstein TB, Stone AB. Long-term fluoxetine treatment of late luteal phase dysphoric disorder. J Clin Psychiatry 1994; 55:332–335.

35. Wood SH, Mortola JF, Chan YF, Moossazadeh F, Yen SS. Treatment of premenstrual syndrome with fluoxetine: a double-blind, placebo-controlled, crossover study. Obstet Gynecol 1992; 80:339–344.

36. Stout AL, Steege JF, Blazer DG, George LK. Comparison of lifetime diagnosis in premenstrual syndrome clinic and community samples. J Nerv Ment Dis 1986; 174:517–521.

37. Stone AB, Pearlstein TB, Brown WA. Fluoxetine in the treatment of late luteal phase dysphoric disorder. J Clin Psychiatry 1991; 52:290–293.

38. Ozeren S, Corakci A, Yucesoy I, Mercan R, Erhan G. Fluoxetine in the treatment of premenstrual syndrome. Eur J Obstet Gynecol Reprod Biol 1997; 73:167–170.

39. Su TP, Schmidt PJ, Danaceau MA, Tobin MB, Rosenstein DL, Murphy DL, Rubinow DR. Fluoxetine in the treatment of premenstrual dysphoria. Neuropsychopharmacology 1997; 16:346–356.

40. Sundblad C, Modigh K, Andersch B, Eriksson E. Clomipramine effectively reduces premenstrual irritability and dysphoria: a placebo-controlled trial. Acta Psychiatr Scand 1992; 85:39–47.

41. Yonkers KA, Gullion C, Williams A, Novak K, Rush AJ. Paroxetine as a treatment for premenstrual dysphoric disorder. J Clin Psychopharmacol 1996; 16:3–8.

42. Yonkers KA, Halbreich U, Freeman E, Brown C, Endicott J, Frank E, Parry B, Pearlstein

T, Severino S, Stout A, Stone A, Harrison W. Sertraline Premenstrual Dysphoric Collaborative Study Group. Symptomatic improvement of premenstrual dysphoric disorder with sertraline treatment: a randomized controlled trial. JAMA 1997; 278:983–988.

43. Pearlstein TB, Stone AB, Lund SA, Scheft H, Zlotnick C, Brown WA. Comparison of fluoxetine, bupropion, and placebo in the treatment of premenstrual dysphoric disorder. Clin Psychopharmacol 1997; 17:261–266.

44. Freeman EW, Rickels K, Sondheimer SJ, Wittmaack FM. Sertraline versus desipramine in the treatment of premenstrual syndrome: an open-label trial. J Clin Psychiatry 1996; 57:7–11.

45. Eriksson E, Hedberg MA, Andersch B, Sundblad C. The serotonin reuptake inhibitor paroxetin is superior to the noradrenaline reuptake inhibitor maprotiline in the treatment of premenstrual syndrome. Neuropsychopharmacology 1995; 12:167–176.

46. Sundblad C, Hedberg MA, Eriksson E. Clomipramine administered during the luteal phase reduces the symptoms of premenstrual syndrome: a placebo-controlled trial. Neuropsychopharmacology 1993; 9:133–145.

47. Halbreich U, Smoller JW. Intermittent luteal phase sertraline treatment of dysphoric premenstrual syndrome. J Clin Psychiatry 1997; 58:399–402.

48. Freeman EW, Rickels K, Sondheimer SJ, Polansky M. A double-blind trial of oral progesterone, alprazolam, and placebo in treatment of severe premenstrual syndrome. JAMA 1995; 274:51–57.

49. Rickels K, Freeman E, Sondheimer S. Buspirone in treatment of premenstrual syndrome. Lancet 1989; i:777.

50. Schmidt PJ, Grover GN, Rubinow DR. Alprazolam in the treatment of premenstrual syndrome: a double-blind, placebo-controlled trial. Arch Gen Psychiatry 1993; 50:467–473.

51. Harrison WM, Endicott J, Nee J. Treatment of premenstrual depression with nortriptyline: a pilot study. Clin Psychiatry 1989; 50:136–139.

52. Dalton K. The Premenstrual Syndrome and Progesterone Therapy. 2d ed. Chicago: Year Book Medical Publishers, 1984.

53. Day J. Danazol and the premenstrual syndrome. Postgrad Med J 1979; 55(suppl 5):87–89.

54. Muse KN, Cetel NS, Futterman LA, Yen SC. The premenstrual syndrome: effects of "medical ovariectomy." N Engl J Med 1984; 311:1345–1349.

55. Mortola JF. Applications of gonadotropin-releasing hormone analogues in the treatment of premenstrual syndrome. Clin Obstet Gynecol 1993; 36:753–763.

56. Hahn PM. Van Vugt DA. Reid RL. A randomized, placebo-controlled, crossover trial of danazol for the treatment of premenstrual syndrome. Psychoneuroendocrinology 1995; 20:193–209.

57. Smith RN, Studd JW, Zamblera D, Holland EF. A randomised comparison over 8 months of 100 micrograms and 200 micrograms twice weekly doses of transdermal oestradiol in the treatment of severe premenstrual syndrome. Br J Obstet Gynaecol 1995; 102:475–484.

58. Mortola JF, Girton L, Fischer U. Successful treatment of severe premenstrual syndrome by combined use of gonadotropin-releasing hormone agonist and estrogen/progestin. J Clin Endocrinol Metab 1991; 72:252A–252F.

59. Mezrow G,. Shoupe D, Spicer D, Lobo R, Leung B, Pike M. Depot leuprolide acetate with estrogen and progestin add-back for long-term treatment of premenstrual syndrome. Fertil Steril 1994; 62:932–937.

60. Halbreich U, Rojansky N, Palter S. Elimination of ovulation and menstrual cyclicity (with danazol) improves dysphoric premenstrual syndromes. Fertil Steril 1991; 56:1066–1069.
61. Wheeler JM, Knittle JD, Miller JD. Depot leuprolide acetate versus danazol in the treatment of women with symptomatic endometriosis: a multicenter, double-blind randomized clinical trial. II. Assessment of safety. The Lupron Endometriosis Study Group. Am J Obstet Gynecol 1993; 169:26–33.
62. Graham CA, Sherwin BB. A prospective treatment study of premenstrual symptoms using a triphasic oral contraceptive. J Psychosom Res 1992; 36:257–266.
63. West CP. Inhibition of ovulation with oral progestins—effectiveness in premenstrual syndrome. Eur J Obstet Gynecol Reprod Biol 1990; 34:119–128.
64. Casson P, Hahn PM, Van Vugt DA, Reid RL. Lasting response to ovariectomy in severe intractable premenstrual syndrome. Am J Obstet Gynecol 1990; 162:99–105.
65. Casper RF, Hearn MT. The effect of hysterectomy and bilateral oophorectomy in women with severe premenstrual syndrome. Am J Obstet Gynecol 1990; 162:105–109.
66. Plouffe L, Jr, Stewart K, Craft KS, Maddox MS, Rausch JL. Diagnostic and treatment results from a southeastern academic center-based premenstrual syndrome clinic: the first year. Am J Obstet Gynecol 1993; 169:295–303.
67. Mitchell ES, Woods NF, Lentz MJ. Differentiation of women with three perimenstrual symptom patterns. Nursing Res 1994; 43:25–30.
68. Yonkers KA. White K. Premenstrual exacerbation of depression: one process or two? J Clin Psychiatry 1992; 53:289–292.
69. McKinlay SM, Brambilla DJ, Posner JG. The normal menopause transition. Maturitas 1992; 14:103–115.
70. Bancroft J, Rennie D, Warner P. Vulnerability to perimenstrual mood change: the relevance of a past history of depressive disorder. Psychosom Med 1994; 56:225–231.
71. Matthews KA, Wing RR, Kuller LH, Meilahn EN, Kelsey SF, Costello EJ, Caggiula AW. Influences of natural menopause on psychological characteristic and symptoms of middle-aged healthy women. J Consult Clin Psychol 1990; 58:345–352.
72. Matthews KA, Wing RR, Kuller LH, Meilahn EN, Plantinga P. Influence of the perimenopause on cardiovascular risk factors and symptoms of middle-aged healthy women. Arch Intern Med 1994; 154:2349–2355.
73. Holte A. Influences of natural menopause on health complaints: a prospective study of healthy Norwegian women. Maturitas 1992; 14:127–141.
74. Abraham S. Llewellyn-Jones D, Perz J. Changes in Australian women's perception of the menopause and menopausal symptoms before and after the climacteric. Maturitas 1994; 20:121–128.
75. Hammar M, Berg G, Fahraeus L, Larsson-Cohn U. Climacteric symptoms in an unselected sample of Swedish women. Maturitas 1984; 6:345–350.

15

Psychiatric Aspects of Cerebral Vascular Disorders

Robert G. Robinson and Sergio Paradiso
University of Iowa College of Medicine
Iowa City, Iowa

Cerebrovascular disease represents one of the major health problems in the United States, with an estimated annual incidence of thromboembolic stroke between 300,000 and 400,000 (1). During the past 30–40 years, however, there has been a steady decline in the incidence of stroke. The age and sex-adjusted annual incidence of stroke in Rochester, Minnesota, dropped from 190 per 100,000 population in 1945–49 to 104 per 100,000 in 1970–74 (2). The decline was presumed to be related to the improved control of hypertension. Nevertheless, among adults over age 50, stroke still remains the third leading cause (behind heart disease and cancer) of mortality and morbidity in the United States.

The psychiatric complications of cerebrovascular disease include a wide range of emotional and cognitive disturbances. Although studies providing empirical data about individual disorders and their relationship to specific types of cerebrovascular disease have begun to emerge only within the last 10 years, these kinds of investigations are essential before we will have a firm empirical data base for our understanding of the clinical manifestations, treatments, and mechanisms of these disorders.

HISTORICAL PERSPECTIVE

The first reports of emotional reactions following brain damage (usually caused by cerebrovascular disease) were made by neurologists and psychiatrists in case descriptions. Although Meyer (3) believed that mental disorders following brain injury were probably the result of an interaction between social, personal, psychological, and biological factors, he proposed that in some cases a relationship might exist between severe mental disorders and specific locations and causes of brain injury. Babinski (4) noted that patients with right hemisphere disease frequently displayed the symptoms of anosognosia, euphoria, and indifference. Bleuler (5) reported that after stroke "melancholic moods lasting for months and sometimes longer appear frequently." Kraepelin (6) hypothesized a causal connection between manic depressive insanity and cerebrovascular disease. He stated that the diagnosis of states of depression may offer difficulties, especially when arteriosclerosis is involved because cerebrovascular disorder may sometimes be an accompanying phenomenon of manic depressive disease but may also itself engender states of depression.

The emotional symptoms associated with brain injury have frequently been attributed to the existence of aphasia (7). In the middle of the nineteenth century, Broca (8) localized the process of speech to the left hemisphere and deduced that the left brain was endowed with different functions than the right brain. Hughlings-Jackson (9) regarded language as an extension of brain function existing in two basic forms: the intellectual (conveying content) and the emotional (expressing feeling). He suggested that these components may be separated by disease.

Goldstein (10) was the first to describe an emotional disorder thought to be uniquely associated with brain disease, which he termed the catastrophic reaction. The catastrophic reaction is an emotional outburst involving various degrees of anger, frustration, depression, tearfulness, refusal, shouting, swearing, and sometimes aggressive behavior. Goldstein ascribed this reaction to the inability of the organism to cope when faced with a serious defect in its physical or cognitive functions. In his extensive studies of brain injuries in war, Goldstein (11) described two symptom clusters: those related directly to physical damage of a circumscribed area of the brain and those related secondarily to the organism's psychological response to injury. Emotional symptoms, therefore, represented the latter category (i.e., the psychological response of an organism struggling with physical or cognitive impairments). The catastrophic reaction will be described in greater detail in a later section of this chapter.

A second emotional abnormality, also thought to be characteristic of brain injury, was the indifference reaction described by Heacen et al. (12) and Denny-Brown et al. (13). The indifference reaction, associated with right hemisphere lesions, consisted of symptoms of indifference toward failures, lack of interest in family and friends, enjoyment of foolish jokes, and minimization of physical difficulties.

Another emotional disorder that has historically been associated with brain injury is pathological laughter or crying. Ironside (14) described the clinical manifestations of this disorder. Patients' emotional displays were characteristically unrelated to their inner emotional state. Crying, for example, may occur spontaneously or after some seemingly minor provocation. This phenomenon has been given various names, such as emotional incontinence, emotional lability, pseudobulbar affect, or pathological emotionalism. Some investigators have differentiated the pseudobulbar disorder, in which there are bilateral brain lesions and subjective feelings of being forced to laugh or cry, from emotional lability, in which there is an easy and sometimes rapid vacillation between laughter and crying. These disorders, however, have never been systematically examined or divided into subcategories based on reliable features such as a characteristic clinical presentation, etiology, or response to treatment. This disorder will also be discussed later in this chapter.

The first systematic study to contrast the emotional reactions of patients with right and left hemisphere brain damage was done by Gainotti (15). He reported that catastrophic reactions were more frequent among 80 patients with left hemisphere brain damage, particularly those with aphasia, than were indifference reactions, which occurred more frequently among 80 patients with right hemisphere brain damage. The indifference reaction was also associated with neglect for the opposite half of the body and space. Gainotti agreed with Goldstein's explanation (11) of the catastrophic reaction as a desperate reaction of the organism confronted with severe physical disability. The indifference reaction, on the other hand, was not as easy to understand. Gainotti suggested that denial of illness and disorganization of the nonverbal type of synthesis may have been responsible for this emotional symptom.

Despite the assertions by Kraepelin (6) and others (e.g., Ref. 16) that emotional disorder may be produced directly by cerebral infarction, many investigators have adopted "psychological" explanations for the emotional symptoms associated with brain injury. Studies examining the emotional symptoms associated specifically with cerebrovascular disease began to appear in the early 1960s. Ullman and Gruen (17) reported that stroke was a particularly severe stress to the organism, as Goldstein (11) had suggested, because the organ governing the emotional response to injury had itself been damaged. Adams and Hurwitz (18) noted that discouragement and frustration caused by disability could themselves impede recovery from stroke. Fisher (19) described depression associated with cerebrovascular disease as reactive and understandable because "the brain is the most cherished organ of humanity." Thus, depression was viewed as a natural emotional response to a decrease in self-esteem from a life-threatening injury and the resulting disability and dependence.

Systematic studies, however, led other investigators, who were impressed by the frequency of association between brain injury and emotional disorders, to hypothesize more direct causal links. In a study of 100 elderly patients with affective disorder, Post (16) stated that the high frequency of brain ischemia associated with first episodes of depressive disorder suggested that the causes for atherosclerosis and depression may be linked. Folstein et al. (20) compared 20 stroke patients with 10 orthopedic patients. Although the functional disability in both groups was comparable, more of the stroke patients were depressed. The authors concluded that "mood disorder was a more specific complication of stroke than simply a response to motor disability."

In conclusion, there have been two primary lines of thought in the study of emotional disorders that are associated with cerebrovascular disease. One attributes emotional disorders to an understandable psychological reaction to the associated impairment; the other suggests a direct causal connection between cerebrovascular disease and neuropsychiatric disorder.

CATEGORIES OF CEREBROVASCULAR DISEASE

The most pragmatic way of classifying cerebrovascular disease is to examine the means by which parenchymal changes in the brain occur. The first of these, ischemia, may occur either with or without infarction of parenchyma and includes transient ischemic attacks (TIAs), atherosclerotic thrombosis, cerebral embolism, and hemorrhage. The last of these, hemorrhage, may cause either direct parenchymal damage by extravasation of blood into the surrounding brain tissue, as in intracerebral hemorrhage (ICH), or indirect damage by hemorrhage into the ventricles, subarachnoid space, extradural area, or subdural area. These changes result in a common mode of expression, defined by Adams and Victor (21) as a sudden, convulsive, focal neurological deficit—or stroke.

Using this categorization (i.e., the means by which parenchymal changes occur), there are four major categories of cerebrovascular disease (Table 1). These include atherosclerotic thrombosis, cerebral embolism, lacunae, and intracranial hemorrhage. In numerous studies of the incidence of cerebrovascular disease (e.g., Ref 1), the ratio of infarcts to hemorrhages has been shown to be about 5:1. Atherosclerotic thrombosis and cerebral embolism each account for approximately one third of all strokes.

Atherosclerotic Thrombosis

Atherosclerotic thrombosis is often the result of a dynamic interaction between hypertension and atherosclerotic deposition of hyaline-lipid material in the walls of peripheral, coronary, and cerebral arteries. Risk factors in the development of atherosclerosis

Table 1   Classification of Cerebrovascular Disease

Ischemic phenomena (85%)
    Infarction
    Atherosclerotic thrombosis
    Cerebral embolism
    Lacunae
    Other causes (arteritis, e.g., infectious or connective tissue disease, cerebral
        thrombophlebitis, fibromuscular dysplasia, venous occlusions)

Transient ischemic attacks

Hemorrhagic phenomena (15%)
    Intraparenchymal hemorrhage
    Primary (hypertensive) intracerebral hemorrhage
    Other causes (hemorrhagic disorders, e.g., thrombocytopenia, clotting disorders, trauma)
    Subarachnoid or intraventricular hemorrhage
    Ruptured saccular aneurysm or arteriovenous malformation
    Other causes
    Subdural or epidural hematoma

---

include hyperlipidemia, diabetes mellitus, hypertension, and cigarette smoking. Athero-matous plaques tend to propagate at the branchings and curves of the internal carotid artery or the carotid sinus, in the cervical part of the vertebral arteries and their junction to form the basilar artery, in the posterior cerebral arteries as they wind around the midbrain, and in the anterior cerebral arteries as they curve over the corpus callosum. These plaques may lead to stenosis of one or more of these cerebral arteries or to complete occlusion. TIAs, defined as periods of transient focal ischemia associated with reversible neurological deficits lasting a few minutes up to 24 hours, almost always indicate that a thrombotic process is occurring. Only rarely is embolism or ICH pre-ceded by transient neurological deficits. Thrombosis of virtually any cerebral or cerebel-lar artery can be associated with TIAs.

Cerebral Embolism

Cerebral embolism, which accounts for approximately one third of all strokes, is usually caused by a fragment breaking away from a thrombus within the heart and traveling up the carotid artery. Less commonly, the source of the embolism may be from an atheromatous plaque within the lumen of the carotid sinus or from the distal end of a thrombus within the internal carotid artery, or it may represent a fat, tumor, or air embolus within the internal carotid artery. The causes of thrombus formation within the heart can include cardiac arrhythmias, congenital heart disease, infectious processes (e.g., syphilitic heart disease, rheumatic valvular disease, and endocarditis), valve pros-theses, postsurgical complications, or myocardial infarction with mural thrombus. Of all strokes, those due to cerebral embolism develop most rapidly.

Lacunae

Lacunae, which account for nearly one fifth of strokes, are the result of occlusion of small penetrating cerebral arteries. They are infarcts that may be so small as to produce no recognizable deficits, or, depending on their location, they may be associated with pure motor or sensory deficits. There is a strong association between lacunae and both atherosclerosis and hypertension, suggesting that lacunar infarction is the result of the extension of the atherosclerotic process into small diameter vessels.

Hemorrhage

Intracranial hemorrhage (ICH) is the fourth most frequent cause of stroke. The main causes of intracranial hemorrhage that present as acute strokes include hypertension, rupture of saccular aneurysms or arteriovenous malformations (AVMs), a variety of hemorrhagic disorders of assorted etiology, and trauma producing hemorrhage. Primary (hypertensive) ICH occurs within the brain tissue. The extravasation of blood forms a roughly circular or oval-shaped mass that disrupts and displaces the parenchyma. Adjacent tissue is compressed, and seepage into the ventricular system usually occurs, producing bloody spinal fluid in more than 90% of the cases. ICHs can range in size from massive bleeds of several centimeters in diameter to petechial hemorrhages of a millimeter or less, most commonly occurring within the putamen, in the adjacent internal capsule, or in various portions of the white matter underlying the cortex. Hemorrhages of the thalamus, cerebellar hemispheres, or pons are also common. Severe headache is generally considered to be a constant accompaniment of ICH, but this occurs in only about 50% of cases. The prognosis for ICH is grave, with 70–75% of patients dying within 1–30 days (21).

Other Types of Cerebrovascular Disease

One of the other causes of cerebrovascular disease is fibromuscular dysplasia, which leads to narrowed arterial segments caused by degeneration of elastic tissue, disruption and loss of the arterial muscular coat, and an increase in fibrous tissue. Inflammatory diseases of the arterial system can also lead to stroke. These include meningovascular syphilis, pyogenic or tuberculous meningitis, temporal arteritis, and systemic lupus erythematosus. There are also many other less common causes of cerebrovascular disease.

PSYCHIATRIC DISORDERS ASSOCIATED WITH CEREBROVASCULAR DISEASE

The emotional disorders that have been associated with cerebrovascular disease are shown in Table 2. The disorder that has received the greatest amount of investigation is poststroke depression.

Poststroke Depression

Probably the most common emotional disorder associated with cerebrovascular disease is depression, which occurs in about 30–50% of patients after acute stroke (22).

Diagnosis

Although some studies of emotional disorders associated with cerebrovascular disease have not used strict diagnostic criteria (23), research diagnostic standards now require that structured interviews and standard diagnostic criteria be used [e.g., DSM-IV (24) or Research Diagnostic Criteria (25)]. The latest criteria published in DSM-IV now categorize poststroke major depression as a "mood disorder due to stroke with major depressive-like episode." For patients with subsyndromal forms of major depression, there are DSM-IV "research criteria" for minor depression (i.e., depression or anhedonia with at least one but fewer than four additional symptoms of major depression). An alternative diagnosis is "mood disorder due to stroke with depressive features," which only requires a predominant mood of depression.

Phenomenology

Robinson and colleagues have carried out two studies examining the phenomenology of poststroke depression (PSD). In the first (26), the frequency of depressive symptoms was compared between a group of 43 patients with major PSD and a group of 43 age-matched patients with "functional" (i.e., no known brain pathology) depression. The main finding was that both groups showed almost identical profiles of symptoms (including symptoms that were not part of the diagnostic criteria) (Fig. 1). More than 50% of the patients who met diagnostic criteria for major PSD reported sadness, anxiety, tension, loss of interest and concentration, sleep disturbances with early morning awakening, loss of appetite with weight loss, difficulty concentrating and thinking, and thoughts of death.

In the second study (27), depressive symptoms among stroke patients were assessed for their specificity for depression (i.e., the frequency of depressive symptoms in patients with an acute stroke and depressed mood were compared to the frequency of these symptoms in acute stroke patients without a depressed mood). In addition, it was also determined whether neuropsychological impairments such as denial or neglect were masking depressive symptoms that would result in a failure to diagnose depression. A consecutive series of 85 stroke patients who acknowledged the presence of a depressed mood (no other symptom was required) were compared with 120 stroke patients without a depressed mood. The study found that, except for early morning awakening, all the affective and autonomic symptoms of depression were significantly more frequent among patients with a depressed mood than among patients without a depressed mood ($p < 0.01$) (Fig. 2). Moreover, the presence of nonspecific symptoms of depression (i.e., the frequency of depressive symptoms in the nondepressed group) may have led to false-positive diagnoses in only 3% of patients, and only 5% of patients had all the symptoms necessary for a diagnosis of major depression except for feelings of sadness (i.e., possible false-negative cases). Therefore, the use of DSM-III criteria in an acutely medically ill population does not appear to produce significant numbers of false-positive or false-negative cases.

In summary, the phenomenology of depressive disorder in stroke patients appears to be virtually identical to that found in patients with primary mood disorders. In addition, the presence of a severe physical illness such as acute cerebral infarction does not appear to lead to significant number of nonspecific depressive symptoms or incorrectly diagnosed cases of depression.

Prevalence

In a study of 103 patients with acute cerebrovascular lesions, Robinson et al. (22) found that 26% of patients who could reliably respond to a verbal interview had the symptom cluster of major depression, and that 20% showed the symptom cluster of minor (dysthymic) depression. Others (28–31) have reported a similar prevalence of depression in stroke patients in a variety of settings including rehabilitation centers, general hospitals, and outpatient clinics. The frequency of depression in community settings, how-

Table 2 Clinical Syndromes Associated with Cerebrovascular Disease

Syndrome	Prevalence (%)	Clinical symptoms	Associated lesion location
Major depression	20	Depressed mood, diurnal mood variation, loss of energy, anxiety, restlessness, worry, weight loss, decreased appetite, early morning awakening, delayed sleep onset, social withdrawal, and irritability	Left front lobe Left basal ganglia
Minor depression	20	Depressed mood, anxiety, restlessness, worry, diurnal mood variation, hopelessness, loss of energy, delayed sleep onset, early morning awakening, social withdrawal, weight loss, and decreased appetite	Right or left parietal and occipital regions
Mania	Unknown, rare	Elevated mood, increased energy, increased appetite, decreased sleep, feeling of well-being, pressured speech, flight of ideas, grandiose thoughts	Right basotemporal or right orbitofrontal lesions
Bipolar mood disorder	Unknown, rare	Symptoms of major depression alternating with mania	Right basal ganglia or right thalamic lesions
Anxiety Disorder	27	Symptoms of major depression, intense worry and anxious foreboding in addition to depression, associated light-headedness or palpitations and muscle tension or restlessness, difficulty concentrating or falling asleep	Left cortical lesions, usually dorsal lateral frontal lobe

Psychotic disorder	Unknown, rare	Hallucinations or delusional	Right temporo-parietal occipital junction
Apathy			
Without depression	22	Loss of drive, motivation, interest, low energy, unconcern	Posterior internal capsule
With depression	11		
Pathological laughing and crying	20	Frequent, usually brief laughing and/or crying; crying not caused by sadness or out of proportion to it; social withdrawal secondary to emotional outbursts	Frequently bilateral hemispheric lesions; Can occur with almost any lesion location
Anosognosia	24–43	Denial of impairment related to motor function, sensory perception, visual perception or other modality with an apparent lack of concern	Right hemisphere and enlarged ventricles
Catastrophic reaction	19	Anxiety reaction, tears, aggressive behavior, swearing, displacement, refusal, renouncement, compensatory boasting	Left anterior-subcortical
Aprosodias			
Motor	Unknown	Poor expression of emotional prosody and gesturing, good prosodic comprehension and gesturing, denial of feelings of depression	Right hemisphere posterior inferior frontal lobe and basal ganglia
Sensory	32–49	Good expression of emotional prosody and gesturing, poor prosodic comprehension and gesturing, difficulty empathizing with others	Right hemisphere posterior inferior parietal lobe and posterior superior temporal lobe

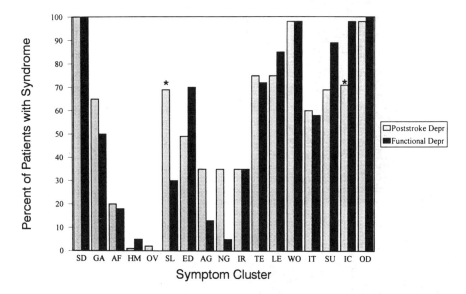

Figure 1 Comparison of symptom profiles in patients with major depression following stroke or functional major depression. The groups are compared in their frequency of syndromes elicited by the Present State Exam. The groups were not significantly different in any syndrome, except slowness (SL) was more frequent in the stroke patients as was loss of interest and concentration (IC) in the functional depression patients. SD = simple depression; GA = general anxiety; AF = affective flattening; HM = hypomania; OV = overactivity; ED = self-depreciation, guilt, lost affect; AG = agitation; NG = self-neglect; IR = ideas of reference; TE = tension; LE = lack of energy; WO = worrying; IT = irritability; SU = social unease; OD = morning depression, appetite loss, early waking, decreased libido. (Adapted from Ref. 26.)

ever, appears to be lower. House et al. (32) found that 11% of stroke patients had major depression and 12% had other depression among 89 community patients, and Burvill et al. (33) found that among 294 community patients in Australia 15% of patients had major depression and 8% had minor depression. The mean frequency of major depression from all reported studies is 20%, while the mean frequency of minor depression is also 20% (34).

Thus, about 40% of patients may develop depression within the first few months after an acute stroke. About half of these will show the symptoms cluster of major depression; the other half will show the symptom cluster of minor depression.

Duration

In a 2-year longitudinal study, a consecutive series of 103 acute stroke patients were prospectively studied (34). At the time of the initial in-hospital evaluation, 26% of the

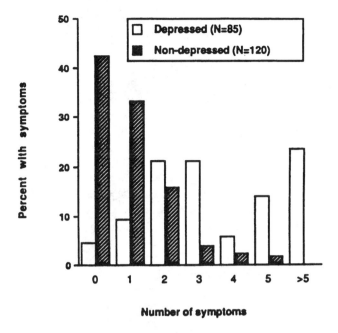

Figure 2 Autonomic and psychological symptoms of depression among patients with depressed mood after stroke. (From Ref. 27.)

patients had the symptom cluster of major depression, whereas 20% had the symptom cluster of minor depression. Although either major or minor depressive disorders was still present in 86% of patients with in-hospital major depression at 6 months follow-up, only one of five patients with major depression continued to have major depression at 1 year follow-up (two cases had minor depression). Patients with minor depression had a less favorable prognosis, with only 40% having no depression at 1 year and 30% having no depression at 2 years follow-up. In addition, about 30% of patients who were not depressed in-hospital became depressed after discharge. Thus, the natural course of major depression appeared to be between 6 months and 1 year, whereas the duration of minor depression was more variable and in many cases the patients appeared to be chronically depressed.

Morris et al. (29) found that among a group of 99 patients in a stroke rehabilitation hospital in Australia, major depression had a duration of 40 weeks, whereas adjustment disorders (minor depression) had a duration of depression of only 12 weeks. These findings confirm the approximately 1-year duration of major depression but suggest that less severe depressive disorders may be more variable in their duration. Astrom et al. (30) found that among 80 patients with acute stroke, 27 developed major depression in hospital or at 3 months follow-up. Of these major depression patients, 15 (60%) had recovered by 1 year follow-up, but by 3 years follow-up only 1 more patient had recovered. Similarly, Burvill et al. (33) found that 54% of 42 patients with major depression at 4 months poststroke had recovered by one year follow-up. Twenty-nine percent continued to have major depression, and 17% had minor depression. This indicates that there may be a minority of patients with either major or minor depression who develop prolonged poststroke depressions.

Several factors have been identified that can influence the natural course of poststroke depression. One is whether the diagnosis is major or minor depression. A second factor is treatment of depression with antidepressant drugs (discussed below). A third factor is lesion location. Starkstein et al. (35) compared two groups of depressed patients: one group ($N = 6$) had recovered from depression by the sixth month poststroke, whereas the other group ($N = 10$) remained depressed at the same time point. There were no significant between-group differences in important demographic variables, such as age, sex, and education, and both groups had similar social functioning and degree of cognitive dysfunction. There were, however, two significant between-group differences. One was lesion location: the recovered group had a higher frequency of subcortical and cerebellar/brain stem lesions; the nonrecovered group had a higher frequency of cortical lesions ($p < 0.01$). Impairments in activities of daily living (ADLs) were also significantly different between the two groups: the nonrecovered group had significantly more severe impairments in ADLs in-hospital than did the recovered group ($p < 0.01$).

In summary, the available data suggest that PSD is not a transient but a long-standing disorder with a natural course of approximately 9–10 months for most major depressions. Depressions lasting more than 2 years, however, do occur in some patients with major or minor depression. Lesion location and severity of associated impairments may influence the longitudinal evolution of these disorders.

Biological Markers

The dexamethasone suppression test (DST) (36) has been investigated as a possible biological marker for functional melancholic depression. Several studies have demonstrated that although there is a statistical association between major PSD and failure to suppress serum cortisol in response to administration of dexamethasone, the specificity of the test has been variable from study to study, and therefore the test does not appear to be diagnostically useful (37–39). In a study of 65 patients whose acute strokes had occurred within the preceding year, Lipsey et al. (38) found that 67% of patients with major depression failed to suppress serum cortisol compared to 25% of patients with minor depression and 32% of nondepressed patients. The sensitivity of the DST for major depression was 67%, but the specificity was only 70%. False-positive tests, found in 30% of patients, seemed to be related to large lesion volumes. Similarly, Reding et al. (39) reported a sensitivity of 47% and a specificity of 87%, with the more extensive strokes likely to lead to an abnormal DST response.

A study by Barry and Dinan (40) examined growth hormone response to desipramine as a biological marker of PSD. They found that growth hormone responses were significantly blunted in patients with PSD, suggesting that diminished α_2-adrenergic receptor function may be an important marker for PSD. The sensitivity of the test was 100%, and the specificity was 75%. Future studies may further examine the validity of the growth hormone response to desipramine as a marker of PSD.

Relationship to Lesion Variables

The first study to report a significant clinical-pathological correlation in poststroke depression was an investigation by Robinson and Szetela (41) of 29 patients with left hemisphere brain injury secondary to stroke ($N = 18$) or traumatic brain injury ($N = 11$). Based on computed tomography (CT) scan localization of the lesion, there was a significant inverse correlation between the severity of depression and the distance of the anterior border of the lesion from the frontal pole ($r = -0.76$) (Fig. 3) This surprising finding led to a number of subsequent examinations of this phenomenon in other populations. Robinson et al. (42) found a significant correlation between severity of depression and proximity of the lesion to the frontal pole in 10 patients with left frontal acute stroke who were right-handed and had no known risk factors for depression ($r = -0.92$, $p < 0.05$).

Several other investigators have also systematically examined the association be-

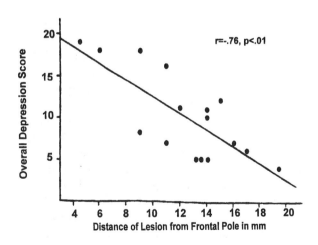

Figure 3 Relationship between severity of depression (as measured by a combined score on the Hamilton, Zung, and Analogue Depression rating scales) and distance of the lesion (either stroke or traumatic brain injury induced) from the frontal pole as measured on CT scan. The closer the anterior border of the lesion was to the frontal pole, the more severe the depressive symptoms. (From Ref. 41.)

tween anterior-posterior lesion location and PSD. Sinyor et al. (23) found a significant inverse correlation between depression scores and distance of the lesion from the frontal pole for a combined group of patients with either left or right hemisphere lesions ($r = -0.47$, $p < 0.05$). Although it was smaller, the correlation was in the same direction as that of the previous study, but was not specific to patients with left hemisphere lesions. Differences in demographic characteristics of the patients and the time since stroke (Sinyor's patients were several months poststroke) may underlie the different results.

Patients with stroke lesions who had been admitted to a rehabilitation center were examined by Eastwood et al. (28). Among patients with left hemisphere lesions, scores on a depression rating scale were significantly correlated with the distance of the lesion from the frontal pole. On the other hand, among patients with right hemisphere lesions, depression scores were not significantly correlated with lesion location. Similarly, Morris et al. (43) found that, after controlling for previous personal and family history of mood disorder, patients with single left hemisphere lesions (but not with right hemisphere lesions) showed a significant inverse correlation between distance of the lesion from the frontal pole and severity of depression. House et al. (32) found a significant, although less robust, correlation between severity of depression as measured by the Beck Depression Inventory (BDI) ($N = 56$) or the Present State Exam (PSE) ($N = 63$) score and proximity of the lesion to the frontal pole for patients with lesions of the right or left hemisphere at 6 months. Finally, Herrmann et al. (31) also found a significant correlation between severity of depression as measured by the Cornell Depression Scale and distance of the lesion to the frontal pole for 20 acute stroke patients with aphasia.

In summary, several studies conducted by different investigators have found that severity of depression during the first few months following stroke is significantly correlated with the distance of the stroke lesion from the frontal pole and that left frontal lesions are usually the most likely lesions to show this relationship. Thus, the location of the lesion along the anterior-posterior dimension appears to be an important variable in the severity of depression following stroke.

A study of 45 patients with single acute stroke lesions restricted to either cortical or subcortical structures in the left or right hemisphere found that 44% of patients with left cortical lesions were depressed, whereas 39% of patients with left subcortical lesions, 11% of patients with right cortical lesions, and 14% of patients with right subcortical lesions were depressed (Fig. 4) (44). Thus, patients who had lesions in the left hemisphere had significantly higher rates of depression than patients with right hemisphere lesions, regardless of the cortical or subcortical location of the lesion. When patients were further divided into those with anterior lesions and posterior lesions, 5 of 5 patients with left cortical lesions involving the frontal lobe had depression as compared to 2 of 11 patients with left cortical posterior lesions. Moreover, 4 of the 6 patients with left subcortical anterior lesions had depression as compared to 1 of 7 patients with left subcortical posterior lesions. Finally, correlations between depression

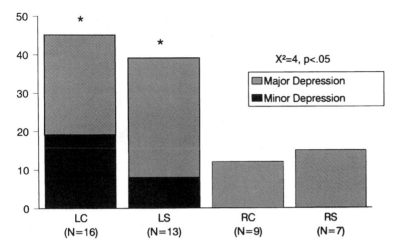

Figure 4   The percentage of major and minor depression in patients with single acute stroke lesions localized on CT scan to involve only cortical (cerebral cortex and/or underlying white matter) or subcortical (subcortical grey nuclei and/or internal capsule) structures. Patients with left cortical or subcortical lesions had a significantly greater frequency of depression than patients with any other lesion location. (From Ref. 44.)

scores and the distance of the lesion from the frontal pole were significant for both patients with left cortical lesions and patients with left subcortical lesions. These relationships were not significant for patients with right hemisphere lesions.

In a subsequent study (45), the relationship between lesions of specific subcortical nuclei and depression was examined. Basal ganglia (caudate and/or putamen) lesions produced major PSD in 7 of 8 patients with left-sided lesions, only 1 of 7 patients with right-sided lesions, and 0 of 10 with thalamic lesions ($p < 0.001$).

Astrom et al. (30) similarly found that among patients with acute stroke, 12 of 14 with left anterior lesions had major depression compared to only 2 of 7 patients with left posterior lesions ($p = 0.017$) and 2 of 23 with right hemisphere lesions ($p < 0.001$). House et al. (46) found only 4 cases of major depression among 40 patients with acute stroke in a community survey and did not find an association with left anterior lesions. Herrmann et al. (31), however, found major depression in 7 of 10 patients with nonfluent aphasia and left anterior lesions compared to 0 of 7 with fluent aphasia and left posterior lesion ($p = 0.0014$), but only during the acute poststroke period.

In summary, the evidence suggests that during the acute stroke period, the frequency of depression is higher among patients with left anterior hemisphere lesions than among patients with right hemisphere lesions. When other confounding factors are removed (e.g., prior lesions and family or personal history of mood disorder), left dorsal lateral frontal cortical and left basal ganglia lesions seem to produce a similar high frequency of major depression that is greater than that for any other lesion location.

Starkstein et al. (47) compared 37 patients with posterior circulation lesions to 42 patients with middle cerebral artery lesions. Patients with posterior circulation lesions were further subdivided into those with hemispheric lesions (temporo-occipital) and those with cerebellar/brain stem lesions. Major or minor depression occurred in 48% of the patients in the middle cerebral artery lesion group and in 35% of patients with cerebellar/brain stem lesions. At 6 months follow-up, frequencies of depression among patients with in-hospital depression were 82% and 20%, respectively. At 1–2 years follow-up, frequencies of depression were 68% and 0%, respectively (Fig. 5). Thus, patients with lesions in the cerebellar/brain stem region had a significantly shorter course of depression. These findings suggest that the mechanism of depression after middle cerebral artery lesions may differ from the mechanism of depression after cerebellar/brain stem lesions. The shorter duration of depression after cerebellar/brain stem lesions may be related to their smaller size and to the possibility that the cerebellar/brain stem lesions produced less injury to the biogenic amine pathways, which have been proposed to play an important role in the modulation of emotions (47).

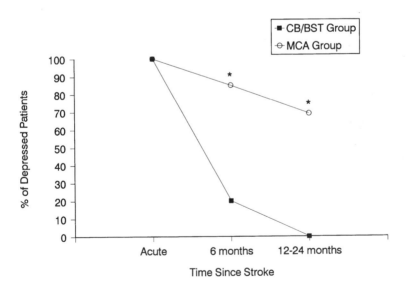

Figure 5 Duration of depression for patients with cerebellar/brain stem (CB/BST) lesions or middle cerebral artery (MCA) lesion. Patients with CB/BST lesions had shorter duration depressive disorders than patients with MCA lesions (From Ref. 47.)

In summary, depressions associated with cerebellar/brain stem lesions appear to be somewhat less frequent and shorter in duration than depressions associated with middle cerebral artery lesions. This may indicate differences in the mechanism of depression associated with these two lesion locations.

In a consecutive series of 93 patients with acute right hemisphere lesions, Starkstein et al. (48) reported that, of 54 patients with positive CT scans, 6 of 9 patients (66%) with major depression and 5 of 8 patients (63%) with minor depression had lesions that involved the parietal lobe, compared to 9 of 25 patients (36%) without mood changes and 1 of 12 patients (8%) with undue cheerfulness. In addition, similar results were reported by Finset (49), who found that patients with lesions in the parietal white matter had a higher frequency of depression than patients with lesions in any other location in the right hemisphere.

Premorbid Risk Factors

Although a significant proportion of patients with left anterior or right posterior lesions developed PSD, not every patient with a lesion in these locations developed a depressive mood. This raises the question of why clinical variability occurs and why some but not all patients with lesions in these locations develop depression.

Starkstein et al. (50) examined these questions by comparing 13 patients with major PSD to 13 stroke patients without depression who had lesions of the same size and location. Eleven pairs had left hemisphere lesions, and 2 pairs had right hemisphere lesions. Damage was cortical in 10 pairs and subcortical in 3 pairs. The groups did not differ on important demographic variables, such as age, sex, socioeconomic status, or education. They also did not differ on family or personal history of psychiatric disorders or neurological deficits. Patients with major PSD, however, had significantly more subcortical atrophy ($p < 0.05$), as measured both by the ratio of third ventricle to brain (i.e., the area of the third ventricle divided by the area of the brain at the same level) and by the ratio of lateral ventricle to brain (i.e., the area of the lateral ventricle contralateral to the brain lesion divided by the brain area at the same level). It is likely that the subcortical atrophy preceded the stroke. Thus, a mild degree of subcortical atrophy may be a premorbid risk factor that increases the risk of developing major depression following a stroke.

In the previously described study of patients with right hemisphere lesions, Starkstein et al. (51) found that patients who developed major depression after a right hemisphere lesion had a significantly higher frequency of family history of psychiatric disorders than did either nondepressed patients with right hemisphere lesions or patients with major depression following left hemisphere lesions. This suggests that a genetic predisposition for depression may play an important role after right hemisphere lesions. Eastwood et al. (28) and Morris et al. (29) have also reported that depressed patients were more likely than nondepressed patients to have either a previous personal history or a family history of psychiatric disorders.

In summary, lesion location is not the only factor that influences the development of PSD. Subcortical atrophy that probably precedes the stroke and a family or personal history of affective disorders also seem to play an important role.

Relationship to Physical Impairment

Both Robinson et al. (22) and Eastwood et al. (28) have reported a low but significant correlation between depression and functional physical impairment (i.e., activities of daily living). This association, however, might be construed as the severe functional impairment producing depression or alternatively the severity of depression influencing the severity of functional impairment. Two recent studies lend support to the latter suggestion.

Sinyor et al. (23) reported that although nondepressed stroke patients showed a slight increase or no change in functional status over time, depressed patients had significant decreases in function during the first month after stroke ($p < 0.05$). In another study, Parikh et al. (52) compared a consecutive series of 63 stroke patients with major or minor depression to nondepressed stroke patients during a 2-year follow-up. Although both groups had similar impairments in ADLs during the time they were in the hospital, the depressed patients had significantly less improvement by 2 years follow-up than the nondepressed patients (Fig. 6). This finding held true after controlling for important variables such as the type and extent of in-hospital and rehabilitation treatment, the size and location of the lesion, the patients' demographic characteristics, the nature of the stroke, the occurrence of another stroke during the follow-up period, and medical history.

In summary, although the correlation between depression and physical impairment after a stroke is not strong, the two variables do appear to interact. The severity of physical impairment may contribute to the development of PSD. However, if depression develops, the patient's physical recovery tends to be retarded for 2 years or more. This finding suggests that the negative effect of depression on physical recovery, especially on ADL, lasts even after the depression has subsided (i.e., major depression tends to spontaneously resolve in most cases within 1 year).

Relationship to Cognitive Impairment

Numerous investigators have reported that elderly patients with functional major depression have intellectual deficits that improve with treatment of depression (53). This issue was first examined in patients with PSD by Robinson et al. (54). Patients with major depression after a left hemisphere infarct were found to have significantly lower (i.e., more impaired) scores on the Mini-Mental State Exam (MMSE) (55) than a comparable group of nondepressed patients. Both the size of the patients' lesions and their depression scores independently correlated with the severity of cognitive impairment.

In a second study (50), stroke patients with and without major depression were matched for lesion location and volume. Ten of 13 patients with major PSD had a

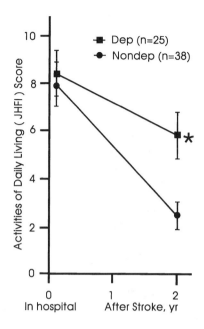

Figure 6 Change in activities of daily living scores (as measured by JHFI) for in-hospital depressed patients (either major or minor depression) and in-hospital nondepressed patients at the time of the in-hospital evaluation and 2 years later. Major or minor depression during the acute stroke period was associated with impaired physical and language recovery 2 years later. (From Ref. 52.)

MMSE score lower than that of their matched control subject, 2 had the same score, and only 1 patient had a higher score ($p < 0.001$). Thus, even when patients were matched for lesion size and location, depressed patients were more cognitively impaired.

In a follow-up study, Bolla-Wilson et al. (56) administered a comprehensive neuropsychological battery and found that patients with major depression and left hemisphere lesions had significantly greater cognitive impairments than nondepressed patients with comparable left hemisphere lesions ($p < 0.05$) (Fig. 7). These cognitive deficits primarily involved tasks of temporal orientation, language, executive motor, and frontal lobe functions. On the other hand, among patients with right hemisphere lesions, patients with major depression did not differ from nondepressed patients on any of the measures of cognitive impairment.

A recent follow-up study by Downhill and Robinson (57) of 140 patients over 2 years following stroke found that major depression was associated with a greater degree of cognitive impairment as measured by MMSE than minor depression or no depression for one year following stroke but only for patients with major depression

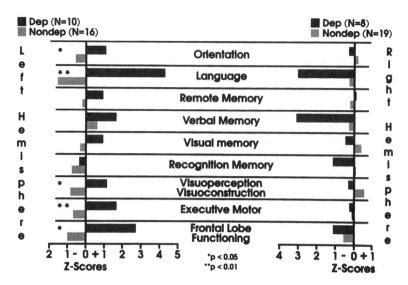

Figure 7   The results of neuropsychological testing in patients with major depression (Dep) or no mood disturbance (Nondep) following a single lesion of the left or right hemisphere. Scores in each cognitive domain were converted to Z-scores so that comparisons could be made across domains. A more positive Z-score indicates a greater degree of impairment. Note that among patients with left hemisphere strokes, patients with major depression were more impaired than the nondepressed in every cognitive domain. Five of these domains reached statistical significance, indicated by asterisks. None of the domains reached significance in the patients with right hemisphere stroke. (From Ref. 34.)

following a left hemisphere lesion. Patients with right hemisphere stroke and minor depression or patients who were 2 years poststroke did not show an effect of depression on cognitive impairment (Fig. 8).

In summary, major depression following a left hemisphere lesion is associated with significant cognitive impairments. Whether these cognitive impairments will improve with treatment of the depression remains to be determined. An uncontrolled study of nortriptyline or fluoxetine in patients with acute poststroke depression found that cognitive function improved with either of the antidepressants over a 6-week treatment period (58).

PSD and Aphasia

In a study of depression among patients with fluent or nonfluent aphasias, Robinson and Benson (59) found that 9 of 17 aphasic patients (53%) were depressed. These findings were similar to the frequencies of major and minor depression found among nonaphasic stroke patients (59). They also found that patients with nonfluent aphasias had a significantly higher frequency of depression than patients with fluent or global aphasia (71% vs. 44% vs. 22%, respectively) ($p < 0.05$). Signer et al. (60) and Herrmann et al. (31) have reported similar findings: depression was present in 63% and 70% of their nonfluent aphasic patients, as compared to 16% and 0% of their fluent aphasic patients, respectively.

Although it may be suggested that the higher frequency of depression among nonfluent aphasic patients was related to their greater awareness of their impairment, in a recent study, Starkstein and Robinson (61) concluded that lesion location was the most important variable in the association between PSD and nonfluent aphasia. In other words, the association between nonfluent aphasia and PSD was explained by the fact that the lesion location that produces nonfluent language may also have produced depression.

Another important issue is how to diagnose depression among patients with severe comprehension deficits. Some authors diagnose depression based only on observed behaviors, such as diminished sleep and food intake, restlessness and agitation, or retarded or tearful behavior (62). However, the sensitivity and specificity of using behavioral observations for the diagnosis of PSD have not been demonstrated. Most investigators have, therefore, excluded patients with severe comprehension deficits.

In conclusion, among patients with dominant hemisphere lesions, the frequency of depression is similar in patients with and without aphasia. Although nonfluent aphasia does not appear to cause depression, aphasia and depression may be produced by lesions of similar anatomical locations (frontal areas of the left hemisphere). Thus, patients with nonfluent aphasia are at higher risk of developing PSD than patients with other types of aphasia.

Mechanism of PSD

Although the cause of PSD remains unknown, one of the mechanisms that has been hypothesized to play an etiological role is dysfunction of the biogenic amine system. The noradrenergic and serotonergic cell bodies are located in the brain stem and send ascending projections through the median forebrain bundle to the frontal cortex. The ascending axons then arc posteriorly and run longitudinally through the deep layers of the cortex, arborizing and sending terminal projections into the superficial cortical layers (63). Lesions that disrupt these pathways in the frontal cortex or the basal ganglia may affect many downstream fibers. Based on these neuroanatomical facts and the clinical findings that the severity of depression correlates with the proximity of the lesion to the frontal pole, Robinson et al. (42) suggested that PSD may be the consequence of severe depletions of norepinephrine and/or serotonin produced by frontal or basal ganglia lesions.

In support of this hypothesis, laboratory investigations in rats have demonstrated that the biochemical response to ischemic lesions is lateralized. Right hemisphere lesions produced depletions of norepinephrine and spontaneous hyperactivity, whereas comparable lesions of the left hemisphere did not (64). More recently, a similar lateralized

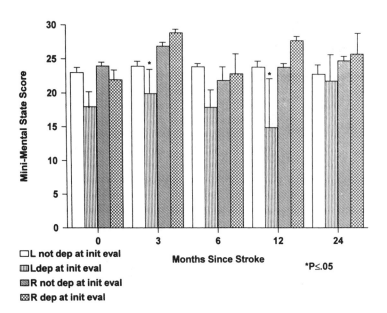

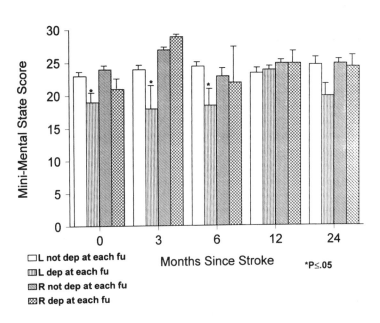

biochemical response to ischemia in human subjects was reported by Mayberg et al. (65). Patients with stroke lesions in the right hemisphere had significantly greater spiperone binding (predominantly 5-hydroxytryptamine type 2[5HT2] receptor binding) in noninjured temporal and parietal cortex than patients with comparable left hemisphere strokes. Patients with left hemisphere lesions, on the other hand, showed a significant inverse correlation between the amount of spiperone binding in the left temporal cortex and depression scores (i.e., higher depression scores were associated with lower serotonin receptor binding).

Thus, a greater depletion of biogenic amines in patients with right hemisphere lesions as compared with those with left hemisphere lesions could lead to a compensatory up-regulation of receptors that might protect against depression. On the other hand, patients with left hemisphere lesions may have moderate depletions of biogenic amines but without a compensatory up-regulation of 5-HT receptors and, therefore, a dysfunction of biogenic amine systems in the left hemisphere. This dysfunction may ultimately lead to the clinical manifestations of depression.

Treatment of PSD

Despite anecdotal reports of the efficacy of tricyclic antidepressants or stimulant medications in the treatment of PSD (66), only three randomized double-blind treatment studies on the efficacy of antidepressant treatment of PSD have been published. The first study (67) examined 14 patients treated with nortriptyline and 20 patients given placebo. The 11 patients treated with nortriptyline who completed the 6-week study showed significantly greater improvement in their scores on the Hamilton Rating Scale for Depression (68) than did 15 placebo-treated patients ($p < 0.01$) (Fig. 9). Successfully treated patients had serum nortriptyline levels between 50 and 150 ng/ml. Three patients experienced side effects (including delirium, confusion, drowsiness, and agitation) that were severe enough to require the discontinuation of nortriptyline. Similarly, Reding et al. (69) reported that patients with PSD (defined by having an abnormal dexamethasone suppression test) taking trazodone had greater improvement in Barthel

---

Figure 8 MMSE scores of patients divided by hemisphere of stroke (L or R) with major depression (dep) or no mood disorder (not dep—excluding patients with minor depression) in-hospital and over 2-year follow-up. The top panel shows scores of in-hospital patients who were depressed and the scores of those same patients (independent of whether they remained depressed) at each follow-up. The bottom panel shows scores of patients with major depression or no mood disorder at each follow-up time point (depressed group changes composition at each follow-up). Cognitive function is significantly more impaired in patients with major depression following left as compared to right hemisphere stroke. The cognitive impairment associated with major depression and left hemisphere stroke lasted for about 1 year. (From Ref. 57.)

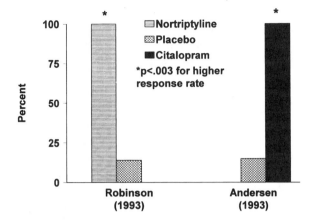

Figure 9 Percentage of patients with >50% reduction in crying episodes or PLACS score using double-blind methodology and either nortriptyline, citalopram, or placebo medication. Both nortriptyline and citalopram produced significantly greater reduction in crying episodes than placebo. (Adapted from Refs. 98 and 99.)

ADL scores (70) than placebo-treated control subjects ($p < 0.05$). A recent double-blind controlled trial using the specific serotonin-reuptake inhibitor (SSRI) citalopram found that Hamilton depression scores were significantly more improved over 6 weeks in patients receiving active ($N = 27$) compared with placebo ($N = 32$) treatment (71) (Fig. 9). At both 3 and 6 weeks, the active group had significantly lower Hamilton scores than the placebo group. This study, for the first time, established the efficacy of SSRIs in the treatment of poststroke depression.

Electroconvulsive therapy (ECT) has also been reported to be effective in treating PSD (72). It causes few side effects and no neurological deterioration. Finally, psychological treatment, including group and family therapy, has also been reported to be useful (73,74). However, controlled studies of these treatment modalities have not been conducted.

Social Factors and PSD

Psychosocial adjustment after stroke is an important issue to consider. Thompson et al. (75) examined 40 stroke patients as well as their caregivers an average of 9 months poststroke. They found that a lack of meaningfulness in life and overprotection by the caregiver were independent predictors of depression. They also found that psychosocial factors could predict depression and motivation in stroke patients. The authors suggested that both cognitive adaptation and social support may be useful approaches in facilitating a patient's ability to cope after a stroke.

Poststroke Mania

Although poststroke mania occurs much less frequently than depression (we have only observed three cases among a consecutive series of more than 300 stroke patients), manic syndromes are sometimes associated with stroke.

Phenomenology of Secondary Mania

Starkstein et al. (45) examined a series of 12 consecutive patients who met DSM-III criteria for an organic affective syndrome, manic type. These patients, who developed mania after a stroke, traumatic brain injury, or tumors, were compared with patients with functional (i.e., no known neuropathology) mania (76). Both groups of patients showed similar frequencies of elation, pressured speech, flight of ideas, grandiose thoughts, insomnia, hallucinations, and paranoid delusions. Thus, the symptoms of mania that occurred after brain damage (secondary mania) appeared to be the same as those found in mania without brain damage (primary mania).

Lesion Location

Cummings and Mendez (77) reported two patients who developed mania after right thalamic stroke lesions. After a review of the literature, they suggested a specific association between secondary mania and lesions in the limbic system or limbic-related areas of the right hemisphere.

Robinson et al. (78) reported on 17 patients with secondary mania. Most of the patients had right hemisphere lesions involving either cortical limbic areas, such as the orbitofrontal cortex and the basotemporal cortex, or subcortical nuclei, such as the head of the caudate and the thalamus. The frequency of right hemisphere lesions was significantly different than that for patients with major depression, who tended to have left frontal or basal ganglia lesions (Fig. 10).

These findings have been replicated in another series of eight patients with secondary mania (79). All eight patients had right hemisphere lesions (seven unilateral and one bilateral injury). Lesions were either cortical (basotemporal cortex in four cases and orbitofrontal cortex in one case) or subcortical (frontal white matter, head of the caudate, and anterior limb of the internal capsule, in three cases, respectively). Positron-emission tomography (PET) scans with [18F]fluorodeoxyglucose (FDG) were carried out in the three patients with purely subcortical lesions. They all showed a focal hypometabolic deficit in the right basotemporal cortex.

In summary, several studies of patients with brain damage have found that patients who develop secondary mania have a significantly greater frequency of lesions in the right hemisphere than patients with depression or no mood disturbance. The right hemisphere lesions that lead to mania tend to be in specific right hemisphere structures that have connections to the limbic system. The right basotemporal cortex appears to be particularly important because direct lesions as well as distant hypometabolic effects (diaschisis) of this cortical region are frequently associated with secondary mania.

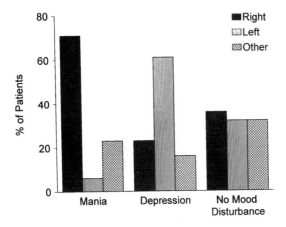

Figure 10 The percentage of patients with mania, major depression, or no mood disorder following brain injury divided by lesion location as visualized on CT scan. Mania was strongly associated with right hemisphere lesions and major depression with left hemisphere injury. (Data from Ref. 34.)

Risk Factors

Not every patient with a lesion in limbic areas of the right hemisphere will develop secondary mania. Therefore, there must be risk factors for this disorder.

In one study, patients with secondary mania were compared to patients with secondary major depression (78). Results indicated that patients with secondary mania had a significantly higher frequency of positive family history of affective disorders than did depressed patients or patients with no mood disturbance ($p < 0.05$). Therefore, it appeared that genetic predisposition to affective disorders may constitute a risk factor for mania.

In another study (76), patients with secondary mania were compared to patients with no mood disturbance who were matched for size, location, and etiology of brain lesion. The groups were also compared with primary mania patients and control subjects. No significant between-group differences were found either in demographic variables or neurological evaluation. Patients with secondary mania, however, had significantly greater degree of subcortical atrophy, as measured by bifrontal and third ventricular to brain ratios, than control patients ($p < 0.001$). Moreover, of the patients who developed secondary mania, those who had a positive family history of psychiatric disorders had significantly less subcortical atrophy than those without such a family history ($p < 0.05$), suggesting that genetic predisposition to affective disorders and brain atrophy may be independent risk factors.

In summary, the relatively rare occurrence of mania after stroke suggests that there are premorbid risk factors that impact on the expression of this disorder. Studies thus far have identified two such factors. One is a genetic vulnerability for affective disorder and the other is a mild degree of subcortical atrophy. The subcortical atrophy probably preceded the stroke, but its cause remains unknown.

Mechanism of Secondary Mania

Several studies have demonstrated that the amygdala (located in the medial portion of the temporal lobe) has an important role in the production of instinctive reactions and the association between stimulus and emotional response (80). The amygdala receives its main afferents from the basal diencephalon (which in turn receives psychosensory and psychomotor information from the reticular formation) and the temporopolar and basolateral cortices (which receive main afferents from heteromodal association areas) (81,82). The basotemporal cortex receives afferents from association cortical areas and the orbitofrontal cortex and sends efferent projections to the entorhinal cortex, hippocampus, and amygdala. By virtue of these connections, the basotemporal cortex may represent a cortical link between sensory afferents and instinctive reactions (83).

A case report (48) suggested that the mechanism of secondary mania was not related to the release of transcallosal inhibitory fibers (i.e., the release of left limbic areas from tonic inhibition due to a right hemisphere lesion). A patient who developed secondary mania after bleeding from a right basotemporal arteriovenous malformation underwent a Wada test before the therapeutic embolization of the malformation. Amytal injection in the left carotid artery did not abolish the manic symptoms (which would be the expected finding if the "release" theory were correct).

In summary, although the mechanism of secondary mania remains unknown, both lesion studies and metabolic studies suggest that the right basotemporal cortex may play an important role. A combination of biogenic amine system dysfunction and release of tonic inhibitory input into the basotemporal cortex and lateral limbic system may lead to the production of mania.

Treatment of Secondary Mania

Although no systematic treatment studies of secondary mania have been conducted, one recent report suggested potentially useful treatment modalities. Bakchine et al. (84) carried out a double-blind, placebo-controlled treatment study in a single patient with secondary mania. Clonidine (0.6 mg/day) rapidly reversed the manic symptoms, whereas carbamazepine (1200 mg/day) was associated with no mood changes and levodopa (375 mg/day) was associated with an increase in manic symptoms. Other treatment modalities, such as anticonvulsants (valproate and carbamazepine), neuroleptics, and lithium therapy, have also been reported to be useful in treating secondary mania (85). None of these treatments, however, has been evaluated in double-blind, placebo-controlled studies.

Poststroke Bipolar Disorder

Although some patients have recurrent manic episodes after brain injury, other manic patients have episodes of depression after brain injury. In an effort to examine which factors are crucial in determining which patients have bipolar as compared with unipolar disorder, Starkstein et al. (86) examined 19 patients with the diagnosis of secondary mania. The bipolar (manic-depressive) group consisted of patients who, after the brain lesion, met DSM-III-R criteria for organic mood syndrome, mania, followed or preceded by organic mood syndrome, depressed. The unipolar mania group consisted of patients who met the criteria for mania described above, not followed or preceded by depression. All patients had CT scan evidence of vascular, neoplastic, or traumatic brain lesion and no history of other neurological, toxic, or metabolic conditions.

The bipolar patients were found to have significantly greater intellectual impairment as measured by MMSE scores than the unipolar mania patients ($p < 0.05$). Almost half of the bipolar patients had recurrent episodes of depression, whereas recurrent episodes of mania occurred in approximately one fourth of patients in both the unipolar and bipolar groups.

Six of the 7 patients with bipolar disorder had lesions restricted to the right hemisphere, which involved the head of the caudate (2 patients), thalamus (3 patients), and dorsolateral frontal cortex and basotemporal cortex (1 patient) (Fig. 11). The remaining patient developed a bipolar illness after surgical removal of a pituitary adenoma. In contrast to the primarily subcortical lesions in the bipolar group, 8 of 12 patients in the unipolar mania group had lesions restricted to the right hemisphere, which involved the basotemporal cortex (6 patients), orbitofrontal cortex (1 patient), and head of the caudate (1 patient). The remaining 4 patients had bilateral lesions

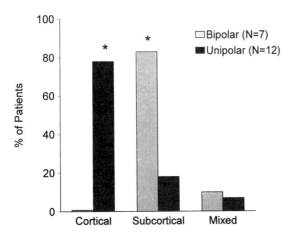

Figure 11   Lesion location in patients with bipolar mood disorder or mania without depression following stroke, traumatic brain injury, or surgical lesions. Patients with bipolar disorder had a significantly greater frequency of subcortical (basal ganglia or thalamus) lesions than patients with mania alone (i.e., unipolar) who had more cortical lesions. Only two patients had mixed cortical and subcortical lesions. *$p < 0.05$. (From Ref. 34.)

involving the orbitofrontal cortex (3 patients) and the orbitofrontal white matter (1 patient).

In summary, this study suggests that among patients with secondary mania, a prior episode of secondary depression may have occurred in about one third of them. Patients with bipolar disorder tend to have subcortical lesions (mainly involving the right head of the caudate or the right thalamus), whereas patients with pure mania tend to show a higher frequency of cortical lesions (particularly in the right orbitofrontal and right basotemporal cortex).

Poststroke Anxiety Disorder

Starkstein et al. (87) examined a consecutive series of patients with acute stroke lesions for the presence of both anxiety and depressive symptoms. Slightly modified DSM-III criteria for "generalized anxiety" disorder (i.e., excluding 6-month duration criteria) were used for the diagnosis of anxiety disorder. The presence of anxious foreboding and excessive worry were required, as were one or more symptoms of motor tension (i.e., muscle tension, restlessness, and easy fatigability), one or more symptoms of autonomic hyperactivity, and one or more symptoms of vigilance and scanning (i.e., feeling keyed up or on edge, difficulty concentrating because of anxiety, trouble falling or staying asleep, and irritability). Of a consecutive series of 98 patients with first-episode acute stroke lesions, only 6 met the criteria for generalized anxiety disorder (GAD) in the absence of any other mood disorder. On the other hand, 23 out of 47 patients with major depression also met the criteria for generalized anxiety disorder. Patients were then divided into those with anxiety only ($N = 6$), anxiety and depression ($N = 23$), depression only ($N = 24$), and no mood disorder ($N = 45$).

The only significant between-group difference in demographic variables was the presence of higher frequency of alcoholism in patients with anxiety only. No significant between-group differences were found in neurological examination. Examination of patients with positive CT scans revealed that anxious-depressed patients had a significantly higher frequency of cortical lesions (16 of 19) than did either the depression-only group (7 of 15), or the control group (13 of 27) (Fig. 12). On the other hand, the depression-only group showed a significantly higher frequency of subcortical lesions compared with the anxious-depressed group. Astrom (88), who examined 71 patients with acute stroke for generalized anxiety disorder, found that the majority of patients with GAD had comorbid major depression. The frequency of GAD with or without depression was about 25% throughout a 3-year follow-up, and the strongest correlates of GAD were right hemisphere lesions, absence of social contacts outside the family, and dependence upon others to perform their activities of daily living. At 3 years follow-up, GAD was associated with both cortical and subcortical atrophy as measured by CT scan.

In summary, the majority of poststroke anxiety disorders were comorbid with depression. Anxiety and depression occurred during the acute poststroke period and were associated with left hemisphere lesions, while anxiety alone was associated with

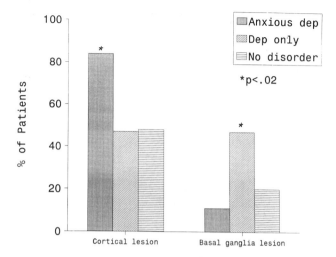

Figure 12   Frequencies of cortical and basal ganglia lesions among poststroke patients with generalized anxiety disorder plus major depression, patients with major depression alone, and patients with no mood or anxiety disturbances. Patients with anxiety plus depression had significantly more cortical lesions than the other groups, and patients with depression only had significantly more basal ganglia lesions than the other groups. (From Ref. 34.)

right hemisphere lesions. About one quarter of patients have GAD up to 3 years following stroke, and both social impairment and physical impairment appear to play a role.

Poststroke Psychosis

In a recent study of psychosis after stroke lesions, Rabins et al. (89) found a very low prevalence of psychosis among stroke patients (only 5 in more than 300 consecutive admissions). All 5 patients, however, had right hemisphere lesions, primarily involving frontoparietal regions. When compared with 5 age-matched patients with cerebrovascular lesions in similar locations but no psychosis, patients with secondary psychosis had significantly greater subcortical atrophy than the controls as manifested by larger frontal horns and area of the lateral ventricle (measured on the side contralateral to the brain lesion). Several investigators have also reported a high frequency of seizures among patients with secondary psychosis (90). These seizures usually started after the brain lesion but before the onset of psychosis. The Rabins et al. study (89) found seizures in 3 of 5 patients with poststroke psychosis, as compared to 0 of 5 poststroke control subjects.

It has been hypothesized that three factors may be important in the mechanism of organic hallucinations, namely a right hemisphere lesion involving the temporoparietal cortex, seizures, and/or subcortical brain atrophy (91).

In conclusion, secondary psychosis is a rare finding in patients with brain injury. They are frequently associated with lesions involving the temporo-parietal junction in the right hemisphere as well as subcortical atrophy or seizure disorder. Treatment has been primarily pharmacologic, utilizing either neuroleptic medication or antiseizure drugs. The mechanism of hallucinations and delusions has not been determined.

Apathy

Apathy is the absence or lack of feeling, emotion, interest, or concern and has been reported frequently among patients with brain injury. Using an apathy scale, Starkstein et al. (92) examined a consecutive series of 80 patients with single stroke lesions and no significant impairment in comprehension. Of 80 patients, 9 (11%) showed apathy as their only psychiatric disorder, while another 11% had both apathy and depression. The only demographic correlate of apathy was age, as apathetic patients (with or without depression) were significantly older than nonapathetic patients. Also, apathetic patients showed significantly more severe deficits in ADLs, and there was a significant interaction between depression and apathy on ADL scores, with the greatest impairment found in patients who were both apathetic and depressed.

Patients with apathy (without depression) showed a significantly higher frequency of lesions involving the posterior limb of the internal capsule as compared with patients with no apathy (92). Lesions in the internal globus pallidus and the posterior limb of the internal capsule have been reported to produce behavioral changes, such as motor neglect, psychic akinesia, and akinetic mutism (93). The ansa lenticularis is one of the main internal pallidal outputs, and it ends in the pedunculopontine nucleus after going through the posterior limb of the internal capsule (94). In rodents, this pathway has a prominent role in goal-oriented behavior (95), and dysfunction of this system may explain the presence of apathy in patients with lesions of the posterior limb of the internal capsule.

Catastrophic Reaction

As mentioned above, catastrophic reaction is a term coined by Goldstein (10) to describe the "inability of the organism to cope when faced with physical or cognitive deficits" and is expressed by anxiety, tears, aggressive behavior, swearing, displacement, refusal, renouncement, and, sometimes, compensatory boasting. Starkstein et al. (96) assessed a consecutive series of 62 patients using the Catastrophic Reaction Scale (CRS), which was developed to assess the existence and severity of the catastrophic reaction. Catastrophic reactions occurred in 12 of 62 consecutive patients (19%) with acute stroke lesions (96).

Three major findings emerged from this study. First, patients with catastrophic reactions were found to have a significantly higher frequency of familial and personal history of psychiatric disorders (mostly depression) than patients without the catastrophic reaction. Second, catastrophic reactions were not significantly more frequent among aphasic (33%) compared with nonaphasic patients (66%). This finding does not support the contention that catastrophic reactions are an understandable psychological response of "frustrated" aphasic patients (15). Third, 9 of the 12 patients with catastrophic reaction also had major depression, 2 had minor depression, and only 1 was not depressed. On the other hand, among patients without catastrophic reaction (i.e., 50 patients), 7 (14%) had major depression, 6 (12%) had minor depression, and 37 (74%) were not depressed. Thus, catastrophic reaction was significantly associated with major depression ($p = 0.0001$).

One may conclude from the above evidence that the catastrophic reaction may have more of a neurophysiological underpinning than just a behavioral response of patients confronted with their limitations. The catastrophic reaction also seemed to characterize a specific type of poststroke major depression (i.e., major depressions associated with anterior subcortical lesions). Anterior brain lesions (both cortical and subcortical) have been consistently associated with poststroke depression. Subcortical damage, however, has usually been hypothesized to underlie the "release" of emotional display by removing inhibitory input to the limbic areas of the cortex (97).

In conclusion, catastrophic reaction occurred in about 20% of stroke patients (96) and was associated with a positive family or personal history of psychiatric disorders. The catastrophic reaction was significantly associated with major depression and may have been mediated by a release of emotional display produced by anterior subcortical lesions.

Pathological Emotions

Emotional lability is a common complication of stroke lesions. It is characterized by sudden, easily provoked episodes of crying, which, although occurring frequently, generally occur in appropriate situations and are accompanied by a congruent mood. Pathological laughing and crying is a more severe form of emotional lability and is characterized by episodes of laughing and/or crying that are not appropriate to the context. They may appear spontaneously or may be elicited by nonemotional events and do not correspond to underlying emotional feelings. Other terms used for these disorders include emotional incontinence or pathological emotions.

Robinson et al. (98) examined the clinical correlates and treatment of emotional lability (including pathological laughter and crying) in 28 patients with either acute or chronic stroke. A Pathological Laughter and Crying Scale (PLACS) was developed to assess the existence and severity of emotional lability.

A double-blind drug trial of nortriptyline versus placebo was conducted. The doses of nortriptyline were 25 mg for 1 week, 50 mg for 2 weeks, 70 mg for 1 week, and 100 mg for the last 2 weeks of the study. Twenty-eight patients completed the 6-week protocol. Patients on nortriptyline ($N = 14$) showed significantly greater improvements in PLACS scores compared with placebo-treated patients ($N = 14$). These differences became statistically significant at 4 and 6 weeks following treatment (Fig. 13).

Although a significant improvement in depression scores was also observed, improvements in PLACS scores were significant for both depressed and nondepressed patients with pathological laughing and crying, indicating that treatment response was not simply related to an improvement in depression.

Andersen et al. (99) has also conducted a double-blind treatment study of pathological emotions following stroke using the SSRI citalopram. This study evaluated 13 patients using a crossover design. All patients on active treatment reported a greater than 50% reduction in the frequency of crying episodes compared to only two during the placebo period. All but 4 of the patients responded within one week of beginning active treatment.

In conclusion, poststroke depression and pathological emotions appear to be independent phenomena, although they may coexist. Moreover, both depression and pathological laughing and crying showed significant improvements following nortriptyline treatment.

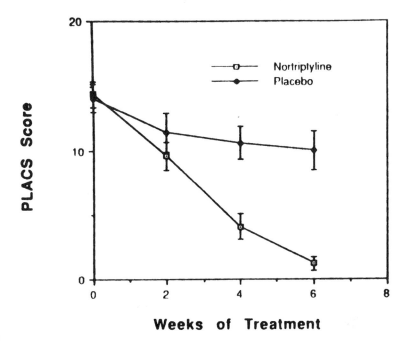

Figure 13 Mean scores of the Pathological Laughing and Crying Scale (PLACS) for patients receiving nortriptyline ($N = 14$) or placebo ($N = 14$). Repeated measure analysis of variances demonstrated significant group by time interaction ($F = 10.2$; $df = 3, 78$; $p < 0.001$). Nortriptyline-treated patients had significantly fewer pathological emotional symptoms at weeks 4 and 6 than placebo-treated patient. (From Ref. 98.)

Aprosodias

The aprosodias have been described by Ross and Mesulam (100) to be abnormalities in the affective components of language, encompassing prosody and emotional gesturing. Prosody can be defined as the "variation of pitch, rhythm, and stress of pronunciation that bestows certain semantic and emotional meaning to speech" (100).

Motor aprosody consists of marked difficulty in spontaneous use of emotional inflection in language (e.g., an absence of normal prosodic variations in speech) or emotional gesturing, while comprehension of emotional inflection or gesturing remains intact. Sensory aprosody, on the other hand, is manifested by intact spontaneous emotional inflection in language and gesturing, while comprehension of emotional inflection or gesturing is markedly impaired. In a manner analogous to the organization of prepositional language in the left hemisphere, both expression and comprehension of emotional inflection have been associated respectively with frontal and temporoparietal regions of the right hemisphere (100).

Starkstein et al. (101) examined prosody comprehension in 59 patients with acute stroke lesions. Using tapes expressing verbal emotion and photos of emotional facial expression, impaired comprehension of emotion was found in a mild form in 10 patients (17%) and in a severe form in 19 patients (32%). Severe aprosody was associated with three clinical variables: neglect for tactile stimulation, lesions of the right hemisphere including the basal ganglia and temporoparietal cortex, and significantly larger third ventricle-to-brain ratio. Although Ross and Rush (102) suggested that patients with sensory aprosody might not be able to recognize their own depressed mood, major depression was found in 2 of 19 (11%) severe aprosody patients and 7 of 30 (23%) nonaprosody patients (difference not significant).

In summary, impairment in the ability to comprehend emotion was found in about one third of patients. It was strongly associated with right hemisphere lesions, subcortical atrophy, and neglect but did not preclude patients from recognizing their own depression.

SUMMARY

Numerous emotional and behavioral disorders occur following cerebrovascular lesions (Table 2). Depression occurs in about 40% of stroke patients, with approximately equal distributions of major depression and minor. These disorders can be successfully treated with tricyclic or SSRI antidepressants.

Mania is a rare complication of stroke. It is strongly associated with right hemisphere damage involving the orbitofrontal cortex, basal temporal cortex, thalamus, or basal ganglia. Risk factors for mania include a familial history of psychiatric disorders and subcortical atrophy. Bipolar disorders are associated with subcortical lesions of the right hemisphere, while right cortical lesions lead to mania without depression.

Anxiety, which is present in about 25% of stroke patients, is associated with depression in the vast majority of cases. Among the few patients with poststroke anxiety and no depression, there is a high frequency of alcoholism and lesions of the right hemisphere.

Apathy is present in about 20% of stroke patients. It is associated with older age, more severe deficits in ADLs, and a significantly higher frequency of lesions involving the posterior limb of the internal capsule.

Catastrophic reactions occur in about 20% of stroke patients. These reactions are not related to the severity of impairments or the presence of aphasia, but may represent a defining symptom for one clinical type of poststroke major depression. Catastrophic reactions are associated with anterior subcortical lesions and may have resulted from a "release" of emotional display in depressed patients.

Psychotic disorders are rare complications of stroke lesions. Poststroke hallucinations are associated with right hemisphere temporoparietal lesions, subcortical brain atrophy, and seizures.

Aprosody occurs in about one third of acute stroke patients and is associated with neglect and right hemisphere lesions. The existence of aprosody, however, does not prevent patients from recognizing their own emotional state.

Pathological laughing and crying is another common complication of stroke lesions that may sometimes co-exist with depression and may be successfully treated with tricyclic antidepressants.

ACKNOWLEDGMENTS

This work was supported in part by National Institute of Mental Health Grants Research Scientist Award MH00163 (to RGR), MH40355, MH52879. The authors thank Thomas R. Price, John R. Lipsey, Rajesh Parikh, Carlos Castillo, Krishna Rao, and Godfrey D. Pearlson, Lynn Book Starr, and Paula Andrezewski, who participated in many of the studies described.

REFERENCES

1. Wolf PA, Dawber TR, Thomas HE, Colton T, Kannel WB. Epidemiology of stroke. In: Thompson RA, Green JR, eds. Advances in Neurology. New York: Raven Press, 1977: 5–19.
2. Garraway WM, Whisnant JP, Furlan AJ, Phillips LH, Kurland LT, O'Fallon WM. The declining incidence of stroke. N Engl J Med 1979; 330:449–452.
3. Meyer A. The anatomical facts and clinical varieties of traumatic insanity. Am J Insanity 1904; 60:373.
4. Babinski J. Contribution a l'etude des troubles mentaux dans l'hemiplegie organique cerebrale (anosognosie). Rev Neurol (Paris) 1914; 27:845–848.
5. Bleuler EP. Textbook of Psychiatry. New York: Macmillan, 1951.

6. Kraepelin E. Manic Depressive Insanity and Paranoia. Edinburgh: E & S Livingstone, 1921.
7. Benson DF. Psychiatric aspects of aphasia. Br J Psychiatry 1976; 123:555–566.
8. Broca P. Sur la faculte du langage article, suuivi d/une observation d'amphemie. Bull Anat Soc (Paris) 1861; 2:330–357.
9. Hughlings-Jackson J. On affections of speech from disease of the brain. Brain 1915; 38: 106–174.
10. Goldstein K. The Organism: A Holistic Approach to Biology Derived from Pathological Data in Man. New York: American Books, 1939.
11. Goldstein K. After Effects of Brain Injuries in War. New York: Grune & Stratton, 1942.
12. Heacen H, deAjuriaguerra J, Massonet J. Les troubles visoconstructifs para lesion parieto occipitale droit. Encephale 1951; 40:122–179.
13. Denny-Brown D, Meyer JS, Horenstein S. The significance of perceptual rivalry resulting from parietal lesions. Brain 1952; 75:434–471.
14. Ironside R. Disorders of laughter due to brain lesions. Brain 1956; 79:589–609.
15. Gainotti G. Emotional behavior and hemispheric side of the brain. Cortex 1972; 8:41–55.
16. Post F. The Significance of Affective Symptoms in Old Age. London: Oxford University Press, 1962.
17. Ullman M, Gruen A. Behavioral changes in patients with stroke. Am J Psychiatry 1960; 117:1004–1009.
18. Adams GF, Hurwitz LM. Mental barriers to recovery from strokes. Lancet 1963; 2:533–537.
19. Fisher SH. Psychiatric considerations of cerebral vascular disease. Am J Cardiol 1961; 7: 379–385.
20. Folstein MF, Maiberger R, McHugh PR. Mood disorder as a specific complication of stroke. J Neurol Neurosurg Psychiatry 1977; 40:1018–1020.
21. Adams RD, Victor M. Principles of Neurology. New York: McGraw-Hill, 1985.
22. Robinson RG, Starr LB, Kubos KL, Price TR. A two year longitudinal study of post-stroke mood disorders: findings during the initial evaluation. Stroke 1983; 14:736–744.
23. Sinyor D, Jacques P, Kaloupek DG, Becker R, Goldenberg M, Coopersmith H. Post-stroke depression and lesion location: an attempted replication. Brain 1986; 109:539–546.
24. American Psychiatric Association. Diagnostic and Statistical Manual of Mental Disorders—DSM-IV. Washington, DC: American Psychiatric Press, Inc., 1994.
25. Spitzer RL, Endicott J, Robins E. Research diagnostic criteria: rationale and reliability. Arch Gen Psychiatry 1978; 35:773–782.
26. Lipsey JR, Spencer WC, Rabins PV, Robinson RG. Phenomenological comparison of functional and post-stroke depression. Am J Psychiatry 1986; 143:527–529.
27. Fedoroff JP, Lipsey JR, Starkstein SE, Forrester A, Price TR, Robinson RG. Phenomenological comparison of major depression following stroke, myocardial infarction or spinal cord lesion. J Affect Disord 1991; 22:83–89.
28. Eastwood MR, Rifat SL, Nobbs H, Ruderman J. Mood disorder following cerebrovascular accident. Br J Psychiatry 1989; 154:195–200.
29. Morris PLP, Robinson RG, Raphael B. Prevalence and course of depressive disorders in hospitalized stroke patients. Int J Psychiatry Med 1990; 20:349–364.
30. Astrom M, Adolfsson R, Asplund K. Major depression in stroke patients: a 3-year longitudinal study. Stroke 1993; 24:976–982.

31. Herrmann M, Bartles C, Wallesch C-W. Depression in acute and chronic aphasia: symptoms, pathoanatomical-clinical correlations and functional implications. J Neurol Neurosurg Psychiatry 1993; 56:672–678.
32. House A, Dennis M, Mogridge L, Warlow C, Hawton K, Jones L. Mood disorders in the year after stroke. Br J Psychiatry 1991; 158:83–92.
33. Burvill PW, Johnson GA, Jamrozik KD, Anderson CS, Stewart-Wynne EG, Chakera TMH. Prevalence of depression after stroke: the Perth Community Stroke Study. Br J Psychiatry 1995; 166:320–327.
34. Robinson RG. The Clinical Neuropsychiatry of Stroke. Cambridge, England: Cambridge University Press, 1998.
35. Starkstein SE, Robinson RG, Price TR. Comparison of spontaneously recovered versus non-recovered patients with post-stroke depression. Stroke 1988; 19:1491–1496.
36. Carroll BJ, Feinberg M, Greden JF, Tarika J, Albala AA, Haskett RF, James NM, Kronfol Z, Lohr N, Steiner M, deVigne JP, Young E. A specific laboratory test for the diagnosis of melancholia: standardization, validation, and clinical utility. Arch Gen Psychiatry 1981; 38:15–22.
37. Finklestein S, Benowitz LI, Baldessarini RJ, Arana GW, Levine D, Woo E, Bear D, Moya K, Stoll AL. Mood, vegetative disturbance, and dexamethasone suppression test after stroke. Ann Neurol 1982; 12:463–468.
38. Lipsey JR, Robinson RG, Pearlson GD, Rao K, Price TR. Dexamethasone suppression test and mood following stroke. Am J Psychiatry 1985; 142:318–323.
39. Reding M, Orto L, Willensky P, Fortuna I, Day N, Steindler SF, Gehr L, McDowell F. The dexamethasone suppression test: an indicator of depression in stroke but not a predictor of rehabilitation outcome. Arch Neurol 1985; 42:209–212.
40. Barry S, Dinan TG. Alpha-2 adrenergic receptor function in post-stroke depression. Psychol Med 1990; 10:305–309.
41. Robinson RG, Szetela B. Mood change following left hemispheric brain injury. Ann Neurol 1981; 9:447–453.
42. Robinson RG, Kubos KL, Starr LB, Rao K, Price TR. Mood disorders in stroke patients: importance of location of lesion. Brain 1984; 107:81–93.
43. Morris PLP, Robinson RG, Raphael B. Lesion location and depression in hospitalized stroke patients: evidence supporting a specific relationship in the left hemisphere. Neuropsychiatr Neuropsychol Behav Neurol 1992; 3:75–82.
44. Starkstein SE, Robinson RG, Price TR. Comparison of cortical and subcortical lesions in the production of post-stroke mood disorders. Brain 1987; 110:1045–1059.
45. Starkstein SE, Boston JD, Robinson RG. Mechanisms of mania after brain injury: 12 case reports and review of the literature. J Nerv Ment Dis 1988; 176:87–100.
46. House A, Dennis M, Warlow C, Hawton K, Molyneux K. Mood disorders after stroke and their relation to lesion location. A CT scan study. Brain 1990; 113:1113–1130.
47. Starkstein SE, Robinson RG, Berthier ML, Price TR. Depressive disorder following posterior circulation compared with middle cerebral artery infarcts. Brain 1988; 111:375–387.
48. Starkstein SE, Berthier PL, Lylyk A, Casasco A, Robinson RG, Leiguarda R. Emotional behavior after a WADA test in a patient with secondary mania. J Neuropsychiatry Clin Neurosci 1989; 1:408–412.
49. Finset A. Depressed mood and reduced emotionality after right hemisphere brain damage. In: Kinsbourne M, ed. Cerebral Hemisphere Function in Depression. Washington, DC: American Psychiatric Press, Inc., 1988:49–64.

50. Starkstein SE, Robinson RG, Price TR. Comparison of patients with and without post-stroke major depression matched for size and location of lesion. Arch Gen Psychiatry 1988; 45:247–252.

51. Starkstein SE, Robinson RG, Honig MA, Parikh RM, Joselyn P, Price TR. Mood changes after right hemisphere lesion. Br J Psychiatry 1989; 155:79–85.

52. Parikh RM, Robinson RG, Lipsey JR, Starkstein SE, Fedoroff JP, Price TR. The impact of post-stroke depression on recovery in activities of daily living over two year follow-up. Arch Neurol 1990; 47:785–789.

53. Wells CE. Pseudodementia. Am J Psychiatry 1979; 136:895–900.

54. Robinson RG, Bolla-Wilson K, Kaplan E, Lipsey JR, Price TR. Depression influences intellectual impairment in stroke patients. Br J Psychiatry 1986; 148:541–547.

55. Folstein MF, Folstein SE, McHugh PR. Mini-Mental State: a practical method for grading the cognitive state of patients for the clinician. J Psychiatr Res 1975; 12:189–298.

56. Bolla-Wilson K, Robinson RG, Starkstein SE, Boston J, Price TR. Lateralization of dementia of depression in stroke patients. Am J Psychiatry 1989; 146:627–634.

57. Downhill JE, Jr, Robinson RG: Longitudinal assessment of depression and cognitive impairment following stroke. J Nerv Ment Dis 1994; 182:425–431.

58. Gonzalez-Torrecillas JL, Mendlewicz J, Lobo A. Effects of early treatment of post-stroke depression on neuropsychological rehabilitation. Int Psychogeriatr 1996; 7:547–560.

59. Robinson RG, Benson DF. Depression in aphasic patients: frequency, severity and clinical-pathological correlations. Brain Lang 1981; 14:282–291.

60. Signer S, Cummings JL, Benson DF. Delusions and mood disorders in patients with chronic aphasia. J Neuropsychiatry Clin Neurosci 1989; 1:40–45.

61. Starkstein SE, Robinson RG. Aphasia and depression. Aphasiology 1988; 2:1–20.

62. Ross ED, Gordon WA, Hibbard M, Egelko S. The dexamethasone suppression test, post-stroke depression, and the validity of DSM-III-based diagnostic criteria. Am J Psychiatry 1986; 143:1200–1201.

63. Morrison JH, Molliver ME, Grzanna R. Noradrenergic innervation of the cerebral cortex: widespread effects of local cortical lesions. Science 1979; 205:313–316.

64. Robinson RG. Differential behavioral and biochemical effects of right and left hemispheric cerebral infarction in the rat. Science 1979; 105:707–710.

65. Mayberg HS, Robinson RG, Wong DF, Parikh RM, Bolduc P, Starkstein SE, Price TR, Dannals RF, Links JM, Wilson AA, Ravert HT, Wagner HN, Jr. PET imaging of cortical S_2-serotonin receptors after stroke: lateralized changes and relationship to depression. Am J Psychiatry 1988; 145:937–943.

66. Finklestein S, Campbell A, Stoll AL, Baldessarini RJ, Stinus L, Pasvitch PA, Domesick VB. Changes in cortical and subcortical levels of monoamines and their metabolites following unilateral ventrolateral cortical. Brain Res 1983; 271:279–288.

67. Lipsey JR, Robinson RG, Pearlson GD, Rao K, Price TR. Nortriptyline treatment of post-stroke depression: a double-blind treatment trial. Lancet 1984; i:297–300.

68. Hamilton M. A rating scale for depression. J Neurol Neurosurg Psychiatry 1960; 23:56–62.

69. Reding JJ, Orto LA, Winter SW, Fortuna IM, DiPonte P, McDowell FH. Antidepressant therapy after stroke: a double-blind trial. Arch Neurol 1986; 43:763–765.

70. Granger CV, Denis LS, Peters NC, Sherwood CC, Barrett JE. Stroke rehabilitation: analysis of repeated Barthel Index measures. Arch Phys Med Rehabil 1979; 60:14–17.

71. Andersen G, Vestergaard K, Lauritzen L. Effective treatment of poststroke depression with the selective serotonin reuptake inhibitor citalopram. Stroke 1994; 25:1099–1104.

72. Murray GB, Shea V, Conn DR. Electroconvulsive therapy for post-stroke depression. J Clin Psychiatry 1987; 47:258–260.

73. Oradei DM, Waite NS. Group psychotherapy with stroke patients during the immediate recovery phase. Am J Orthopsychiatry 1974; 44:386–395.

74. Watzlawick P, Coyne JC: Depression following stroke: brief, problem-focused family treatment. Family Proc 1980; 19(1):13–18.

75. Thompson SC, Sobolew-Shobin A, Graham MA, Jenigion AS. Psychosocial adjustment following stroke. Social Sci Med 1989; 28:239–247.

76. Starkstein SE, Pearlson GD, Boston J, Robinson RG. Mania after brain injury: a controlled study of causative factors. Arch Neurol 1987; 44:1069–1073.

77. Cummings JL, Mendez MF. Secondary mania with focal cerebrovascular lesions. Am J Psychiatry 1984; 141:1084–1087.

78. Robinson RG, Boston JD, Starkstein SE, Price TR. Comparison of mania with depression following brain injury: causal factors. Am J Psychiatry 1988; 145:172–178.

79. Starkstein SE, Mayberg HS, Berthier ML, Fedoroff P, Price TR, Dannals RF, Wagner HN. Secondary mania: neuroradiological and metabolic findings. Ann Neurol 1990; 27:652–659.

80. Gloor P. Role of the human limbic system in perception, memory and affect: lessons for temporal lobe epilepsy. In: Doane BK, Livingston KE, eds. The Limbic System: Functional Organization and Clinical Disorders. New York: Raven Press, 1986:159–169.

81. Beck E. A cytoarchitectural investigation into the bondaries of cortical areas 13 and 14 in the human brain. J Anat 1949; 83:145–147.

82. Crosby E, Humphrey T, Laner E. Correlative Anatomy of the Nervous System. New York: MacMillan, 1962.

83. Goldar JC, Outes DL. Fisiopatologia de la desinhibicion instintiva. Acta Psiquiatr Psicol Am Lat 1972; 18:177–185.

84. Backchine S, Lacomblez L, Benoit N, Parisot F, Chain F, Lhermitte F. Manic-like state after orbitofrontal and right temporoparietal injury: efficacy of clonidine. Neurology 1989; 39:778–781.

85. Starkstein SE, Robinson RG. The role of the frontal lobes in affective disorder following stroke. In: Levin H, Eisenberg HM, Benton AL, eds. Frontal Lobe Function and Dysfunction. New York: Oxford University Press, 1991:288–303.

86. Starkstein SE, Fedoroff JP, Berthier MD, Robinson RG. Manic depressive and pure manic states after brain lesions. Biol Psychiatry 1991; 29:149–158.

87. Starkstein SE, Cohen BS, Fedoroff P, Parikh RM, Price TR, Robinson RG. Relationship between anxiety disorders and depressive disorders in patients with cerebrovascular injury. Arch Gen Psychiatry 1990; 47:785–789.

88. Astrom M. Generalized anxiety disorder in stroke patients: a 3-year longitudinal study. Stroke 1996; 27:270–275.

89. Rabins PV, Starkstein SE, Robinson RG. Risk factors for developing atypical (schizophreniform) psychosis following stroke. J Neuropsychiatry Clin Neurosci 1991; 3:6–9.

90. Levine DN, Finklestein S. Delayed psychosis after right temporoparietal stroke or trauma: relation to epilepsy. Neurology 1982; 32:267–273.

91. Starkstein SE, Robinson RG, Berthier ML. Post-stroke delusional and hallucinatory syndromes. J Neuropsychiatry Neuropsychol Behav Neurol 1992; 5:114–118.

92. Starkstein SE, Fedoroff JP, Price TR, Leiguarda R, Robinson RG. Apathy following cerebrovascular lesions. Stroke 1993; 24:1625–1630.

93. Helgason C, Wilbur A, Weiss A, Redmond KJ, Kinsbury NA. Acute pseudobulbar mutism due to discrete bilateral capsular infarction in the territory of the anterior choroidal artery. Brain 1988; 111:507–519.

94. Nauta WJH. Reciprocal links of the corpus striatum with the cerebral cortex and the limic system: a common substrate for movement and thought? In: Mueller J, ed. Neurology and Psychiatry: A Meeting of Minds. Basel: S. Karger, 1989: 43–63.

95. Bechara A, van der Kooy D. The tegmental pedunculopontine nucleus: a brainstem output of the limbic system critical for the conditioned place preferences produced by morphine and amphetamine. J Neurosci 1989; 9:3440–3449.

96. Starkstein SE, Fedoroff JP, Price TR, Leiguarda R, Robinson RG. Catastrophic reaction after cerebrovascular lesions: frequency, correlates, and validation of a scale. J Neurol Neurosurg Psychiatry 1993; 5:189–194.

97. Ross ED, Stewart RS. Pathological display of affect in patients with depression and right frontal brain damage. J Nerv Ment Dis 1987; 175:165–172.

98. Robinson RG, Parikh RM, Lipsey JR, Starkstein SE, Price TR. Pathological laughing and crying following stroke: validation of measurement scale and double-blind treatment study. Am J Psychiatry 1993; 150:286–293.

99. Andersen G, Vestergaard K, Riis J. Citalopram for post-stroke pathological crying. Lancet 1993; 342(8875):837–839.

100. Ross ED, Mesulam MM. Dominant language functions of the right hemisphere: prosody and emotional gesturing. Arch Neurol 1979; 36:144–148.

101. Starkstein SE, Fedoroff JP, Price TR, Leiguarda RC, Robinson RG. Neuropsychological and neuroradiological correlates of emotional prosody comprehension. Neurology 1994; 44:515–522.

102. Ross ED, Rush AJ. Diagnosis and neuroanatomical correlates of depression brain damaged patients. Arch Gen Psychiatry 1981; 38:1344–1354.

16

Traumatic Brain Injury

Ricardo E. Jorge and Robert G. Robinson

University of Iowa College of Medicine
Iowa City, Iowa

INTRODUCTION

Associations between traumatic brain injury (TBI) and a variety of neuropsychiatric disorders have been reported in the medical literature for many years. Adolf Meyer (1), for example, identified a number of disorders, which he referred to as the "traumatic insanities," and proposed associations between these disorders and specific lesion locations. Hillbom (2) studied 415 patients with wartime head injuries and emphasized the importance of frontal lesions in the pathogenesis of psychiatric and behavioral disturbances, particularly if they were located in the left hemisphere. In his classical study on the Oxford collection of head injury records, Lishman (3) analyzed potential etiological factors involved in the development of psychiatric disturbances following traumatic brain injury. These studies stressed the importance of biological variables such as the extent of brain damage, lesion location, and the presence of posttraumatic epilepsy in determining the type and duration of psychiatric disorder.

Relatively few studies, however, have examined the prevalence of specific mood disorders associated with TBI and their effect on outcome variables. Issues such as the prevalence of major depressive disorder following TBI, clinical variables that predict the development of major depression, the natural course of post-TBI major depression, and the influence of mood disorders on the longitudinal evolution of post-TBI physical and intellectual impairments are largely unexplored and deserve further research endeavor.

EPIDEMIOLOGY OF TRAUMATIC BRAIN INJURY

In the United States, the annual incidence of traumatic brain injury can be conservatively estimated as 200 per 100,000 population (4). This figure includes new cases of TBI leading either to immediate brain death or admission to a hospital.

The epidemiological data suggest that most of these injuries occur among adolescents and young adults, with a second peak occurring among elderly subjects (5). There is also a significant gender difference. Males have consistently shown two to three times the frequency of brain injury as do females (5). African Americans have higher rates of traumatic brain injury than other groups, a fact that may be explained by increased firearm exposure and higher homicide rates for this group (6).

Low socioeconomic status constitutes an independent risk factor for TBI. This association remains significant when controlling for race and ethnicity variables (7).

The single greatest risk factor for TBI is alcohol/drug use and alcohol/drug disorder. Close to one third of brain injury patients have an identifiable alcohol problem before trauma, and more than 50% are intoxicated at the time of the injury (8).

Transport-related causes (i.e., motor vehicle accidents and pedestrians hit by vehicles) are the most important form of exposure, particularly in younger patients. Falls are the second prevalent cause, showing a strong association with older age (4).

There is also a sustained increment in the relative frequency of brain injuries secondary to assault (specially penetrating injuries involving firearm use) as well as sports-and recreation-related injuries (9).

According to the U.S. National Hospital Discharge Survey of 1992, of those cases identified by brain injury as the principal diagnosis, 31% were further categorized as concussions, 20% as skull fractures (i.e., involving the vault, base, or other locations), 15% as intracranial hemorrhage, 9% as cerebral laceration and contusion, and the remaining 25% as nonspecific intracranial injury (10).

Approximately 80% of hospitalized brain injuries are considered mild, 10% are moderate, and 10% are severe (4). Case-fatality rate estimates vary from 3 to 8% among different U.S. incidence studies (4). Since 1979, however, the death rate associated with traumatic brain injury has decreased from 24.6 to 19.3 per 100,000 population per year. This is probably due to multiple interventions, including legislation, improved vehicle braking systems, passive-restraint systems, and enhanced neurosurgical intensive care (9).

Unfortunately, the aforementioned reduction in mortality rates may be mirrored by an increase in the number of TBI survivors with some type of chronic disability. The incidence of new disabilities from brain injuries may be estimated as 33 per 100,000 population per year or approximately 83,000 new disabled patients each year (4).

Although huge, the financial burden from TBI is difficult to estimate. Total costs for all head injuries occurring in 1985 were estimated to be $37.8 billion. About 65% of these costs were assigned to patients who survived the traumatic event; the remainder were related to head injury deaths (11).

CLINICAL FEATURES

Acute Behavioral Syndromes

Head injury encompasses a wide range of severity, from patients who die at the moment of trauma to those that do not require medical evaluation or assistance. Most patients admitted to the hospital with a head trauma diagnosis have mild brain injury. A minority of these mildly affected patients will develop acute complications (e.g., brain swelling, intracranial infection) or prolonged postconcussional symptoms (12). Furthermore, neuroradiological studies (CT, MRI) have established the presence of structural brain lesions in some mild head injury patients who have not experienced clinical complications (13).

The most consistent effect of head injury is impairment of consciousness, ranging from transient confusion to protracted coma. The Glasgow Coma Scale (GCS) is commonly used to grade the severity of traumatic brain injury (14). The scale gives a quantitative estimate of level of consciousness and neurological status based on patterns of eye opening, as well as best verbal and motor responses. GCS scores between 13 and 15 are considered indicative of mild brain injury, scores between 9 and 12 are indicative of moderate head injury, and scores between 3 and 8 indicate severe injury.

The early phase of recovery from TBI is characterized by disorientation, confusion, and impaired memory function. Apathetic withdrawal, agitation, or severe delirium may also be observed in these patients.

Duration of posttraumatic amnesia (PTA) has been another widely used measure of TBI severity. PTA is usually assessed using the Galveston Orientation and Amnesia Test (GOAT), which evaluates orientation to person, place, and time, as well as awareness of the accident and its consequences (15).

Duration of PTA has proved to be a good predictor of the degree of disability (16), vocational outcome (17), and the occurrence of personality change following TBI (18). During PTA, clinical descriptions of TBI patients overlap with those of delirium. Delirium is characterized by disorientation, prominent attentional deficits, amnesic dysfunction, vasoconstrictive impairment, and disorders in high-order thinking. In addition, patients may present with perceptual disturbances (e.g., illusions or hallucinations), delusional thoughts, psychomotor agitation or retardation, affective lability, and neuro-vegetative symptoms (e.g., tachycardia, hypertension, diaphoresis, and sleep-wake cycle disruption). Delirium usually has an acute onset and a fluctuating course. It is more frequently observed in severe TBI cases. Geriatric age, coexistent severe medical disease, polypharmacy, basal ganglia, and right hemisphere lesions have been also proposed as significant risk factors (19).

Chronic Behavioral Consequences of Traumatic Brain Injury

Cognitive Disorders

Cognitive disturbances are among the most important sequelae observed in the long-term follow-up of survivors of severe traumatic brain injury.

Levin et al. (20) reported on the cognitive outcome of 127 severe brain-injured patients who were capable of completing serial neuropsychological assessments during a one-year follow-up period (i.e., excluding those patients with persistent vegetative state or with very severe intellectual impairment). At a year follow-up, the brain-injured patients showed slower information processing and impaired memory function when compared with a neurologically intact control group. In contrast, linguistic and visuo-spatial abilities were found to be within the normal range (20).

Patients with mild and moderate head injuries may also show cognitive impairment following brain trauma. These patients complain of lack of concentration and memory deficits during the first weeks following TBI. However, spontaneous recovery is the rule for the vast majority of these patients (21,22).

Attentional deficits are among the most frequent neuropsychological symptoms that may be observed following resolution of posttraumatic amnesia. Attention consists of multiple processes subserved by interrelated neural networks. TBI patients may present with restricted attention span and slowed information processing. The most consistent findings, however, are associated with performance in most demanding tasks (e.g., in divided attention paradigms such as the Paced Auditory Serial Addition Task) (23). These processes are related to the functioning of a central executive system that integrates ongoing information with both long-term memory data and the individual's goals. Prefrontal circuits are essential components of the distributed networks that constitute the neural substrate of this executive system (24).

Linguistic competence is also frequently affected by traumatic brain injury. Approximately one third of severely brain-injured patients admitted to a rehabilitation facility showed fluent (51%), nonfluent (35%), or global aphasic syndromes. Aphasia, however, tends to resolve in the majority of these patients during the first year following the traumatic event (25). If language is assessed using the traditional neurological concepts of fluency, comprehension, repetition, and naming, anomia constitutes the most prevalent long-term linguistic deficit following trauma.

TBI patients may also have high-order language alterations and present with a defective narrative discourse, a lack of semantic coherence, aprosodia, and impaired language pragmatics. All of these result in an impoverished language and a reduced communication proficiency (26). Memory functions are distinctively impaired in TBI patients. Memory deficits are the more frequent cognitive disturbance reported by patients and relatives in the chronic phase of traumatic brain injury. Memory dysfunction is characterized by both anterograde and retrograde deficits, faulty sequencing of events, and inefficient encoding and storage strategies. The involvement of both prefrontal and medial temporal structures (e.g., the hippocampus) in these patients may represent the organic correlate of this particular neuropsychological profile (27).

Finally, a prominent defect in control and executive functions has been consistently described in patients surviving severe head injury. When confronted with a demanding environment, the adaptive functioning of TBI patients is often impaired. In this situation, the patient is affected by lack of initiative, rigid thinking, and faulty problem-solving ability (28). Executive functions include goal formulation, planning, selection of adequate response patterns, and monitoring of ongoing behavior.

Deficits in these functions are difficult to identify using standard psychometric testing. Several neuropsychological tasks, however, were specifically designed to quantify these deficits. These include the Wisconsin Card Sorting Test, the Tower of London Test, and the Trail Making Test. Once again, the executive dysfunction observed in

TBI patients is strongly associated with the selective involvement of fronto-subcortical pathways (28). In contrast to what happens with memory and control functions, visuospatial and praxic abilities are basically preserved during the chronic phase of traumatic brain injury. This finding may be explained by the relative indemnity of posterior association cortices. Unawareness or denial of deficits is a cognitive disorder frequently observed in TBI patients, particularly in those who have suffered extensive frontal lobe damage (29). Unawareness of deficits constitutes a severe behavioral sequel that impedes realistic goal setting and interferes with the rehabilitation process.

Dementia Following Traumatic Brain Injury

Dementia is a syndrome defined by the impairment of memory and at least another cognitive domain in the absence of an alteration of consciousness. The cognitive defect must have a significant impact on the social and occupational functioning of the involved subject. The DSM-IV classification system introduces the category dementia due to head trauma in order to classify those cases in which dementia is etiologically related to traumatic brain damage. Dementia due to head trauma is characterized by prominent memory and executive dysfunction, with roughly conserved visuospatial, praxic, and primary linguistic functions. In addition, these patients may be severely apathetic and evidence markedly slow information processing. The physical examination, in turn, may reveal the presence of extrapyramidal signs (30).

TBI may uncover a subjacent dementing illness in elderly subjects. On the other hand, a chronic subdural hematoma may present as a progressive dementia in this age group (31). There is also some evidence that the occurrence of previous traumatic episodes constitute a risk factor for the development of Alzheimer's disease (32).

Personality Changes

Traumatic brain injury patients may experience significant personality changes. These patients had been described as irritable, childish, inconsiderate, anxious, or aggressive. They lack foresight and misjudge the consequences of their actions. Disinhibition is a frequent and striking clinical feature that may lead to antisocial behavior. On the other hand, such patients may become apathetic, abulic, and withdrawn (33). Blumer and Benson (34) grouped these changes into two distinct syndromes: a pseudo-depressed personality syndrome, which is characterized by apathy and blunted affect, and a pseudopsychopathic personality syndrome portraying disinhibition, egocentricity, and sexual inappropriateness as its outstanding features. DSM-IV defines personality change due to traumatic brain injury as a persistent personality disturbance that represents a change from the individual's previous personality profile (or a deviation from normal development in children) and is attributable to the physiopathological changes produced by brain trauma. The disturbance must not occur exclusively during the course of delirium and cannot be diagnosed if dementia is present. In addition, the disturbance must not be better accounted for by another mental disorder (e.g., mood disorder or substance abuse). DSM-IV further categorizes this condition into the following subtypes: labile (if the predominant symptom is affective lability), disinhibited, aggressive, apathetic, paranoid, combined, and an unspecified (other) type (e.g., personality changes associated with a seizure disorder). The clinical syndrome is usually determined by premorbid personality features, psychosocial factors, and the extent and location of brain damage.

Disinhibition, antisocial conduct, and hypersexuality have been linked to the occurrence of orbitofrontal lesions (35), apathy, and abulia to medial frontal lesions, while aggression and poor impulse control have been described in patients with anterior temporal lesions (36). Traditional personality-assessment instruments such as projective tests or the Minnesota Multiphasic Personality Inventory (MMPI) have been used among TBI patients with conflicting results (37). The Neurobehavioral Rating Scale was specifically designed to assess and quantify personality and behavioral changes in this population (38).

NEUROPATHOLOGY

Closed Versus Penetrating Injury

At a first glance, head injuries may be divided into closed or penetrating injuries, accounting for the integrity of meningeal coverings following trauma. Missile wounds are the most frequent cause of penetrating brain injuries. They tend to produce discrete lesions and may be complicated by infection or hemorrhage. On the other hand, motor vehicle accidents are the most frequent cause of closed trauma, which represent the majority of traumatic brain injuries. Diffuse brain damage is a prominent feature of their pathophysiology, determining the clinical course and long-term outcome.

Primary Versus Secondary Brain Damage

Primary brain damage is largely effected by contact and inertial forces that occur at the time of injury. Contact forces result in laceration of the scalp, skull fractures, intracranial hemorrhages, contusions, and intracerebral hemorrhages. Inertial loading consists of acceleration/deceleration and rotational forces, which result in diffuse axonal injury and eventually acute subdural hematoma from the tearing of subdural bridging veins (39).

Secondary brain damage is produced by pathological processes that are initiated at the moment of injury but span a variable period following the traumatic episode. These include brain damage secondary to ischemia (e.g., resulting from associated hypotension and/or hypoxia), brain swelling, raised intracranial pressure (with consequent reduction of cerebral perfusion pressure), and infection (40).

Focal Lesions

Contusions and lacerations generally occur at the surface of the brain, are more prominent at the crest of cerebral gyri, and have a special predilection for the frontal and temporal poles, the orbitofrontal cortex, and the inferolateral aspect of the temporal lobe. Lacerations are usually accompanied by extracerebral hemorrhages (burst lobe). The selective damage of limbic and para-limbic cortical areas involved in emotional processing is associated with the occurrence of behavioral and psychiatric disturbances.

Bleeding may occur into the epidural space (i.e., between the skull and the dura), the subdural space (i.e., between the dura and the arachnoid), or the subarachnoid space. Epidural hematomas are generally associated with skull fracture and are more frequently encountered in the temporal region or the posterior fossa. Subdural hematomas usually affect the fronto-temporo-parietal convexity, are more frequent than epidural hematomas, and have an increased morbidity and mortality. Both types of collections, however, may present with significant mass effect that progressively distorts and compresses the adjacent brain, constituting a surgical emergency. Subarachnoid hemorrhage is highly prevalent among severe head injury patients. It may be occasionally associated with arterial vasospasm, a dreaded vascular complication occurring during the first week following brain trauma.

Intracerebral hemorrhages are often multiple, involving the frontal and temporal lobes and basal ganglia, and may have a delayed onset (i.e., hours or days after trauma).

Focal ischemic damage may result from traumatic vascular lesions (e.g., arterial dissection, vascular distortion and compression, venous thrombosis) or from arterial vasospasm (39).

Diffuse Axonal Injury

Diffuse axonal injury (DAI) involves widespread damage to axons but is preferentially evident within the corpus callosum, thalamus, and dorsolateral quadrants of upper brain stem. Pathologic processes include fragmentation of the axolemma, axonal transport disruption, axonal bulb formation, astrogliosis, and microglial activation. Although usually associated with immediate and persistent coma, lesser degrees of axonal disruption may be seen in patients with a lucid interval or even in patients who suffered mild brain injuries (41). Axonal pathology may determine functional disconnection between cortical and subcortical areas. Moreover, the involvement of ascending aminergic pathways may be related to the occurrence of psychiatric complications (e.g., major depression, apathetic syndromes).

Diffuse Ischemic Damage

Diffuse ischemic damage (DID) is highly prevalent among patients with severe head injuries. Graham et al. (42) reported severe ischemic damage in 27% of their 151 pathologically examined cases, moderately severe ischemic damage in 43%, and mild damage in another 30% of cases. Ischemic damage was more frequently observed in the hippocampus and the basal ganglia than in the cerebral cortex and cerebellum (42). These changes enabled early recognition and vigorous treatment of hypoxia and hypotension during patient transportation and upon admission to critical care units.

A CT-based classification scheme was proposed by investigators of the Traumatic

Coma Data Bank project (43). Criteria are defined along neuropathological and severity dimensions. They are based on the presence of diffuse or mass (focal) lesion patterns on CT scans. Diffuse lesions are further categorized according to the grade of compression of mesenchephalic cisterns and the amount of displacement of midline structures. Focal lesions are defined by their size and by the completion of surgical evacuation procedures. The influence of these different patterns of injury on the long-term neurobehavioral outcome of TBI patients has not been definitively determined. Previous studies have stressed the importance of diffuse brain injury as a predictor of long-term disability of TBI patients (44). On the other hand, focal lesions were associated with a more favorable prognosis. The antecedent of diffuse ischemic damage has been associated with a poor cognitive outcome at 1-year follow-up (45). A more recent study, however, did not find significant differences in neuropsychological outcome between two groups of severe TBI patients with focal or diffuse patterns of injury (46). Furthermore, we must emphasize that both focal and diffuse lesions coexist in most traumatic brain-injured patients.

NEUROCHEMICAL CHANGES FOLLOWING TBI

During the last decade, intensive research has been conducted on the complex neurochemical changes occurring after brain trauma. This was conducted with the hope of identifying interventions that could modify the pathologic processes resulting in diffuse neuronal death. For example, there is evidence of increased functional activity of basal forebrain cholinergic systems after TBI. Pathologic excitation of basal forebrain nuclei following acetylcholine release may result in structural damage of these nuclei and persistent behavioral deficits (47,48).

Traumatic brain injury acutely activates the sympathoadrenonmedullary axis as well as ascending catecholaminergic pathways. Circulating levels of catecholamines show a significant correlation with TBI severity as measured by Glasgow Coma Scale scores (49). In addition, activation of serotonergic systems has been suggested to play a role in posttraumatic metabolic dysfunction (50). The neurotoxic effect of the excitatory amino acids (EAA) glutamate and aspartate has been studied at length. Overactivity of EAA neurotransmitter systems plays a role in neuronal damage associated with diverse types of injury. This would be mediated through changes in the membrane conductance of sodium and calcium ions (51). In addition, traumatic injury is associated with the formation of highly reactive oxygen free radicals, which in turn will effect the peroxidation of cell membranes, cytosolic proteins, and nucleic acids (52). There is also evidence of the activation of complement proteins as well as different cytokines such as interleukin 1b and tumor necrosis factor (53,54). TBI patients may present with structural and functional changes of the hypothalamic-pituitary axis. Hormonal responses to trauma include increases in adrenocorticotropin and cortisol, growth hormone, and prolactin levels. In contrast, gonadotropins, sex steroid hormones, and thyroid hormone concentrations decrease. The presence of elevated prolactin levels is strongly associated with hypothalamic damage (55). Prigatano hypothesized that changes in adrenocortico-tropic hormone (ACTH) and cortisol levels that occur in TBI patients may mediate changes in mood (56). Corticotropin-releasing hormone is also involved in adaptation to acute stress and may also be responsible for certain features of anxiety and depressive disorders (57).

The impressive body of empirical research accumulated during recent years has provided theoretical support for the clinical testing of diverse therapeutic strategies such as EAA receptor blockade or the use of free radical scavengers (39). The magnitude, regional distribution, and relationship of the temporal course of these neurochemical changes to mood disorders remain largely unexplored and constitute an interesting field for further investigation.

OUTCOME OF TBI

The study of the long-term outcome of TBI patients involves the longitudinal analysis of neurological, neuropsychological, psychiatric, and psychosocial variables. Some of these variables are readily operationally defined, while others are more elusive and diffi-cult to quantify. The Glasgow Outcome Scale (GOS) has been widely used as a measure of the long-term outcome of TBI patients (58). It consists of five levels of outcome: death, persistent vegetative state, severe disability (conscious but dependent in activities of daily living), moderate disability (disabled but living independently), and good recov-ery (mild neuropsychiatric sequelae but able to resume an otherwise normal life). Al-though crude, the scale is appreciated for both its validity and high reproducibility. The long-term outcome of TBI patients is primarily related to severity of brain injury. In addition, the type and location of the intracranial lesion as well as the efficacy of acute medical and surgical treatments may have a decisive impact on it (59–61).

Outcome is also influenced by concurrent factors, which include age (62), socio-economic status, educational level, previous psychiatric disorders (e.g., history of alcohol and/or drug abuse, personality disorders), and premorbid social functioning levels (63). Finally, the quality and extent of rehabilitation services and the availability of social and vocational support also play a significant role in TBI outcome. The NIH Traumatic Coma Data Bank was initiated by the National Institute of Neurological Disorders and Stroke in order to characterize the natural history of traumatic head injury and to evaluate the determinants of recovery (64). Of 746 severely head-injured patients stud-ied in this cohort, 243 patients (32.5%) died, 315 patients (42%) were either severely disabled or in a vegetative state, 138 (18%) had moderate disability, and the remaining 50 (7%) had a good recovery as measured by the GOS at the time of hospital discharge (65).

Rimel et al. (21) analyzed the outcome of 170 patients with moderate head inju-ries at 3 months following traumatic brain injury. According to the GOS, 38% of moderate head injury patients made a good recovery, 49% were left with moderate disability, and 10% had severe disability. The mortality rate was 3%. The same authors found that the majority of mild head injury patients (78%) made a good recovery, 22% were left with moderate disability, and no patients experienced severe disability (22). As we have seen, cognitive and behavioral disturbances constitute important sequelae observed in the long-term follow-up of survivors of traumatic brain injury. The question is, how do these behavioral deficits express themselves in terms of disability? Deficits in cognition and personality contribute more to disability than other neurological deficits (e.g., hemiparesis) (66). The full impact of traumatic brain injury is perhaps manifested in social and vocational adjustment. Many patients are unable to return to work or to resume academic activities. In addition, those who do return frequently have to take less demanding jobs with reduced responsibilities and lower compensation (67). Ruff et al. (68) analyzed predictors of psychosocial outcome following severe head trauma. They reported that 18% of former workers had returned to gainful employment and 62% of former students had returned to school by 6 months follow-up. For those not back to work or school at 6 months, 31% of former workers and 66% of former students had returned by 12 months. The three most significant predictors for returning to work or school were age, intact verbal abilities, and speed of information processing. In their series of moderate head injury patients, Rimel et al. (21) reported that 69% of patients who had been gainfully employed before the injury were unemployed at 3 months follow-up. In contrast to mild head injury patients, socioeconomic and demographic factors were not significantly associated with unemployment. Significant predictors were related, however, to the severity of brain injury (e.g., length of coma or length of posttraumatic amnesia) (21). Furthermore, behavioral changes associated with TBI may disrupt interpersonal relationships and pose a great burden on family members (66). During the first year after injury, more than two thirds of relatives experienced moderate to severe degrees of burden as a consequence of the behavioral changes in their family member (69). Five years after the injury, the percentage of impeded relatives augmented to 90% (67). Consistent with these findings, Livingston et al. reported that about a quarter of family primary caregivers were depressed at 6 and 12 months following TBI (70).

In summary, patients and families may be confronted with behavioral problems, social isolation, and unemployment long after TBI. Thus, it is not surprising that psychosocial adjustment and community reentry have become the targets of rehabilitation efforts. The patient's motivation as well as awareness of cognitive and physical impairments proved to have a significant influence upon rehabilitation outcome (71). In addition, a history of alcohol and/or drug abuse may be also significantly associated with a poor outcome (8).

DEPRESSIVE DISORDERS

Mood and anxiety disorders have been found to be frequent complications of TBI. The presence of mood and anxiety disorders has also been found to play a relevant role in shaping long-term outcome. Dimken and Reitan (72) reported on the longitudinal evolution of emotional functions (measured using MMPI scores) in a consecutive series of 27 TBI patients followed for 18 months. They concluded that emotional disturbances tend to decline over time after injury and that they are associated with the presence of neuropsychological impairment. On the other hand, Fordyce et al. (73) found significantly higher MMPI depression scores in the chronic stage of TBI (i.e., 6 months after brain injury) than in the more acute stages. The prevalence of depressive disorders following TBI has varied dramatically from 6 to 77% (74–76). McKinlay et al. (77) reported indirect evidence of a depressed mood in about half of their patients at 3, 6, or 12 months following severe brain injury. Kinsella et al. (78) reported in a series of 39 patients within 2 years of severe brain injury that 33% were classified as depressed and 26% as suffering from anxiety.

Schoenhuber and Gentili found depressive symptoms in 39% of 103 patients with mild head injury interviewed at one-year follow-up and concluded that these patients have an increased risk of developing depression compared to an appropriate control group (79). More recently, Gualtieri and Cox estimated that the frequency of major depression in traumatic brain-injured patients lies between 25 and 50% (80). The variability in the reported frequency of depressive disorders, particularly major depression, may be due to the lack of uniformity in the psychiatric diagnosis. Most of the previously mentioned studies relied on rating scales (e.g., MMPI) or relatives' reports rather than on structured interviews and established diagnostic criteria (e.g., DSM-IV or DSM-III-R). Fedoroff et al. (81) examined the prevalence, duration, and clinical correlates of mood and anxiety disorders in a group of 66 patients admitted to the Shock Trauma Center of the Maryland Institute of Emergency Medical Services System (MIEMSS) with traumatic brain injury.

The patients were mostly white males of lower socioeconomic classes in their third decade. The principal cause of brain injury was motor vehicle accidents. The majority of patients (68%) had moderate brain injuries, 11 patients (17%) suffered severe brain injuries, and 10 patients (15%) were categorized as mild head injuries. Almost a third of these patients (30%) had a history of alcohol and/or drug abuse, and 11 patients (17%) had a personal history of psychiatric disorder (i.e., excluding alcoholism and/or drug abuse). Patients were evaluated during their in-hospital period and at 3, 6, and 12 months following brain injury. A semi-structured psychiatric interview was conducted using a modified version of the Present State Exam (PSE) (82). The PSE was modified to elicit symptoms related to mood and anxiety disorders. Affective disturbances were diagnosed according to DSM-III-R criteria (83). Quantitative depression ratings were obtained using the Hamilton Depression Rating Scale (HDRS) (84). Cognitive function was measured using the Mini-Mental State Exam (MMSE) (85), and impairment of activities of daily living was measured using the John Hopkins Functioning Inventory (JHFI) (86). Quantitative assessments of social functioning were made using the Social Functioning Exam (SFE) and the Social Ties Checklist (STC) (87). Follow-up data was obtained in 58 out of the 66 initially admitted patients (88%). Furthermore, 52 patients (79%) completed three out of four evaluations. There were no significant differences between the follow-up ($n = 58$) and the dropout ($n = 8$)

groups in background characteristics, initial psychiatric variables, severity of brain injury, or type and location of brain damage.

In the acute stage of TBI (i.e., approximately one month after brain injury), 17 of 66 patients (26%) developed major depression and another two patients (3%) developed minor (dysthymic) depression (81). Jorge et al. (88) cross-sectionally analyzed this data at the 3-, 6-, and 12-month evaluations. The prevalence of major depression during the year following traumatic brain injury remained stable at 25% with some patients recovering from major depression and other patients developing delayed-onset depressions (88). Minor depression was diagnosed in another eight patients during the course of the year (Fig. 1).

Of the 17 acutely depressed patients, seven (41%) also met DSM-III-R criteria for generalized anxiety disorder (GAD), while none of the 47 nondepressed patients met criteria for GAD (89). There were also 11 patients who developed major depression at some point during the follow-up period (i.e., 4 patients at 3 months, 4 patients at 6 months, and 3 patients at 12 months after brain injury). Thus, 28 of the 58 patients (47%) with follow-up data met DSM-III-R criteria for major depression at some time during the first year after the traumatic episode (90).

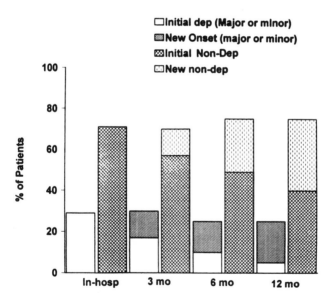

Figure 1 The percentage of patients initially evaluated while hospitalized for acute traumatic brain injury who were depressed or nondepressed at 3, 6, or 12 months follow-up. After the initial evaluation, patients whose depression had resolved were called new nondepressed, while nondepressed patients who became depressed were called new-onset depression. Note that the number of originally depressed patients declined over time, although the total depressed stayed fairly constant.

In addition to the frequency of depressive disorders, another important aspect of post-TBI mood disorders is their duration. Affective disorders may be transient syndromes lasting for a few weeks or persistent disorders lasting for many months (Fig. 2) (91).

Previous investigators have suggested that transient disorders may be associated with neurophysiological disturbances (e.g., neurochemical changes in the injured brain), whereas prolonged disorders may be reactive psychological responses to physical or cognitive impairment (92–94). Jorge et al. found that patients who developed major depression during the acute period had an estimated mean duration of depression of 4.7 months, with a minimum of 1.5 months and a maximum of 12 months. Seven patients developed transient depressive syndromes of less than 3 months duration (i.e., approximately 6 to 8 weeks), while another seven patients developed more prolonged depressive syndromes lasting 6 months or more. In addition, two patients had recurrent depressions with major depression in hospital, no depression at the 3- or 6-month evaluation, and major depression again at 1-year follow-up (88). In addition, anxious depressions had a significantly longer duration than nonanxious depressions. Anxious depression had a median duration of 7.5 months, while nonanxious depressions had a median duration of 1.5 months (Fig. 2) (89). Delayed-onset major depressions, in turn, had an estimated mean duration of 4.0 months (90).

In summary, major depression appeared to have a natural course of about 4–5

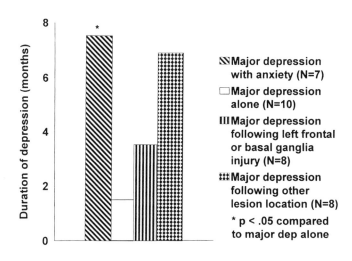

Figure 2   The duration of major depression in patients with major depression following acute traumatic brain injury. Patients with major depression plus generalized anxiety disorder had significantly longer duration depressions than patients with major depression alone. Patients with left frontal or basal ganglia lesions also tended to have shorter-duration depressions than patients with other lesions.

months following TBI. Some patients developed transient depressive disorders of 6 or 8 weeks duration, while others had depressions lasting up to a year.

Diagnosis

The general diagnostic category for post-TBI depressive disorders is mood disorder due to a general medical condition (TBI), and the pertinent subtypes are (1) with major depressive-like episode (if the full criteria for a major depressive episode are met) and (2) with depressive features (prominent depressed mood, but full criteria for a major depressive episode are not met). This diagnostic category, however, requires that the depressive disorder is judged to be a physiological consequence of the medical condition (e.g., TBI). If DSM-IV criteria are to be used in TBI patients, one of the basic issues that must be addressed is the specificity of symptoms on which these diagnostic criteria are based. For example, symptoms of major depression such as sleep, appetite, or libido changes may occur in patients with TBI as a consequence of brain injury or as a nonspecific consequence of an acute medical illness. Consequently, major depressive disorder could be systematically overdiagnosed. On the other hand, patients may deny the presence of a depressed mood as part of a general unawareness of deficit or a denial syndrome. This could result in underdiagnosis of depression. In an effort to examine this issue, the 52 post-TBI patients previously described were longitudinally examined for specificity of symptoms of depression (95). Depressive symptoms were divided into "autonomic" and "psychological" subtypes using the distinctions proposed by Davidson and Turnbull (96). Their frequency was analyzed in patients who presented with a depressed mood compared to those without a depressed mood.

Among patients who acknowledged a depressed mood, the mean frequency of autonomic symptoms was 2.7 (SD = 1.4) and of psychological symptoms was 3.1 (SD = 1.9). This was more than three times higher than the frequency of autonomic [0.8 (SD = 0.8)] and psychological [0.9 (SD = 0.9)] symptoms in patients who denied having a depressed mood.

The psychological symptoms that discriminated depressed from nondepressed patients at both the initial evaluation and at 1-year follow-up were related to changes in self-attitude (e.g., feeling of hopelessness, suicidal ideation, self-deprecation, and lack of self-confidence). The only autonomic symptom that distinguished depressed from nondepressed patients over one year was lack of energy (i.e., subjective anergia). Autonomic symptoms such as decreased appetite and weight loss, initial insomnia, and diurnal mood variation (with morning depression) appeared to be significantly associated with depression only during the initial or 3-month evaluation, not at 1-year follow-up. On the other hand, loss of libido, early morning awakening, difficulty concentrating, and inefficient thinking distinguished depressed from nondepressed patients only after 6 months or a year had elapsed. Finally, increased appetite, weight gain, and hypersomnia did not discriminate between depressed and nondepressed groups at any time (Table 1).

Anxiety symptoms were significantly associated with depression during the first

Table 1 Percentage of 66 Traumatic Brain Injury Patients With or Without Depressed Mood Presenting with DSM-III-R Symptoms for Major Depressive Disorder

DSM-III-R symptoms	Initial evaluation		6-Month follow-up		1-Year follow-up	
	Depressed	Nondepressed	Depressed	Nondepressed	Depressed	Nondepressed
Depressed mood	100	0[a]	100	0[a]	100	0[a]
Loss of interest/Anhedonia	11	6	25	10	45	3[a]
Weight loss/Loss of appetite	37	11[a]	17	6	18	3
Weight gain/Increased appetite	5	7	8	3	18	0
Insomnia	53	26	67	16[a]	50	6[a]
Hypersomnia	32	34	17	23	19	0
Psychomotor agitation	32	4[a]	8	11	20	4
Psychomotor retardation	11	9	8	7	20	0
Anergia	58	26[a]	50	13[a]	45	9[a]
Feelings of worthlessness	5	2	50	6[a]	55	0[a]
Guilt	37	11[a]	54	16[a]	18	0
Diminished ability to think or concentrate	84	60	58	23	55	6[a]
Suicidal ideation	16	0[a]	24	0[a]	27	0[a]

[a] $p < 0.05$.

6 months following closed head trauma. At 1-year follow-up, the frequency of anxiety symptoms was not significantly different in patients with or without depressed mood. The fact that symptoms that were specific to depression changed over the course of the first year following TBI suggests that the nature of post-TBI depressions may change over time. Since there are depressive symptoms that are not specific to depression, the questions arises whether existing DSM criteria for major depression should be modified? (This issue was discussed in Chapter 2 on diagnosis in patients with physical illness.) If we required the presence of at least three specific symptoms (including depressed mood) for diagnosing major depression, standard DSM-III-R criteria would have a 100% sensitivity and 94% specificity at the initial evaluation, 88% sensitivity and 94% specificity at 3 months, 91% sensitivity and 96% specificity at 6 months, and 80% sensitivity and 100% specificity at one-year follow-up. Thus, the standard diagnostic criteria (DSM-III-R) have a high sensitivity and specificity for identifying depressed patients when compared with alternative specific symptom diagnostic criteria and may, therefore, be used for the diagnosis of major depression in the TBI population.

The differential diagnosis of post-TBI major depression includes adjustment disorder with depressed mood, apathy, emotional lability, and posttraumatic stress disorder. Patients with adjustment disorders develop short-lived and relatively mild emotional disturbances within 3 months of a stressful life event. Although they may present with depressive symptoms, they do not meet DSM-IV criteria for major depression. Posttraumatic stress disorder occurs following an unusually severe distressing event. It is characterized by symptoms of reexperiencing the trauma, ranging from transient flashbacks or vivid nightmares to severe dissociative states in which the patient behaves as if he or she is actually living the traumatic event. In addition, patients typically avoid all the circumstances related to the trauma and become withdrawn and emotionally blunted.

Emotional lability is characterized by the presence of sudden and uncontrollable affective outbursts (e.g., crying or laughing), which may be congruent or incongruent with the patient's mood and which occur spontaneously or triggered by minor stimuli. It lacks the pervasive alteration of mood as well as the specific vegetative symptoms associated with a major depressive episode. Emotional lability, however, may respond to treatment with antidepressants.

Finally, TBI patients may present with apathetic syndromes that interfere with the rehabilitation process (97). Apathy is frequently associated with psychomotor retardation and emotional blunting. Some patients have, however, a depressed mood. Although apathy is frequently associated with frontal lobe damage, the relationship between apathy and the type, extent, and location of traumatic brain injury has not been systematically studied.

Mechanism of Depression

Previous clinical and epidemiological studies have stressed that several premorbid factors may be relevant to the etiology of post-TBI mood disorders. Previous psychiatric disorder, for instance, has been implicated as a risk factor for receiving head injury (98). In the previously cited study of 66 acute TBI patients (81), patients with acute onset major depression ($n = 17$) did not differ from nondepressed patients ($n = 47$) with respect to demographic variables, type or severity of brain injury, family history of psychiatric disorder, or the degree of physical or cognitive impairment. There was, however, a significantly greater frequency of previous personal history of psychiatric disorders in the major depressed group. There was not, on the other hand, a significant difference between groups in the frequency of personal history of alcohol or other substance abuse (Fig. 3).

Major depressed patients had significantly poorer premorbid social functioning (as measured by initial SFE scores) than the nondepressed group (81). In addition, cross-sectional analysis at 3-, 6-, and 12-month follow-up evaluations showed that poor social functioning was the strongest clinical correlate of major depression (88). On the other hand, major depression was not significantly associated with the degree of cognitive impairment (as measured by MMSE scores).

Lishman (3) reported that several years after penetrating brain injury depressive symptoms were more common among patients with right hemisphere lesions. Depressive symptoms were also most frequent among patients with frontal and parietal lesions than among patients with other lesion locations. Grafman et al. (100) also reported that several years following penetrating head injury, depressive symptoms were more frequently associated with penetrating injuries involving the right hemisphere

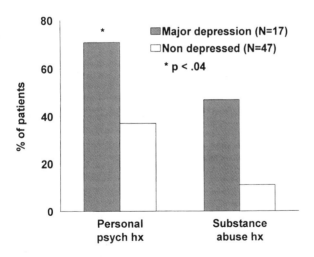

Figure 3 The association of major depression following traumatic brain injury with prior personal or prior history of substance abuse (alcohol was most frequent substance of abuse). Although both risk factors showed similar associations with depression, only psychiatric history reached statistical significance.

(right orbitofrontal lesions) than with any other lesion location. Among the 66 acute TBI patients previously described, 42 (64%) had a diffuse pattern of brain injury on their CT scans and 24 (36%) had focal lesions. Among the 42 patients with diffuse injury, 11 (17% of total) had normal CT scans. Among the 24 patients with focal injury, the lesion was surgically evacuated in 12 patients (18% of total). (Nine of these 12 patients had an acute subdural hematoma, 2 patients had an epidural hematoma, and 1 patient underwent a right temporal lobectomy following a burst lobe injury.) The remaining 12 patients (18%) had brain contusions greater than 25 cc on their CT scans. In addition, 3 of these patients had associated small extraparenchymal hemorrhages (2 subdural and 1 epidural) that did not require surgery. There were no significant differences between major depressed and nondepressed groups in the frequency of diffuse or focal patterns of injury. In addition, there were no significant between-group differences in the frequency of extraparenchymal hemorrhages, contusions, intracerebral or intraventricular hemorrhages, hydrocephalus, or CT findings suggestive of brain atrophy.

A logistic regression model showed that major depression following acute traumatic brain injury was associated with the presence of left dorsolateral frontal and/or left basal ganglia lesions and, to a lesser extent, with right hemisphere and parieto-occipital lesions (Fig. 4) (81). The association between left anterior lesions and major depression held up only during the initial evaluation. Furthermore, five of eight acutely depressed patients (62.5%) with left anterior lesions had depressive syndromes that

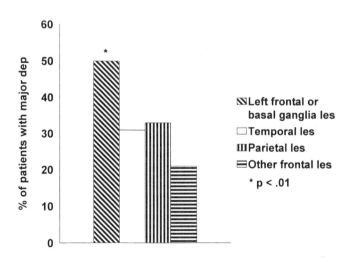

Figure 4 The percentage of patients with various lesion locations who had major depression during the initial in-hospital evaluation following traumatic brain injury. Patients with left frontal or left basal ganglia lesions were significantly more likely to develop major depression than patients with any other lesion location.

lasted only about 1.5 months. These transient depressions were also associated with diffuse patterns of brain injury and left subcortical involvement (89). These results are consistent with our previous findings in stroke patients of an increased frequency of depression among patients with left anterior hemisphere lesions (101). Left dorsolateral frontal cortex and left basal ganglia may be strategic locations for the disruption of ascending aminergic pathways and their related behavioral functions. Depressions after the acute TBI period were not related to the presence of specific lesion locations. They were associated, however, with a personal history of psychiatric disorder and with poor social functioning levels (90). Thus, psychosocial factors appeared to be more important in the chronic stage.

In summary, some acute-onset depressions appear to be related to lesion characteristics and may have their etiology in biological responses of the injured brain. Left dorsolateral frontal and left basal ganglia lesions were strongly associated with major depression during the initial in-hospital evaluation and may represent strategic lesion locations that elicit biochemical responses that ultimately lead to the clinical manifestation of depression. By 3 months follow-up, however, the major correlates of depression were previous history of psychiatric disorder and impaired social functioning. Thus, prolonged or delayed-onset depressions may be mediated by psychosocial factors, suggesting psychological reaction as a possible mechanism.

Secondary Mania

Secondary manic and hypomanic states have been reported in a number of organic disorders such as thyroid disease (102), uremia (103), vitamin B_{12} deficiency (104), or following open heart surgery (105). Mania has also been associated with brain tumors (106), CNS infections (107), stroke (108), and traumatic brain injury (109). Shukla et al. (110) reported on 20 patients who developed manic syndromes after closed head trauma. They found a significant association between mania and the presence of posttraumatic seizures, predominantly of the partial complex type (temporal lobe epilepsy). They also found no association with a family history of bipolar disorder among 85 first-degree relatives (110). Starkstein et al. (111) reported on 25 patients with manic syndromes secondary to cerebrovascular, traumatic, or neoplastic brain lesions. Secondary manic patients had a significantly greater frequency of right hemisphere lesions, particularly in specific limbic-related areas such as basotemporal or orbitofontal cortices, thalamus, or basal ganglia compared to depressed patients or controls (106,111). In addition, both a family history of mood disorder and the presence of subcortical atrophy were identified as probable risk factors for the development of mania following brain injury (112).

We have also studied the prevalence of manic syndromes among the 66 patients with acute TBI patients previously described (113). Of the original 66 patients, six patients (9%) developed secondary mania at some point during the 1-year follow-up period (i.e., five patients at 3 months and one patient at 6 months after brain injury). Manic episodes that met DSM-III-R diagnostic criteria were short-lasting (approximately 2 months). The presence of an expansive mood (without fulfilling criteria for mania or hypomania), however, had a mean duration of 5.7 months. Secondary mania was not related to the type or severity of brain injury, degree of physical or intellectual impairment, level of social functioning, or presence of family or personal history of psychiatric disorder. In addition, mania was not associated with the development of posttraumatic epilepsy. Mania following TBI, however, was associated with the presence of basotemporal polar lesions. The development of abnormal electrical activation patterns in limbic networks, functional changes in aminergic inhibitory systems, and the presence of aberrant regeneration pathways may play a role in the genesis of these syndromes (113).

Post-TBI mania is now diagnosed by DSM-IV as mood disorder due to a general medical condition, with manic or with mixed features. As in the case of depressive disorders, the general code for the medical condition should be noted on Axis III. Diagnosis should not be made if the mood disturbance occurs only during a course of delirium. Delirium is characterized by sudden onset, fluctuating course, disorientation, and prominent attentional deficits. In addition, the diagnosis requires the presence of clinical evidence of a medical or metabolic derangement (e.g., urinary tract infection or hyponatremia). The differential diagnosis of manic syndromes following TBI should include:

1. Substance-induced mood disorder, which may occur following intoxication or withdrawal from different drugs. It is especially important in TBI patients, who frequently have a history of substance abuse and who are also often medicated with psychotropic drugs for their medical condition. Substance-induced mood disorder is usually uncovered by a careful clinical interview and/or toxicological screening.
2. Psychosis associated with epilepsy is more frequently observed among patients with epileptic foci located in limbic or para-limbic cortices. Psychotic episodes may be temporally linked to seizures or may have a more prolonged interictal course. In the latter case, the clinical picture is characterized by the presence of partial and/or complex-partial seizures and of a schizoaffective syndrome. Electroencephalographic and functional neuroradiological studies (e.g., SPECT and PET) will usually define ictal and interictal disturbances.
3. TBI patients may show personality changes that include mood instability, paranoid ideation, poor control over aggression, as well as disinhibited behavior and hypersexuality. These patients lack, however, the pervasive alteration of mood that characterizes secondary manic syndromes.

Relationship of Mood Disorders to Outcome

In a study of 66 acute TBI patients followed over 1 year, factors were identified that contributed to poor outcome in social functioning, activities of daily living, or intellectual function (114). In a first analysis, the amount of improvement or deterioration in social, ADL, and cognitive function was measured in 52 of these 66 patients during the 1-year follow-up. Change was estimated for each patient using a simple linear regression of time (months postinjury) on each of three impairment scales (MMSE, JHFI, and SFE). The slope (B) was taken as the degree of change that individual showed on that scale. Negative slopes for JHFI and SFE and a positive slope for MMSE reflected recovery. Poor outcome was defined by identifying patients who (1) had a deteriorating slope in the linear regression of time on SFE, JHFI, or MMSE scores and (2) fell outside the interquartile range (p75–p25). Eleven patients (21%) fulfilled these criteria for SFE, 7 (13%) for JHFI, and 11 (21%) for MMSE. The rest of the patients (e.g., 52 − 11 = 41 for SFE) constituted the control groups. At the time of the initial evaluation, 13 of the 52 patients (25%) with adequate follow-up data were diagnosed as having major depression. One patient had minor depression, and the remaining 38 patients (73%) were nondepressed. It was assumed that the effect of depression on long-term outcome would only be identifiable in depressive disorders with a longer course. Thus, patients with prolonged major depression (i.e., 6 months or longer) constituted the major depression group. One patient with a bipolar disorder and five patients with secondary mania constituted the mania group. Finally, 19 patients who did not develop an affective disturbance during the entire course of the study constituted the nonaffective disorder (Non-AD) group. There was a significant association between poor psychosocial outcome (i.e., worsening Social Functional Exam scores over time) and the presence of major depression. Patients with short-term depression (i.e., less than 3 months) recovered like nondepressed patients. There was also an association between poor activities of daily living outcome and major depression. Half of the patients with major depression and initial ADL impairment had poor outcomes, whereas none of the patients without affective disorders had a poor ADL outcome. The presence of mood disorders did not appear to influence the patient's cognitive outcome as measured by MMSE scores.

In summary, although patients with moderate head injuries may present with relatively mild physical impairments, they may experience behavioral disorders that have a significant impact on the extent and quality of their interpersonal relationships and on their community reentry. Major depression appeared to have a deleterious effect on both psychosocial and activities of daily living outcome. Since depressive disorders tend to resolve by one year, depression might negatively influence patient participation in rehabilitation efforts early during their course of recovery, thus leading to poor recovery even when the depression is over.

Treatment of Mood Disorders

Patients with brain injury are more sensitive to the side effects of medications, especially psychotropics. Silver and Yudofsky proposed several general guidelines to their use in this population (115). Doses of psychotropics must be prudently increased, minimizing side effects (i.e., start slow, go slow). The patient must receive, however, an adequate therapeutic trial with regard to dosage and duration of treatment. Brain-injured patients must also be frequently reassessed in order to determine changes in treatment schedules. Special care must be taken in monitoring drug interactions. Finally, if there is evidence of a partial response to a specific medication, augmentation therapy is warranted, considering mechanisms of action and side effects of the second drug. To our knowledge, there have been no double-blind, placebo-controlled studies of the efficacy of pharmacological treatments of depression in traumatic brain injured patients. Selection among competing antidepressants is usually guided by their side effect profiles. Mild anticholinergic activity, minimal lowering of seizure threshold and low sedative effects are the most important factors to be considered in the choice of an antidepressant drug in this population (116). Tricyclic antidepressants (TCAs) have important anticholinergic effects that may interfere with cognitive and memory functions. In addition, they may lower the seizure threshold. If, however, a decision is made to administer TCAs, nortriptyline (starting at 10 mg/day) constitutes a reasonable alternative, provided that blood levels and toxic effects are carefully monitored (115). Serotonin selective re-uptake inhibitors (SSRIs) are antidepressants which appear to have a less adverse effect profile (117). The most common side effects include headache, gastrointestinal complaints, and insomnia. Diminished libido and sexual dysfunction may be an additional concern. Fluoxetine (starting at 10 mg/day), sertraline (starting at 25 mg/day) or paroxetine (starting at 5–10 mg/day) are among the most useful drugs in this group. Trazodone is an alternative antidepressant that also inhibits serotonin reuptake. Treatment is started at low doses (50–100 mg) at bedtime following a snack. Dose may be gradually increased every 3–4 days up to 400 mg. The most troublesome side effects are sedation and orthostatic hypotension (118). There are case reports of successful treatments of post-TBI depression with psychostimulants (119). These include dextroamphetamine (8–60 mg/day), methylphenidate (10–60 mg/day), and pemoline (56.25 to 75 mg/day). They are given twice a day, with the last dose at least 6 hours before sleep in order to prevent initial insomnia. Treatment is begun at lower doses which are then gradually increased. Patients taking stimulants need close medical control to prevent abuse or toxic effects. The most common side effects are anxiety, dysphoria, headaches, irritability, anorexia, insomnia, cardiovascular symptoms, dyskinesias, or even psychotic symptoms (118,120). There is also some evidence of the clinical efficacy of dopamine agonists (e.g., bromocriptine or lisuride) in patients with poor motivation and frontal lobe deficits (121,122).

Electroconvulsant (ECT) therapy is not contraindicated in TBI patients and may be considered if other methods of treatment prove unsuccessful. ECT should be administered with the lowest possible effective energy, using pulsatile currents, with an interval of 2 to 5 days between treatments and a reduced number of treatments for a complete course (four to six) (115). Nondominant unilateral ECT is preferred.

Buspirone, a drug that has an agonist effect on 5-HT1 receptors and an antagonist effect on D2 dopaminergic receptors, has proved to be a safe and efficacious anxiolytic. Initial dosing is 15 mg/day given in three divided doses, and it may gradually be increased (5 mg every 4 days) to up to 60 mg/day. The most common side effects are dizziness and headaches (123).

Finally, social intervention and adequate psychotherapeutic support may play important roles in the treatment of depression following traumatic brain injury (124,125). There have been no systematic studies of the treatment of secondary mania. There are, however, several reports of potentially useful treatment modalities. Bakchine et al. (126) conducted a double-blind, placebo-controlled study, in a single patient with secondary mania following TBI. Clonidine (600 µg/day) was effective in reverting manic symptoms; carbamazepine (1200 mg/day) did not elicit mood changes; and l-dopa/benzeraside (375 mg/day) resulted in an increase of manic symptoms. Lithium (112), carbamazepine (127), and valproate (128) therapies have also been reported to be efficacious in individual cases. Lithium has been reported to impair cognitive performance in traumatic-brain-injured patients (129). In addition, it may lower seizure threshold. Some authors limit its use to patients in whom bipolar disorder preceded the onset of TBI (115). Carbamazepine (CBZ) should be gradually increased to obtain therapeutic blood levels (8 to 12 µg/ml). Complete blood counts should be obtained every 2 weeks for the first 2 months of therapy and every 3 months thereafter. Liver function tests should be obtained every 3 months. Frequent side effects include sedation, dry mouth, gastrointestinal upset, drowsiness, impaired concentration, ataxia, nystagmus, and rash. Severe complications include pancytopenia, aplastic anemia, and cholestatic jaundice.

Valproic acid is progressively increased from 500 mg/day up to the dose necessary to obtain plasma levels between 50 and 100 µg/ml. The maximum recommended dose is 60 mg/kg/day divided into two to four doses. Valproic acid has potentially serious side effects. These include hepatotoxicity ranging from a discrete elevation of transaminases and serum ammonia levels to irreversible liver failure. Hemorrhagic pancreatitis has also been reported. Less serious side effects include drowsiness, tremor, gastritis, and increased weight. Liver function tests and serum amylase levels should be monitored.

As we have already mentioned, emotional lability may respond to treatment with antidepressants (130–132). There is, however, a great variability in treatment response among brain-injured patients, with some showing a rapid response at relatively low doses and others requiring more time and a full-dose schedule. It might be emphasized, however, that pharmacological treatments of post-TBI mood disorders need to be adequately examined in controlled treatment trials.

CONCLUSION

In summary, mood disorders are a frequent complication of TBI and may play an important role in shaping long-term outcome. The reported frequency of depressive disorders following TBI has varied from 6% to 77%. In a study using structured interviews and DSM-III-R criteria to ascertain the prevalence of mood disorders, 17 of 66 patients (26%) developed major depression during the acute stage of TBI (i.e., approximately 1 month after brain injury). There were also 11 patients who developed delayed-onset major depression at some point during a 1-year follow-up period. Thus,

47% of patients with follow-up data developed major depression during the first year after the traumatic episode. Major depression appeared to have a natural course of 4 to 5 months following TBI.

When compared with their nondepressed counterparts, major depressed patients did not show significant differences in demographic variables or in the type or severity of brain injury. There was, however, significantly greater frequency of previous personal history of psychiatric disorders and poorer premorbid social functioning in the major depressed group. During a 1-year follow-up study, poor social functioning proved to be the strongest clinical correlate of major depression. There was also a significant association between poor psychosocial outcome and the presence of major depression. Furthermore, major depression appeared to have a deleterious effect on activities-of-daily-living outcome.

There is empirical evidence supporting an association between post-TBI depression and specific lesion locations. In our series, major depression following acute TBI was associated with the presence of left dorsolateral frontal and/or left basal ganglia lesions. Late-onset depressions were associated, however, with a personal history of psychiatric disorder and with poor social functioning. Thus, psychosocial factors appear to be more important in the chronic stage of TBI.

Secondary mania and hypomanic states have also been associated with TBI. We found that six of 66 TBI patients (9%) developed secondary mania at some point during the first year following TBI. Although manic episodes were short-lasting (approximately 2 months), the presence of an expansive mood had a mean duration of 5.7 months. Secondary mania was not related to the type or severity of brain injury, the presence of posttraumatic epilepsy, the degree of physical or intellectual impairment, level of social functioning, or the presence of family or personal history of psychiatric disorder. Secondary mania was, however, associated with the presence of basotemporal lesions.

There is a paucity of systematic studies of the pharmacological treatment of mood disorders following TBI. Selection among competing antidepressants is usually guided by their side-effect profiles. Mild anticholinergic activity, minimal lowering of seizure threshold, and low sedative effects are the most important factors to be considered in the choice of an antidepressant drug in this population. Tricyclic antidepressants (TCAs) have important anticholinergic effects that may interfere with cognitive and memory functions. In addition, they may lower the seizure threshold. Serotonin-selective reuptake inhibitors (SSRIs) are antidepressants that appear to have a less adverse side-effect profile. Fluoxetine, sertraline, and paroxetine are among the most useful drugs in this group.

Lithium, carbamazepine, and valproate therapies have been reported to be efficacious in individual cases of secondary mania. Lithium, however, has been reported to impair cognitive performance in traumatic-brain-injured patients. In addition, it may lower seizure threshold. Some authors limit its use to patients in whom bipolar disorder preceded the onset of TBI.

Future research should establish the efficacy or lack of efficacy of various modalities of treatment for depression or mania following TBI. Further research is also needed to identify the mechanisms of psychiatric disorders following TBI and to document their impact on short- and long-term recovery from brain injury.

REFERENCES

1. Meyer A. The anatomical facts and clinical varieties of traumatic insanity. Am J Insanity 1904; 60:373–441.
2. Hillbom E. After-effects of brain injuries. Acta Psychiatr Neurol Scand 1960; 142(suppl): S1–S195.
3. Lishman WA. Brain damage in relation to psychiatric disability after head injury. Br J Psychiatry 1968; 114:373–410.
4. Kraus JF, Sorenson SB. Epidemiology. In: Silver JM, Yudofsky SC, Hales RE, eds. Neuropsychiatry of Traumatic Brain Injury. Washington, DC: American Psychiatric Press, 1994:3–42.
5. Klauber MR, Barret-Connor E, Marshall LF, et al. The epidemiology of head injury: a prospective study of an entire community: San Diego County, California, 1978. Am J Epidemiol 1981; 113:500–509.
6. Sosin DM, Sacks JJ, Smith SM. Head injury associated deaths in the United States from 1979 to 1986. JAMA 1989; 262:2251–2255.
7. Kraus JF, Black MA, Hessol N, et al. The incidence of acute brain injury and serious impairment in a defined population. Am J Epidemiol 1984; 119:186–201.
8. Miller NS. Alcohol and drug disorders. In: Silver JM, Yudofsky SC, Hales RE, eds. Neuropsychiatry of Traumatic Brain Injury. Washington, DC: American Psychiatric Press, 1994:471–498.
9. Sosin DM, Sniezek JE, Waxweiler RJ. Trends in death associated with traumatic brain injury, 1979 through 1992: success and failure. JAMA 1995; 273:1778.
10. Graves EJ. Vital and Health Statistics: Detailed Diagnosis and Procedures. National Hospital Discharge Survey, 1992. Washington DC: Centers for Disease Control and Prevention, National Center for Health Statistics, 1994.
11. Max W, Mac Kenzie E, Rice D. Head injuries: costs and consequences. J Head Trauma Rehab 1991; 6:76–91.
12. Jennett B. Epidemiology of head injury. J Neurol Neurosurg Psychiatry 1996; 60:362–369.
13. Jenkins A, Teasdale GM, Hadley MDM, et al. Brain lesions detected by magnetic resonance imaging in mild and severe head injuries. Lancet 1986; ii:445–446.
14. Teasdale GM, Jennett B. Assessment of coma and impaired consciousness: a practical scale. Lancet 1974; ii:81–84.
15. Levin HS, O'Donnell VM, Grossman RG. The Galveston orientation and amnesia test. J Nerv Ment Dis 1979; 167:675–684.
16. Jennett B, Snoek J, Bond MR, et al. Disability after severe head injury: observations on the use of the Glasgow Outcome Scale. J Neurol Neurosurg Psychiatry 1981; 44:285.
17. Oddy M, Humphrey M, Uttley D. Subjective impairment and social recovery after closed head injury. J Neurol Neurosurg Psychiatry 1978; 41:611.
18. King NS. Emotional, neuropsychological, and organic factors: their use in the prediction

of persisting postconcussion symptoms after moderate and mild head injuries. J Neurol Neurosurg Psychiatry 1996; 61:75–81.

19. Trzepacz PT. Delirium. In: Silver JM, Yudofsky SC, Hales RE, eds. Neuropsychiatry of Traumatic Brain Injury. Washington, DC: American Psychiatric Press, 1994:189–218.

20. Levin HS, Gary HE, Eisenberg HM, et al. Neurobehavioral outcome 1 year after severe head injury: experience of the Traumatic Coma Data Bank. J Neurosurg 1990; 73:699–709.

21. Rimel RW, Giordani B, Barth JT, et al. Moderate head injury: completing the clinical spectrum of brain trauma. Neurosurgery 1982; 11:344–351.

22. Rimel RW, Giordani B, Barth JT, et al. Disability caused by minor head injury. Neurosurgery 1981; 9:221–228.

23. Gronwall D. Advances in the assessment of attention and information processing after head injury. In: Levin HS, Grafman J, Eisenberg HM, eds. Neurobehavioral Recovery from Head Injury. Oxford: Oxford University Press, 1987.

24. Gronwall D, Wrightson P. Memory and information processing capacity after closed head injury. J Neurol Neurosurg Psychiatry 1981; 44:889.

25. Sarno MT, Buonaguro A, Levita E. Characteristics of verbal impairment in closed head injury patients. Arch Phys Med Rehabil 1986; 67:400.

26. Novoa OP, Ardila A. Linguistic abilities in patients with prefrontal damage. Brain Lang 1987; 30:206.

27. Squire LR, Zola-Morgan S. The medial temporal lobe memory system. Science 1991; 253:1380.

28. Levin HS, Goldstein FC, Williams DH, et al. The contribution of frontal lobe lesions to the neurobehavioral outcome of closed head injury. In: Levin HS, Einsenberg HM, Benton AL, eds. Frontal Lobe Function and Dysfunction. New York: Oxford University Press, 1991.

29. Prigatano GP. The relationship of frontal lobe damage to diminished awareness: studies in rehabilitation. In: Levin HS, Einsenberg HM, Benton AL, eds. Frontal Lobe Function and Dysfunction. New York: Oxford University Press, 1991.

30. Levin HS, Goldstein FC. Closed head injury and Alzheimer's disease: epidemiologic, neurobehavioral and neuropathologic links. J Int Neuropsychol Soc 1995; 1:183.

31. Jennett B. Head injuries. In: Caird FI, Littleton MA, eds. Neurological Disorders in the Elderly. Woburn, MA: John Wright & Sons, 1982.

32. Van Duijn CM, Tanja TA, Haaxma R, et al. Head trauma and the risk of Alzheimer's disease. Am J Epidemiol 1992; 135:775–782.

33. Macmillan MB. A wonderful journey through skulls and brains: the travels of Mr. Gage's tamping iron. Brain Cogn 1986; 5:67.

34. Blumer D, Benson DF. Personality changes with frontal and temporal lobe lesions. In: Blumer D, Benson DF, eds. Psychiatric Aspects of Neurological Disease. New York: Grune & Stratton, 1975.

35. Benton AL. The prefrontal region: its early history. In: Levin HS, Einsenberg HM, Benton AL, eds. Frontal Lobe Function and Dysfunction. New York: Oxford University Press, 1991.

36. Tonkonogy TM. Violence and temporal lobe lesions: head CT and MRI data. J Neuropsychiatry Clin Neurosci 1991; 3:189–196.

37. O'Shanick GJ, O'Shanick AM. Personality and intellectual changes. In: Silver JM, Yudofsky SC, Hales RE, eds. Neuropsychiatry of Traumatic Brain Injury. Washington, DC: American Psychiatric Press, 1994.

38. Levin HS, High WM, Goethe KE, et al. The Neurobehavioral Rating Scale: assessment

of the behavioral sequelae of head injury by the clinician. J Neurol Neurosurg Psychiatry 1987; 50:183.

39. Graham DI, McIntosh TK. Neuropathology of brain injury In: Evans RW, ed. Neurology and Trauma. Philadelphia: WB Saunders, 1996:53–90.

40. Chesnut RM. Secondary brain insults after head injury: clinical perspectives. New Horizons 1995; 3:366–375.

41. Adams JH, Graham DI, Murray LS, et al. Diffuse axonal injury due to non missile head injury in humans: an analysis of 45 cases. Ann Neurol 1983; 12:557–563.

42. Graham DI, Adams JH, Doyle D. Ischaemic brain damage in fatal non missile head injuries. J Neurol Sci 1978; 39:213–234.

43. Marshall LF, Marshal SB, Kauber MR, et al. A new classification of head injury based on computer tomography. Neurosurgery 1991; 75(suppl):14–20.

44. Katz DI. Neuropathology and neurobehavioral recovery from closed head injury. J Head Trauma Rehabil 1992; 7:1–15.

45. Levin HS. Neurobehavioral recovery. central nervous system status report. J Neurotrauma 1992; 1(suppl):S359–S373.

46. Wilson JTL, Hadley DM, Wiedmann KD, et al. Neuropsychological consequences of two patterns of brain damage shown by MRI in survivors of severe head injury. J Neurol Neurosurg Psychiatry 1995; 59:328–333.

47. Lyeth BG, Hayes RL. Cholinergic and opiod mediation of traumatic brain injury. J Neurotrauma 1992; 9:S463–S474.

48. Schmidt RH, Grady MS. Loss of forebrain cholinergic neurons following fluid-percussion injury: implications for cognitive impairment in closed head injury. J Neurosurg 1995; 83: 496–502.

49. Hamill RW, Woolf PD, McDonald JV, Lee LA, Kelly M. Cahecholamines predict outcome in traumatic brain injury. Ann Neurol 1987; 21:438–443.

50. Pappius HM, Dadoun R. Effect of injury on the indoleamines in cerebral cortex. J Neurochem 1987; 49:321–325.

51. Choi D. Calcium mediated neurotoxicity: relationship to specific channel types and its role in ischemic damage. Trends Neurosci 1989; 11:21–26.

52. Kirsch JR, Helfaer M, Lange DG, et al. Evidence for free radical mechanisms of brain injury resulting from ischemia/reperfusion-induced events. J Neurotrauma 1992; 9:S157–S164.

53. Woodroofe MN, Sarna GS, Wadhwa M, et al. Detection of interleukin 1 and interleukin 6 in adult rat brain following mechanical injury, by in vivo microdialysis: evidence for a role for microglia in cytokine production. J Neuroimmunol 1991; 33:227–236.

54. DeKosky ST, Styren SD, O'Malley ME, et al. Interleukin-1 receptor antagonist suppresses neurotrophin response in injured rat brain. Ann Neurol 1996; 39:123–127.

55. Woolf PD. Hormonal responses to trauma. Crit Care Med 1992; 20:216–226.

56. Prigatano GP. Psychiatric aspects of head injury: problems areas and suggested guidelines for research. In: Levin HS, Grafman J, Eisenberg HM, eds. Neurobehavioral Recovery from Head Injury. Oxford: Oxford University Press, 1987:215–232.

57. Nemeroff CB. New vistas in neuropeptide research in neuropsychiatry: focus on corticotropin-releasing-factor. Neuropsychopharmachology 1992; 6:69–75.

58. Jennett B, Bond M. Assessment of outcome after severe brain damage: a practical scale. Lancet 1977; i:480–484.

59. Katz DI, Alexander MP. Traumatic brain injury: predicting course of recovery and outcome for patients admitted to rehabilitation. Arch Neurol 1994; 51:661–670.

60. Gennareli TA, Spielman GM, Langfitt TW, et al. Influence of the type of intracranial lesion on outcome from severe head injury: a multicenter study using a new classification system. J Neurosurg 1982; 56:26–32.
61. Luerssen TG, Marshall LF. The medical management of head injury. In: Braakman R, ed. Handbook of Clinical Neurology. Vol. 13 (57): Head Injury. Amsterdam: Elsevier Science Publishers, 1990.
62. Vollmer DG, Torner JC, Jane JA, et al. Age and outcome following traumatic coma: why do older patients fare worse? J Neurosurg 1991; 75:S37–S49.
63. Levin HS, Hamilton WJ, Grossman R. Outcome after head injury. In: Braakman R, ed. Handbook of Clinical Neurology. Vol 13 (57): Head Injury. Amsterdam: Elsevier Science Publishers, 1990.
64. Marshall LF, Becker DP, Bowers SA, et al. The National Traumatic Coma Data Bank: design, purpose, goals and results. J Neurosurg 1983; 59:276–284.
65. Marshall LF, Eisenberg HM, Jane JA, et al. The outcome of severe closed head injury. J Neurosurg 1991; 75:S28–S36.
66. Thomsen IV. Late outcome of very severe blunt head trauma: a 10–15 year second follow-up. J Neurol Neurosurg Psychiatry 1984; 47:260–268.
67. Brooks N, Campsie L, Symington C, et al. The five year outcome of severe head injury: a relative's view. J Neurol Neurosurg Psychiatry 1986; 49:764–770.
68. Ruff RM, Marshall LF, Crouch J, et al. Predictors of outcome following severe head trauma: follow-up data of the Traumatic Coma Data Bank. Brain Injury 1993; 7:101–111.
69. Brooks DN, McKinlay W. Personality and behavioral change after severe blunt head injury, a relative's view. J Neurol Neurosurg Psychiatry 1983; 46:336–344.
70. Livingston MG, Brooks KN, Bond MR. Three months after severe head injury: psychiatric and social impact on relatives. J Neurol Neurosurg Psychiatry 1985; 48:870–875.
71. Prigatano GP. Disturbances of self-awareness of deficit after traumatic brain injury. In: Prigatano GP, Schacter DL, eds. Awareness of Deficit After Brain Injury: Clinical and Theoretical Issues. New York: Oxford University Press, 1991.
72. Dimken S, Reitan RM. Emotional sequelae of head injury. Ann Neurol 1977; 2:492–494.
73. Fordyce DJ, Rouche JR, Prigatano GP. Enhanced emotional reactions in chronic head trauma patients. J Neurol Neurosurg Psychiatry 1983; 46:620–624.
74. Rutherford WH, Merrett JD, McDonald JR. Sequelae of concussion caused by minor head injuries. Lancet 1977; i:1–4.
75. Levin HS, Grossman RG. Behavioral sequelae of closed head injury: a quantitative study. Arch Neurol 1978; 35:720–727.
76. Varney NR, Martzke JS, Roberts RJ. Major depression in patients with closed head injury. Neuropsychology 1987; 1:7–9.
77. McKinlay WW, Brooks DN, Bond MR, Martinage DP, Marshall MM. The short term outcome of severe blunt head injury as reported by the relatives of the head injury person. J Neurol Neurosurg Psychiatry 1981; 44:527–533.
78. Kinsella G, Moran C, Ford B, et al. Emotional disorder and its assessment within the severe head injured population. Psychol Med 1988; 18:57–63.
79. Schoenhuber R, Gentili M. Anxiety and depression after mild head injury: a case control study. J Neurol Neurosurg Psychiatry 1988; 51:722–724.
80. Gualtieri CT, Cox DR. The delayed neurobehavioral sequelae of traumatic brain injury. Brain Injury 1991; 5:219–232.

81. Fedoroff JP, Starkstein SE, Forrester AW, et al. Depression in patients with acute traumatic brain injury. Am J Psychiatry 1992; 149:918–923.
82. Wing JK, Cooper E, Sartorius N. Measurement and Classification of Psychiatric Symptoms. Cambridge: Cambridge University Press, 1974.
83. American Psychiatric Association. Diagnostic and Statistical Manual of Mental Disorders. 3rd ed. Washington, DC: American Psychiatric Press, 1987.
84. Hamilton M. A rating scale for depression. J Neurol Neurosurg Psychiatry 1960; 23:56–62.
85. Folstein MF, Folstein SE, McHugh PR. Mini-Mental State: a practical method for grading the cognitive state of patients for the clinician. J Psychiatr Res 1975; 12:189–198.
86. Robinson RG, Szetela B. Mood change following left hemispheric brain injury. Ann Neurol 1981; 9:447–453.
87. Starr LB, Robinson RG, Price TR. Reliability, validity, and clinical utility of the social functioning exam in the assessment of stroke patients. Exp Aging Res 1983; 9:101.
88. Jorge RE, Robinson RG, Arndt SV, et al. Depression following traumatic brain injury: a 1 year longitudinal study. J Affect Dis 1993; 27:233–243.
89. Jorge RE, Robinson RG, Starkstein SE, et al. Depression and anxiety following traumatic brain injury. J Neuropsychiatry Clin Neurosci 1993; 5:369–374.
90. Jorge RE, Robinson RG, Arndt SV, et al. Comparison between acute and delayed onset depression following traumatic brain injury. J Neuropsychiatry Clin Neurosci 1993; 5: 43–49.
91. Grant I, Alves W. Psychiatric and psychosocial disturbances in head injury. In: Levin HS, Grafman J, Eisenberg HM, eds. Neurobehavioral Recovery from Head Injury. Oxford: Oxford University Press, 1987:232–261.
92. Lishman WA. Physiogenesis and psychogenesis in the post-concussional syndrome. Br J Psychiatry 1988; 153:460–469.
93. Van Zomeren AH, Saan RJ. Psychological and social sequelae of severe head injury. In: Braakman R, ed. Handbook of Clinical Neurology. Vol 13. (57): Head Injury. Amsterdam: Elsevier Science Publishers, 1990:397–420.
94. Silver JM, Yudofsky SC, Hales RE. Depression in traumatic brain injury. Neuropsychiatry Neuropsychol Behav Neurol 1991; 4:12–23.
95. Jorge RE, Robinson RG, Arndt SV. Are depressive symptoms specific for a depressed mood in traumatic brain injury? J Nerv Ment Disord 1993; 181:91–99.
96. Davidson J, Turnbull CD. Diagnostic significance of vegetative symptoms in depression. Br J Psychiatry 1986; 148:442–446.
97. Marin RS, Fogel BS, Hawkins J, et al. Apathy: a treatable syndrome. J Neuropsychiatry Clin Neurosci 1995; 7:23–30.
98. Selzer ML, Rogers JE, Kern S. Fatal accidents: the role of psychopathology, social stress, and acute disturbances. Am J Psychiatry 1968; 124:1028–1036.
99. Finset A. Depressed mood and reduced emotionality after right hemisphere brain damage. In: Kinsbourne M, ed. Cerebral Hemisphere Function in Depression. Washington, DC: American Psychiatric Press, 1988.
100. Grafman J, Vance SC, Swingartner H, et al. The effects of lateralized frontal lesions on mood regulation. Brain 1986; 109:1127–1148.
101. Robinson RG, Starr LB, Kubos KL, Rao K, Price TR. Mood disorders in stroke patients: importance of location of lesion. Brain 1984; 197:81–93.
102. Corn TH, Checkley SA. A case of recurrent mania with recurrent hyperthyroidism. Br J Psychiatry 1983; 143:74–76.

103. Thomas CS, Neale TJ. Organic manic syndrome associated with advanced uremia due to polycystic kidney disease. Br J Psychiatry 1991; 158:119–121.
104. Goggans FC. A case of mania secondary to vitamin B_{12} deficiency. Am J Psychiatry 1984; 141:300–301.
105. Isles LJ, Orrell MW. Secondary mania after open-heart surgery. Br J Psychiatry 1991; 159:280–282.
106. Robinson RG, Boston JD, Starkstein SE, et al. Comparison of mania with depression following brain injury: causal factors. Am J Psychiatry 1988; 145:172–178.
107. Thienhaus OJ, Khosla N. Meningeal cryptococosis misdiagnosed as a manic episode. Am J Psychiatry 1984; 141:1459–1460.
108. Cummings JL, Mendez MF. Secondary mania with focal cerebrovascular lesions. Am J Psychiatry 1988; 141:1084–1087.
109. Bamrah JS, Johnson J. Bipolar affective disorder following head injury. Br J Psychiatry 1991; 158:117–119.
110. Shukla S, Cook BL, Mukherjee S, et al. Mania following head trauma. Am J Psychiatry 1987; 144:93–96.
111. Starkstein SE, Mayberg HS, Berthier ML, et al. Secondary mania: neuroradiological and metabolic findings. Ann Neurol 1990; 27:652–659.
112. Starkstein SE, Pearlson GD, Boston JD, et al. Mania after brain injury: a controlled study of causative factors. Arch Neurol 1988; 44:1069–1073.
113. Jorge RE, Robinson RG, Starkstein SE, et al. Secondary mania following traumatic brain injury. Am J Psychiatry 1993; 150:916–921.
114. Jorge RE, Robinson RG, Arndt SV, et al. Influence of major depression on 1-year outcome in patients with traumatic brain injury. J Neurosurg 1994; 81:726–733.
115. Silver JM, Yudofsky SC. In: Silver JM, Yudofsky SC, Hales RE, eds. Neuropsychiatry of Traumatic Brain Injury. Washington, DC: American Psychiatric Press, 1994:3–42.
116. Silver JM, Hales RE, Yudofsky SC. Psychopharmacology of depression in neurologic disorders. J Clin Psychiatry 1990; 51:33–39.
117. Cassidy JW. Fluoxetine: a new serotonergically active antidepressant. J Head Trauma Rehab 1989; 4:67–69.
118. Zasler ND. Advances in neuropharmacological rehabilitation for brain dysfunction. Brain Injury 1992; 6:1–14.
119. Gualtieri CT. Pharmacotherapy and the neuro-behavioral sequelae of traumatic brain injury. Brain Injury 1988; 101–129.
120. Kraus MF. Neuropsychiatric sequelae of stroke and traumatic brain injury: the role of psychostimulants. Int J Psychiatry Med 1995; 25:39–51.
121. Powell JH, Al-Adawi S, Morgan J, et al. Motivational deficits after brain injury: effects of bromocriptine in 11 patients. J Neurol Neurosurg Psychiatry 1996; 60:416–421.
122. Barret K. Treating organic abulia with bromocriptine and lisuride: four single case studies. J Neurol Neurosurg Psychiatry 1991; 54:718–721.
123. Gualtieri CT. Buspirone: Neuropsychiatric effects. J Head Trauma Rehabil 1991; 6:90–92.
124. Prigatano GP. disordered mind, wounded soul: the emerging role of psychotherapy in rehabilitation after brain injury. J Head Trauma Rehab 1991; 6:1–10.
125. Sbordone RJ. Psychotherapeutic treatment of the client with traumatic brain injury: a conceptual model. In: Kreutzer JS, Wehman P, eds. Community Integration Following Traumatic Brain Injury. Baltimore: Paul H Brookes Publishing, 1990.

126. Backchine S, Lacomblez L, Benoit N, et al. Manic like state after orbitofrontal and right temporoparietal injury: efficacy of clonidine. Neurology 1989; 39:777–781.

127. Bouvy PF, van de Wetering BJM, Meerwaldt JD, et al. A case of organic brain syndrome following head injury successfully treated with carbamazepine. Acta Psychiatr Scand 1988; 77:361–363.

128. Pope HG, McElroy SL, Satlina, et al. Head injury, bipolar disorder and response to valproate. Compr Psychiatry 1988; 29:34–38.

129. Hornstein A, Seliger G. Cognitive side effects of lithium in closed head injury [letter]. J Neuropsychiatry Clin Neurosci 1989; 1:446–447.

130. Schiffer RB, Hendon RM, Rudick RA. Treatment of pathological laughing and weeping with amitriptyline. N Engl J Med 1985; 312:1480–1482.

131. Seliger G, Hornstein A, Flax J, et al. Fluoxetine improves emotional incontinence. Brain Injury 1992; 6:267–270.

132. Robinson RG, Parikh RM, Lipsey JR, et al. Pathological laughing and crying following stroke: validation of a measurement scale and a double blind study. Am J Psychiatry 1993; 150:286–293.

17

Epilepsy

Howard A. Ring
St. Bartholomew's and the Royal London School of Medicine
London, England

HISTORICAL BACKGROUND

In 1866, long before the advent of electroencephalography, Hughlings Jackson described epilepsy as "sudden, excessive, rapid and local discharges of the grey matter." This description remains relevant, but in recent years confusion surrounding the various diagnostic schemes applied to epilepsy has been reduced by the development by the International League Against Epilepsy, (ILAE) of classifications of epileptic seizures (Table 1) and, separately, of epilepsies and epileptic syndromes (Table 2) (1). The distinction between seizures and syndromes emphasizes the important point that an individual epileptic syndrome involves more than just seizure type and frequency and may also include etiology, precipitating factors, age of onset, chronicity, and associated difficulties. These additional factors are also important because they define more widely the range of problems that may be faced by patients.

The association between epilepsy and behavioral or psychiatric symptomatology has been noted since the time of ancient Greece, when Hippocrates described a relationship between epilepsy and what was subsequently termed melancholia (2). In the Middle Ages the occurrence of seizures was at times considered to be evidence of demonic or more rarely divine possession. In the nineteenth century with the development of a more scientific approach to the treatment of epilepsy, interactions between seizures and mental states were discussed in textbooks of the time. However, the historical legacy of fear and ignorance that has surrounded people with epilepsy continues to some extent up to the present day, leading to the persistence of social stigmatization, which contributes to the psychological and social stresses experienced by those with epilepsy.

Table 1 International League Against Epilepsy Classification of
Epileptic Seizures (abbreviated)

1. Focal (partial, local) seizures
   A. Simple partial seizures
      With motor symptoms
      With somatosensory or special sensory symptoms
      With autonomic symptoms or signs
   B. Complex partial seizures
      With simple onset followed by impairment of consciousness
      With impairment of consciousness at onset
   C. Partial seizures evolving to secondarily generalized seizures
      (tonic-clonic, tonic, or clonic)
2. Generalized seizures
   A. Absence seizures
   B. Myoclonic seizures
   C. Clonic seizures
   D. Tonic seizures
   E. Tonic-clonic seizures
   F. Atonic seizures

AN ILLUSTRATIVE CASE HISTORY

Sam is a 30-year-old man of normal intelligence living with his parents. There is no
family history of epilepsy or psychiatric disorder. At the age of 10 months he suffered
from sustained febrile convulsions requiring hospital admission. He made a good recovery and was well until the age of 13, when he started experiencing episodes characterized
by several minutes of apparent unawareness of his environment, wandering around
picking at his clothing and making chewing movements. After several of these episodes
he was diagnosed as suffering from epilepsy. Electroencephalographic investigation revealed a left temporal lobe epileptic focus, and later structural brain imaging suggested
damage in the region of the left hippocampus.

At the age of 13 Sam was commenced on antiepileptic medication and over the
intervening years has never been without seizures for more than about 3 months. He
has generally experienced three to four fits per month. At the age of 19 he experienced
his first secondarily generalized tonic-clonic seizure and since then has on average had
one of these per month. He has been prescribed a total of seven different agents and
at times has been on as many as three different antiepileptics at one time. Following
the development of seizures his school initially requested his parents to withdraw him.
It was only after sustained pressure from his parents that it was agreed that he could
remain there. During his adolescence he occasionally missed time from school because
of ill health but no more than his peers. However, his life became more isolated. He
was invited to friends' homes less often, participated less in extracurricular activities,

Table 2 International League Against Epilepsy Classification of Epilepsies (abbreviated)

1. Generalized
   Idiopathic generalized epilepsies with age-related onset
      Benign neonatal convulsions
      Childhood absence epilepsy
      Juvenile myoclonic epilepsy
      Other idiopathic generalized epilepsies
   Cryptogenic or symptomatic generalized epilepsies
      West's syndrome
      Lennox-Gastaut syndrome
   Symptomatic generalized epilepsies with nonspecific etiology
2. Localization-related
   Idiopathic with age-related onset
      Benign epilepsy with centrotemporal spikes
   Symptomatic
      Epilepsia partialis continua
      Temporal lobe epilepsies
      Frontal lobe epilepsies
      Parietal lobe epilepsies
      Occipital lobe epilepsies
3. Epilepsies and syndromes undetermined as to whether focal or generalized
4. Special syndromes
   Febrile convulsions
   Seizures occurring only when there is an acute metabolic or toxic event related to, e.g.,
      alcohol, eclampsia

and during these was escorted by his parents or older brother. His school work deteriorated some what, and though he completed his school education he did so with less success than might have been predicted. He initially had difficulty obtaining employment and for several years held temporary jobs stacking shelves in supermarkets. In his mid-twenties he attended a course that gave him a qualification and experience as an assistant librarian and has held several such posts since then. However, he has not worked for the last 2 years. His had his first girlfriend at the age of 19. He has had three girlfriends and a sexual relationship with one of these, who also had epilepsy. He does not currently have a girlfriend.

Sam was first seen by a psychiatrist when he was 22 years old. This was following an overdose of his antiepileptic medication taken in the context of several weeks of deepening depression after the break-up of the relationship with his first girlfriend, during which time he had also stopped taking his daily prescribed medication. His mood subsequently improved following some cognitive therapy. He remained in good mental health until the age of 29, when, at a time when his seizures had become less severe and less frequent, he became suspicious that his neighbors were poisoning his drinking water. He started drinking only canned drinks, subsequently complained to his parents, and, just prior to his referral to psychiatric services, approached his neighbors to ask them why they were doing this to him. On mental state examination he was found to have a number of persecutory delusions. No history of hallucinations could be elicited and he appeared to be euthymic. He had no insight and initially refused all offers of medication or hospitalization. However, with the support of his parents a course of neuroleptic medication was instituted. Within 4 weeks his psychotic phenomena had receded.

This history makes the point that psychopathology developing in people with epilepsy can be related to various pressures and predisposing factors. A diagnosis of epilepsy may lead to reduced social life and activities. Both frequent seizures and the medication used to control them often have adverse effects on cognitive function. Suffering from a chronic illness in adolescence may lead to great pressures on the individual and his or her family and is occasionally associated with periods of poor compliance with necessary medical regimens. There are increased rates of suicide and attempted suicide in people with epilepsy. However, in addition to the psychosocial difficulties, epilepsy is associated with biological disturbances of brain functioning that at times appear to be directly related to the development of psychiatric symptomatology.

PSYCHIATRIC DISORDERS IN PATIENTS WITH EPILEPSY

Depression

Prevalence of Depression in Epilepsy

Depression is a clinically important concomitant of epilepsy. However, minor degrees of depression and anxiety are common in everyday life, and it can be difficult to know when such states should be defined as an illness, hence becoming an appropriate target for medical intervention. A common approach is to say that whenever the mental state is sufficiently disturbed to disrupt the normal daily functioning of that particular individual, then an illness has developed. General diagnostic systems, such as ICD-10 and DSM-IV, provide clinical criteria that must be met in order for a particular diagnosis to be made. With respect to epilepsy, in DSM-IV the situation is more complex because the available diagnoses for somebody with depression and epilepsy are "mood disorder due to epilepsy" or "adjustment disorder with depressed mood." The former assumes a biological link between the medical and the emotional state, and the latter describes a psychological response occurring within 3 months of the onset of a stressor (in this case epilepsy or possibly individual seizures). Hence postictal and interictal depressions may be classified as different conditions, based on unproven assumptions regarding the relationship between seizure activity and mood disturbance.

It is difficult to draw specific conclusions about the frequency of anxiety and depression in patients with epilepsy. There have been very few studies investigating the absolute prevalence of psychiatric morbidity in epilepsy in the community. An American study examined patients attending vocational services for the disabled (3). Although only 35% of those sent a questionnaire responded, of these 175 subjects, 24% agreed with a description of themselves as feeling unhappy most of the time. A significantly lower proportion (12%) of a "comparably disabled" control population of those without epilepsy attending the same services described themselves in this way.

Two British studies have assessed patients with epilepsy registered with a number of primary health care family doctors. In a sample of 218 patients, Pond et al. (4) recorded psychological difficulties in 29%. In half of these the difficulties were "neurotic" in nature. Twenty-five years later Edeh and Toone (5), in a similar community-based survey of 88 patients, recorded neurotic depression in 22% of their sample.

It has been reported that in those with epilepsy, the highest frequency of psychiatric morbidity is seen in institutionalized patients and those attending clinics specializing in the treatment of intractable seizure disorders (6). Although a proportion of this group will have severe psychopathology, there also appear to be higher levels of more minor psychiatric symptoms in these patients with poorly controlled epilepsy. In a Canadian study of a consecutive series of patients with intractable epilepsy presenting for consideration of neurosurgical treatment, it was found that 45% were identified by the General Health Questionnaire (GHQ) as having psychiatric disorders (7). These patients were studied in an interictal state. The GHQ is a screening measure of nonpsychotic emotional illness that has been validated in patients with medical problems. The patients scored most highly on subscales measuring anxiety and somatic concerns. These results are supported by those from another study, also using the GHQ, but performed in a different country (England rather than Canada). This work (8) studied patients with chronic epilepsy attending an outpatient clinic. Like Manchanda et al. (7), these authors also observed that 45% of their subjects met the criteria for psychiatric caseness, scoring particularly highly on subscales measuring anxiety, depression, and hysteria.

The importance of understanding depression in epilepsy is highlighted when the frequency of suicide and parasuicide in this population is considered. Barraclough (9), reviewing 11 previous studies, reported a suicide rate five times that in the general population. Mathews and Barabas (10) reviewed eight studies and noted a suicide rate in epilepsy patients of 5% compared to 1.4% in control populations. In patients with temporal lobe epilepsy, the relative risk is even greater. There is also an increased risk of parasuicide, particularly of overdoses.

Mania is rare in association with epilepsy. Williams (11) described elation in just 3 of 2000 patients. The few cases reported in the literature are in the form of anecdotal accounts of individual cases.

Hence there is clear evidence that depression is more common in those with epilepsy than in the population at large. The observation that it is also more common in these patients than in comparably disabled nonepileptic subjects suggests that in some patients the cerebral pathophysiology of epilepsy may have a specific role in the biological etiology of their depression.

Clinical Manifestations of Depression in Epilepsy

Patients may experience either depression or anxiety separately, but they often occur together, and when relatively mild the symptoms can be difficult to distinguish from each other. Both states may develop in association with disruptions to the life of the patient related to their epilepsy, but equally these symptoms may start without the development of any changes in life circumstances, epilepsy, or antiepileptic medication. Once established, these mental states can be experienced as preoccupations with aspects of epilepsy or as intrusive and pervasive free-floating emotions.

In some patients with more severe anxiety there may be associated episodes of hyperventilation, which can be mistaken for seizures by both patients and doctors.

When suffering mild anxiety or depression, a patient's daily functioning and sleep may be normal or impaired to a small degree. In general, greater functional impairment is associated with more severe psychopathology. Clinical observation suggests that when patients are depressed or anxious, they may be more likely to report side effects from their antiepilepsy medication.

Because an epileptic seizure is an event defined in time, many authors have used temporal definitions to characterize different associations between epilepsy and affective disturbance. The most common temporal separation is into prodromal, peri-ictal, and interictal periods. The peri-ictal period includes the aura, the ictus itself, and the immediate postictal period.

Prodromal Phenomena

The prodrome, occurring hours to days before a seizure, was investigated by Blanchet and Frommer (12), who report a prospective study in which 27 patients with epilepsy self-rated their moods using personal feelings scales and recorded life events on a daily basis for at least 56 days. During this time 13 patients had at least one seizure. The authors observed that in these the mean ratings of mood on 8 of the 10 scales showed a decline on the day(s) preceding the seizure and an increase after the seizure. In 4 patients the mean depression scale rating on the day preceding the seizure was significantly lower than the mean rating on normal days. Although an increase in negative life events was reported by patients whose mood fell before seizures, this correlation was not significant.

There are several possible explanations for the association between lowered mood ratings and the subsequent occurrence of seizures. Lower mood may be a symptom of the prodromal phase of seizure activity, initiated by the same biological processes that bring about the seizure. Alternatively, it may be that the mood change itself precipitates a seizure.

Peri-Ictal Phenomena

The aura is the earliest stage of subjective awareness of seizure activity. Many different sensations have been recorded. Taylor and Lochery (13) investigated 215 aura experiences in 88 patients with temporal lobe epilepsy. They recorded details of auras of various complexities and types, but it is noteworthy that although there were 24 experiences of "epigastric fear," there were no reports of any other affective states.

Williams (11) investigated emotional phenomena in 2000 patients with epilepsy and found that 100 of them reported an emotion as part of the "epileptic experience." As in the study by Taylor and Lochery (13), the most commonly reported emotion was fear, occurring in Williams's sample in 61% of the 100 patients with emotional phenomena. On some occasions this fear was quite pervasive, with psychic and somatic features. In contrast to this, depression was reported less often, in just 21% (i.e., in 1% of the whole group). However, Williams observed that when depression did occur it tended to last longer than the other peri-ictal phenomena, persisting for up to several days after the ictus. This was interpreted as being akin to naturally occurring depression, which tends to be self-sustaining.

Depression occurring as a postictal phenomenon is, however, well recognized. It characteristically lasts longer than other postictal states and at times may be severe and associated with suicidal behavior (14). In other patients the mood change is less profound but may still occur after most seizures. Case descriptions give a clear impression that the period of depression is more than just an understandable emotional reaction to the advent of a seizure, suggesting instead a biological link with the seizure process.

Thus peri-ictal depression, although it does occur, is not common but is characterized by a greater persistence than other postictal emotional phenomena. It is interesting to note that depressive auras appear to be particularly rare, whereas fear is more common.

Interictal Phenomena

Several studies have investigated the phenomenology of interictal depression. Mendez et al. (15) compared 20 depressed epileptic inpatients to 20 nonepileptic depressed subjects. Both groups met DSM-III criteria for major depression. All the patients had endogenous features of depression—anergia, anhedonia, appetite, and sleep disturbance—but the authors concluded that the major distinguishing characteristics of the depressed patients with epilepsy with respect to the nonepileptic group were a chronic dysthymic background, a relative lack of neurotic traits such as somatization or self-pity, and a history of periods of agitated peri-ictal psychotic behavior.

The depressive phenomenology of a larger group of epileptic patients meeting Research Diagnostic Criteria for major depressive disorder was described by Robertson et al. (16). These authors assessed 66 patients using clinical examination and a number of standardized rating scales. In this study patients obtained very high state and trait anxiety scores. The authors suggest that the high level of state anxiety may have been due to the depression, since it decreased significantly during a 6-week double-blind, placebo-controlled antidepressant trial.

Etiology of Depression in Epilepsy

There are no clearly established mechanisms by which epilepsy may bring about clinical depression. Just as depression is a heterogeneous condition, so it is likely that various factors combine in different ways in different patients with epilepsy to generate particular forms of associated depressive illness. However, based on clinical and experimental observations, it is possible to explore possible etiological elements common across patients.

A variety of seizure and treatment variables have been explored, and in general little consensus has been reached with regard to biological etiologies. It appears that a temporal lobe focus is more likely to be associated with depression, but seizure frequency may not be. As discussed below, certain antiepileptic regimens may be associated with the development of depression.

The social sequelae of having epilepsy were present more than 2000 years ago, when Hippocrates referred to the condition as the "scared disease." Since that time much has been written on the social stigmatization of those with epilepsy. Even in our own more enlightened times this stigmatization persists. The most powerful means of reducing this prejudice is the education of the public about the realities of epilepsy. Such education for families of those with epilepsy will reduce the stresses within some of these families that may contribute to the development of depression.

In a postictal study of almost 200 patients who had only recently learned that they had epilepsy, having been diagnosed within the previous 3 years, the greatest concern, in 80%, was fear of seizures. The second most common concern was of stigma at work, in 69% (17). These concerns were greater in those with a higher frequency of seizures, demonstrating that in the early stages of epilepsy the psychosocial effects are related to the severity of the medical condition. The authors of this study go on to conclude that this suggests that the stigmatizing effects of receiving the label of epilepsy are less than those associated with continuing symptoms. The authors also point out that in order to gain an insight into how an increasingly chronic course of epilepsy affects the development of psychosocial difficulties and the sense of being stigmatized, a prospective long-term follow-up of their cohort will be required.

At the other end of the clinical spectrum, in patients who have been seizure-free on medication for some time, the psychosocial outcomes of discontinuing antiepileptic medication have also been investigated. A randomized parallel-group prospective study of patients who were either slowly withdrawn or who continued their standard treatment regimens has been reported (18). It was found that although seizure recurrence on withdrawal was, not surprisingly, associated with increased measures of distress, so was just continuing the medication. This latter finding may relate to the feelings among some well-controlled patients that, even though they were seizure-free, continuing therapy implied continuing epilepsy. These observations suggest some enduring stigma associated with the diagnosis and that some psychosocial benefit may be gained by withdrawing these drugs in those for whom the risk of relapse after cessation of antiepileptic agents appears low.

An interesting aspect of this study by Jacoby et al. (18) is that it specifically considered aspects of psychosocial distress in patients whose epilepsy was well controlled. Most published studies have examined patients with intractable epilepsy. Overall, in this study of people who had been seizure-free for at least 2 years, the patients appeared well adjusted to living with epilepsy, with few problems in daily life. Because those whose epilepsy is in remission constitute the largest proportion of people with epilepsy, this finding of generally good adjustment is an important and positive observation.

Psychoses in Epilepsy

Prevalence of Psychoses in Epilepsy

Although it is unclear from epidemiological studies whether there is an overall excess of psychosis considering all people with epilepsy, clinical case series indicate that psychosis is a significant problem in patients attending specialized epilepsy centers. This suggests that risk factors for the development of psychosis may be related to a complicated, chronic, and treatment-resistant condition, which is the type of epilepsy often found in patients attending specialist units. A number of authors have reported an increase of schizophrenia-like psychoses in epilepsy patients, especially in those suffering from temporal lobe epilepsy.

Over the years there has been some confusion with respect to the various patterns of psychosis observed in people with epilepsy. The clearest classification method, and the one with most value with respect to etiological and treatment considerations, is to consider psychoses not by the precise phenomenological characteristics of the psychotic experiences but rather, as is also the case for depression, to classify the psychoses of epilepsy in relation to whether the psychotic symptoms occur in association with seizures, soon after the cessation of seizure activity, or during the interictal period.

Clinical Manifestations of Psychosis in Epilepsy

Ictal Psychoses

Prolonged focal and generalized nonconvulsive epileptic activity lasting several hours or days may present with psychotic symptoms. Generalized nonconvulsive status is characterized by altered or narrowed consciousness. Patients are disorientated and apathetic. Contact with the environment is partially preserved, and patients are often able to perform simple tasks. Positive psychotic symptoms such as delusions and hallucinations occur in only some of these patients, as they may in some patients with complex partial status. Temporal and frontal foci have been associated with complex partial status and psychotic phenomena. Treatment of the status has been reported to lead to rapid resolution of the abnormal mental state (19). Simple focal status or aura continua may cause complex hallucinations, thought disorders, and affective symptoms, but insight is usually maintained, and true psychoses emerging from such a state have not been described.

Postictal Psychoses

Most postictal psychoses are precipitated by a series of generalized seizures or following an episode of status epilepticus. More rarely, psychoses occur after single grand mal seizures or following series of complex partial seizures. Postictal psychoses account for approximately 25% of psychoses in epilepsy. Logsdail and Toone (20) noted a higher frequency of postictal psychosis in patients with focal epilepsies and complex partial seizures. In most patients there is a characteristic lucid interval lasting from 1 to 6 days between the epileptic seizures and onset of psychosis, which may lead to an incorrect diagnosis.

The psychopathology of postictal psychosis is variable, but most patients present with abnormal mood and paranoid delusions (20). Some patients are confused throughout the episode, others present with fluctuating impairment of consciousness and orientation, and sometimes there is no confusion at all. Psychotic symptoms spontaneously remit within days or weeks, often without need for additional neuroleptic treatment. However, in some cases chronic psychoses develop from recurrent and even a single postictal psychosis.

Interictal Psychoses

Interictal psychoses occur between seizures and cannot directly be linked to the ictus. They are less frequent than peri-ictal psychoses and account for 10–25% of epileptic psychoses. Interictal psychoses are, however, clinically more significant in terms of severity and duration than peri-ictal psychoses, which usually are short-lasting and often self-limiting.

Although the phenomenology of postictal psychoses is often described as schizophreniform, in fact the published accounts describe various presentations. The preservation of warm affect and a high frequency of delusions and religious mystical experiences have been noted, and some authors have stressed the rarity of negative symptoms and the absence of formal thought disorder. Others have reported that visual hallucinations were more prominent than auditory hallucinations and that delusions were less well organized. Phenomenology apart, Glithero and Slater argued that long-term prognosis of psychosis in epilepsy was better than that of schizophrenia. In a follow-up study on his patients he found that chronic psychotic symptoms tended to remit and personality deterioration was rare (21). Other authors also described outcome to be more favorable and long-term institutionalization to be less frequent than in schizophrenia.

Etiology of Psychoses in Epilepsy

Although the etiology of epileptic psychoses remains unknown, a number of studies have investigated possible risk factors that may contribute to the development of such symptoms. There is no convincing evidence for a significant role for genetic factors. Most authors do not find any evidence for an increased rate of psychiatric disorders in relatives of epilepsy patients with psychoses.

With respect to the role of duration of epilepsy, the interval between age at onset of epilepsy and age at first manifestation of psychosis has been very similar across several series, being in the region of 11–15 years. Although it has been suggested that this interval is the result of limbic kindling associated with seizures ultimately leading to the dysfunction that brings about psychosis, it has been more convincingly argued by some authors that the supposedly specific interval represents an artifact. They noted that the observed interval had a wide range and that it was significantly shorter in patients with later onset of epilepsy and that there is a tendency in the general population for the peak age of onset of epilepsy to be earlier than that of schizophrenia.

There is better evidence that the type of epilepsy is related to the risk of developing a psychosis. There is an excess of temporal lobe epilepsy in most case series of patients with epilepsy and psychosis. A summary of the data of 10 studies revealed that 217, or 76%, of 287 such patients suffered from temporal lobe epilepsy (22), and there is evidence from several studies that focal seizure symptoms that indicate ictal mesial temporal or limbic involvement are overrepresented in patients with psychosis. There is a general consensus that psychoses are very rare in patients with neocortical extratemporal epilepsies.

There are several studies showing that psychoses in generalized epilepsies differ from psychoses in temporal lobe epilepsy. The former are more likely to be short-lasting and confusional. Schneiderian first-rank symptoms and chronicity are more frequent in patients with temporal lobe epilepsy.

The strongest risk factors for psychosis in epilepsy are those that indicate severity of epilepsy. These are long duration of active epilepsy, multiple seizure types, and a history of status epilepticus.

Left lateralization of temporal lobe dysfunction or temporal lobe pathology as a risk factor for schizophreniform psychosis was originally suggested by Flor-Henry (23). The literature has been summarized by Trimble (19). In a synopsis of 14 studies with 341 patients, 43% had left, 23% right, and 34% bilateral abnormalities, representing a clear bias towards left lateralization. However, lateralization of epileptogenic foci has not been confirmed in all controlled studies.

Some reports have suggested an antagonism between epilepsy and psychosis. These led von Meduna to introduce convulsive therapy for the treatment of schizophrenia. In the 1950s Landolt (24) published a series of papers on patients who had epilepsy who became psychotic when their seizures were under control. He defined forced normalization as "the phenomenon characterised by the fact that, with the recurrence of psychotic states, the EEG becomes more normal, or entirely normal as compared with previous and subsequent EEG findings." Forced normalization was thus essentially an EEG phenomenon. The clinical counterpart of this process, in which patients become psychotic when their seizures became controlled, with the psychosis subsequently resolving with return of seizures, has been described as alternative psychosis.

These phenomena have now been well documented. The EEG does not need to become "normal," but rather may just show a decrease in interictal disturbances. The clinical presentation may not necessarily be a psychosis. In childhood or in the mentally handicapped aggression and agitation are common. Other manifestations may include depression, mania, and anxiety states. The psychotic episodes may last days or weeks. They may be terminated by a seizure, after which the EEG abnormalities then return. More recently forced normalization has been reported in association with the barbiturates, benzodiazepines, ethosuximide, and vigabatrin. It has been observed that recurrence of seizures may be associated with a great improvement in mental state, and Reynolds (25) has suggested that it may therefore be justifiable in such patients to reduce antiepileptic therapy temporarily with the aim of allowing the occurrence of one or more seizures.

Aggressive Disorders and Episodic Dyscontrol

The association between violent behavior and epilepsy has a long and controversial history. Although prison surveys indicate that more prisoners have epilepsy than would be expected from population statistics, closer examination reveals that they are not any more likely to be associated with violent crime (26). Nevertheless, in recent times the issue has been reexamined, in part driven by the use of epileptic automatisms as a legal defense against charges of crimes of violence.

An international workshop was convened to consider the nature of aggression during epileptic seizures (27). This group observed that the peri-ictal aggressive acts that they studied appeared suddenly, without evidence of planning, lasting an average of 29 seconds and occurring during complex partial seizures. The behavior was attributed to ictal fear or in response to being restrained. The authors concluded that directed aggression during seizures was rare and that committing murder or manslaughter during random and unsustained psychomotor automatisms was a "near impossibility." In their paper they propose several criteria to help determine whether a violent crime was the result of an epileptic seizure.

In a detailed study of five patients with temporal lobe epilepsy and a history of violent behavior, Devinsky and Bear (28) also concluded that ictal violence was rare. They observed that the more frequent, clinically important aggressive behaviors did not occur during the ictal period.

The study of interictal violence brings more emphasis to the consideration of variables not directly associated with the epileptic process. Mendez et al. (15) studied 44 patients with epilepsy who presented for psychiatric evaluation because of violent behavior and compared them with 88 nonviolent control patients with epilepsy. They found that the groups did not differ on seizure variables or EEG findings. On the other hand, the group with a history of violent behavior were more likely to be young men with cognitive impairment and other psychopathology such as psychosis.

Although aggressive behavior is not uncommon in society, some individuals present with a repeated history of sudden, brief and uncontrollable outbursts of violence, often with minimal provocation. Such attacks may be associated with the intake of small amounts of alcohol. After these outbursts of what have been described as episodic dyscontrol, the individual may express remorse.

The association of episodic dyscontrol with epilepsy has been based on the suggestion that epilepsy can occur without seizures but with behavioral disturbance. This idea has developed from the concept of masked or larval epilepsy, which originated in the nineteenth century from the writings of Morel (29).

Bach-y-Rita et al. (30) described 130 patients presenting with violent behavior in whom the pattern of disturbance was one of episodic dyscontrol. Seven of these patients had a known history of temporal lobe epilepsy, and a total of 25 out of the 130 subjects reported a seizure at some time. However, the authors made the point that multiple neurological and social factors could interact to produce this pattern of disturbance. This conclusion is supported by observations that after specifically excluding patients with epilepsy, men with episodic violent behavior similar to that described by Bach-y-Rita and colleagues can be found.

The precise status of episodic dyscontrol as a discrete entity currently remains unclear, as do possible associations with other pathological processes. Overall, it appears that temporal lobe EEG abnormalities are associated with episodic dyscontrol in both those with and without epilepsy (31), suggesting that feelings of dyscontrol and rage are primarily associated with discharges in the amygdala and hippocampus (32).

Although, as discussed above, aggressive behavior conforming to the pattern of episodic dyscontrol should probably be considered as quite distinct from a diagnosis of epilepsy, it has been successfully treated with carbamazepine (33). Indeed, for some time carbamazepine has been noted to be useful in reducing the number of aggressive episodes in violent psychiatric patients without EEG abnormalities.

IMPACT OF PSYCHIATRIC ILLNESS ON THE MANAGEMENT OF EPILEPSY

The development of psychiatric symptoms places additional burdens on those with epilepsy, their families, and their doctors. Pharmacological control of epilepsy is dependent on patients complying accurately with their prescribed anticonvulsant regimens. However, there are various ways in which psychopathology may interfere with compliance. Depression can lead to apathy and self-neglect, including ceasing to take medication, and may also be associated with a decrease in memory and concentration abilities leading to mistakes in the taking of medication. Postictal psychotic states may be associated with confusion, interfering with the ability to follow what are often quite complicated treatment regimes. More sustained psychotic states, both postictal and interictal, may be associated with persecutory delusions, which can lead to the patient stopping medication, for instance, because they believe they are being poisoned. Disturbances in regular antiepileptic treatment generally lead to an increase in seizure frequency. As described above, this increase in seizure frequency may in turn be associated with the development or worsening of psychopathology, leading to a vicious circle of deteriorating seizure control and subsequent further increase in psychiatric symptomatology.

The effect of this deterioration in state may be to prevent a person who had previously been living independently from continuing to do so. The combination of declining seizure control and worsening mental state places increased burdens on caregivers and doctors at a time when their support is most needed. In addition, this combination of symptoms may be particularly difficult to deal with, in that those most comfortable at coping with seizures may be perturbed by the associated psychiatric symptoms and vice versa. Not only health care professionals may find the development of psychiatric symptoms in a person with epilepsy difficult to handle. Both seizures and mental illness are, in the eyes of the general public, strongly stigmatized conditions. Hence those people displaying this combination of symptoms not uncommonly feel particularly marginalized from society at large, even when their more troubling symptoms have abated.

The treatment of psychopathology in people with epilepsy is particularly complicated by the fact that the majority of psychotropic medications lower the seizure threshold, increasing the likelihood of the patient having a seizure, even when using standard therapeutic doses. This is discussed further below.

Another distinct area in which the development of psychiatric symptoms may directly interfere with treatment of epilepsy is when psychiatric symptoms develop directly as a result of the effects of antiepileptic medications. There are reports of a wide range of behavior disturbances, aggression, depression, and psychotic symptoms developing in association with prescription of various antiepilepsy drugs. There are anecdotal reports of the development of mental symptoms associated with most if not all antiepileptic drugs; in some there are more reports than in others. Phenobarbitone, vigabatrin, clobazam, and ethosuxemide have been reported to be associated with an increase in depressive symptoms. Occasionally the development of treatment-related psychiatric symptoms leads to a need to discontinue that particular agent. There is some evidence that those with a previous history of psychiatric illness are more likely to develop anticonvulsant-related psychopathology.

EFFECT OF PSYCHOTROPIC DRUGS ON PSYCHIATRIC DISORDER AND ITS MANAGEMENT

The first stage in treating psychiatric states that may develop in patients with epilepsy is awareness of the possibility that such symptoms can develop. This ongoing vigilance, together with an understanding of the ways in which individual personal factors, a diagnosis of epilepsy, and abnormalities of mental state may interact, will guide the approach to treatment.

Compliance with treatment regimens is important for the optimal control of epilepsy, and even in the absence of additional psychopathology this is an issue. When patients are also suffering from a psychiatric disorder, then compliance with the demands of treatment may be worse. An important determinant of compliance is the quality of the doctor-patient relationship, and it is therefore important that this element of care be specifically addressed. Any approach to management should always include education and support of patients and their families. This will help patients to follow treatment recommendations. Consideration of these issues will also help to ensure good communication between health care professionals and patients so that patients feel that the issues that are important to them are as much a focus of treatment as, for instance, the doctor's concern about drug-related side effects or seizure frequency.

When managing psychopathology in people with epilepsy, while the psychiatric symptoms themselves will often need to be treated actively, the antiepileptic treatment may also require modification. For instance, a patient can become depressed because his or her seizure control has recently deteriorated, causing increased disruption to daily activities. In these circumstances, optimizing antiepileptic drug use to reduce seizure frequency may be the best treatment for the depression, as well as for the epilepsy. Similarly, a patient who develops persecutory delusions in the context the recent development of serial or very frequent seizures needs his or her epilepsy treatment improved as a matter of urgency. In this case a cessation of seizure activity will often be associated with amelioration of the abnormal mental state.

In treating the psychiatric conditions that may arise in association with epilepsy, a variety of outcome measures must be considered. These include the change in detectable psychopathology, effects on seizure frequency, and overall quality of life. A treatment can have a variable effect across these areas. For instance, treating depression with an antidepressant that lowers the seizure threshold, thereby provoking more seizures, may lead to a decrease in quality of life despite a reduction in depressive symptomatology. Alternatively, some patients may prefer the risk of more seizures if their depression can be treated. Hence, for each individual patient, not only the current clinical state but also the broader psychosocial situation must be assessed. Only then can an optimal treatment package be developed.

Depression

Particular pharmacotherapies of epilepsy may themselves lead to psychopathology and will therefore need to be reconsidered. There is evidence that the use of both phenobarbitone and of polypharmacy in the management of epilepsy are associated with an increased incidence of depression. In general, changing anticonvulsant medication from these regimens to, where possible, the use of carbamazepine as monotherapy may be associated with a decrease in depression. Carbamazepine, which like the tricyclic antidepressants has a tricyclic structure, has been known for some years to have an antidepressant effect in patients with primary depression as well as in those with epilepsy and depression (34).

In view of the interplay of psychosocial and biological factors in the genesis of anxiety and depression, several authors have pointed out the value of including the appropriate type of psychotherapy within the overall management plan. Cognitive strategies can be used to treat mild to moderate degrees of depression as well as generalized anxiety disorder and agoraphobia. These approaches, based on work by Beck, have as the main focus of treatment the identification, by the patient with the help of the therapist, of anxious or depressive cognitions and "thinking errors" such as arbitrary inference of ambiguous situations and overgeneralizing of negative events. Having recognized these phenomena, patients are taught to switch to more helpful thoughts and reactions in response to negative or stressful situations such as a seizure. Self-help groups may be helpful, particularly in dealing with symptoms of dysthymia, as opposed to more severe depression (35). Such groups have also helped patients to reduce anxieties by providing a forum for sharing problem-solving strategies relating to many aspects of daily living with epilepsy. In other circumstances, support and possibly advocacy for the patient in areas such as employment or housing may be more appropriate than a more formal medical intervention in reducing symptoms of anxiety and depression. A thorough assessment of not only the patient's mental state but also their psychosocial environment will indicate whether such socially orientated interventions are called for.

In the more severe depressive illnesses that can develop in people with epilepsy, antidepressant treatment and occasionally electroconvulsive therapy may be indicated. In addition, and importantly, suicidal behavior is a well-recognized feature of depression in people with epilepsy, therefore an early part of management should be to decide about the level of any suicidal risk and to adjust subsequent placement and treatment accordingly. Considering pharmacotherapy, antidepressants have been reported to lower the seizure threshold. The use of tricyclic and related antidepressants and selective serotonin-reuptake inhibitors has been associated with occurrence of seizures in people without epilepsy, although the frequency of this effect has been difficult to establish. It appears that a significant proportion of those experiencing antidepressant-related seizures have a predisposing factor, such as a previous seizure, ongoing alcohol withdrawal, or various additional medications. In the case of imipramine, the most widely studied tricyclic, a recent review observed that the literature reported seizure rates between 0.3 and 0.6% at effective doses (36). Higher doses may be associated with further increased rates. Lithium also has pro-convulsant potential. The risk of this may be less with monoamine oxidase inhibitors. Although clear findings are limited, there is evidence that these agents may also be associated with increased seizure frequency in people with epilepsy. It has been suggested that those with a family history of epilepsy may be more likely to develop a seizure in association with the use of a tricyclic antidepressant (37). It is also important to bear in mind the problem of drug interactions between antidepressants and anticonvulsants. Nevertheless, many patients with depression and epilepsy benefit from antidepressant medication, and, provided the small risk of exacerbating seizures is considered, there is no general contraindication to their use.

Although there is limited experience with the use of electroconvulsive therapy in epilepsy, Betts (38) reports that it causes no problems and points out that in severe drug-resistant depression (38) with the attendant risk of suicide, it may be life-saving.

Psychoses

The general principles underlying the management of psychoses developing in people with epilepsy are in many ways similar to those discussed with respect to depression. Attention should be paid to the increased burden that the development of psychotic symptoms will place on patients and their carers. Compliance with antiepileptic medication should be assessed and drug interactions between antiepileptic and antipsychotic medication considered. Patients recovering from the psychotic episode may become concerned that they are developing a mental illness, and this may lead to the development of depression or suicidal thoughts. Those developing a chronic psychotic state will require the full range of psychiatric and psychosocial support.

The treatment of peri-ictal psychoses will largely be aimed at terminating seizure activity. Postictal psychoses may be short-lived and self-limiting. In these cases, and because this state may be associated with postictal confusion, an important treatment priority is to keep the patient safe. This will involve skilled nursing care and may also require the use of sedating medication. If postictal psychotic features persist and in the case of interictal psychoses, neuroleptics are often indicated. As with antidepressants, the use of antipsychotics must be tempered with particular caution given the potential for interactions with antiepileptics and the effect of neuroleptics on lowering the seizure threshold. Phenothiozenes are more likely to provoke seizures than butyrephenones, and a number of reports describe the effective use of haloperidol, sulpiride, and pimozide. There is less experience with the newer atypical neuroleptics, but several reports describe increased seizure activity in patients prescribed clozapine.

REFERENCES

1. ILAE. Commission on Classification and Terminology of the International League Against Epilepsy. Proposal for revised classification of epilepsies and epileptic syndromes. Epilepsia 1989; 30:389–399.
2. Lewis AJ. Melancholia: a historical review. J Ment Sci 1934; 80:1–42.
3. Mendez MF, Cummings JL, Benson F. Depression in epilepsy: significance and phenomenology. Arch Neurol 1986; 13:766–770.
4. Pond D, Bidwell B, Stein L. A survey of 14 general practices. Part 1: medical and demographic data. Psychiatr Neurol Neurochirurg 1960; 63:217–236.
5. Edeh J, Toone BK. Antiepileptic therapy, folate deficiency, and psychiatric morbidity: a general practice survey. Epilepsia 1985; 26:434–440.
6. Stevens JR. Psychiatric aspects of epilepsy. J Clin Psychiatry 1988; 49(suppl):49–57.
7. Manchanda R, Schaefer B, McLachlan RS, Blume WT. Interictal psychiatric morbidity and focus of epilepsy in treatment-refractory patients admitted to an epilepsy unit. Am J Psychiatry 1992; 149:1096–1098.
8. Kogeorgos J, Fonagy P, Scott DF. Psychiatric symptom patterns of chronic epileptics attending a neurological clinic: a controlled investigation. Br J Psychiatry 1982; 140:236–243.
9. Barraclough B. Suicide and epilepsy. In: Reynolds EH, Trimble MR, eds. Epilepsy and Psychiatry. Edinburgh: Churchill Livingstone, 1981:72–76.
10. Mathews WS, Barabas G. Suicide and epilepsy: a review of the literature. Psychosomatics 1981; 22:515–524.
11. Williams D. The structure of emotions reflected in epileptic experiences. Brain 1956; 79:29–67.

12. Blanchet P, Frommer GP. Mood change preceeding epileptic seizures. J Nerv Ment Dis 1986; 174:471–476.
13. Taylor DC, Lochery M. Temporal lobe epilepsy; origin and significance of simple and complex auras. J Neurol Neurosurg Psychiatry 1987; 50:673–681.
14. Betts TA. Depression, anxiety and epilepsy. In: Reynolds EH, Trimble MR, eds. Epilepsy and Psychiatry. Edinburgh: Churchill Livingstone, 1981:60–71.
15. Mendez MF, Doss RC, Taylor JL. Interictal violence in epilepsy—relation to behavior and seizure variables. J Nerv Ment Dis 1993; 181:566–569.
16. Robertson MM, Trimble MR, Townsend HRA. Phenomenology of depression in epilepsy. Epilepsia 1987; 28:364–372.
17. Chaplin JE, Yepez-Lasso R, Shorvon SD, Floyd M. National general practice study of epilepsy: the social and psychological effects of a recent diagnosis of epilepsy. Br Med J
18. Jacoby A, Johnson A, Chadwick A. Psychosocial outcomes of antiepileptic drug discontinuation. Epilepsia 1992; 33:1123–1131.
19. Trimble MR. Interictal psychoses of epilepsy. In: Smith DB, Treiman DM, Trimble MR, eds. Advances in Neurology. New York: Raven Press, 1991:143–152.
20. Logsdail SJ, Toone BK. Postictal psychoses. A clinical and phenomenological description. Br J Psychiatry 1988; 152:246–252.
21. Glithero E, Slater E. The schizophrenia-like psychoses of epilepsy. IV Follow-up record and outcome. Br J Psychiatry 1963; 109:134–142.
22. Trimble MR. The Psychoses of Epilepsy. New York: Raven Press, 1991.
23. Flor-Henry P. Psychosis and temporal lobe epilepsy: A controlled investigation. Epilepsia 1969; 10:363–395.
24. Landolt H. Serial electroencephalographic investigations during psychotic episodes in epileptic patients and during schizophrenic attacks. In: Lorentz de Haas AM, ed. Lectures on Epilepsy. Amsterdam: Elsevier, 1953:91–133.
25. Reynolds EH. The pharmacological management of epilepsy associated with psychological disorders. Br J Psychiatry 1982; 141:549–557.
26. Gunn J, Bonn J. Criminality and violence in epileptic prisoners. Br J Psychiatry 1971; 118:337–343.
27. Delgado-Escueta AV, Mattson RH, King L, et al. The nature of agression during epileptic seizures. N Engl J Med 1981; 305:711–716.
28. Devinsky O, Bear D. Varieties of aggressive behavior in temporal lobe epilepsy. Am J Psychiatry 1984; 141:651–656.
29. Trimble MR, Ring HA, Schmitz B. Neuropsychiatry of the epilepsies. In: Fogel BS, Schiffer RB, eds. Neuropsychiatry: A Comprehensive Textbook. Baltimore: Williams and Wilkins, 1996.
30. Bach-y-Rita G, Lion JR, Climent CE, Ervin FR. Episodic dyscontrol: a study of 130 violent patients. Am J Psychiatry 1971; 127:1473–1478.
31. Trimble MR. Biological Psychiatry. Chichester: John Wiley & Sons, 1988.
32. Heath RG. Psychosis and epilepsy: similarities and differences in the anatomic-physiologic substrate. In: Koella WP, Trimble MR, eds. Temporal Lobe Epilepsy, Mania and Schizophrenia and the Limbic System. Basel: Karger, 1982:106–116.
33. Lewin J, Sumners D. Successful treatment of episodic dyscontrol with carbamazepine. Br J Psychiatry 1992; 161:261–262.
34. Post RM, Uhde TW, Roy-Byrne PP, Joffe RT. Antidepressant effects of carbamazepine. Am J Psychiatry 1986; 143:29–34.

35. Becu M, Becu N, Manzur G, Kochen S. Self-help epilepsy groups: an evaluation of effect on depression and schizophrenia. Epilepsia 1993; 34:841–845.

36. Rosenstein DL, Nelson JC, Jacobs SC. Seizures associated with antidepressants: a review. J Clin Psychiatry 1993; 54:289–299.

37. Edwards JG. Antidepressants and seizures: epidemiological and clinical aspects. In: Trimble M, ed. The psychopharmacology of epilepsy. Chichester: John Wiley & Sons, 1985:119–139

38. Betts TA. Depression, anxiety and epilepsy. In: Reynolds EH, Trimble MR, eds. Epilepsy and Psychiatry. Edinburgh: Churchill Livingstone, 1981:60–71.

18

Alzheimer's Disease and Other Dementias

Neal G. Ranen* and Barry W. Rovner

Jefferson Medical College
Thomas Jefferson University
Wills Geriatric Psychiatry Program
Philadelphia, Pennsylvania

Approximately 8–10% of people over 65 years of age have dementia, and perhaps an equal number have subclinical cognitive impairment. About a third of these latter individuals will be recognized as demented within 2 years. In special populations, such as nursing home residents, the prevalence of dementia is even higher and has been estimated to be approximately 80%. Despite the high rate of dementia in those over 65, it remains underdiagnosed (1). Although there are no treatments for the underlying pathology of the majority of dementias, there are effective symptomatic treatments for the psychiatric aspects of these diseases, which can reduce morbidity among both patients and caregivers.

HISTORICAL OVERVIEW AND CASE ILLUSTRATION

Alois Alzheimer first described the clinical symptoms and pathology of the disease that came to bear his name in 1907. He described a woman who died in her fifties, had early prominent psychotic features, and experienced rapid cognitive decline (2). Alzheimer went on to describe the presence of "miliary foci" in the cerebral cortex that "represent the sites of deposition of a peculiar substance." Today, we know these foci to be the amyloid neuritic plaques that form the characteristic pathology of Alzheimer's disease.

---

* *Current affiliation:* Health Pathways of Albright Care Services, York, and Penn State College of Medicine, Hershey, Pennsylvania.

The case described by Alzheimer is somewhat atypical both in the early age of onset and in the prominent, early delusional thought content and rapid cognitive decline. Perhaps more typical is the case of Mrs. S., an 81-year-old woman whose cognitive decline had a slow insidious onset and a gradually progressive course. Her initial symptoms eluded detection by the family physician for several years, in part because the family explained away the patient's problems. Her history was remarkable for both a family and personal history of major depression. She had been treated with monthly psychotherapy for 30 years prior to evaluation, but her last "nervous breakdown" was 40 years earlier. Past medical history was remarkable for hypertension, a myocardial infarction 20 years previously, a left carotid bruit, and hypothyroidism.

The patient arrived with her husband, sister, and daughter, all of whom gave a different history. The sister denied the presence of any cognitive problems, attributing everything to marital difficulties and an unforgiving husband; the husband attributed her behaviour solely to depression; and the daughter firmly believed that there was a physical basis to the patient's decline. Overall, it was ascertained that she had been declining cognitively for the previous 5 years, with problems with memory and orientation. She began to call people by the wrong name and was unable to identify her grandchildren in pictures. She increasingly relinquished her usual responsibilities to the husband, who eventually took over management of the household. Friends began calling the daughter to report that the patient seemed confused. The patient also had become more apathetic and hypersomnolent. She had occasional tearful episodes and refused to join activities even when prompted. She was eating less than usual and had lost several pounds. The Mini Mental Status Examination score was 18/30, losing points for orientation, recall, naming, comprehension, and copy design. Magnetic resonance imaging (MRI) scan revealed scattered white matter lesions, but no frank stroke. Thyroid-stimulating hormone, B_{12}, and RPR levels were normal.

The initial impression was probable Alzheimer's disease with depressive symptoms. The patient was treated with an antidepressant, and her appetite and energy improved but her apathy did not. She would, however, become interested in activities when prompted and participated well in a structured psychosocial day program. As the disease progressed, she began to wander more at night, often compelled by the thought that her home was actually not her home. Although she and her husband had remained sexually active, she would rebuff her husband's advances because she did not recognize him and thought that it was improper for another man to share her bed. Because of her deterioration in self-care and dangerous behavior, such as leaving the stove on, she required nursing home placement.

DIAGNOSIS OF ALZHEIMER'S DISEASE

In many ways this case represents both a classic example of Alzheimer's disease and a dilemma in differential diagnosis. It also highlights the psychiatric aspects of the disease. Alzheimer's disease is defined clinically as a gradually progressive accumulation of cognitive deficits, usually beginning with memory impairment (amnesia) and later manifesting aphasia (language disturbance), apraxia (impaired ability to carry out motor activities, such as dressing and bathing, despite intact motor functions), and agnosia (failure to recognize or identify objects despite intact sensory functions). This constellation of deficits is sometimes referred to as the four As. Disturbances in executive functioning (planning, organizing, sequencing, and abstracting) as well as poor insight, depression, and apathy can begin in the early stages of the disease. These symptoms continue into the middle stage of the disease, when additional behavioral and psychiatric disturbances, such as agitation and delusions, may occur. Some patients with Alzheimer's disease will manifest "catastrophic reactions," which are overwhelming emotional responses to relatively minor stresses, such as changes in routine or environment. Some patients exhibit a period of agitation during the evening hours, which is referred to as "sundowning." Later in the disease, neurological symptoms such as rigidity, myoclonus, worsening gait disturbance, and primitive release reflexes are more evident. Duration of disease is typically 8–12 years from onset.

The MRI scan in Alzheimer's disease may reveal nonspecific diffuse atrophy. The classic pattern on SPECT scan, which measures cerebral blood flow, consists of bitemporoparietal hypoperfusion. Although there is a relationship between brain atrophy and intellectual decline in Alzheimer's disease (3), the correlation is not clinically significant enough for any one individual to enable a clinician to make a diagnosis based on the scan alone.

To meet DSM-IV criteria for dementia (see Table 1), the cognitive deficits must result in an impairment in functioning (4). NINCDS criteria for probable Alzheimer's disease (see Table 2) is similar to the DSM-IV criteria in requiring that the cognitive deficits not be due to any other conditions, such as multiple strokes, or systemic conditions such as B_{12} deficiency known to cause dementia (5).

Patients or other informants may initially (and mistakenly) describe their cognitive decline as having an acute onset related to a psychosocial event, such as the death of a spouse. However, further questioning often reveals a true gradual onset with merely an unmasking of the cognitive deficits with loss of supportive compensation by a caregiver.

DIFFERENTIAL DIAGNOSIS OF ALZHEIMER'S DISEASE

The differential diagnosis of dementia is quite broad (see Table 3). However, many of the causes of dementia are due to systemic or neurological diseases that are readily distinguishable from Alzheimer's disease. Perhaps the most common cause of dementia after Alzheimer's disease is multi-infarct or vascular dementia. A diagnosis of vascular dementia requires the presence of focal neurological signs and multiple cortical or strategic subcortical lesions on brain imaging. There is an emerging consensus that vascular dementia is overdiagnosed. This occurs particularly if a patient has risk factors for vascular disease and scattered periventricular white matter changes on MRI. Such

Table 1   DSM-IV Diagnostic Criteria for Dementia of the Alzheimer's Type

A. The development of multiple cognitive deficits manifested by both of the following:
   1. Memory impairment (impaired ability to learn new information or to recall previously learned information
   2. One (or more) of the following cognitive disturbances:
      a. Aphasia (language disturbances)
      b. Apraxia (impaired ability to carry out motor activities despite intact motor function)
      c. Agnosia (failure to recognize or identify objects despite intact sensory function)
      d. Disturbance in executive functioning (i.e., planning, organizing, sequencing, abstracting)
B. The cognitive deficits in criteria A1 and A2 each cause significant impairment in social or occupational functioning and represent a significant decline from a previous level of functioning.
C. The course is characterized by gradual onset and continuing cognitive decline.
D. The cognitive deficits in criteria A1 and A2 are not due to any of the following:
   1. Other central nervous system conditions that cause progressive deficits in memory and cognition (e.g., cerebrovascular disease, Parkinson's disease, Huntington's disease, subdural hematoma, normal-pressure hydrocephalus, brain tumor)
   2. Systemic conditions known to cause dementia (e.g., hypothyroidism, vitamin B_{12} or folic acid deficiency, niacin deficiency, hypercalcemia, neurosyphilis, HIV infection)
   3. Substance-induced conditions
E. The deficits do not occur exclusively during the course of a delirium.
F. The disturbance is not better accounted for by any another Axis I disorder (e.g., major depressive disorder, schizophrenia).

changes are often described as "periventricular white matter ischemic changes," reflexively leading to a diagnosis of vascular dementia even though there are no frank strokes. Most studies have found no association between white matter hyperintensities and neuropsychological performance in healthy patients unless the lesions are extensive. White matter abnormalities are seen in approximately one third of patients with Alzheimer's disease and should not by themselves dissuade the physician from that diagnosis. Typically, vascular dementia presents with truly abrupt onset and stepwise deterioration, consistent with accumulating vascular events. Certainly, vascular and Alzheimer's pathology can coexist, since both are common conditions in advanced age.

Lewy body disease (LBD) as an etiology for dementia has become increasingly appreciated (6). There are multiple forms of LBD, including pure LBD and the Lewy body variant of Alzheimer's disease, where both Lewy body and Alzheimer pathology coexist. Lewy body dementia is classically characterized by the presence of extrapyramidal symptoms or marked sensitivity to developing extrapyramidal symptoms on neuroleptic (antipsychotic) medication. In contrast to Alzheimer's disease, such patients present with early rather than late neurological symptoms. These patients characteristically

Table 2   NINCDS-ADRDA Criteria for Clinical Diagnosis of Alzheimer's Disease

I.   The criteria for the clinical diagnosis of probable Alzheimer's disease include:
  Dementia established by clinical examination and documented by the Mini-Mental
    Test, Blessed Dementia Scale, or some similar examination, and confirmed by
    neuropsychological tests
  Deficits in two or more areas of cognition
  Progressive worsening of memory and other cognitive functions
  No disturbance of consciousness
  Onset between the ages of 40 and 90 years, most often after age 65
  Absence of systemic disorders or other brain diseases that in and of themselves could
    account for the progressive deficits in memory and cognition
II. The diagnosis of *probable* Alzheimer's disease is supported by:
  Progressive deterioration of specific cognitive functions, such as language (aphasia),
    motor skills (apraxia), and perception (agnosia)
  Impaired activities of daily living and altered patterns of behavior
  Family history of similar disorders, particularly if confirmed neuropathologically
  Laboratory results of:
    Normal lumbar puncture as evaluated by standard techniques
    Normal pattern of nonspecific changes in EEG, such as increased slow-wave activity
    Evidence of cerebral atrophy on CT with progression documented by serial
      observation.
III. Other clinical features consistent with the diagnosis of *probable* Alzheimer's disease,
    after exclusion of causes of dementia other than Alzheimer's disease, include:
  Plateaus in the course of progression of the illness
  Associated symptoms of depression, insomnia, incontinence, delusions, illusions,
    hallucinations, catastrophic verbal, emotional, or physical outbursts, sexual
    disorders, and weight loss
  Other neurological abnormalities in some patients, especially with more advanced
    disease and including motor signs such as increased muscle tone, myoclonus, or
    gait disorder
  Seizures in advanced disease
  CT normal for age
IV. Clinical diagnosis of *possible* Alzheimer's disease:
  May be made on the basis of the dementia syndrome, in the absence of other
    neurologic, psychiatric, or systemic disorders sufficient to cause dementia, and in the
    presence of variation in the onset, in the presentation, or in the clinical course
  May be made in the presence of a second systemic or brain disorder sufficient to
    produce dementia, which is not considered to the cause of the dementia
  Should be used in research studies when a single, gradually progressive severe cognitive
    deficit is identified in the absence of other identifiable cause.
V.   Criteria for diagnosis of *definite* Alzheimer's disease are:
  The clinical criteria for probable Alzheimer disease, and histopathologic evidence
    obtained from a biopsy or autopsy.

Table 3   Differential Diagnosis of Alzheimer's Disease

Vascular disease
Lewy body dementia
Parkinson's disease
Frontotemporal dementia (e.g., Pick's disease)
Huntington's disease
Normal pressure hydrocephalus
Delirium, including chronic drug intoxication
Alcoholic dementia
Metabolic disorders, including vitamin B_{12} deficiency, hypothyroidism
Infectious causes, including HIV, neurosyphilis, and bacterial meningitis
Major depression

have prominent psychiatric symptomatology and delirium-like spells in the course of their progressive decline.

Estimates of the prevalence of dementia in Parkinson's disease have ranged from 20 to 60% of cases. The dementia of Parkinson's disease has been referred to as a "subcortical" dementia because it has less striking symptoms attributable to the cerebral cortex (e.g., aphasia or agnosia). Instead, initial cognitive changes involve loss of cognitive speed and flexibility and disturbances in planning and organizing. Although memory is impaired, recognition is relatively preserved; therefore, patients may respond to cues.

Other less common causes of dementia include normal pressure hydrocephalus (NPH) and Pick's disease. NPH classically presents as a triad of dementia, gait disturbance, and urinary incontinence. Central ventricular enlargement with a periventricular "halo effect" is seen on MRI. Pick's disease (or lobar degeneration) is a frontotemporal dementia and is characterized by early psychiatric symptomatology, particularly disinhibition and coarsening of personality. MRI scan may reveal isolated frontal or temporal degeneration, and SPECT may demonstrate frontal or temporal lobar hypoperfusion.

Also important in the differential diagnosis of Alzheimer's disease is the dementia of depression (previously termed "pseudodementia"). Some elderly patients with severe depression have cognitive deficits; they usually resolve with resolution of the other depressive symptoms. Nonetheless, dementia of depression may not simply be a benign reversible condition, as it is associated with an increased future risk for dementia, predominantly Alzheimer's disease (7).

It is important to differentiate delirium from dementia and to identify delirium when it occurs in patients with dementia. Delirium is a disturbance in attention/level of consciousness due to exogenous causes such medications and comorbid medical problems, such as urinary tract infections, abnormal blood sugar, or pneumonia. The patient who presents with an unexpected rapid deterioration of cognition along with a waxing and waning level of consciousness or significant disturbance of the sleep/wake cycle should be evaluated for delirium.

RISK FACTORS AND PROTECTIVE FACTORS

Perhaps the most important risk factors for Alzheimer's disease are genetic ones (8). The genetics of Alzheimer's disease can be divided into two categories: autosomal dominant genetic mutations and the genetic susceptibility factor associated with particular forms of a protein known as apolipoprotien E (ApoE). Gene mutations on chromosomes 1, 14, and 21 have been shown to cause Alzheimer's disease. Such autosomal dominant genetic mutations account for a minority of all cases of Alzheimer's disease, however, and are most important as causes of early onset disease. Mutations in the amyloid precursor protein (APP) gene (found on chromosome 21) are the best characterized and lead to abnormal accumulation of beta-amyloid, which is a primary component of amyloid neuritic plaques. Interest in chromosome 21 arose from the observation that patients with Down syndrome, or trisomy 21, developed Alzheimer's disease pathology at an early age.

The risk associated with certain forms of the gene that codes for APOE, found on chromosome 19, is a factor in a many cases of Alzheimer's disease. ApoE is found in three forms: ApoE 2, ApoE 3, and ApoE 4. ApoE is involved in cholesterol transport and is a known risk factor for coronary artery disease. Individuals with two copies of ApoE 4 (homozygous) have approximately an 80% likelihood of developing Alzheimer's disease by age 80 and have an earlier age of onset. One copy of ApoE 4 also yields an increased, but less higher, risk. There is, however, a lack of association between E-4 and Alzheimer's disease in some populations, such as African Americans, Amish, and Finnish centenarians. There is also evidence that ApoE 2 may be protective. The mechanism is unknown, but it has been suggested that E2 binds to tau protein, preventing neurofibrillary tangle formation, and that E4 binds to amyloid, enhancing plaque formation.

Risk factors (other than genetic factors) for Alzheimer's disease include older age and head injury (especially if associated with an ApoE 4 allele). Possible protective factors appear to include lifetime use of nonsteroidal anti-inflammatory drugs, steroids, estrogen replacements, and antioxidants such as vitamins E and C. There is also evidence that premorbid brain size is a determinant of reserve capacity against intellectual decline in Alzheimer's disease (3).

DIAGNOSTIC EVALUATION

Early in the course of the disease, patients are often unaware of their deficits. Therefore, the dementia evaluation begins with a thorough history provided by informants as well as the patient. This is accomplished by interviewing informants separately from the patient, as informants may be reluctant to report behavioral disturbances, particularly aggressiveness, in the presence of the patient. A thorough mental status exam should be performed, including a cognitive screening examination. Cognitive screening scales such as the Mini Mental Status Examination (MMSE) (9) are helpful in following the patient's course longitudinally. Cognitive evaluation should include testing of orientation, attention, memory, recall, and language, including both expressive language such as naming, and writing, and receptive language, such as understanding spoken and written commands. Constructional ability is assessed by having the patient copy a diagram. Testing of apraxia can also include asking the patient to mimic hand movements or demonstrate how they comb their hair or brush their teeth. Clock drawing can be useful in assessing executive functions, such as planning and sequencing, and hemineglect. In addition, an assessment of general intellectual functioning, including knowledge of current events, as well as assessment of insight, judgment, and ability to abstract, should be undertaken. The presence of noncognitive psychiatric features, such as depression and delusions, should also be assessed. A neurological examination should be performed, looking for focal or extrapyramidal signs.

Laboratory evaluation should include screening for reversible causes of dementia such as vitamin B_{12} deficiency, thyroid abnormalities, neurosyphilis (RPR), a complete blood count, and chemistry screening (10). Neuroimaging may be performed, particularly if there is a specific indication, such as focal neurological deficits.

GENERAL MANAGEMENT STRATEGIES

Once the etiology of the dementia has been established, management of the patient begins. Reversible causes of dementia should be treated as indicated. Currently, the core component of the management of nonreversible causes of dementia consists of minimizing excess disability, such as addressing emotional and behavioral complications, devising a schedule or routine of constructive activities, and maximizing physical health otherwise. Even though most patients and families prefer a cure, minimizing excess disabilities is the strategy behind care of most common chronic diseases. At present, the greatest opportunities for intervention and the alleviation of patient suffering, family burden, and societal costs are within the domains of the behavioral and psychological signs and symptoms. However, with advances in our understanding of the pathophysiology, research is being directed to finding specific treatments for the disease, and already, medications working at the neurotransmitter level are available (see below).

There are some important caveats to appreciate in the longitudinal management of patients with Alzheimer's disease. As indicated above, the first is to appreciate that a patient's judgment, memory, and insight are impaired so that others need to be available to provide information on daily functioning. Second, although mortality is increased, disease progression is highly variable, often depending on the quality of care a patient receives. Third, medications should be reviewed regularly because adverse drug reactions are common, particularly with medications with anticholinergic properties. Tune et al. (11) performed a study of anticholinergic activity of commonly used drugs and found such activity surprisingly common.

Fourth, regular health maintenance visits should be scheduled to discuss issues of safety, advanced directives, and contingency plans for expected progression of the disease. Fifth, cormorbid conditions should be aggressively treated. These conditions, including delirium, urinary tract infections, pneumonia, and pulmonary embolus, occur at higher rates in patients with dementia, and prolonged recovery is the norm.

Finally, caregivers should be trained in strategies to manage behavioral disturbances, such as appreciating irritability as a symptom of the disease and not fueling the patient's irritability by arguing with them over matters of no consequence. Support groups are often helpful in this regard and should be encouraged to minimize isolation, to develop adaptive coping skills, and to access community resources. Caregiver interventions have been found to significantly delay nursing home placement (12).

RECOGNITION AND MANAGEMENT OF SPECIFIC PSYCHIATRIC/BEHAVIORAL SYNDROMES

Common psychiatric/behavioral disturbances in Alzheimer's disease include depression, apathy, psychosis, irritability and agitation, and other behavioral problems such as driving impairment.

Depression

Although major depression in its full form is uncommon, depressive symptoms such as anhedonia and amotivation are common.

The prevalence of depression among patients with Alzheimer's disease is highly variable, depending on patient samples and diagnostic criteria (13). Alzheimer's patients with dysthymia (or minor depression) tend to have onset of their affective symptoms in the early stages of dementia (14). In contrast, about one half of Alzheimer's patients with major depression experienced onset of the mood disorder prior to the onset of dementia. A prior history of depression (15), younger age of onset of Alzheimer's disease (16), and female gender (17,18) have been reported as possible risk factors for depression in patients with Alzheimer's disease. Although frank mania is rare, elation has been reported in up to 20% of Alzheimer's patients (19).

Depressed Alzheimer's patients have greater impairment in activities of daily living (ADLs) compared to nondepressed Alzheimer's patients matched on age, physical mobility, and degree of cognitive impairment. Furthermore, Rovner et al. (20) found that major depression increased one-year mortality in nursing home residents, the majority of whom (59%) were demented.

There are some clues as to the biochemical basis of depression in Alzheimer's disease. Zweig et al. (21) reported more severe neuronal loss in both the locus coeruleus and the dorsal raphe nucleus in depressed versus nondepressed patients with Alzheimer's disease, demonstrating abnormalities in production of biogenic amines as important in the development of depression in Alzheimer's disease. In contrast, relative preservation of the cholingeric system has been seen in depressed versus nondepressed Alzheimer's patients (22).

Rather than prominent self-reproach/guilt and difficulties with concentration, more reliable indicators of depression in Alzheimer's disease include nonverbal manifestations of dysphoria such as irritability, demandingness, dependency behavior, and complaining (23). This is consistent with the diminished insight and relative lack of appreciation that Alzheimer's patients have for their illness (anosagnosia) and their internal mood state even in earlier stages of the disease (24).

Antidepressants are effective in treating depression in Alzheimer's disease (25). However, one study (26) found that euthymic Alzheimer's patients receiving imipramine exhibited a mild decline in cognition, suggesting that antidepressants with strong anticholinergic effects should be avoided.

The consensus practice guidelines for treatment of Alzheimer's disease (25) suggests that selective serotonin-reuptake inhibitors (sertraline, fluoxetine, paroxetine) are the most appropriate first-line agents, although the secondary amine tricyclic antidepressants (nortriptyline, desipramine), or newer agents such as bupropion or venlafaxine, may also be useful.

There are case studies supporting the safety and efficacy of electroconvulsive therapy in the treatment of depression in patients with Alzheimer's disease (27), especially those who had been unresponsive or intolerant to antidepressant medications. Twice rather three times weekly and unilateral rather than bilateral treatments may decrease the risk of delirium.

Apathy

Important in the differential diagnosis of depression in Alzheimer's disease is primary apathy. Such amotivational states are common (28) and result in the lack of spontaneous initiation of activity by the patient. However, when apathetic patients are actively engaged and continually prompted, they can derive enjoyment from activities. Apathy can be a source of conflict when caregivers believe the patient is physically capable of activities but "won't" do them.

Treatments for apathy are not well documented, but dopaminergic agents such as psychostimulants, bupropion, bromocriptine, and amantadine may be helpful.

Delusions and Hallucinations

Hallucinations and delusions are common in Alzheimer's disease and typically begin in the mid and latter states of the disease (29).

Delusions affect between 30 and 50% of Alzheimer's patients (13,30). The most frequent delusions involve false beliefs of theft, infidelity of the spouse, abandonment, feeling the house is not one's home, persecution, phantom boarder, and the Capgras phenomenon, which consists of believing that someone close to the patient is an identical appearing impostor (31). There is some evidence that Alzheimer's patients with delusions decline more rapidly cognitively than those without (32). Hallucinations are less common, seen between 9 and 20% of patients. Visual hallucinations are most common, followed by auditory hallucinations.

Hallucinations and delusions are most appropriately treated with antipsychotic medication. Traditional antipsychotic agents such as haloperidol or thioridazine are effective but have the attendant extrapyramidal adverse effects, which occur more frequently in elderly and demented populations. Such extrapyramidal side effects can be an increased source of morbidity, including predisposing the patients to falls. Patients may be more apathetic on these medications, which can contribute to incontinence. The conventional antipsychotic agents are also associated with tardive dyskinesia, for which the elderly, women, and individuals with dementia are at increased risk. The newer "atypical" neuroleptics such as clozapine, risperidone, and olanzepine have the advantage of reduced extrapyramidal effects and possibly tardive dyskinesia. However, with risperidone, and perhaps olanzepine, extrapyramidal symptoms are dose dependent and may appear at higher doses. Very low starting doses are recommended in this population, for example, haloperidol 0.5 mg, thioridazine 10 mg, risperidone 0.5 mg, clozaril 6.25–12.5 mg, and olanazepine 2.5–5 mg per day. Although clozapine is less likely to be associated with extrapyrmadial reactions, it is associated with sedation, postural hypotension, and elevated seizure risks, carries a risk of agranulocytosis, and requires weekly blood monitoring.

Irritability, Agitation, and Aggressiveness

Agitation and particularly aggressive behavior can be seen in patients with Alzheimer's disease. Increased irritability and aggressive behavior occur in 30–50% of Alzheimer's patients (33). Aggressive behavior is more frequent in dementia with psychosis (24,35,36). "Agitation" may consist of increased motor activity or loud, repetitive, distressed verbalizations. It is important to specify which behaviors are being observed and under what circumstances the behaviors occur when a patient is said to be "agitated." Catastrophic reactions occur when a demented patient is faced with a task that overwhelms their cognitive abilities. Because of the deficits in cognition, they are predisposed to catastrophic reactions when they are unable to complete a task that others press them to do. When overwhelmed, they become agitated or "catastrophic."

Prior to initiating treatment with medication, identifying why a patient is agitated is important. Is it because a caregiver is hurrying the patient or pushing him beyond his capabilities? Is it because the patient is bored and restless? Is the patient depressed and anxiously pacing, or delusional and fearing assault? Is a urinary tract infection present, or is the patient in pain from arthritis, an impaction, or dental disease? The clinician should undertake this kind of differential reasoning before proceeding immediately to a medication.

If there is not an easily identified cause of agitation and aggressiveness, it can be difficult to treat, and for this reason nearly every medication in the psychiatric pharmacopoeia has been tried. Antipsychotic agents remain the best documented for agitation and are used as described above for delusions and hallucinations. Benzodiazepines appear to perform better than placebo but not as well as antipsychotics in treating behavioral symptoms (25). Side effects of benzodiazepines include sedation, worsening cognition, delirium, increased risk of falls, and paradoxical excitement. The anticonvulsants carbamazepine and valproate have been reported to be effective, as have certain serotoninergic agents such as trazodone, buspirone, and selective serotonin-reuptake inhibitors, such as sertraline. Medroxyprogesterone and depot leuprolide may have a role in treating disinhibited sexual behavior, particularly aggressive sexual behavior in male patients with dementia.

Driving

Even mild dementia can pose a legitimate driving concern. Mildly affected Alzheimer's patients were shown to have lower driving scores when matched on MMSE scores to patients with vascular dementia and diabetes mellitus. Overall, there is a correlation between MMSE score and driving (37). However, in the office setting such a correlation is not clinically useful because the MMSE may be insensitive both to some retained skills and to serious attentional impairments and reduced reaction time. Tests of selective attention and working memory have been associated with driving scores. Unfortunately, there are no simple screening tests of level of cognitive impairment that indicate when driving is unsafe. Passing a driving test is not necessarily indicative of how a patient will perform on his or her own, because a person being tested is often prompted as to what to do by the instructor.

There is a strong consensus that demented patients with moderate impairment should not drive. This includes patients who cannot perform moderately complex tasks, such as preparing simple meals or performing household chores. Often caregivers will overestimate the patient's driving performance and may have a vested interest in the patient continuing to drive. The physician should consult the laws in their state regarding reporting of unsafe drivers.

TREATMENTS AIMED AT COGNITIVE DECLINE

Cholinesterase Inhibitors

There are currently two FDA approved medications for the treatment of Alzheimer's disease: donepezil and tacrine (38). Both are cholinesterase inhibitors and thereby increase the availability of acetylcholine by blocking its breakdown in the synaptic cleft. Both medications were demonstrated in large double-blind, placebo-controlled, randomized studies to confer modest improvements in cognition and global function. Donepezil, a piperidine-based compound, is structurally distinct from tacrine, an acridine-based molecule. Donepezil has the advantage of fewer adverse effects, including the absence of hepatocellular toxicity, and therefore carries no requirement for blood monitoring. Use of cholinesterase inhibitors has been associated with delay in nursing home placement (39) and improvements in behavior (40) as well as cognition. Lewy body dementia may also respond to cholinergic therapies (41). The most common adverse effects of these medications stem from their cholinergic properties and include adverse gastrointestinal effects (more common with tacrine than donepezil) including nausea, vomiting, and diarrhea, bradycardia, increased gastric acid secretion, which may be a concern in those with a history of peptic ulcer disease or those taking nonsteroidal anti-inflammatory agents, and potential interaction with anesthetic muscle relaxants. Tacrine is started at 10 mg four times a day and can be increased every 6 weeks by 10 mg four times a day. Best results are obtained at higher doses, with 160 mg a day optimal if tolerated. Donepezil is started at 5 mg PO qhs, with current recommendations to increase the dose if tolerated to 10 mg after 4–6 weeks (38).

Estrogen-Replacement Therapy

Women on estrogen-replacement therapy (ERT) have a lower incidence of Alzheimer's disease, and if they do develop the disease, they do so at a later age. The longer the duration of use of estrogen, the lower the apparent risk of Alzheimer's disease. There is preliminary evidence that treatment of Alzheimer's disease with ERT may improve cognitive functioning and may enhance the effect of cholinesterase inhibition (25).

Studies are ongoing investigating the use of steroids and nonsteroidal anti-inflammatory drugs in the treatment of Alzheimer's disease.

Vitamin E

Alpha-tocopherol (vitamin E), at doses of 2000 IU a day, and the selective monoamine oxidase inhibitor selegiline were reported to delay progression to predetermined endpoints, such as institutionalization, in patients with moderate-severity Alzheimer's disease (42). However, these findings have been viewed with caution on a number of levels, including that the findings were seen only after post hoc statistical adjustment, that there was no effect on cognitive scales, and that combined treatment with vitamin E and selegiline yielded no additive benefit (43).

CONCLUSION

Appropriate recognition of Alzheimer's disease and its attendant psychiatric/behavioral syndromes can reduce avoidable morbidity among both patients and caregivers. Further information and support for patients and their family members or other caregivers can be obtained from the Alzheimer's Association (phone 1-800-621-0379).

REFERENCES

1. Callahan M, Hendrie HC, Tierney WM. Documentation and evaluation of cognitive impairment in elderly primary care patients. Ann Intern Med 1995; 122:422–429.
2. Alzheimer A. Uber eine eigenartige Erkankung der Hirnrinde. Allg Z Psychiatrie 1907; 64:146.
3. Mori E, Hirono N, Yamashita H, Imamura T, Ikejiri Y, Ikeda M, Kitagaki H, Shimomura T, Yoneda Y. Permorbid brain size as a determinant of reserve capacity against intellectual decline in Alzheimer's disease. Am J Psychiatry 1997; 154:18–24.
4. American Psychiatric Association. Diagnostic and Statistical Manual of Mental Disorders. 4th ed. Washington, DC: APA, 1994.
5. McKhan G, Drachman D, Folstein M, Katzman R, Price D, Stadlan EM. Clinical diagnosis of Alzheimer's disease: report of the NINCDS-ADRDA Work Group under the auspices of Department of Health and Human Services Task Force on Alzheimer's Disease. Neurology 1984; 34(7):939–944.
6. McKeith IG, Fairbairn AF, Perry RH, Thompson P. The clinical diagnosis and misdiagnosis of senile dementia of Lewy body type (SDLT). Br J Psychiatry 1994; 165:324–332.
7. Devanand DP, Sano M, Ming-Xin T, Taylor S, Gurland BJ, Wilder D, Stern Y, Mayeux R. Depressed mood and incidence of Alzheimer's disease in the elderly living in the community. Arch Gen Psychiatry 1996; 53:175–182.
8. Mukaetova-Ladinka EB, Roth M. Alzheimer's disease—new approaches to old problems. Int Rev Psychiatry 1995; 7:419–435.
9. Folstein MF, Folstein SE, McHugh PR. "Mini-Mental State": a practical method for grading the cognitive state of patients for the clinician. J Psychiatr Res 1975; 2:189–198.
10. Okagaki JF, Alter M, Byrne TN, Daube JR, Franklin G, Frishberg BM, Goldstein ML, Greenberg MK, Lanska DJ, Mishra S, Odenheimer GL, Paulson G, Pearl RA, Rosenberg JH, Sila C, Stevens JC. Practice parameter for diagnosis and evaluation of dementia. Neurology 1994; 44:2203–2206.
11. Tune L, Carr S, Hoag E, Cooper T. Anticholinergic effects of drugs commonly prescribed for the elderly: potential means for assessing risk of delirium. Am J Psychiatry 1992; 149: 1393–1394.
12. Milletman MS, Ferris SH, Shulman E, Steinberg G, Levin B. A family intervention to delay nursing home placement of patients with Alzheimer disease. JAMA 1996; 76:1752–1731.
13. Wragg RE, Jeste DV. Overview of depression and psychosis in Alzheimer's disease. Am J Psychiatry 1989; 146:577–587.
14. Migliorelli R, Teson A, Sabe L, Petracchi M, Leiguarda R, Starkstein S. Prevalence and correlates of dysthymia and major depression among patients with Alzheimer's disease. Am J Psychiatry 1995; 152:37–44.
15. Pearlson GD, Ross CA, Lohr WD, Rovner BW, Chase GA, Folstein MF. Association between family history of affective disorder and the depressive syndrome of Alzheimer's disease. Am J Psychiatry 1990; 147(4):452–456.

16. Rovner BW, Broadhead J, Spencer M, Carson K, Folstein MF. Depression and Alzheimer's disease. Am J Psychiatry 1989; 146(3):350–353.
17. Reifler BV, Larson E, Teri L, Poulsen M. Dementia of the Alzheimer's type and depression. J Am Geriatr Soc 1986; 34(12):855–859.
18. Lazarus L, Newton N, Cohler B, Lesser J, Schweon C. Frequency in presentation of depressive symptoms in patients with primary degenerate dementia. Am J Psychiatry 1987; 144:41–45.
19. Cummings JL, Victoroff JI. Noncognitive neuropsychiatric syndromes in Alzheimer's disease. Neuropsychiatry Neuropsychol Behav Neurol 1990; 3:140–158.
20. Rovner BW, German PS, Brant LJ, Clark R, Burton L, Folstein MF. Depression and mortality in nursing homes. JAMA 1991; 265(8):993–996.
21. Zweig RM, Ross CA, Hedreen JC, Steele C, Cardillo JE, Whitehouse PJ, Folstein MF, Price DL. Neuropathology of aminergic nuclei in Alzheimer's disease. Prog Clin Biol Res 1989; 371:353–365.
22. Zubenko GS, Moossy J, Kopp U. Neurochemical correlates of major depression in primary dementia. Arch Neurol 1990; 47:209–214.
23. Vida S, Des Rosiers P, Carrier L, Gautheir S. Prevalence of depression in Alzheimer's disease and validity of research diagnostic criteria. J Geriatr Psychiatry Neurol 1994; 7(4): 238–244.
24. Reed RR, Jagust WI, Goulter I. Anosagnosia in Alzheimer's disease: relationships to depression; cognitive function and cerebral perfusion. J Clin Exp Neuropsychol 1993; 15:231–244.
25. American Psychiatric Association Work Group on Alzheimer's Disease and Related Dementias. Practice guideline for the treatment of patients with Alzheimer's disease and other dementias of late life. Am J Psychiatry 1997; 154(suppl):5.
26. Teri L, Reifler BV, Veith RC, Barnes R, White E, McLean P, Raskind M. Imipramine in the treatment of depressed Alzheimer's patients: impact on cognition. J Gerontol 1991; 46(6):372–377.
27. Price TRP, McAllister TW. Safety and efficacy of ECT in depressed patients with dementia: a review of clinical experience. Convuls Ther 1989; 5:61–74.
28. Rubin E, Morris J, Berg L. The progression of personality changes in senile dementia of the Alzheimer's type. J Am Geriatr Soc 1989; 35:721–725.
29. Rosen J, Zubenko GS. Emergence of psychosis and depression in the longitudinal evaluation of Alzheimer's disease. Biol Psychiatry 1991; 29:224–232.
30. Cummings JL, Miller B, Hill MA, Neshkes R. Neuropsychitric aspects of multi-infarct dementia and dementia of the Alzheimer's type. Arch Neurol 1987; 44(4):389–393.
31. Reisberg B, Borenstein J, Salob SP, Ferris SH, Franssen E, Georgotas A. Behavioral symptoms in Alzheimer's disease: phenomenology and treatment. J Clin Psychiatry 1987; 48(suppl):9–14.
32. Drevets WC, Rubin EH. Psychotic symptoms and the longitudinal course of senile dementia of the Alzheimer's type. Biol Psychiatry 1989; 25:39–48.
33. Patel V, Hope T. Aggressive behavior in elderly people with dementia: a review. Int Geriatr Psychiatry 1993; 8:457–472.
34. Deutsch LH, Bylsma FW, Rovner BW, Steele C, Folstein MF. Psychosis and physical aggression in probable Alzheimer's disease. Am J Psychiatry 1991; 148:1159–1163.
35. Flynn FG, Cummings JL, Gornbein J. Delusions in dementia syndromes: investigation of behavioral and neuropsychological correlates. J Neuropsychiatry Clin Neurosci 1991; 3: 364–370.

36. Aarsland D, Cummings JL, Yenner G, Miller B. Relationship of aggressive behavior to other neuropsychiatric symptoms in patients with Alzheimer's disease. Am J Psychiatry 1996; 153:243–247.

37. Fox GK, Bowden SC, Bashford GM, Smith DS. Alzheimer's disease and driving: prediction and assessment of driving performance. JAGS 1997; 45:949–953.

38. Doraiswamy PM. Current cholinergic therapy for symptoms of Alzheimer's disease. Primary Psychiatry 1996; (Nov.):56–68.

39. Knopman D, Schneider L, Davis K, Talwalker S, Smith F, Hoover T, Gracon S. Long-term tacrine (Cognex) treatment: effects on nursing home placement and mortality. Neurology 1996; 47:166–171.

40. Kaufer DI, Cummings JL, Christine D. Effect of tacrine on behavioral symptoms in Alzheimer's disease: an open-label study. J Geriatr Psychiatry Neurol 1996; 9:1–6.

41. Perry EK, Haroutunian V, Davis KL, Levy R, Lantos P, Eagger, S, Honavar M, Dean A, Griffiths M, McKeith IG. Neocortical cholinergic activities differentiate Lewy body dementia from classical Alzheimer's disease. Neuroreport 1994; 5(7):747–749.

42. Sano M, Ernesto C, Thomas RG, Klauber MR, Schafer K, Grundman M, Woodbury P, Growdon J, Cotman CW, Pfeiffer E, Schneider LS, Thal LJ. A controlled trial of selegiline, alpha-tocopherol, or both as treatment for Alzheimer's disease. N Engl J Med 1997; 336:1216–1222.

43. Drachman DA, Leber P. Treatment of Alzheimer's disease—searching for a breakthrough, settling for less. N Engl J Med 1997; 336:1245–1247.

19

Sleep Disorders

Gabriele M. Barthlen*
Mount Sinai Medical Center
New York, New York

HISTORICAL BACKGROUND

Historically few physiological conditions have received as much attention by poets, novelists, scholars, and scientists as sleep. Ancient medical papyruses of Egypt, written around 1350 B.C., contain information on the interpretation of dreams, which were regarded as being contrary predictions; e.g., a dream about death meant a long life. The Egyptians drank wine and other alcoholic beverages to treat insomnia. Other remedies included medicinal plants, particularly the opium poppy, and scopolamine derived from the nightshade.

Chinese remedies for excessive sleepiness included ephedra, a stimulant containing ephedrine, and the medical herb ginseng, used for stimulation and sedation. Sleep was regarded by the Chinese as a state of unity with the universe and therefore very important for health.

Hippocrates, who wrote more than 70 books covering all aspects of medicine, wrote around 400 B.C.: "In whatever disease sleep is laborious, it is a deadly symptom." He used narcotics derived from the opium poppy for insomnia.

The Bible emphasizes the importance of sleep and rest. The essential elements for good sleep were believed to be hard work, a clear conscience, freedom from anxiety, and trust in Jehovah (1).

The Jewish physician Moses Ben Maimon, better known as Maimonides (1200 A.D.), cast the first rules on how much sleep is needed: "It is sufficient for a person to sleep one third of a 24 hour period, which is 8 hours. He should arise from his bed before sunrise" (2).

---

* *Current affiliation*: Freiburg University Medical Center, Freiburg, Germany.

Sleep was depicted poetically by Shakespeare in the seventeenth century (*Macbeth*, 1605):

Sleep that knits reveled of care
The death of each day's life, sore labour's bath.
Balm of hurt minds, great nature's second course chief nourisher.

Another passage by Shakespeare suggests that the playwright himself may have suffered from insomnia:

O Sleep, O Gentle Sleep,
Nature's soft nurse, how have I frightened thee
That thou no more wilt weigh my eyelids down,
and steep my senses with forgetfulness.

The neurologist Thomas Willis (1621–1695) described restless legs syndrome, nightmares, and insomnia. He recognized that caffeine can prevent sleep and that excessive sleepiness was not a disease but primarily a symptom. He devoted four chapters to disorders producing sleepiness and insomnia in his book *The Practice of Physick* (1692). He discovered that a laudanum solution of powdered opium was effective in treating restless legs syndrome.

In the seventeenth and eighteenth centuries, several sleep theories emerged, such as sleep being due to congestion of cerebral blood vessels or, alternatively, due to cerebral anemia. Other theories were that an alteration in the transference of information by neural glia could explain sleep or that sleep was due to an expansion of neuronal processes. Chemical theories were that sleep was caused by lack of oxygen or by an accumulation of lactic acid or toxic waste products. Behavioral theories included that sleep was due to the loss of peripheral stimuli.

The first medication introduced specifically as a hypnotic was bromide in 1853; it was followed by paraldehyde, urethan, and sulfonal. The first description of narcolepsy was given by Jean Baptiste Edouard Gelineau (1828–1906). Obstructive sleep apnea syndrome and Pickwick's syndrome was first depicted in 1836 by Charles Dickens (1812–1870). He described Joe, a fat boy, who was always excessively sleepy in his *Posthumous Papers of the Pickwick Club*. William Hill observed in 1889 that upper airway obstruction contributed to "stupidity" in children.

In the twentieth century, the focus shifted towards dreams and their significance. "The interpretation of dreams is the royal road to knowledge of the part the conscience plays in mental life" Sigmund Freud wrote in *The Interpretation of Dreams* in 1905. He also recognized that paralysis of skeletal muscles during dream sleep prevented the dreamer from acting out dreams.

During the twentieth century the ascending reticular activating system was described, REM sleep was differentiated from non-REM sleep, and it was recognized that serotonin containing neurons of the raphe nucleus were important in the maintenance of sleep. The "biological clock" was placed in the anterior ventral hypothalamus, which was subsequently called the suprachiasmatic nucleus. In the 1960s barbiturates were replaced by benzodiazepines, the use of which has declined since the 1980s because of increased awareness of their disadvantages. Insomnia became recognized as a symptom rather than a diagnosis.

In the 1960s Fredrick Snyder recognized and promoted the importance of psychiatric disorders in sleep medicine, especially depression, in the sense that troubled minds have troubled sleep and troubled sleep causes troubled minds. Behavioral techniques such as stimulus control and sleep restriction therapy were developed, and circadian rhythm disturbances such as jetlag and shift work were recognized as chronobiological disorders.

Organized sleep disorders medicine in the United States began with the founding of the Association for the Psychophysiological Study of Sleep in 1961, which is now called the Association of Professional Sleep Societies (APSS).

CASE PRESENTATION

The following case description depicts physical and psychiatric comorbidity.

A 37-year-old morbidly obese man presented with sleep onset insomnia, early morning awakening, and difficulty breathing when sleeping. He had a history of depression (never treated with antidepressants) and was considered to have an anxiety disorder treated with diazepam (Valium, 5–10 mg) every evening. He had been taking Valium for over 6 months and reported rebound insomnia and nervousness when not taking the drug.

On examination, he weighed 291 pounds and was 72″ tall. Respiratory rate was 20 breaths per minute and labored. He showed an anxious and depressed affect and was irritable, but formal mental status testing was normal. Neurological examination was normal. He was excessively sleepy and started snoring whenever left sitting alone.

Diagnostic polysomnography showed a sleep latency of 0.5 minutes (normal = 10–20), and absent rapid eye movement (REM) sleep (normal = 20% REM sleep). The respiratory disturbance index (RDI) was 40, indicating complete cessation or a partial decrease of breathing 40 times an hour (<5 is normal). Baseline oxygen saturation during wakefulness was 88%, and minimum oxygen saturation was 76% during respiratory events. Awake pCO_2 was 58. He had taken Valium 5 mg before the study night. Subsequently he underwent his first therapeutic continuous positive airway pressure (CPAP) and bi-level positive airway pressure (BiPAP) titration. CPAP and BiPAP are forms of noninvasive ventilation, where compressed room air is delivered through a nasal mask, splinting the upper airway open. Posttherapy polysomnography (PSG) showed an RDI of only 3 with an inspiratory BiPAP pressure of 9 cm H_2O and an expiratory pressure of 6 cm H_2O. However, mean oxygen saturation during respiratory events remained 82%. That night, he slept for 350 minutes but insisted that he hardly slept at all.

The patient subsequently underwent repeat overnight CPAP/BiPAP titrations, with supplementary oxygen up to 2.5 liters per minute. During his last titration, with

BiPAP at an inspiratory pressure of 16 cm H_2O and an expiratory pressure of 14 cm H_2O, with supplementary oxygen at 1 liter per minute, his blood oxygen saturation remained above 90%. Clinically, he was more alert and less irritable after treatment nights, but continued to complain of sleep onset and sleep maintenance insomnia despite normal objective sleep efficiencies.

Despite being warned that he should under no circumstances take any central nervous system (CNS) and respiratory depressants such as benzodiazepines, he continued to take these medications and managed to obtain prescriptions from other physicians. He also was only poorly compliant with CPAP/BiPAP, using the device only twice a week.

Subsequently, he had several emergency room admissions for acute respiratory distress, requiring intubation on one occasion. These admissions were always precipitated by discontinued use of CPAP/BiPAP while using only supplementary oxygen at night, and taking diazepam (Valium) or lorazepam (Ativan) in the evening.

Discussion

This patient presents with several psychiatric issues: anxiety, benzodiazepine addiction, depression, as well as noncompliance with vital medical treatment. He takes benzodiazepines for anxiety, already a controversial indication. In addition, these drugs are contraindicated in patients with obesity-hypoventilation (Pickwick's) syndrome and sleep apnea syndrome, such as in our patient. Pickwickian patients already hypoventilate at baseline; any CNS depressant such as benzodiazepines or alcohol will worsen this condition.

Pathophysiologically, obstructive sleep apnea is due to compromise and abnormal collapsibility of the oropharyngeal space. Medications that further decrease muscle tone, such as benzodiazepines, will increase oropharyngeal collapsibility and depress respiratory drive, resulting in more severe apneas. In addition, this patient had central apneas, which will be prolonged with use of CNS depressants. Physicians prescribing these medications should be more aware of this potentially dangerous situation, as they may put the patient at risk for fatal respiratory depression during sleep. This is exemplified in our patient, whose medical conditions comprise obesity-hypoventilation syndrome, obstructive and central sleep apnea syndrome, as well as hypoxia and hypercarbia.

He also suffers from depression but has refused pharmacological antidepressant treatment. Antidepressants do not impair ventilatory drive. Thus, treatment with an antidepressant with additional anxiolytic action, such as doxepin, would have benefited this patient. It is even conceivable that he might have become more compliant with CPAP/BiPAP treatment, once his depressive symptoms (which included apathetic inertia) were alleviated.

His continued noncompliance with vital respiratory support (CPAP/BiPAP) as well as chronic benzodiazepine intake was felt to possibly represent parasuicidal tendencies; it had been stressed to the patient that he was at a substantial risk every night to die in his sleep. He was well aware that conditions associated with sleep apnea syndrome and nocturnal hypoxemia are cardiac arrhythmias, stroke, myocardial infarction, pulmonary hypertension, and sudden death. His inability to fully comprehend the consequences of noncompliance with therapy may have been due to the cognitive deficits known to occur in sleep apnea patients (4).

In addition to his psychiatric diagnoses, the patient suffers from "sleep state misperception syndrome," a condition in which patients mainly remember the time spent awake at night and do not correctly perceive sleep time. This syndrome can occur when sleep continuity is severely disrupted by multiple awakenings and electrocortical arousals. When not receiving nasal CPAP or BiPAP, our patient experienced more than 200 awakenings and arousals every night, which usually occurred at termination of apneic and hyponeic events. Rather than having the underlying nocturnal breathing disorder treated, the patient used these sleep disruptions as another excuse to take benzodiazepines.

PREVALENCE, CLINICAL MANIFESTATION, AND CLINICAL CORRELATION OF PSYCHIATRIC ILLNESSES IN PATIENTS WITH SLEEP DISORDERS

Polysomnography, Description of Methods

Once a patient is clinically suspected to suffer from one of the 84 currently classified sleep disorders (5), he or she will undergo polysomnography. This diagnostic test consists of continuous noninvasive nocturnal measurement of multiple physiological parameters including cerebral electrical activity (EEG) and eye movements (electro-oculogram, EOG) to correctly identify sleep stages, nasal-oral airflow, as well as chest and abdominal respiratory effort to assess respiration, oximetry to collect oxygen saturation measurements, an EKG to monitor cardiac function, and surface leg electromyography (EMG) to monitor limb activity.

Anxiety and Sleep

Patients with an acute anxiety disorder complain of sleep onset and sleep maintenance insomnia, which may be attributed to apprehensive expectations and fear. Once insomnia is chronic, an almost inevitable dread of the next poor night will create a vicious circle, as the patient has become conditioned to associate nighttime with being awake. Polysomnography reveals a long sleep latency, decreased sleep efficiency, increased amounts of stages 1 and 2 (light sleep), and decreased amounts of slow wave (deep) sleep. REM sleep (dream sleep)–related abnormalities have not been demonstrated in patients with anxiety disorder (6).

Treatment of insomnia using behavioral techniques and psychotherapy is often helpful. Antidepressants have also been used successfully (7).

Depression and Sleep

Many of the neurochemical and physiological processes involved in the regulation of sleep are also involved in the regulation of mood. Subjectively, patients with depression often complain of fragmented sleep, with difficulties falling asleep, frequent awakenings, and—the hallmark sleep disturbance in depression—early morning awakenings. Depressed patients also more often report frightening dreams involving scenes of pursuit, abandonment, or physical harm.

On polysomnography, patients show a prolonged sleep latency (>20 minutes), a short REM latency (<45 minutes), increased REM sleep early in the night, high REM density (increased amounts of eye movements during REM sleep), early morning awakening, and decreased slow wave sleep. Sleep pathology is more prominent during acute depression; however, many electrophysiological abnormalities remain during remission. Interestingly, most antidepressants have profound REM-suppressing properties, and selective REM deprivation (by awakening the patient after 3 or 4 hours of sleep) resulted in one study in a significant improvement of mood on the subsequent day (8).

Conversely, a variety of sleep disorders may lead to secondary depression. The following sleep disorders, to name just a few, have been associated with a depressed mood in patients with no previous history of depression: sleep apnea syndrome (SAS), periodic limb movements in sleep (PLMS), and bruxism (tooth grinding).

Patients with obstructive sleep apnea syndrome often present with depressed mood, decreased interest in the environment, and decreased libido. These changes may be due to the frequent nocturnal awakenings associated with sleep apnea or—less likely—due to nocturnal hypoxemia.

Another condition commonly associated with depression is insomnia, which in turn is often a presenting symptom in depressed patients. In fact, any sleep disorder associated with frequent nocturnal awakenings, be it PLMS, bruxism, or very heavy snoring, may lead to a dysphoric mood on the subsequent day. This is presumably due to unrestful sleep, frequent arousals, and decreased amounts of slow wave sleep (which has been attributed restorative function, as evidence by growth hormone excretion occurring almost exclusively during slow wave sleep). In patients with "atypical depression" hypersomnia may rarely occur.

Before initiating treatment in a depressed patient who presents with significant complaints about sleep, a thorough evaluation by a sleep specialist should be considered. In many cases, a sleep study is warranted to rule out co-existing organic pathology, which could aggravate or contribute to the patient's depressed mood. Appropriate treatment of such pathology, such as noninvasive nocturnal ventilation with CPAP or BiPAP (for sleep apnea syndrome), dopamine agonists (for PLMS), or a dental appliance (for bruxism) will facilitate response to treatment of the underlying depression.

In patients who have insomnia due to an endogenous depression, use of an antidepressant with sedating properties, for example, amitryptiline, doxepine, or trazodone, may alleviate their sleep disturbance. In seasonal affective disorder, or winter depression, light therapy may be effective (7).

Drug Dependency and Sleep

Benzodiazepines are among the most commonly prescribed medications in the world and are often used for anxiety disorders and insomnia. Eleven percent of the U.S. population took anxiolytics in 1980. Of the adult population, 1.6% has used benzodiazepines for a year or longer. Physical benzodiazepine dependence has been amply demonstrated in both animals and humans. Tolerance often develops, efficacy is lost, and especially the long-acting agents can have carry-over effects during the day, resulting in drowsiness, decreased concentration, and impaired daytime performance.

Withdrawal from benzodiazepines often results in reemergence of insomnia and, if withdrawn abruptly, causes rebound insomnia, which is worse than the original condition. Upon withdrawal, new signs and symptoms may emerge, such as confusion, anxiety, headaches, tremor, dysphoria, and, rarely, hallucinations and tinnitus. In susceptible patients, seizures have been precipitated by abrupt benzodiazepine withdrawal. During withdrawal, patients demonstrate severe sleep onset and sleep maintenance insomnia and REM sleep rebound on polysomnography, which is often subjectively experienced as nightmares.

Detoxification of benzodiazepines is facilitated by gradual tapering over several weeks, or switching from a short half-life to a long half-life benzodiazepine, such as clonazepam, before discontinuation. Other strategies for detoxification include use of a beta-adrenergic receptor antagonist such as propanolol, reduction of adrenergic transmission with clonidine, and use of the anticonvulsant carbamazepine (Tegretol). Barbiturate detoxification is carried out similarly.

A condition in which benzodiazepines and other central nervous system depressants are frankly contraindicated is the obesity-hypoventilation syndrome (Pickwick's syndrome). Patients with this disease already suffer from impaired gas exchange, and any CNS depressant medication will impair respiratory drive (which is generated though hypoxemia as well as hypercarbia).

Another condition adversely affected by benzodiazepines is sleep apnea syndrome, be it the obstructive, mixed, or central type. Obstructive sleep apnea syndrome is worsened by benzodiazepines and alcohol, as these agents have muscle-relaxing properties. Central apneas will worsen, too, as CNS depressants decrease respiratory drive (9).

Insomnia and Associated Conditions

Insomnia is the subjective impression of having difficulties falling asleep or staying asleep. Transient insomnia, which often is situational, is defined as lasting up to one week, short-term insomnia weeks to months, and chronic insomnia more than 3 months. Most patients presenting to a sleep center suffer from chronic insomnia. Daytime effects of insomnia are fatigue, difficulty concentrating, a depressed mood, and irritability (10).

Despite subjective reports of daytime impairment, there is often no objective decline of cognitive or locomotive skills. Furthermore, insomniacs as a group are not sleepier than normal subjects during the day when objective measurements of "sleepiness" such as the Multiple Sleep Latency Test (MSLT) is used. During the MSLT, patients are given five nap opportunities during the day at 2-hour intervals, and objective sleep latency is measured polysomnograpically. In a recent study (11) insomniacs actually had increased MSLT values. These insomniacs displayed increased tension and confusion, decreased vigor, personality disturbance, and subjective overestimation of poor sleep. In addition, they had increased body temperature and increased 24-hour whole body metabolic rate.

Although many patients with severe depression or anxiety have disrupted sleep, most patients with insomnia do not have a psychiatric disorder. Insomnia is usually a manifestation of another sleep disorder, a medical disorder, psychiatric disorder, behavioral factors, circadian rhythm disorders, or a primary sleep pathology (e.g., periodic limb movements in sleep or sleep apnea syndrome).

Medical Conditions

Any condition producing pain such as arthritis or sciatica can lead to difficulty sleeping. Patients with pulmonary disease such as asthma often have disturbed sleep; so do patients with neurological disorders like Parkinson's disease. Medications used to treat these conditions such as theophylline in patients with asthma or L-dopa in patients with Parkinson's disease may worsen sleep quality, as they have stimulating properties.

Psychiatric Conditions

Most depressed patients have insomnia, and it is often the presenting symptom. Other psychiatric disorders presenting with profound insomnia include anxiety disorder, obsessive compulsive disorder, and panic disorder.

In mania, duration of sleep is reduced, sometimes to extremes such as 2 or 3 hours, and latency to REM sleep may be shortened. However, most patients do not complain of insomnia. In the acute phase of their illness, schizophrenic patients suffer from sleep maintenance insomnia, and polysomnography may show reduced amounts of REM sleep and slow wave sleep.

Behavioral Conditions

Insomnia can develop when a person engages in stimulating activities before bedtime such as working, watching a stimulating movie, or studying. Other factors that may lead to poor sleep are chronic stress, caffeine use late at night, daytime naps, leaving the TV or radio on throughout the night, exercising late in the evening, and not adhering to regular bed and wake times. In addition, drugs such as caffeine, cocaine, and alcohol may disrupt sleep. Cocaine, a potent central nervous system stimulant, is associated with severe sleep onset and sleep maintenance insomnia.

Circadian Rhythm Disorders

These conditions result from abnormal timing of sleep. Delayed sleep phase syndrome is commonly seen in young adults, who often cannot fall asleep until two, three, or four o'clock in the morning, and then sleep until noon. If they have to retire at hours prior to their preferred sleep time, they often exhibit severe sleep onset insomnia with a sleep latency of several hours duration. Treatment for this condition consists of chronotherapy, which is carried out by delaying the bed time by 3 hours every day (e.g., having a patient go to bed at 6 a.m. on treatment day one, at 9 a.m. on day two, etc.), until the desired bed and sleep time (e.g., midnight) is reached. The patient then needs to adhere strictly to this newly established desired bedtime in order to stabilize his or her "internal clock", a cell group in the hypothalamus called the suprachiasmatic nucleus. Additional measures to consolidate the new sleep-wake schedule are bright light exposure in the morning after awakening (e.g., 3000–5000 lux for 30 minutes) and avoidance of bright light in the afternoon and evening (e.g., by wearing sunglasses later in the day).

Advanced sleep phase syndrome is commonly seen in the elderly. They often retire early, and are wide awake at two or three in the morning. Although they may have slept for six or seven hours, they subjectively have the impression that they did not sleep much during the night, as waking up at two or three in the morning is not socially acceptable. Therapy consists of bright light exposure in the afternoon (e.g., 3000–5000 lux for 30 minutes) in order to delay sleep onset, keeping regular bed and rise times, and avoiding daytime naps.

Another circadian rhythm disorder associated with insomnia is often seen in shift workers. When changing schedules, shift workers may develop insomnia, as the internal clock needs several days to adjust to the new schedule. Subjects adjust easier if the new shift is phase-delayed (i.e., changing from an afternoon to a night shift, rather than changing from a night to an afternoon shift). People who are "night owls," have a natural tendency to go to bed late and thus adjust more easily to night shifts. Workers under 50 years of age also seem to have fewer problems with shift changes.

Jetlag syndrome is a circadian rhythm disorder caused by desynchronization of the internal clock and external "zeitgebers" (time cues). Airplane passengers adjust more easily when they are not sleep deprived prior to the trip, when they fly west, when time zone changes do not exceed 3 hours, and when they have already changed their sleep-wake schedule in the old time zone to match the new time zone. Once at the new destination, it is important to adhere to the local social and environmental zeitgebers.

Primary Sleep Pathology

Sleep apnea syndrome, periodic limb movements in sleep, and bruxism are conditions that can awaken a patient repeatedly during the night and result in insomnia.

A patient with SAS can have up to 200–300 apneic episodes in one night. Because most apneas terminate with electrocortical arousals, 200–300 nocturnal arousals or awakenings will occur. Treatment consists of noninvasive ventilation with nasal CPAP, palatal surgery such as uvulopalatopharyngoplasty (UPPP), or a mandibular advancement device to increase the posterior pharyngeal space. Weight loss, positional training (not sleeping in the supine position, where apneas are usually more severe), and avoidance of CNS depressants such as sedatives, hypnotics, and alcohol will facilitate sleep normalization.

Similarly, PLMS are frequently associated with arousals, resulting in disrupted sleep continuity. PLMS are involuntary leg movements, occurring sometimes every minute, but only at night. Walking results in lessening or abolition of these movements. Movements may or may not be associated with an electrocortical arousal, and sleep is less disturbed when patients have isolated leg movements only, without associated emergence of an alpha or beta pattern on EEG.

A related disorder, restless legs syndrome (RLS), is commonly seen in patients with PLMS. Both PLMS and RLS are frequently seen in older people. They may also be associated with anemia, uremia, or peripheral neuropathy. RLS is characterized by an uncomfortable tingling or burning sensation in the legs, which is relieved by moving the affected limb. Patients with RLS and insomnia should be evaluated polysomnographically in a sleep center, as over 90% of RLS patients suffer from PLMS.

Patients with bruxism and insomnia should also be evaluated polysomnographically. If the individual episodes of tooth-grinding are associated with electrocortical arousals, treatment with a biteplate should be initiated.

Subjective Insomnia/Sleep State Misperception Syndrome

Most insomniacs exaggerate the severity of their sleep problem; they overestimate the time it takes them to fall asleep (sleep latency) and underestimate the total amount of sleep. Over 10% of patients who were evaluated at a sleep center for a complaint of insomnia were found to have normal sleep (11).

Sleep in the Elderly

Sleep in the older population is often characterized by disrupted sleep, decreased sleep time, and increased daytime sleepiness. Basic sleep need seems to be the same, but sleep ability becomes impaired with age. Sleep becomes lighter in the elderly, who often lack slow wave sleep (deep sleep); they awaken more often and feel less rested in the morning. This is often compensated for by staying in bed longer or taking daytime naps. Insomnia is more prevalent in the older population, as are primary sleep pathologies such as SAS, RLS, and PLMS.

Treatment of Insomnia

Treatment should be aimed at the primary cause of the sleep disturbance. Once the underlying medical, neurological, or psychiatric disorder is treated, sleep usually also improves. Isolated psychophysiological insomnia is treated with behavioral measures, which at times may be accompanied by short-term use of hypnotics. Agents that are short acting, such as triazolam, that have little effect on sleep architecture, such as zolpidem, or that have sedating and anxiolytic properties, such as doxepin or trazodone, can be tried.

Behavioral Treatment

General rules that need to be enforced with patients are commonly referred to as "sleep hygiene." Each of these recommendations needs to be discussed with the patient, and a copy of the guidelines listed in the Appendix could be given at the end of the sleep consultation.

In case these general rules for sleep hygiene are not sufficient, behavioral treatment approaches should be tried. A successful concept called "sleep restriction therapy" or "sleep consolidation therapy" consists of restricting the patient's total bed time to the amount of hours he or she is able to sleep. For example, if the patient reports a total sleep time of 5 hours in a 24-hour period, time allowed in bed should be restricted to 5 hours. After a few nights, the patient will learn that only 5 hours are available for him to sleep and sleep becomes consolidated. This concept also includes mild sleep deprivation, as 5 hours of sleep are usually not enough. Once the patient sleeps solidly for those 5 hours, total time allowed in bed can be gradually extended by 30-minute periods until the patient starts complaining of insomnia again (When starting this program, the total hours allowed in bed should not be less than 4.)

Other concepts such as progressive muscle relaxation, electromyographic biofeedback, self-hypnosis, cognitive refocusing, guided imaginery, meditation techniques, and experimentally nocturnal rocking (13) have been tried with modest success. Another approach is stimulus control, based on the theory that insomnia resuts from negative conditioning of the bedroom or sleep environment. It teaches the patient to associate the bedroom with relaxation and sleep.

Pharmacological Treatment

Most medications used to promote sleep are members of the benzodiazepine group, such as triazolam, temazepam, or lorazepam. Nonbenzodiazepine agents include zolpidem, trazodone, or doxepine. An accepted indication for the use of pharmacotherapy is treatment of short-term insomnia, which should not exceed 2 weeks (with the exception of doxepine and trazodone, which are allowed for longer use). If long-term insomnia is present, medical or psychiatric illness can usually be determined during a detailed interview by a sleep specialist and is often confirmed by polysomnography (14).

IMPACT OF PSYCHIATRIC ILLNESS ON THE MEDICAL MANAGEMENT AND COURSE OF SLEEP DISORDERS

Using our case study as an example, this patient carries several psychiatric diagnoses—anxiety, depression and drug dependency—all of which adversely affect his serious organic sleep disorder (obesity-hypoventilation syndrome as well as obstructive and central sleep apnea syndrome).

The patient insisted that he needed antianxiety medication, which would also treat his self-perceived insomnia, and he was able to obtain benzodiazepines from several different physicians. His noncompliance with sleep apnea therapy (nasal noninvasive ventilation with CPAP and BiPAP) put him at great danger for life and led to numerous emergency room and intensive care unit admissions. It is conceivable that his noncompliance with treatment and inability to understand the consequences was partially caused by nocturnal and diurnal hypoxemia and hypercarbia. Another reason for impaired daytime cognition could be his frequent apnea-related nocturnal awakenings, leading to excessive daytime sleepiness. It is also conceivable that his continued use of benzodiazepines led to impaired daytime cognition through accumulation of the drug.

The following measures might have achieved better results in this patient:

1. More stress on weight loss. Losing a substantial amount of weight would have helped treat his obesity-hypoventilation syndrome, as well as sleep apnea syndrome. In his case, a physician-supervised weight loss program, possibly aided by anorectics, should have been initiated.
2. Better education about the necessity of noninvasive nocturnal ventilation.
3. Intensive education about the potential lethal effects of CNS depressants.
4. Closer psychiatric guidance and supervision. The patient should have been encouraged to follow up closely with supportive psychotherapy, which may have enhanced compliance.
5. Only one physician prescribing medications. Ideally, this should have been a psychiatrist with expertise in sleep medicine.
6. Prescribing agents with only minimal effects on respiratory drive. If a sleep-inducing agent were to be used, a nonbenzodiazepine drug such as zolpidem should have been considered. Another option could have been antidepressants such as doxepine or trazodone.
7. Use of anxiolytic agents that do not affect ventilation. Medications such as buspirone should have been considered.
8. Use of two different antidepressants. An agent with alerting properties such as fluoxetine could have been given in the morning, and a sedating antidepressant such as doxepine in the evening. This combination has been useful in patients with excessive daytime sleepiness and nocturnal insomnia.

GENERAL EFFECTS OF PSYCHIATRIC MEDICATIONS ON SLEEP

We will now review commonly used psychiatric medications other than hypnotics and anxiolytics and their effect on sleep.

Antidepressants

These agents include the tricyclic components, tetracyclics, and monoamineoxydase inhibitors and reduce REM sleep regardless of their pharmacologic composition. Impaired performance and daytime drowsiness are likely to arise with antidepressants having a sedative profile, such as amitriptyline or doxepin. On the other hand, zimelidine and nomifensine (neither available in the United States) may improve daytime psychomotor and cognitive function.

Most antidepressants worsen, or even cause PLMS, with the possible exemption of buproprione. PLMS are often subclinical, with the sleeper not being aware of their presence. However, a bed partner may have observed rhythmic twitching or movement of the legs. On polysomnography, periodic limb movements in sleep are readily evident as rhythmic increases of the anterior tibialis muscle tone, often associated with an electrocortical arousal. Thus, if a patient treated with antidepressants (including selective serotonin-reuptake inhibitors) develops sleep onset and maintenance insomnia associated with daytime fatigue and sleepiness, he should be evaluated for the presence of PLMS. The patient should also be asked if he has developed an irresistable urge to move his legs when lying in bed (RLS), a condition frequently seen in patients who have PLMS.

Antidepressants with alerting and stimulating properties such as fluoxetine or monoamine oxidase inhibitors can cause insomnia.

Lithium

Therapeutic doses of lithium increase the latency to or suppress REM sleep. Slow wave sleep is usually increased, and wakefulness may be reduced. During the daytime, patients subjectively often report poor concentration and cognitive impairment, particularly during the early stages of treatment.

Neuroleptics

Neuroleptics do not characteristically affect sleep, although some tend to decrease wakefulness and increase slow wave sleep. The incidence of sedation varies. The butyrophenones are least likely to elicit drowsiness, as compared to the phenothiazines, which have sedating properties.

Stimulants

Tea and caffeinated coffee both contain caffeine, which is also used in many over-the-counter medications including pain killers, appetite suppressants, and tonics for fatigue. Caffeine leads to increased wakefulness, reduced slow wave sleep (deep sleep), and reduced total sleep time.

Other stimulants include the amphetamines, which have been used in the treatment of attention deficit disorder, narcolepsy, fatigue, depressed mood, and behavioral problems. Amphetamines increase wakefulness and delay the onset of REM sleep. Pemoline (Cylert) has only minimal effects on sleep, but as with all central nervous stimulants, ingestion within a few hours of sleep should be avoided.

Anorectics

Drugs enhancing catecholamine activity are often used to depress appetite. The central stimulant action of these drugs is inseparable from their anorectic properties, so insomnia is a frequent side effect. As an exception, fenfluramine, although chemically related to the amphetamines, is associated with sedation.

PREVALENCE OF SLEEP DISORDERS ASSOCIATED WITH MENTAL DISORDERS

Psychoses

Most psychotic patients experience some degree of sleep disruption during exacerbation of their illness.

Mood Disorders

At least 90% of patients with mood disorders have sleep disturbances at some time. Point prevalence for major depression is about 6%, with a lifetime risk for major depression of 15–20%. The lifetime risk for bipolar disorder is approximately 1%.

Anxiety Disorders

Sleep disorders appear to be common in patients with anxiety.

Panic Disorders

Panic disorder has a prevalence of 0.5–1%. Many patients have some degree of sleep disturbance, but the exact prevalence of sleep disturbance among patients with panic disorder is unknown.

Alcoholism

Sleep disturbances are common among alcoholics. They may occur early in the course of excessive alcohol intake, culminate when alcohol abuse peaks, and continue after discontinuation. Sleep disturbances such as frequent nocturnal awakenings and typically early morning awakenings may last for many years during the long-term abstinence period.

SUMMARY

The importance of sleep and dreaming is documented by extensive writing on sleep throughout the ages. Recent studies have underscored the relationship of sleep problems to medical disorders, psychiatric disorders, prescription and over-the-counter drugs, including caffeine, alcohol and drug abuse, as well as poor sleep hygiene. Psychiatric illnesses frequently produce sleep complaints and disturbances of sleep physiology. Chronic benzodiazepine use for insomnia lacks efficacy but is difficult to discontinue once initiated. Primary sleep disorders can induce depressive syndromes. Diagnosis and management of sleep problems often requires the expertise of sleep specialists working in a collaborative environment with psychiatrists and other physicians.

APPENDIX: HANDOUT FOR PATIENTS

General Rules For Good Sleep

Falling asleep: If you are having trouble falling asleep, get out of bed and do something else. Preferably, move to another room and return to bed only when you feel sleepy.

Establish a bedtime routine such as reading, taking a warm shower or bath, or resting quietly.

Stress: Almost everyone experiences an occasional night of lost or disturbed sleep. It is a natural, perhaps adaptive, response to acute stress.

Naps: If you are having trouble falling asleep at night, avoid naps during the day. It is particularly important not to nap in the evening.

Getting up: No matter how poorly you have slept the night before, always set your alarm to arise at the same time each morning.

Exercise: Regular exercise can be an effective aid to sleep. However, do not exercise strenuously in the late afternoon or evening.

Noises: Loud noises may disturb sleep even if you are unaware of waking or do not remember the noise in the morning. These disturbances can reduce restful sleep. If you sleep near excessive noise, try special noise-insulation windows, heavy curtains in the bedroom, or earplugs to protect the amount of restful sleep you get. White noise machines have been used by some people to muffle intermittent background sounds.

Hunger: Hunger may disturb sleep. A light evening snack seems to help people get to sleep. The protein L-tryptophane, which is concentrated in milk, has sleep-promoting properties. Thus, try to drink a large glass of milk before bedtime.

Food and drinks: Various drinks and foodstuffs stimulate the body and disturb sleep. Avoid coffee, tea, caffeinated cola, and spicy foods near bedtime. Avoid late heavy meals.

Sleep quality and quantity: Everyone has a unique sleep pattern. Some adults need 10 hours a night; others need only 5. Most people function best with approximately 8 hours of sleep.

Symptom of a medical problem: Excessive sleepiness or fatigue may signal a medical or psychiatric disorder, such as sleep apnea or depression. It is important to get a proper diagnosis and treatment of the underlying cause of a chronic sleep disturbance.

Pregnancy: Excessive sleepiness during the first 3 months of pregnancy is normal. You may also develop an irresitable urge to move your legs when lying down, called "restless legs syndrome."

Medications/Alcohol: Although an occasional sleeping pill may be of some benefit, chronic (nightly) use of sedatives may be dangerously addictive after a few weeks. Long-term nightly use of sleeping pills can actually hinder good sleep. Natural sleep is the best sleep. Sleeping medications should be used with caution and only for the short-term management of a sleep complaint. Do not self-medicate or increase the dosage yourself. If you feel that your medication is losing its effect, report this to your doctor.

Sleeping medications depress the central nervous system, as does alcohol. Excessive alcohol consumption together with sleeping pills is extremely hazardous and potentially fatal. These agents are particularly dangerous if you have sleep apnea, as they cause further impairment of breathing.

If your doctor prescribes a sleep medication, ask for clear directions and information about the particular drug. Some sleeping pills have a prolonged effect and can impair your coordination and driving skills the following day.

Although alcohol may help to induce sleep, it interferes with good sleep quality and causes frequent and early awakenings (12).

REFERENCES

1. Ecclesiastes 5:12; Psalms 3:5, 4:8; Proverbs 3:24–26.
2. Misheneh Torah, Hilchotch de'oth. Chapter 4.
3. Thorpy MJ, Yager J. The Encyclopedia of Sleep and Sleep Disorders. New York: Facts on File, 1990.
4. Kotterba S, Duchna HW, Widdig W, Raschke K, Blombach S, and Bax K. Kognitive Defizite bei Patienten mit obstruktiver Schlafapnoe und chronisch obstruktiver Atemwegs-erkrankung. Akt Neurol 1996; 23:13.
5. Association of Professional Sleep Societies. International Classification of Sleep Disorders; Diagnostic and Coding Manual. Diagnostic classification steering committee, 1990.
6. Reynolds CF, Shaw Dh, Newton TF. EEG in outpatients with generalized anxiety disorders; a preliminary comparison with primary depression. Psychiatry Res 1985; 12:251–259.
7. Barthlen GM, Stacy C. The dyssomnias, parasomnias, and sleep disorders associated with medical and psychiatric diseases. Mount Sinai J Med 1994; 6(2):139–159.
8. Buysse DJ, Reynolds CF, Kupfer DJ. In: Carskadon MA, ed. Encyclopedia of Sleep and Dreaming. New York: Macmillan, 1993.
9. Gillin JC. Sleep and psychoactive drugs of abuse and dependence. In: Kryger MH, Roth T, Dement WC, eds. Principles and Practice of Sleep Medicine. 2nd ed. Philadelphia: WB Saunders, 1993.

10. Bonnet MH, Arand DL. Sleep loss in aging (review). Clin Geriatr Med 1989; 5(2):405–420.
11. Colman M, Roffwarg H, Kennedy S, Guilleminault C, Cinque J, Cohn M, Karacan I, Kupfer D, Lemmi H, Miles L, Orr W, Phillips E, Roth T, Sassin J, Smith F, Weitzman E, Dement W. Sleep wake disorders based on a polysomnographic diagnosis; a national cooperative study. JAMA 1982; 247:997–1003.
12. Project Sleep. National Program on Insomnia and Sleep Disorders, March 1996.
13. Barthlen GM, Lund R, Ruether E. Augmentation of slow wave sleep and reduction of arousals in adults with chronic insomnia by all-night rocking in a swing bed. In: Koella WP, Rüther E, Schultz H, eds. Sleep '84. Stuttgart, Germany: Gustav Fischer, 1985:403–405.
14. Stepanski EJ. Insomnia. In: Carscadon MA, ed. Encyclopedia of Sleep and Dreaming. New York: Macmillan, 1993.

20

Migraine and Other Headache Disorders

Kathleen R. Merikangas, Denise J. Stevens, and James R. Merikangas
Yale University School of Medicine
New Haven, Connecticut

HISTORICAL BACKGROUND

Headache syndromes are widespread disorders that cause substantial impairment in occupational and social functioning. The most prevalent headache syndromes include migraine and tension-type headache. Although not as common, other chronic pain conditions associated with psychopathology include posttraumatic headache and trigeminal neuralgia.

Numerous clinical, epidemiological, and anecdotal studies have examined the association between migraine and psychopathology. Over 50 years ago, clinicians involved in the treatment of migraine were aware of a set of characteristic features of migraineurs including anxiety, depression, and social fears. Wolff (1) was so convinced of this constellation of attributes that he is often credited as being the initiator of the concept of the "migraine personality." However, more careful inspection of his description reveals that the characteristics of "extreme physical fatigue, apathy, and anxious anticipation" are more akin to psychiatric symptoms than personality traits. Earlier descriptions of these characteristics can also be found throughout the clinical literature. The most common features of these descriptions are depression characterized by anergia and anxiety disorders, particularly panic disorder and phobia. The contemporary equivalent to these features is the "atypical" subtype of depression.

The purpose of this chapter is to: 1) provide background on the definition, magnitude, and risk factors of the major headache syndromes; 2) describe appropriate clinical evaluation and differential diagnosis of headache; 3) summarize evidence for the association between headache syndromes and psychiatric disorders; and 4) review the treatment of persons with headache syndromes and psychiatric disorders.

CASE EXAMPLE

A 37-year-old divorced mother of two small children had seen a neurologist for persistent throbbing headaches that were accompanied by nausea and dizziness. She was treated with propranolol but had little relief. Because of increasing depression, she sought psychiatric treatment with the encouragement of her treating neurologist, who suggested that the headaches were psychosomatic, caused by her recent divorce and subsequent coping problems. On interview she did indeed appear depressed, but she stated that she actually felt better after the divorce and was convinced that her depression was the result rather than the cause of the headaches.

She had no previous history of migraine and during previous depressive episodes had had no headaches. On neurological examination there were no abnormalities and her laboratory profile was unremarkable. A CT scan of the brain demonstrated a parasagittal meningioma the size of a walnut. This was removed with no complications and no subsequent neurological deficits. Both the headache and the depression resolved with no pharmacological treatment.

DEFINITIONS

The International Headache Society (IHS) (2) introduced a new headache classification system in 1988 in order to provide specific operational criteria for the major headache syndromes and to facilitate international standardization of the diagnostic nomenclature for headache syndromes. The criteria are intended to be applied to classify headache subtypes based on information obtained from a history, a physical and neurological examination, and appropriate laboratory investigations. In this system note that there is no category for "psychosomatic" or "psychogenic" headache because there has never been a valid demonstration that mental illness or life stress causes headaches. This chapter describes the most frequent primary headache syndromes, namely, migraine, tension-type headache, cluster headache, and posttraumatic headache. The remainder of the headache subtypes described in the IHS system are secondary to a variety of acute and chronic conditions. It is essential to evaluate multiple causes of headache for a thorough clinical evaluation of headache as described below. The bulk of this chapter will focus on migraine since this is the most common headache syndrome and there is abundant research on the links between migraine and psychiatric disorders.

Table 1 International Headache Society Criteria for Migraine Without Aura

A. At least five attacks
B. Duration between 4 and 72 hours
C. At least two of the following:
 1. Unilateral
 2. Pulsating pain
 3. Moderate to severe intensity
 4. Worsening with exertion
D. One of the following:
 1. Nausea or vomiting
 2. Photophobia and phonophobia

Source: Ref. 2.

Migraine

Migraine is a complex debilitating condition characterized by either the presence or absence of aura symptoms. Migraine presentation is multifaceted with symptoms emanating from multiple systems, including vascular, neurological, gastrointestinal, endocrine, and visual manifestations. These symptoms may be accompanied by a variety of changes in behavior and cognition, including mood alterations and confusion. Historically, the usual definitions of migraine included the presence of cyclic headaches associated with a variety of gastrointestinal and neurological symptoms.

The IHS criteria for migraine with and without aura are presented in Tables 1 and 2. The core features of most definitions of migraine include recurrent headache accompanied by gastrointestinal symptoms such as nausea or vomiting and hyperesthesia manifested by photophobia or phonophobia. The headache generally has a pulsatile or throbbing quality and therefore is exacerbated by routine physical activity involving

Table 2 International Headache Society Criteria for Migraine with Aura

A. At least two attacks that fulfill criteria in B and C
B. At least three of the following characteristics:
 1. One or more completely reversible aura symptoms that indicate focal cerebral cortical or brain stem dysfunction (or both)
 2. At least one aura symptom develops gradually over >4 minutes or two or more symptoms occur in succession
 3. No aura symptom lasts >60 minutes
 4. Headache follows aura in <1 hour
C. No evidence of related organic disease

Source: Ref. 2.

movement of the head and is often unilateral. The new classification of migraine by the IHS no longer includes the common classic distinction; instead, migraine is separated by the presence or absence of aura symptoms (reversible neurological dysfunction).

The classification of migraine has been complicated by the following phenomena: the co-occurrence of multiple headache syndromes within individual persons; the tendency for headache characteristics to change across the life span; the effects of professional and self-treatment of headache in obscuring the manifestations of the underlying headache syndromes(s); and the lack of generalizability of treated samples from which the diagnostic criteria were derived.

Tension-Type Headache

The definition of tension-type headache according to IHS criteria is presented in Table 3. Briefly, tension headache is characterized by episodes of bilateral pain lasting several

Table 3   International Headache Society Diagnostic Criteria for Tension-Type Headache

I. Episodic tension-type headache
    A. At least 10 previous headache episodes fulfilling criteria B–D listed below; number of days with such headache: 180/year
    B. Headache lasting from 30 minutes to 7 days
    C. At least two of the following pain characteristics:
        1. Pressing/tightening (nonpulsating) quality
        2. Mild or moderate intensity
        3. Bilateral location
        4. No aggravation by walking stairs or similar routine physical activity
    D. Both of the following:
        1. No nausea or vomiting (anorexia may occur)
        2. Absence of photophobia and phonophobia, or presence of one but not the other
II. Chronic tension-type headache
    A. Average headache frequency > 15 days/month for >6 months (180 days/ year), fulfilling criteria B–D listed below
    B. At least two of the following pain characteristics:
        1. Pressing/Tightening quality
        2. Mild or moderate severity
        3. Bilateral location
        4. No aggravation by walking stairs or similar routine physical activity
    C. Both of the following:
        1. No vomiting
        2. No more than one of the following: nausea, photophobia, or phonophobia

Source: Ref. 2.

days at a time. It is distinguished from migraine headache by its generally longer duration, the lack of pulsating quality of the pain, the lack of worsening with physical activity, and the absence of gastrointestinal concomitants. However, migraine and tension-type headache may often coexist, either simultaneously or alternating over time. It is no longer believed that tension-type headache results from muscle tension. Indeed, neck pain may result from head movement to reduce headache pain.

Cluster Headache

Cluster headache is a distinct syndrome characterized by frequent attacks (often several per day) over a 1- to 2-month period, separated by headache-free intervals for as long as 1 or 2 years. Although it is commonly grouped with migraine, current evidence including epidemiological data, treatment response, and clinical features suggests that cluster headache may comprise a distinct syndrome.

Cluster refers to a "clustering in time," with the headache bouts occurring every day to several times a day over a period of days to weeks, followed by a lengthy headache-free interval. Cluster headache is generally retro-orbital in location and is accompanied by autonomic changes such as lacrimation, rhinorrhea, erythema of the eye, and agitation. Patients with cluster headache do not retire to dark rooms and lie down to avoid the stimulation but may in fact do quite the opposite, appearing almost manic in their agitation. The pain can be so intense that the sufferer may appear to be psychotic because of the screaming and thrashing that may be associated with the pain.

Chronic paroxysmal hemicrania is a type of cluster headache specifically responsive to treatment with indomethacin and characterized by many daily focal attacks of pain lasting for short periods, generally about 15 or 20 minutes per attack.

Posttraumatic Headache

Posttraumatic headache is variable in symptom presentation, severity, and duration. The key symptoms include a headache following head trauma accompanied by a loss of consciousness, posttraumatic amnesia, and abnormal laboratory tests. Although headache following a traumatic head injury has often been attributed to emotional factors, empirical evidence suggests that emotional factors are more likely to be a sequela rather than a cause of posttraumatic headache. Nevertheless, the etiology of posttraumatic headache is unknown. The major hypotheses of the pathogenesis of posttraumatic headache include cerebral edema, cortical spreading depression, innate vulnerability to cerebral vasospasm, and transient elevation of intracranial pressure. There is no direct relationship between the prevalence or chronicity of posttraumatic headache and several indicators of severity of head injury including duration of unconsciousness, posttraumatic amnesia, electroencephalographic abnormalities, presence of skull fracture, or the presence of blood in the cerebrospinal fluid. There appears to be an inverse relationship between the severity of the head injury development of post–head injury headache;

posttraumatic headache is more common after injuries that do *not* result in skull fracture.

The onset of typical migraine attacks following acute head trauma occurs so frequently that it has been hypothesized that head trauma serves as a trigger for migraine in persons with underlying susceptibility to migraine. There is a substantial body of literature suggesting that individuals with either a personal or family history of migraine are particularly susceptible to headache following head trauma. Moreover, relatives of posttraumatic migraine subjects have an increased prevalence of neurological symptoms, suggesting a propensity to neurological manifestations of migraine.

PREVALENCE

Epidemiological studies have shown that approximately 60% of persons in the general population report a history of severe headaches. Migraine without aura and tension-type headache are the most common headache syndromes in the general population. The lifetime prevalence of migraine derived from systematic population surveys is about 12% (3–6). Epidemiological studies that have applied the IHS criteria reveal lifetime prevalence rates of approximately 6% among men (range 4% to 19%) and 17% among women (range 8% to 29%). The severity of migraine ranges from mild to near total disability. Over 80% of those with migraine report some degree of disability. A significant aspect of the impact of migraine that is often neglected is the degree to which migraine is associated with occupational and social impairment. Missed work or school days and impairment in familial and social relationships approximate that of other serious chronic diseases but are rarely recognized (9,10).

Migraine is more common among women and persons between the ages of 20 and 45 years, and the incidence decreases after the fourth decade of life. Migraine may often begin in childhood when boys and girls are equally likely to suffer from migraine headache. Migraine in childhood is more likely to be associated with gastrointestinal complaints, particularly episodic bouts of stomach pain, vomiting, or diarrhea, and the duration is shorter than that commonly observed in adults. In women, migraine is strongly associated with reproductive system function, with increased incidence during puberty and the first trimester of pregnancy, and it is associated with exogenous hormone use. After menopause, the frequency of migraine attacks generally decreases dramatically, unless estrogen-replacement therapy is administered.

A family history of migraine is one of the most potent and consistent risk factors for migraine. Although migraine has been postulated to have an autosomal dominant mode of transmission, recent reviews of the genetic studies of migraine indicate that its mode of transmission has not been well established. A substantial proportion of migraine patients have no family history of this condition (7).

The course of migraine is highly variable. In general, both the frequency and duration of migraine decrease at midlife in both men and women, and the symptomatic manifestations may change substantially over time.

Compared to studies of migraine, far fewer studies have investigated the epidemiology and risk factors associated with tension-type headache (13,15–17). The prevalence of tension-type headache has been estimated to range from approximately 30% to 80% depending on the definitions used. It is difficult to arrive at true estimates of the prevalence of tension-type headache given that migraine and tension-type headaches may co-occur in the same individual. Tension-type headaches are also more common in women and young adults, but there is a less steep decrement in prevalence with age.

Although posttraumatic headache is quite rare in the general population (i.e., about 1% lifetime prevalence), it is quite common among those with a history of a concussion or head injury (32). The estimates of the prevalence of severe and chronic headache following severe head injury based on retrospective data range from 28% to 62%. Children and young adults appear to be particularly susceptible to the development of headache after head trauma. The results of prospective studies of the incidence of headache following severe head injury, usually defined as postconcussion headache, reveal that approximately 50% of each series of admissions continue to suffer from headache at the time of discharge from the index admission, with a gradual dissipation to 20% at 1 year. Persistence of headache has been related to female sex, age over 45, the presence of dizziness, lack of skull fracture, intracranial hematoma, disorders of smell, hearing, or vision, depression, and impaired concentration.

Cluster headache has a very low population prevalence (less than 1% of the general population) and occurs nearly exclusively in males (16). The age at onset of cluster headache is somewhat later than that of migraine and tension-type headache; the first attack of cluster usually begins in the late 20s or 30s and may recur intermittently throughout life. Risk factors include smoking and heavy alcohol use.

DIFFERENTIAL DIAGNOSIS AND CLINICAL EVALUATION

A very skillful workup is essential because headache is such a nonspecific complaint with an enormous number of etiologies ranging from the trivial to the acutely life-threatening. A thorough examination should include a description of the type and location of pain, timing, precipitants, prodromal events, and associated symptoms. The following factors are important to determine in order to define whether the headache is migrainous: 1) onset, 2) frequency, 3) location, 4) duration, 5) quality, 6) severity, 7) precipitants, 8) precursors, 9) triggers, 10) phenomena that worsen or relieve the pain, 11) warning signs, 12) prodromal events, 13) specific symptoms including visual changes, gastrointestinal symptoms, or neurological symptoms, 14) sensitivity to light, noise, sounds, or touch, 15) mood changes, and 16) cognitive changes. In addition, it is important to obtain a detailed family history, description of course, and a history of previous evaluation and treatment. Differential diagnosis of headache is based on a neurological examination to rule out pathognomonic signs that might indicate other brain disorders.

In addition to a history and physical examination, laboratory studies are critical when metabolic, structural, vascular, or other sources of headache are suspected. Even if the results are negative and do not uncover a metabolic, endocrine, or autoimmune etiology, this information may serve as a baseline for subsequent drug therapy. Application of the HIS criteria requires that all the potential causes of headache be considered. The diagnosis of headache requires the exclusion of other conditions, including structural lesion, vascular formation, viral or bacterial meningitis, or encephalitis, intracranial abscess or hemorrhage, cerebral contusion, metabolic disorders (urea cycle disorders, aminoacidopathies, mitochondrial disorders), pseudotumor cerebri, vasculitis, brain tumors, sinusitis, or ocular disorders, any of which may be concurrent rather than causal.

An image of the brain is mandatory for the evaluation of patients with severe or persistent headache, the "first" or "worst" headache, or when a subdural hematoma is suspected. Magnetic resonance imaging (MRI) is indicated when hydrocephalus, brain tumor, sinusitis, vasculitis, or posterior fossa lesions are suspected or when exposure to electromagnetic radiation is contraindicated. X-rays of the jaw and cervical spine are useful to rule out malocclusions and degenerative changes.

COMORBIDITY OF HEADACHE SYNDROMES AND PSYCHIATRIC DISORDERS

Evidence and Magnitude of Comorbidity

There is now substantial evidence that corroborates early anecdotal clinical descriptions regarding the co-occurrence of migraine with depression and anxiety. Numerous studies of depression in clinical samples of migraine patients and the converse have been conducted. Associations between the two disorders are consistently found, irrespective of the index disorder for which the subjects sought treatment (8). Studies of clinical samples reveal that approximately 40% of patients in treatment for migraine have a lifetime history of depression or an anxiety disorder.

The results of studies of community samples are summarized in Table 4 (11,12,14,26,27,29,31,36). Rates of depression among subjects with migraine in community studies range from 15 to 60%, depending upon the definition of depression

Table 4   Association (Odds Ratio) Between Migraine with Depression and Anxiety: Community Studies

Authors (Ref.)	N	Depression	Anxiety
Merikangas et al. (36)	115	2.9	—
Merikangas et al. (11,31)	591	2.2	2.7
Stewart et al. (14)	10,169	—	5.3
Breslau et al. (26,29)	1,007	3.6	1.9
Moldin et al. (27)	914	2.1	2.1
Merikangas et al. (12)	1,218	3.0	2.8

employed. There is remarkable similarity in the magnitude of the association between depression and migraine across the five studies. The odds ratios across studies were nearly identical, despite the variation in the subjects characteristics, geographic site, and specific assessments of migraine and depression. These findings exclude sampling as a source of bias in the co-occurrence of depression and migraine reported in previous clinical samples. The relationship between migraine and anxiety disorders has also been investigated because of the well-known association between depression and anxiety. When examined alone, anxiety disorders are also associated with migraine in both clinical and community studies, as shown in Table 4.

Devlen (24) investigated anxiety and depression symptoms among migraine sufferers ascertained from both the community and a large sample of headache clinics. The findings revealed that both anxiety and depression are common among migraine sufferers, irrespective of the source of ascertainment. Unfortunately, these scores were not reported for community subjects without migraine, so the significance of these proportions could not be determined. However, the simultaneous association with all of these disorders needs to be examined systematically. In our clinic, two-thirds of the patients seeking treatment for migraine report a lifetime history of an affective or anxiety disorder (25).

Evidence for an association between migraine and the bipolar subtype of depression is particularly strong. Samples of adults (18) and children (48) in treatment for bipolar disorder, as well as epidemiological studies (11,12,31), support an even stronger association between migraine with bipolar spectrum disorder (major depression with either manic or hypomanic episodes).

Strong associations also emerged between depressive disorder and both self-reported migraine/cluster headache and frequent severe headaches among the relatives who were evaluated in a large collaborative family study of depressives and controls (27). Comorbidity of migraine and major depression was much greater among those persons who had been treated for depression (i.e., adjusted odds ratio of 2.6) than those who had not (i.e., adjusted odds ratio of 1.6). This confirms the above-cited bias that occurs in clinical samples of individuals with depression.

The association between headaches and several subtypes of depression was also examined in a large-scale epidemiological study of the U.S. adult population (28). Similar to the study of Moldin et al. (27), standardized diagnostic criteria were employed for depressive syndromes, but the measure of headache was derived from the subject's report of excessive or frequent headache. Significant associations emerged for all the major psychiatric syndromes including major depressive disorder (odds ratio = 2.6), dysthymia (odds ratio = 2.2), panic disorder (odds ratio = 2.1), somatization disorder (odds ratio = 3.3), and alcoholism (odds ratio = 1.5). Similar to the other epidemiological studies, these associations should be interpreted with caution because the study was not designed specifically to address these questions. Thus, correction for chance associations in such a large study would be necessary.

Finally, there is also some elevation in drug abuse among subjects with headaches of all types and migraine in particular. In most cases, this appears to be a consequence of medications used to alleviate migraine, particularly those that include barbiturates or sedatives. In contrast, although narcotics are often used to treat migraine, there is little evidence that this leads to high rates of dependence among patients with headache.

Incidence and Order of Onset

Longitudinal studies may be employed to identify sources of comorbidity by studying the stability of expression of an index disorder either with or without the comorbid disorders over the long-term course. The prospective design enables elucidation of the causal relationship between the index disorder and the comorbid disorder and the risk factors and sequelae of each condition. Homogeneous subtypes of these conditions may also be identified according to their patterns of longitudinal course.

Two epidemiological studies have studied the order of onset of depression, anxiety, and migraine. The results of a prospective longitudinal cohort study of young adults in Zurich, Switzerland, revealed that the onset of anxiety disorders tended to *precede* that of migraine in about 80% of the cases of migraine with comorbid anxiety/depression, and that the onset of depression followed that of migraine in three-quarters of the comorbid cases (11).

Retrospective data from a community survey in Detroit, Michigan, produced strikingly similar findings. The associations between migraine, anxiety, and depression were not only of the same magnitude, but also the order of onset of the three conditions was the same, with anxiety in childhood and adolescence followed by migraine and then depression in adulthood (26). More recent evaluation of the prospective data from the Detroit Area Survey provided evidence that support a bidirectional influence between migraine and major depression, with each disorder increasing the risk for the first onset of the other (29).

Comorbidity may be an important source of heterogeneity in studies of biochemical or psychophysiological parameters or treatment outcome. For example, studies of tyramine conjugation deficit among subjects with migraine and tension-type headache stratified by major depression revealed that subjects with both migraine and depression had lower urinary excretion of tyramine than subjects with migraine alone or controls (30).

Comorbidity of Psychiatric Disorders and Other Headache Subtypes

Despite the commonly held belief that depression and anxiety are most strongly associated with tension-type headache, evidence from both clinical and community samples suggests that comorbidity between affective and anxiety disorders is far greater for migraine than for tension-type headache (31). In a study of a community sample in Zurich, Switzerland, the results showed that comorbidity was greatest for subjects with migraine with aura, intermediate for those with migraine without aura, and lowest for those with tension-type headache alone. Thus, the IHS description of anxiety and depression as possible etiological factors for tension-type headache does not appear to be well based.

Cluster headache, which is predominant in males, does not seem to be associated systematically with either anxiety state of depression. However, there is evidence from clinical studies that alcohol triggers cluster attacks and that cluster headache may be more common among those with alcoholism.

Finally, posttraumatic headache is often associated with depression that occurs after the acute injury. Like migraine, it is postulated that severe head trauma may uncover innate vulnerability to depression or migraine in susceptible individuals (32).

The tendency for multiple subtypes of headache to co-occur must also be considered in the evaluation of psychiatric comorbidity. Ham et al. (33) inspected differences in symptoms of depression and anxiety among patients with combined headache (i.e., migraine and tension-type), posttraumatic headache, nonheadache pain syndromes, and controls. The results revealed no differences in symptom ratings of either anxiety or depression between the specific subtypes of headache or low back pain group, yet all differed significantly from nonheadache controls. These findings are particularly meaningful in light of the work of Holm et al. (34), who describe the need to control for confounding between somatic symptoms of depression and headache in studies of their association.

Von Korff et al. (35) conducted a questionnaire study of members of a local health maintenance organization in order to gain understanding of the longitudinal course of affective disorders and migraine. Their results indicated that subjects with depressive symptoms were not more likely to exhibit an increased incidence of all pain syndromes, but rather, appeared to be specific to frequent and/or severe headaches or chest pain.

Causal Mechanisms

One of the most important recent developments in research regarding psychiatric disorders and migraine is the focus on gaining understanding of possible mechanisms for the role of psychological factors in headache rather than on only examining their co-occurrence. There are two possible explanations for the relationship between migraine and depression/anxiety: 1) migraine and depression/anxiety share common underlying pathological mechanisms; or 2) migraine and depression/anxiety are causally related, either with migraine causing depression/anxiety, or the converse. Evidence for these explanations may be derived from follow-up studies, which demonstrate the course and precursors of the conditions; neurobiological studies and challenge paradigms, which identify common underlying susceptibility and etiological factors; and family studies, which can investigate the coaggregation of the two conditions.

Patterns of cosegregation of migraine and depression have been examined in three separate family studies conducted by the same research group (12,31,36). In the first two studies, which employed the family-history method, patterns of cosegregation of migraine and depression were investigated in the relatives of probands with depression (31,36) and in the third the relatives of probands with migraine (12). The results of both studies indicated that migraine and depression share a syndromic relationship, representing manifestation of the same disease, as opposed to their representing distinct diseases resulting from the same underlying etiology (31,36). The results of both studies indicated that migraine and depression share a syndromic relationship, representing manifestation of the same disease, as opposed to their representing distinct diseases resulting from the same underlying etiological factors.

Familial patterns of expression of migraine and psychopathology were recently reported for a large family study of probands with migraine, depression or anxiety, and controls (12). Associations between migraine and psychiatric disorders in the 1218 first-degree relatives revealed that migraine was strongly associated with both the affective and anxiety disorders, with the greatest associations emerging for the bipolar subtype of depression and for agoraphobia and panic subtypes of anxiety disorders. The patterns of transmission of migraine with major depression and anxiety were consistent with a transmissible association between depression and migraine and a nontransmissible association between anxiety and migraine. That is, probands with depression had an increased risk of migraine in their relatives, whereas probands with anxiety did not. The transmissible association between depression and migraine was most strongly attributable to the bipolar subtype of depression. This suggests that migraine and depression may have a partially shared underlying diathesis.

When taken together, evidence from prospective epidemiological and family studies reveals that migraine and anxiety/affective disorders are strongly associated in the general community and in families of probands with these disorders; this association is strongest for depression of the atypical subtype and phobic anxiety syndromes; and the onset of anxiety disorders generally *precedes* that of migraine, thereby suggesting that these conditions may comprise early manifestations of a syndrome characterized by concomitant expression of anxiety, affective disorders and migraine over the lifetime course. In contrast, the onset of depression may occur either prior to or after the onset of migraine.

The most likely explanation for the above findings is that the combination of these disorders comprises a subtype of either migraine or depression/anxiety in which symptoms of all of these disorders are manifest at some point during the longitudinal course. Because disturbances in the same neurochemical systems have been implicated in migraine, depression, and anxiety disorders, perturbation of a particular system or systems may produce symptoms of all three conditions, thereby producing one syndrome rather than three discrete entities. Support of this interpretation derives from a large-scale epidemiological study in the United States in which persons with a history of migraine who no longer suffered from episodic attacks of headache continued to have significantly more depression than those without a history of migraine.

MEDICAL MANAGEMENT OF HEADACHE SYNDROMES AND COMORBID PSYCHIATRIC DISORDERS

The findings described above underscore the importance of systematic assessment of depression and anxiety in persons with migraine. If there is a subtype of migraine associated with anxiety and depression, it is critical to treat the entire syndrome rather than limiting the treatment goal to headache cessation. The use of prophylactic medications with lassitude, fatigue, or depression as a side effect should be avoided, if possible; if not, careful clinical evaluation of the above-cited manifestations of depression including anergia, hypersomnia, and irritability should be monitored.

In general, comorbid depression and anxiety are more important in the selection of migraine prophylaxis than in the treatment of an acute attack of migraine. When nonpharmacological approaches have failed and the frequency and severity of migraine attacks lead to impairment in functioning, preventative treatment is indicated. The beta-blockers are currently the most popular treatment choice in migraine prophylaxis (37–39). However, the effect of this class of drugs is moderate at best. No study has reported complete elimination of migraine; however, the average duration and severity are reduced by 50% in most subjects (39,40). Moreover, anhedonia, irritability, and lassitude, which may emerge after variable periods of time, are major side effects of beta-blockers (40). Thus, clinicians should be cautious in prescribing these agents to patients with a history of depression. In contrast, patients with high levels of autonomic anxiety may actually benefit from this class of drugs.

Given the overlap of symptoms of the actual migraine episode, including acute changes in energy, appetite, mood, and level of anxiety, and those on the anxiety/depression spectrum, which has been found to occur between episodes of migraine, it is not surprising that similar pharmacological agents have been successfully employed in the treatment of migraine and the anxiety/depression syndrome. Table 5 shows the antidepressants that have been shown to reduce both affective disorders and migraine. The antidepressant drugs, particularly those of the tricyclic class, have often been shown to be superior to the above-cited "first-line" agents of migraine treatment. Amitriptyline alone and amitriptyline with beta-blockers have been found in comparative trials to yield a >50% response in more than 70% of the subjects (41–44). This is the highest treatment response rate of any of the prophylactic agents for migraine. However, patients often report excessive sedation from tricyclic agents. Ziegler and colleagues (44) reported the results of a comparative crossover trial of propranolol and amitriptypline in migraine prophylaxis. Whereas amitriptyline reduced the severity, frequency, and duration of headache attacks, propranolol only reduced the severity of attacks. No corre-

Table 5 Antidepressant Treatment of Affective Disorders and Migraine

Drug	Trade name	Daily dose (mg)	Ref.
Amitriptyline	Elavil, Endep	10–150	41–44
Doxepin	Sinequan, Adapin	10–150	61
Phenelzine	Nardil	15–60	25,45,46
Divalproex sodium	Depakote	250–2000	58–60

lation between efficacy and blood levels or other physiological changes was found. Amitriptyline was more effective in females, whereas males were equally responsive to the two agents. The findings were particularly intriguing because depression was not correlated with preferential response to amitriptyline.

Although less widely studied, the monoamine oxidase inhibitors (MAOIs) have also been reported to be efficacious in the treatment of migraine headache, particularly in patients who have been unresponsive to first-line prophylactic treatment including the beta-adrenergic blocking agents, ergot compounds, and prostaglandin inhibitors (47). Several uncontrolled trials of MAOIs in the treatment of migraine have reported success in migraine prophylaxis (25,49–53). Nearly 30 years ago, Anthony and Lance (45) published an uncontrolled study that employed 45 mg of phenelzine per day for periods of up to 2 years and reported a reduction in the frequency of migraine of at least 50% in 80% of the subjects. In a recent review of prophylactic treatment of migraine, Daroff and Whitney (46) declared that phenelzine may be the most efficacious antimigraine agent.

Combinations of the above classes of drugs have also been used for patients who fail to respond to first-line treatments. Tricyclics plus beta-blockers and tricyclics plus MAOIs are often used concomitantly in the preventive treatment of severe migraine (53). However, caution should be exercised when combining these two drugs, given the potential for interaction.

Merikangas and Merikangas (25) recently reported the results of a 1-year open trial comparing the efficacy of phenelzine, atenolol, and their combination in the prophylactic treatment of 63 adults with migraine headache. Phenelzine either alone or in combination with atenolol led to a greater than 75% reduction in the severity and frequency of migraine attacks in 70% of the subjects, whereas only 35% of the subjects on atenolol alone reported a decrease of this magnitude. The psychiatric syndromes were also effectively treated by phenelzine alone or in combination with a beta-blocker. The results also demonstrated the safety of the concomitant administration of MAOIs and beta-blockers, with the combination of the two drugs actually leading to a decrease in the side effects associated with either drug alone.

Systematic clinical interviews revealed that the majority of the migraine patients had a history of either major depression or an anxiety disorder. The MAOIs have been shown to have superior efficacy to the tricyclics in the treatment of anergic depression with concomitant anxiety, particularly social phobia (54,55). Given reports of their efficacy in several uncontrolled studies, they should also be considered in treating patients with severe migraine with the above-cited psychiatric features. However, there is a clear need for controlled trials of traditional antimigraine agents that stratify patients by the presence of depression/anxiety.

Another medication that has been used to treat both migraine and mood disorders and panic disorder is valproate, which is currently a first-line treatment for bipolar affective disorder (56). Recent evidence reveals that valproate may be effective in migraine prophylaxis as well (59,60). Thus, valproate may be the treatment of choice in patients with migraine and depression with bipolarity or recurrent depression.

There is an amazing lack of evidence regarding the efficacy of other antidepressants in the treatment of migraine. One controlled study reported that doxepin was effective in treating patients with mixed vascular and tension-type headache (61). Another study actually integrated depressive symptom ratings in the choice of pharmacotherapy of tension-type headache. Manna et al. (62) employed a crossover clinical trial design to compare the efficacy of fluvoxamine and mianserin in the treatment of tension-type headache. The findings indicated that the latter agent was more effective in the treatment of mild tension-type headache with prominent depressive symptoms, whereas fluvoxamine was superior for patients with more severe headache without concomitant depression. Anecdotal evidence suggests that the selective serotonin-reuptake inhibitors and trazodone may exacerbate migraine; however, systematic studies are indicated (63). Use of tricyclic antidepressants other than amitriptyline should be encouraged since this agent is the most sedating of all of the drugs in this class. The secondary amines (e.g., nortriptyline and desipramine) appear to be equally efficacious in the treatment of depression but have fewer side effects than do the parent tertiary amines (e.g., amitriptyline, imipramine) (57). However, the relative efficacy of tricyclic antidepressants in migraine prevention has not been examined. In general, the doses of antidepressants that have been studied in migraine prophylaxis are far lower than those employed in the treatment of depression.

SUMMARY

The association between migraine and depression/anxiety, particularly in light of the findings from prospective data, warrants further study to determine whether depression can be used as an index of a discrete syndrome. Studies that differentiate pure migraine from migraine associated with affective and anxiety disorder on such domains as psychophysiology and brain imaging are indicated. In fact, failure to discriminate between migraine with and without concomitant depression could obscure the results of studies across all domains of migraine research, including studies of pathophysiology, treatment response, biological markers, and genetics.

These findings also underscore the importance of complete neurological and psychiatric evaluation of subjects with migraine. Serious depression and anxiety disorders may not be obvious and are often uncovered with probing by an experienced clinician. This is particularly applicable to depression of the atypical variety or one that is chiefly characterized by irritability or anhedonia, rather than sadness and dysphoria. In addition, symptoms of anxiety and phobic states may not be apparent in a clinical situation. There is an urgent need for recognition of depression and anxiety in individuals with migraine and the integration of this information into treatment decisions.

REFERENCES

1. Wolff HG. Personality features and reactions of subjects with migraine. Arch Neurolog Psychiatry 1937; 37:895–921.

2. International Headache Society. Classification and diagnostic criteria for headache disorders, cranial neuralgias, and facial pain. Cephalalgia 1988; 7:1–96.
3. Waters WE, O'Connor PJ. Prevalance of migraine. J Neurol Neurosurg Psychiatry 1975; 38:613–616.
4. Crisp AH, Kalucy RS, McGuinness B, Ralph PC, Harris G. Some clinical, social and psychological characteristics of migraine subjects in the general population. Postgrad Med J 1977; 53:691–697.
5. Linet M, Stewart W. Migraine headache: epidemiologic perspectives. Epidemiol Rev 1984; 6:107–139.
6. Stewart WF, Shechter A, Rasmussen BK. Migraine prevalence: a review of population based studies. Neurology 1994; 44(6 suppl 4):17–23.
7. Merikangas KR. Genetic epidemiology of migraine. In: Sandler M, Collins GM, eds. Migraine: A Spectrum of Ideas. Oxford: Oxford University Press, 1990:40–50.
8. Merikangas KR, Angst J. Depression and migraine. In: Sandler M, Collins GM, eds. Migraine: A Spectrum of Ideas. Oxford: Oxford University Press, 1990:248–258.
9. Stang PE, Osterhaus JR, Celentano DD. Migraine: patterns of healthcare use. Neurology 1994; 44(6 suppl 4):47–55.
10. Lissovoy G, Lazarus SS. The economic cost of migraine: present state of knowledge. Neurology 1994; 44(6 suppl 4):56–62.
11. Merikangas KR, Angst J, Isler H. Migraine and psychopathology: results of the Zurich cohort study of young adults. Arch Gen Psychiatry 1990; 47:849–853.
12. Merikangas KR. Sources of genetic complexity of migraine. In: Sandler M, Ferrari M, Harnett S, eds. Migraine Pharmacology and Genetics. London: Altman, 1996:254–281.
13. Merikangas KR, Whitaker AE, Isler H, Angst J. The Zurich Study XXIII: epidemiology of headache syndromes in the Zurich cohort study of young adults. Eur Arch Psychiatry Clin Neurosci 1994; 244:145–152.
14. Stewart W, Linet M, Celentano D. Migraine headaches and panic attacks. Psychosom Med 1989; 51:559–569.
15. Edmeads J, Findlay H, Tugwell PL, Pryse-Phillips W, Nelson RF, Murray TJ. Impact of migraine and tension-type headache on life-style, consulting behavior, and medication use: a Canadian population survey. Can J Neurol Sci 1993; 20:131–137.
16. Rasmussen BK, Jensen R, Schroll M, Olesen J. Epidemiology of headache in a general population: a prevalence study. J Clin Epidemiol 1991; 44:1147–1157.
17. Rasmussen, B.K. Migraine and tension-type headache are separate disorders. Cephalalgia 1996; 16:217–223.
18. Cassidy WL, Flanagan NB, Spellman ME. Clinical observations in manic-depressive disease. JAMA 1957; 164:1535–1546.
References 19–23 deleted in proof.
24. Devlen J. Anxiety and depression in migraine. J Royal Soc Med 1994; 87:338–341.
25. Merikangas KR, Merikangas JR. Combination monoamine oxidase inhibitor and betablocker treatment of migraine, with anxiety and depression. Biol Psychiatry 1995; 38:603–610.
26. Breslau N, Davis GC. Migraine, physical health and psychiatric disorder: a prospective epidemiologic study in young adults. J Psychiatr Res 1993; 27:211–221.
27. Moldin SO, Scheftner WA, Rice JP, Nelson E, Kneacvich MA, Akiskal H. Association between major depressive disorder and physical illness. Psychol Med 1993; 23:755–761.
28. Kroenke K, Price RK. Symptoms in the community: prevalence, classification, and psychiatric comorbidity. Arch Intern Med 1993; 153:2474–2480.

29. Breslau N, Davis GC, Schultz LR, Peterson EL. Migraine and major depression: a longitudinal study. Headache 1994; 34:387–393.
30. Merikangas KR, Stevens DE, Merikangas JR, Katz CBS, Glover V, Cooper MA, Sandler M. Tyramine conjugation deficit in migraine, tension-type headache and depression. Biol Psychiatry 1995; 38:730–736.
31. Merikangas KR, Merikangas JR, Angst J. Headache syndromes and psychiatric disorders: association and familial transmission. J Psychiatr Res 1993; 27:197–210.
32. Merikangas KR, Angst J. Post-traumatic headache in the Swiss male cohort study. Swiss Arch Neurol Psychiatry 1996; 147:105–108.
33. Ham LP, Andrasik F, Packard RC, Bundrick CM. Psychopathology in individuals with post-traumatic headaches and other pain types. Cephalalgia 1994; 14:118–126.
34. Holm JE, Penzien DB, Holroyd KA, Brown TA. Headache and depression: confounding effects of transdiagnostic symptoms. Headache 1994; 34:418–423.
35. Von Korff M, Le Resche L, Dworkin SF. First onset of common pain symptoms: a prospective study of depression as a risk factor. Pain 1993; 55:251–258.
36. Merikangas KR, Risch NJ, Merikangas JR, Weissman MM, Kidd KK. Migraine and depression: association and familial transmission. J Psychiatr Res 1988; 22:119–129.
37. Daroff RB, Whitney CM. Treatment of vascular headaches. Headache 1986; 26:470–472.
38. Tfelt-Hansen P. Efficacy of β-blockers in migraine: a critical review. Cephalalgia 1986; 6: 15–24.
39. Anthony, M. Review of beta-adrenoceptor blocking agents in migraine. In: Carroll JD, Pfaffenrath V, Sjaastad O, eds. Migraine and Beta-Blockade. Molndal, Sweden: AB Hassle, 1988:193–199.
40. Peatfield RC, Fozard JR, Rose FC. Drug treatment of migraine. In: Rose FC, ed. Handbook of Clinical Neurology. Vol 48. Amsterdam: Elsevier, 1986:173–216.
41. Gomersall JD, Stuart A. Amitriptyline in migraine prophylaxis: changes in pattern of attacks during a controlled clinical trial. J Neurol Neurosurg Psychiatry 1973; 36:684–690.
42. Couch JR, Ziegler DK, Hassanein R. Amitriptyline in the prophylaxis of migraine: effectiveness and relationship of antimigraine and antidepressant effects. Neurology 1976; 26: 121–127.
43. Couch JR, Hassanein R. Amitriptyline in migraine prophylaxis. Arch Neurol 1979; 36: 695–699.
44. Ziegler DK, Hurwitz A, Preskorn S, Hassanein R, Seim J. Propranolol and amitriptyline in prophylaxis of migraine: pharmacokinetic and therapeutic effects. Arch Neurol 1993; 50:825–830.
45. Anthony M, Lance JW. Monoamine oxidase inhibition in the treatment of migraine. Arch Neurol 1969; 21:263–268.
46. Daroff RB, Whitney CM. Treatment of vascular headaches. Headache 1986; 26:470–472.
47. Raskin NH. Headache. 2d ed. New York: Churchill-Livingstone, 1988.
48. Younes RP, Delong GR, Neiman G, Rosner B. Manic-depressive illness in children: treatment with lithium carbonate. J Child Neurol 1986; 1:364–368.
49. Kimball RW, Friedman AP, Vallejo E. Effects of serotonin in migrainous patients. Neurology 1960; 10:107–111.
50. Dalsgaard-Neilson AT. Behandling af migraine-patienter med niamid. Ugeskr Laeger 1962; 124:10–11.
51. Michelacci S, Franchi G. Treatment of vascular headaches. Minerva Med 1962; 53:1521–1523.
52. Perrault M. Migraines sevères, M.A.O.-I's et methysegide. Prog Med 1963; 11:413–422.

53. White K, Simpson G. The combined use of MAOIs and tricyclics. J Clin Psychiatry 1984; 45:67–69.

54. Quitkin FM, Harrison W, Stewart JW, et al. Response to phenelzine and imipramine in placebo nonresponders with atypical depression. Arch Gen Psychiatry 1991; 48:319–323.

55. Liebowitz MR, Gorman JM, Fyer AJ, et al. Pharmacotherapy of social phobia: an interim report of a placebo-controlled comparison of phenelzine and atenolol. J Clin Psychiatry 1988; 49:252–257.

56. Pope HG, McElroy SL, Keck PE, Hudson JI. Valproate in the treatment of acute mania. Arch Gen Psychiatry 1991; 48:62–68.

57. Keck PE, Merikangas KR, McElroy SL, Strakowski SM. Diagnostic and treatment implications of psychiatric comorbidity with migraine. Ann Clin Psychiatry 1994; 6:165–171.

58. Sorensen KV. Valproate: a new drug in migraine prophylaxis. Acta Neurol Scand 1988; 78:346–348.

59. Hering R, Kuritzky A. Sodium valproate in the prophylactic treatment of migraine: a double blind study versus placebo. Cephalalgia 1992; 12:81–84.

60. Mathew NT, Spaer JR, Silberstein SD, Rankin L, Markley HC, Solomon S, Rapoport AM, Silber CJ, Denton RL. Migraine prophylaxis with divalproex. Arch Neurol 1995; 52: 281–286.

61. Moreland TJ, Storli OV, Mogstad TE. Doxepin in the prophylactic treatment of mixed vascular and tension headache. Headache 1979; 19:382–383.

62. Manna V, Bolino F, DiCicco L. Chronic tension-type headache, mood depression and serotonin: therapeutic effects of fluvoxamine and mianserine. Headache 1993; 34:44–49.

63. Workman EA, Tellian F, Short D. Trazodone induction of migraine headache through mCPP. Am J Psychiatry 1992; 149:712–713.

21

Parkinson's Disease

Sergio E. Starkstein and Gustavo Petracca
Raúl Carrea Institute of Neurological Research–FLENI
Buenos Aires, Argentina

INTRODUCTION

Parkinson's disease (PD) is a neurodegenerative disorder characterized by tremor, muscle rigidity, bradykinesia, and postural instability. PD usually starts at middle or late life and has a gradual and chronic progression. Other characteristic symptoms of the disease are fatigue, diminution in automatic movements, masked facial expression, monotonous voice, constipation, and decreased sexual drive.

A wide variety of psychiatric disorders may be present in PD such as depression, anxiety, emotional lability, and medication-induced psychotic disorders. In this chapter, we will discuss the prevalence, clinical manifestations, and main correlates of the most frequent psychiatric disorders found in PD. We will examine how these psychiatric disorders impact on the medical management and course of PD and review the usefulness of different therapeutic modalities.

DEPRESSION IN PARKINSON'S DISEASE

Clinical Vignette

O. B. is a 74-year-old engineer who was referred to the neurology clinic of our institute because of gait problems and falling episodes. His motor problems had started one year before, when he noticed more rigidity in his right upper and lower limbs and a tendency to fall toward the right. On neurological examination he showed hypophonia, slight loss of facial expression, intermittent resting tremor in his right hand, mild cogwheel rigidity restricted to the right side, mild slowing on finger tapping, hand movements, and leg agility, moderately stooped posture, slow shuffling gait, and mild postural instability. The patient reported that several years before the onset of the motor problems he became more apathetic and lost interest in his everyday activities. At the onset of extrapyramidal signs he also developed a depressive mood, and at the time of the neuro-psychological evaluation he reported feeling sad most of the time, with difficulties falling asleep, loss of interest in activities of daily living, worrying about minor matters, difficulties in concentration, and loss of energy and libido. He was diagnosed as having PD and major depression, and he was started on levodopa (Madopar 125 mg q.i.d.) and nortriptyline (with an initial dosage of 25 mg/day and reaching a dosage of 75 mg/day after 2 weeks). Two months later O. B. showed marked improvements in both his motor impairments and his mood disorder.

Historical Background

In 1817 James Parkinson (1) described a group of patients who were so demoralized by the disease that they refused treatment. In 1924, Janet (2) explicitly recognized the association between depression and PD and explained the mood disorder as secondary to psychological trauma. More recently, Mindham (3) proposed that depression in PD should be considered an understandable consequence of the progressive physical impairment. PD itself was proposed to result from a "perfectionist personality" or from "suppressed hostility" before the biological basis of the disease were discovered (4).

Prevalence of Depression in PD

Although several studies have examined the prevalence of depressive disorders in PD, important methodological aspects should be first considered. Some authors reported a very high prevalence of depression—e.g., 90% in Mindham's study (1)—but in these studies patients were mostly selected from admissions to psychiatric units. Other studies found a lower prevalence of depressive disorders, although in most of those studies depression was diagnosed based on a cut-off score on a depression scale and not on standardized diagnostic criteria (5).

Only a few studies have examined the prevalence of depression using semi-structured psychiatric interviews. In a study that included a consecutive series of 105 patients who were seen in a neurology clinic for regular follow-up visits, we found that 20% of the patients had major depression and 21% had minor (dysthymic) depression (6). Moreover, 20% of the 63 patients who were not depressed at the psychiatric evaluation reported a history of depression. Brown and McCarthy (7) examined 40 patients with PD using the Present State Exam and found a high frequency of simple depression, tension, irritability, worrying, and loss of interest and concentration. Seventy percent of patients had at least one of these symptoms, and 55% had two or more.

Several authors assessed the frequency of depression in multicenter samples or patients living in the community. Davous et al. (8) examined the prevalence of depression among 506 PD patients attending the neurology services in French General Hospitals. Depression was diagnosed based on the Montgomery-Asberg Scale scores. Definite or probable depression was present in 33% of the patients, and 9% had a severity score suggestive of major depression. Hantz et al. (9) assessed the prevalence of depression among most PD patients living in a defined metropolitan area using the 30-item General Health Questionnaire and the Structured Clinical Interview for DSM-III-R (SCID). They found a prevalence of mood and anxiety disorders of 6.8% and a rate of major depression of 2.7%. In a community-based study that included 245 patients with PD, Tandberg et al. (10) found mild depression in 45%, moderate depression in 5%, and major depression in 7.7% of the patients. In this study patients were assessed with both the Montgomery-Asberg Scale and the Beck Depression Inventory.

In conclusion, the prevalence of depression in PD may vary according to sampling methods and case ascertainment. Among community-dwelling patients mild depressions are very frequent, whereas major depression is less prevalent. Among patients attending a neurology clinic for follow-up visits, the prevalence of major depression is higher.

Clinical Manifestations of Depression in PD

One important issue is how to diagnose depression in patients whose neurological disease may also feature "depressive-like" symptoms, such as slowness, masked facial expression, and a soft and monotonous voice. To examine the sensitivity and specificity of psychological and autonomic symptoms of depression in PD, we assessed 33 PD patients who reported a depressed mood and compared them with a group of PD patients who did not report depression (6). Both groups were matched for severity of the disease, duration of illness, age, and education. The depressed group reported more severe autonomic symptoms of depression such as anxiety, loss of appetite, early and middle insomnia, and loss of libido. On the other hand, there were no significant between-group differences on early morning awakening and anergia and retardation. Moreover, all of the psychological symptoms of depression, such as worrying, brooding, loss of interest, suicidal ideation, social withdrawal, self-depreciation, and ideas of reference were significantly more frequent in the depressed than in the nondepressed groups. We also found that the presence of at least three affective and three autonomic symptoms of depression had a sensitivity of 96% and a specificity of 100% for the diagnosis of major depression (based on DSM-III diagnostic criteria), whereas the sensitivity and specificity for both major or minor depression was 88% and 97%, respectively. Several authors have also demonstrated that affective and autonomic symptoms are common features of depression in PD, and Huber et al. (11) reported that whereas affective and autonomic symptoms may be seen at all stages of the illness, autonomic (vegetative) symptoms of depression are primarily observed in the late stages of the disease.

Sleep disorders and pain are frequent complaints among PD patients. We examined the association between depression, sleep problems, and pain in a consecutive series of 79 PD patients using specific sleep and pain questionnaires (12). We found that depression accounted for most of the variance in the correlation with sleep disturbances and pain, and sleep problems and pain were most severe among PD patients with major depression. Whereas PD patients with minor depression showed significantly more severe sleep problems than PD patients without depression, no significant between-group difference was found in the severity of pain. Similar to patients with "primary" (i.e., no known brain injury) depression, PD patients with depression showed a significantly shorter rapid eye movement latency than nondepressed PD patients (13).

In DSM-IV (14), depression in PD is diagnosed using the criteria for "Mood Disorder Due to a General Medical Condition" (Table 1), which specifies two diagnoses: one with depressive features (if the predominant mood is depressed but the full criteria for a major depressive episode are not met), the other with major depressive-like episode (if the full criteria for a major depressive episode are met [except Criterion D]).

Few studies have formally examined the long-term evolution of depressive symptoms in PD. Depression may start before the onset of motor symptoms (15), and we reported that 29% of 21 PD patients with major depression were depressed before the onset of motor symptoms (6). On the other hand, we also found that only 5% of patients with minor depression and 2.7% of patients without depression had a history of depressive mood before the onset of motor symptoms, suggesting that minor but not major depression may be related to the development of the motor symptoms of PD.

To examine longitudinal changes in the prevalence of depression we followed our sample of 105 PD patients over a 1-year period (16). We found that 56% of the patients with initial major depression still had major depression at the follow-up evaluation, 33% had minor depression, and 11% were not depressed. Among patients with minor depression at the initial evaluation, 26% still had minor depression at the follow-up evaluation, 11% had major depression, and 63% were not depressed ($\chi^2 = 11.5$; $p < 0.001$). Finally, among patients without depression at the initial evaluation, 82%

Table 1 Diagnostic Criteria for Mood Disorder Due to Parkinson's Disease

---

A. A prominent and persistent disturbance in mood predominates in the clinical picture and is characterized by either (or both) of the following:
   1. Depressed mood or markedly diminished interest or pleasure in all, or almost all, activities
   2. Elevated, expansive, or irritable mood
B. There is evidence from the history, physical examination, or laboratory findings that the disturbance is the direct physiological consequence of Parkinson's disease.
C. The disturbance is not better accounted for by another mental disorder.
D. The disturbance does not occur exclusively during the course of a delirium.
E. The symptoms cause clinically significant distress or impairments in social, occupational, or other important areas of functioning.

Source: Adapted from Ref. 14.

were not depressed at the 1-year follow-up and the remaining 18% had minor depression.

In conclusion, both affective and autonomic symptoms of depression in patients with PD occur in the context of a depressive syndrome and not as a symptom of PD. The use of standardized criteria such as in the DSM-IV may help to obtain valid and reliable diagnoses of depression in PD. Whereas major depression may start before the onset of the motor symptoms and may have a long duration (>1 year), minor depression usually starts after the onset of motor symptoms and has a shorter duration.

Clinical Correlates of Depression in PD

Depression may impair the quality of life, cognitive abilities, and physical functions of PD patients, and several studies have examined this possibility. Most of them showed a significant correlation between depression scores and deficits in activities of daily living (ADLs) (see Ref. 5 for a review), but whether deficits in ADLs produce depression or depression produces further deficits in ADLs could not be determined. Thus, in our longitudinal 1-year follow-up study, we examined a consecutive series of patients with PD and either major, minor, or no depression. We found that major depressed PD patients had a significantly greater decline in ADLs than PD patients with either minor or no depression. Moreover, PD patients with major depression had a significantly faster progression along the stages of the illness than minor or nondepressed PD patients.

Depression may also impact upon the cognitive functioning of PD patients. In our initial study of a consecutive series of 105 PD patients, we found that those with major depression ($n = 21$) had significantly lower Mini-Mental State Exam (MMSE) scores than those with either minor ($n = 20$) or no depression ($n = 64$) (17). Moreover, when we calculated a multiple regression analysis between MMSE scores and age, duration of illness, age at onset, levodopa dosage, depression scores, deficits in ADLs, and scores of tremor, rigidity, and akinesia, the variable that showed the most significant correlation with MMSE score was depression (i.e., the higher the depression scores, the more severe the cognitive impairment).

Since the MMSE is a rather crude measure of cognitive functions, we assessed depressed and nondepressed PD patients using a comprehensive neuropsychological battery (18). PD patients with major depression ($n = 15$) were matched for age, education, and stage of illness with nondepressed PD patients. The main finding was that patients with major depression had significantly more severe deficits than nondepressed PD patients on neuropsychological tasks related to frontal lobe functions (e.g., Wisconsin Card Sorting Test, Verbal Fluency, Design Fluency, and section B of the Trail Making Test). On the other hand, no significant differences were found between PD patients with minor or no depression, demonstrating that the cognitive impairments related to depression in PD were restricted to those patients with major depression and mainly consisted of deficits on frontal lobe–related tasks.

This finding raised the question of whether the cognitive deficits found in major-depressed PD patients are fully explained by the presence of depression or result from an interaction between depression and the neuropathology of PD. Thus, in a recent study we compared 31 nondepressed patients with PD, 19 major-depressed patients with PD, 27 major-depressed patients without PD, and 13 age-comparable normal controls for the presence of neuropsychological deficits (19). Both patients and controls were assessed with a structured psychiatric interview and a comprehensive neuropsychological battery. We found that major depressed patients with or without PD showed significantly more severe deficits on tests of verbal fluency and auditory attention than nondepressed patients with PD or age-comparable normal controls (Figure 1). However, PD patients with major depression showed significantly more severe deficits on tasks of concept formation and set switching than the other three groups (Figure 2). Thus, whereas some neuropsychological deficits in depressed patients with PD may be explained by the presence of depression itself, deficits in concept formation and set switching may be related to neuropathological changes specific to PD with major depression.

Another important issue is whether depression in PD predicts further cognitive decline. To examine this issue, we assessed 92 PD patients divided into those with major, minor, and no depression who were followed during a 1-year period (16). We found that whereas major-depressed PD patients showed a significant decline in MMSE scores, no significant changes were found among PD patients with either minor or no depression.

Recent studies have examined metabolic correlates of depression in PD. Mayberg et al. (20) found that depressed patients with PD had significantly lower metabolic activity in the inferior frontal cortex and head of the caudate as compared to nondepressed PD patients matched for age and severity of motor deficits. Ring et al. (21) reported that depressed PD patients had significantly lower frontomedial and cingulate metabolic activity than nondepressed PD patients with a comparable severity of PD. Moreover, this metabolic change was similar to that found in patients with primary (i.e., no known brain injury) depression. In a recent study, Mayberg et al. (22) examined brain metabolic changes in depressed PD patients before and after fluoxetine treatment. They found that mood improvement after active treatment was associated with significant metabolic increments in the dorsal frontal cortex, and this increase was a normalization of an abnormal metabolic pattern. They also found a significant metabolic decrease in ventral paralimbic areas, although, in this case, the metabolic change was not a normalization of an abnormal metabolic pattern. On the other hand, nonresponders to fluoxetine treatment had *increased* metabolism in these ventral paralimbic areas, suggesting that metabolic changes in these regions may play a critical role in the antidepressant effect of fluoxetine.

Mayeux et al. (23) reported decreased concentrations of the serotonin metabolite 5-hydroxyindoleacetic acid (5-HIAA) in depressed as compared to nondepressed patients with PD. Recent studies demonstrated a selective modulation of activity of mesocorticolimbic dopaminergic neurons by serotonergic afferents to the ventral tegmental area (where most of the dopaminergic fibers to cortico-limbic areas originate) (24).

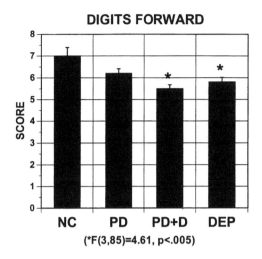

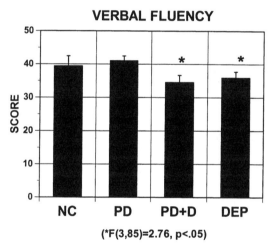

Figure 1 Patients with major depression—with (PD+D) or without (DEP) PD—had significantly lower scores than normal controls (NC) or nondepressed patients with PD (PD). *F = ANOVA.

Lesions of the median and dorsal raphe nuclei (which give rise to most cortical serotonergic fibers) decrease dopaminergic utilization in the prefrontal cortex. Thus, deficits in more than one biogenic amine system may underlie the production of depression in PD.

Few studies have examined the motor correlates of depression in PD. In a recent study we compared 78 patients with "classic" PD (i.e., patients featuring tremor, rigidity, and akinesia), and 34 patients with the akinetic-rigid variant of PD (i.e., without

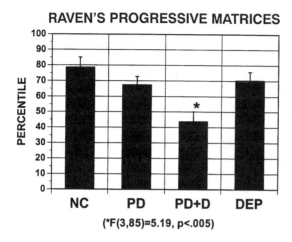

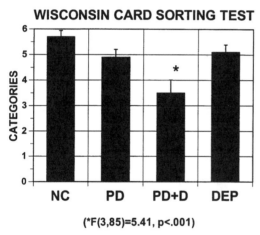

Figure 2   Major depressed patients with PD showed significantly lower scores than the other three groups.

tremor) (25). While there were no significant between-group differences in demographic variables and severity of the disease, patients with akinetic-rigid PD had a significantly higher prevalence of major depression than patients with the classical variant (38% vs. 15%, respectively; $p < 0.01$) (Fig. 3). Since akinetic-rigid PD has been associated with dysfunction of frontomedial regions, our finding provides further support for the hypothesis of frontal dysfunction among PD patients with major depression.

In conclusion, important clinical differences between major and minor (dysthymic) depression in PD were demonstrated. Whereas major depression was significantly associated with more severe cognitive impairments (primarily involving deficits in fron-

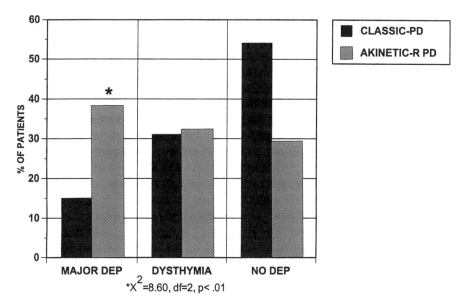

Figure 3   Patients with akinetic-rigid PD had a significantly higher prevalence of major depression than patients with classic PD.

tal lobe–related functions), minor depression was not associated with significant intellectual impairments. Moreover, while patients with major depression showed a significant cognitive and motor decline over a one-year period, no significant declines were found among PD patients with minor or no depression. Finally, whereas PD patients with the akinetic-rigid variant showed a significantly higher prevalence of major depression than PD patients with the classical variant, the prevalence of minor depression was similar. Thus, major depression in PD may result from both a relatively more severe disruption of meso-cortico-limbic dopaminergic pathways and an abnormal coupling between frontal dorsal and ventral areas, whereas minor depression in PD may be an emotional reaction of predisposed individuals to the physical burden of the disease.

Treatment of Depression in PD

Antidepressant drugs are the most common treatment modality for depression in PD. While there are few adequate controlled studies of antidepressants in PD, they demonstrated the usefulness of imipramine, desipramine, and nortriptyline in the treatment of depression (26). Nortriptyline may be started with a dose of 10–25 mg/day and gradually increased by 3–4 days until 70–75 mg/day is reached. While the most common side effects of tricyclic drugs among PD patients are dry mouth, constipation, and orthostatic hypotension, other side effects of these medications include sedation, increased intraocular pressure in patients with narrow angle glaucoma, urinary reten- tion, delirium, and visual blurring. Tricyclic antidepressants delay cardiac conduction and are contraindicated in patients with heart blocks or conduction abnormalities, se- vere arrhythmias, or a recent myocardial infarction. Whereas monoamine oxidase inhib- itors such as phenelzine have been demonstrated to be useful antidepressants in PD, concerns about causing a hypertensive crisis when using levodopa with a nonselective MAOI have limited their use. Finally, the usefulness of selective serotonin-reuptake inhibitors such as fluoxetine and sertraline among depressed PD patients has yet to be demonstrated through controlled studies, although their lack of anticholinergic side effects suggests an important role for these drugs in PD.

Several studies have demonstrated significant mood improvements in PD patients after electroconvulsive therapy (ECT) (27,28). Moreover, there are reports of significant improvements in motor symptoms such as rigidity and bradykinesia, as well as a signifi- cant reduction of the "on-off" phenomenon in patients with severe PD treated with ECT. However, in most studies no significant correlations were found between the improvement of parkinsonian symptoms and mood changes after electroconvulsive therapy (ECT). Finally, cognitive therapy may also play an important role for at least some depressed patients with PD (perhaps those with minor depression), but this possi- bility has not been empirically examined.

ANXIETY IN PD

In a recent study, Menza et al. (29) found that 28% of 42 consecutive patients with PD met DSM-III-R criteria for anxiety disorders, while another 40% had some anxiety symptoms. This prevalence of anxiety disorders was significantly higher than that found in a group of patients with severe osteoarthritis and similar functional deficits. Other studies using population norms or patients with multiple sclerosis as controls also re- ported a higher prevalence of anxiety among patients with PD (30).

Anxiety in PD may not be an isolated finding, since in the study by Menza et al. (29) 92% of PD patients with anxiety symptoms were also depressed, and 49% of the variance of anxiety scores was explained by depression. Other important variables such as stage and duration of illness, levodopa dosage, and severity of disability did not correlate significantly with anxiety scores.

Several studies examined the prevalence of panic attacks in PD. Vazquez et al. (31) reported recurrent panic attacks in 24% of 131 patients with PD. They found that PD patients with panic attacks had a significantly younger age at onset of PD, had more severe gait problems, higher scores of depression and anxiety, and were on higher doses of levodopa. An important finding was that about 90% of the panic attacks appeared in the off state and improved with levodopa, suggesting that panic attacks in PD may be a manifestation of the dopaminergic disturbance and not an isolated psychi- atric phenomenon. In a recent study, Siemers et al. (32) examined the association between anxiety disorders and motor performance in PD. They also found higher anxiety scores in the off as compared to the on state, and there also was a significant correlation between anxiety scores and motor disability. They also found that anxiety trait scores were significantly correlated with duration of illness and depression scores. In a recent study, Maricle et al. (33) found that levodopa infusion in eight PD patients produced a progressive increase in tapping speed, mood elevation, and anxiety reduction. These motor and behavioral effects were dose dependent and were not obtained with placebo infusion.

Whereas the mechanism of anxiety in PD is still unknown, Iruela et al. (34) suggested that panic attacks in PD may result from a disinhibition of the locus coeruleus due to low dopaminergic tone, which may produce an abnormal increase of central noradrenergic transmission. In conclusion, most studies suggest that anxiety (as a trait) is significantly associated with the presence of depression, but changes in anxiety may also be related to fluctuations in motor performance.

PSYCHOSIS IN PD

While psychotic signs such as hallucinations, delusions, and delirium have been frequently reported in PD, these behavioral disorders are usually produced by antiparkinsonian medication in patients with advanced motor impairments. Anticholinergic drugs, amantadine, and dopaminergic agonists have all been reported to produce significant psychotic symptoms (35).

Visual hallucinations are among the most frequent medication-induced side effects. Most patients report seeing animals or people but are usually aware that this represents an abnormality (i.e., hallucinosis), although some patients may suffer true hallucinations. Delusions were reported to be present in 3–30% of PD patients (35). As with hallucinations, delusions are most frequent among elderly PD patients with severe motor problems and cognitive deficits (36).

Psychotic symptoms usually improve with dosage reduction or withdrawal of the offending medication. However, most PD patients cannot tolerate the reduction of dopaminergic agonists and may require the use of antipsychotic drugs.

While neuroleptics are the drugs most widely used to treat psychosis, they are usually associated with prominent extrapyramidal side effects and may not be well tolerated by most PD patients. However, the recent development of antipsychotic drugs with few or no affinity for dopaminergic receptors involved in PD allow a better treatment of psychotic disorders in PD. The atypical antipsychotic clozapine is usually started at a small dosage (e.g., 25–50 mg/day) since most PD patients respond to these low dosages (37). Since this drug may produce bone marrow suppression, hematological monitoring is required. Olanzapine (38) is another atypical antipsychotic with a high affinity for dopaminergic D4 and serotonergic receptors. While its clinical profile is similar to clozapine, it does not produce granulocytopenia. A recent open-label study using olanzapine (38) (1–15 mg/day) in 15 PD patients with drug-induced psychosis demonstrated a significant decrement of psychotic symptoms (mainly delusions and hallucinations) without worsening of extrapyramidal symptoms.

A recent study examined the usefulness of ondansetron (39) (a 5-HT$_3$ receptor antagonist) in the treatment of 16 PD patients with psychosis. A daily dose of 12–24 mg resulted in a moderate to marked improvement in measures of visual hallucinations, paranoid delusions, confusion, and global functional impairment. Ondansetron was well tolerated by most patients and did not produce worsening of parkinsonian symptoms.

PATHOLOGICAL AFFECT IN PARKINSON'S DISEASE

Emotional lability is the sudden onset of laughing or crying episodes that the patient is unable to suppress, which generally occurs in appropriate situations and is accompanied by a congruent alteration of mood (e.g., depression in patients with crying episodes). On the other hand, pathological laughing or crying are sudden episodes that do not correspond to an underlying emotional change. "Pathological affect" refers to patients with either emotional lability or pathological laughing or crying.

While pathological affect is a well-known finding among patients with PD, this phenomenon has not been examined in a systematic way. In a recent study (40) we examined a consecutive series of 89 patients with PD using the Pathological Laughing and Crying Scale (PLACS). We found that 42 of the 89 patients (47%) showed pathological affect: 41 patients had crying episodes, and only one patient had laughing episodes. Based on psychiatric findings, 25 patients (61%) had emotional lability (i.e., depression and pathological affect-crying), whereas the remaining 16 (39%) patients had pathological crying. We also found that patients with emotional lability had a significantly higher prevalence of major depression and more severe cogwheel rigidity, postural problems, and gait impairments than depressed PD patients without emotional lability.

CONCLUSIONS

Depression, anxiety, pathological affect, and psychotic disorders such as delusions and hallucinations are frequently found among patients with PD. Cross-sectional studies demonstrated depression in about 40% of the patients [half with major and half with minor (dysthymic) depression]. Major depression was associated with more severe cognitive impairments, was more prevalent among patients with the akinetic-rigid variant of PD, and was associated with a faster progression of the illness. Depression in PD may be successfully treated with antidepressant drugs. Anxiety disorders are also prominent in PD, although they may be part of a broader depressive syndrome. While panic attacks have also been reported in PD, they are almost exclusively present in the "off" states and may result from neurochemical disturbances specific to PD. Psychotic disorders, such as delusions, hallucinations, and delirium are frequent among older patients with prominent cognitive impairments. Psychotic disorders are usually produced by the antiparkinsonian medications (mainly anticholinergic drugs and dopaminergic agonists) and may be effectively treated with the newer atypical antipsychotic drugs. Finally, emotional lability is a frequent finding in PD and is significantly associated with major depression.

ACKNOWLEDGMENTS

This chapter was partially supported by grants from the Raúl Carrea Institute of Neurological Research, the CONICET, and the Fundación Pérez Companc.

REFERENCES

1. Parkinson J. An Essay on the Shaking Palsy. London: Sherwood, Neely & Jones, 1817.
2. Janet P. Leçons sur les Maladies du Système Nerveux. Paris: Delahaye, 1924.
3. Mindham RHS. Psychiatric symptoms in parkinsonism. J Neurol Neurosurg Psychiatry 1970; 33:188–191.
4. Dakof GA, Mendelsohn GA. Parkinson's disease: the psychological aspects of a chronic illness. Psychol Bull 1986; 99:375–387.
5. Starkstein SE, Mayberg HS. Depression in Parkinson's disease. In: Starkstein SE, Robinson RG, eds. Depression in Neurologic Disease. Baltimore: Johns Hopkins University Press, 1993.
6. Starkstein SE, Preziosi TJ, Bolduc PL, Robinson RG. Depression in Parkinson's disease. J Nerv Ment Dis 1990; 178:37–41.
7. Brown RG, McCarthy B. Psychiatric morbidity in patients with Parkinson's disease. Psychol Med 1990; 20:77–87.
8. Davous P, Auquier P, Grignon S, Neukirch HC. A prospective study of depression in French patients with Parkinson's disease: the Depar study. Eur J Neurol 1995; 2:455–461.
9. Hantz P, Caradoc-Davies G, Caradoc-Davies T, Weatherall M, Dixon G. Depression in Parkinson's disease. Am J Psychiatry 1994; 151:1010–1014.
10. Tandberg E, Larsen JP, Aarsland D, Cummings JL. The occurrence of depression in Parkinson's disease. Arch Neurol 1996; 53:175–179.
11. Huber SJ, Freidenberg DL, Paulson GW, Shuttleworth EC, Christy JA. The pattern of depressive symptoms varies with progression of Parkinson's disease. J Neurol Neurosurg Psychiatry 1990; 53:275–278.
12. Starkstein SE, Preziosi TJ, Price TR. Sleep disorders, pain and depression in Parkinson's disease. Eur Neurol 1991; 31:359–365.
13. Kostick VS, Susic V, Przedborski S, Sternic N. Sleep EEG in depressed and nondepressed patients with Parkinson's disease. J Neuropsychiatr Clin Neurosci 1991; 3:176–179.
14. APA Diagnostic and Statistical Manual of Mental Disorders. 4th ed. Washington, DC: American Psychiatric Press, 1994.

15. Santamaría J, Tolosa E, Valles A. Parkinson's disease with depression: a possible subgroup of idiopathic parkinsonism. Neurology 1986; 36:1130–1133.
16. Starkstein SE, Mayberg HS, Preziosi TJ, Robinson RG. A prospective longitudinal study of depression, cognitive decline, and physical impairments in patients with Parkinson's disease. J Neurol Neurosurg Psychiatry 1992; 55:377–382.
17. Starkstein SE, Preziosi TJ, Forrester AW, Robinson RG. Specificity of affective and autonomic symptoms of depression in Parkinson's disease. J Neurol Neurosurg Psychiatry 1990; 53:869–873.
18. Starkstein SE, Preziosi TJ, Berthier ML, Bolduc PL, Mayberg HS, Robinson RG. Depression and cognitive impairment in Parkinson's disease. Brain 1989; 112:1141–1153.
19. Kuzis G, Sabe L, Tiberti C, Leiguarda R, Starkstein SE. Cognitive functions in major depression and Parkinson's disease. Arch Neurol 1997; 54:982–986.
20. Mayberg HS, Starkstein SE, Sadzot B, Preziosi T, Andrezejewski PL, Dannals RF, Wagner HN, Robinson RG. Selective hypometabolism in the inferior frontal lobe in depressed patients with Parkinson's disease. Ann Neurol 1990; 28:57–64.
21. Ring HA, Bench CJ, Trimble MR, Brooks DJ, Frackowiak SJ, Dolan RJ. Depression in Parkinson's disease: a positron emission study. Br J Psychiatry 1994; 165:333–339.
22. Mayberg HS, Mahurin RK, Brannan SK. Parkinson's depression: discrimination of mood-sensitive and mood-insensitive cognitive deficits using fluoxetine and FDG-PET. Neurology 1995; 45:A166.
23. Mayeux R, Stern Y, Cote L, Williams JBW. Altered serotonin metabolism in depressed patients with Parkinson's disease. Neurology 1984; 34:642–646.
24. Meltzer HY, Lawy MT. The serotonin hypothesis of depression. In: Meltzer HY, ed. Psychopharmacology: The Third Generation of Progress. New York: Raven Press, 1987.
25. Starkstein SE, Petracca G, Chemerinski E, Tesón A, Sabe L, Merello M, Leiguarda R. Depression in classic vs. akinetic-rigid Parkinson's disease. Movement Disord 1998; 13: 29–33.
26. Klaasen T, Verhey FRJ, Sneijders GHJM., Rozendaal N, de Vet HCW, van Praag HM. Treatment of depression in Parkinson's disease: a meta-analysis. J Neuropsychiatr Clin Neurosci 1995; 7:281–286.
27. Burke WJ, Peterson J, Robin EH. Electroconvulsive therapy in the treatment of combined depression in Parkinson's disease. Psychosomatics 1988; 29:341–346.
28. Douyon R, Serby M, Klutchko B. ECT and Parkinson's disease revisited: a "naturalistic" study. Am J Psychiatry 1989; 146:1451–1455.
29. Menza MA, Robertson-Hoffman DE, Bonapace AS. Parkinson's disease and anxiety: comorbidity with depression. Biol Psychiatry 1993; 34:465–470.
30. Henderson R, Kurlan R, Kerson JM. Preliminary examination of the comorbidity of anxiety and depression in Parkinson's disease. J Neuropsychiatr Clin Neurosci 1992; 4:257–264.
31. Vazquez A, Jimenez-Jimenez FJ, Garcia-Ruiz P, Garcia-Urra D. "Panic attacks" in Parkinson's disease: a long-term complication of levodopatherapy. Acta Neurol Scand 1993; 87: 14–18.
32. Siemers ER, Shekhar A, Quaid K, Dickson H. Anxiety and motor performance in Parkinson's disease. Movement Disord 1993; 8:501–506.
33. Maricle RA, Nutt JG, Valentine RJ, Carter JH. Dose-response relationship of levodopa with mood and anxiety in fluctuating Parkinson's disease: a double-blind, placebo-controlled study. Neurology 1995; 45:1757–1760.

34. Iruela LM, Ibañez-Rojo V, Palanca I, Caballero L. Anxiety disorders and Parkinson's disease. Am J Psychiatry 1992; 149:719–720.
35. Naimark D, Jackson E, Rockwell E, Jeste DV. Psychotic symptoms in Parkinson's disease patients with dementia. J Am Geriatr Soc 1996; 44:296–299.
36. Fernandez W, Stern G, Lees AJ: Hallucinations and parkinsonian motor fluctuations. Behav Neurol 1992; 5:83–86.
37. Chacko RC, Hurley RA, Harper RG, Jankovic J, and Cardoso F. Clozapine for acute and maintenance treatment for psychosis in Parkinson's disease. J Neuropsychiatr Clin Neurosci 1995; 7:471–475.
38. Wolters EC, Jansen ENH, Tuynman-Qua HG, Bergmans PLM. Olanzapine in the treatment of dopaminomimetic psychosis in patients with Parkinson's disease. Neurology 1996; 47:1085–1087.
39. Zoldan J, Friedberg G, Livneh M, Melamed E. Psychosis in advanced Parkinson's disease: treatment with Ondansetron, a 5-HT3 receptor antagonist. Neurology 1995; 45:1305–1308.
40. Petracca G, Chemerinski E, Merello M, Leiguarda R, Starkstein SE. Prevalence and correlates of pathological affect in PD. In preparation.

22

Disorders Affecting Psychotropic Absorption, Metabolism, and Toxicity

Vicki L. Ellingrod
University of Iowa College of Pharmacy
Iowa City, Iowa

INTRODUCTION

Prescribing psychotropic medications in medically ill populations requires a deep understanding of the pharmacokinetic changes that can occur. Additionally, careful risk-benefit assessment needs to be conducted to determine if the usage of these medications is appropriate given the patient's current medical condition. Special considerations important in this population include (1):

1. Potential drug-drug interactions can occur between medications used for psychiatric illness and medications used for medical illness.
2. Impairment in renal and hepatic functioning may alter psychotropic drug pharmacokinetics.
3. The incidence of adverse drug reactions from the psychotropic medications may aggravate preexisting medical conditions.

The first consideration is beyond the scope of this chapter and is discussed elsewhere in this publication. The others are the basis for understanding medication use in the medical psychiatry population. Changes in pharmacokinetics can affect the mechanism and time course of a drug's absorption, distribution, metabolism, or excretion, with the overall effect being alterations in the drug's intensity, duration of action, or time to onset of effect (2). This chapter will serve primarily as a basic overview of some of the pharmacokinetic changes seen in the internal medicine/psychiatry population. Often the medical literature for this patient population is lacking. Scientific studies for psychotropic medication are often not conducted in such a specialized group of patients. Thus, some of the information and clinical recommendations contained in this chapter are based on theoretical or potential changes of pharmacokinetic parameters often seen in the medically ill. When possible, specific pharmacokinetic changes are mentioned, but often this is not possible due the diversity seen in the internal medicine psychiatry population. Also, medical illnesses vary in their severity and do not consistently affect drug pharmacokinetics consistently. With this in mind, the clinician is reminded that each patient should be evaluated on an individual basis with appreciation of basic pharmacokinetic principles related to drug therapy and their medical illness.

PHARMACOKINETICS

Absorption

Absorption is defined as a process in which an unchanged drug proceeds from the site of administration to the site of measurement within the body, which is most commonly the blood or plasma (2). Most psychotropic drugs are absorbed either by oral or intramuscular routes. Other routes of administration that involve absorption, but are not often used for psychotropic medications, include sublingual, buccal, subcutaneous, dermal, pulmonary, and rectal routes. Drugs that are administered intravenously do not undergo adsorption since they are administered directly into the blood stream. Several factors affect the absorption of a drug from its site of administration. The percent of drug that is absorbed depends on whether the drug is an acid or a base, the lipophilic properties of the drug, the physiology of the gastrointestinal tract, and the amount of drug that is metabolized by the liver before reaching systemic circulation. Each of these concepts will be independently discussed.

The stomach is the location in which oral dosage forms of drugs are put into solution so that they can be absorbed. In an acidic environment drugs that are weak acids are in a nonionic state and have a higher absorption rate than drugs that are weak bases and in an ionized state. Weak bases are absorbed later in the small bowel, where the environment is more basic (3). Good examples of psychotropic medications that are weak bases are the phenothiazines, tricyclic antidepressants, and many benzodiazepines (4). These medicines are absorbed in the small bowel in an unionized state. If changes occur in stomach and intestinal pH due to medical illness or concurrent medications, the absorption of these weak acids and weak bases may increase or decrease depending on the situation (5). Alterations in absorption due to changes in pH can potentially occur in many situations. Examples include patients who are achlorhydric, patients receiving medications to suppress acid secretion, patients with renal dysfunction since higher gastric pHs may be produced, and patients with chronic obstructive pulmonary disease (COPD) since hypoxia can alter the pH balance (6). It has also been shown that women have less stomach acid secretion than men, although the data is conflicting (3). The true clinical significance of these changes is not known, but gender differences may explain why a greater therapeutic effect of certain medications may be seen in women (3). Aside from these medical conditions that alter stomach and intestinal pH, another factor that may affect drug absorption is excessive vomiting. This condition primarily affects only orally absorbed medications since absorption cannot occur if the stomach contents are emptied prematurely. An alternative to oral administration of medication in this situation is intramuscular, sublingual, or intravenous administration.

The amount of drug absorbed is not dependent on only the acid and base properties of each compound. Another contributing factor to the overall absorption is the drug's lipophilicity, or ability to pass though lipid membranes. Since the gut is lined in epithelium with tight junctions, absorption of most drugs is accomplished by lipid diffusion. This diffusion from administration site to blood stream is based upon a concentration gradient guiding drug permeation. This condition is satisfied when a drug is given by any of the routes of administration listed previously that require absorption. When a drug is given intramuscularly it is already in solution. The extent of absorption then depends on the degree of lipophilicy. A high degree of lipid solubility relative to aqueous solubility is needed for this diffusion, although too low an aqueous solubility is undesirable since the drug must be in an aqueous solution to be absorbed. Chemically each drug has a pKa value. This pKa is the pH at which the concentrations of the ionized and un-ionized forms are equal. Because lipophilicity is a characteristic of each specific drug, changes in physiological conditions relative to medical illness may not be clinically significant. The degree of lipid solubility for each medication may become relevant in patients with impaired drug absorption, since a drug's pKa, acid-base properties, and pH at the site of absorption all play a part in drug permeation (7).

After a drug is put into a solution, the next step in absorption is transit through the small intestine. The rate of gastric emptying as well as total transit time in the small intestine can significantly influence the absorption of psychotropic medication (4). There are several medical conditions and medications that can delay or increase the rate of gastric emptying and transit time. Gastroparesis is probably the most encountered medical condition since it results in a slowing of gastric emptying and a delayed or slower transit time in the intestine. The overall result of these changes may not be an overall decrease in absorption, but a delay in the time it takes to completely absorb a drug. Changes in gastric emptying and transit time are often associated with disease such as diabetes mellitus, atrophic gastritis, gastric cancer, pyloric stenosis, pancreatitis, migraine, and gastric ulcer (4). Additionally, physiological changes in gastrointestinal structure that occur with short bowel syndrome, gastrectomy, and gastroplasty can also cause malabsorption problems (8). Since very little has been researched about the use of psychotropic medications in these three special cases, we can only conclude that the potential for decreased drug absorption is present and act accordingly. To overcome this potential problem, the author has four recommendations based on her clinical practice and experience: (1) the use of parenteral medications on a short-term basis, if available, since the gastrointestinal track is not involved in their absorption, (2) the use of rectal medications, if possible, based on patient anatomy and availability of this dosage form, (3) the use of medications that have a "therapeutic range" such that monitoring serum concentrations of the medications can be used to determine the extent of drug absorption, and (4) dosing the medications based solely on clinical response, which may involve administering doses that are higher than are usually used due to decreased absorption of the preparation. Although the use of parenteral medications would be optimal in these situations since gastrointestinal absorption is not a factor, clinically this is not feasible on a long-term basis and thus may be only useful in situations where the medications may be used on a short-term basis such as delirium. Additionally, many of the psychotropic medications are not available in an injectable dosage form, which would preclude using them in this fashion. Each one of these recommendations may apply to certain cases more than others, but may be tried if conventional dosing of psychotropic drugs in these conditions fails due to malabsorption.

In addition to physical states that alter absorption, medications that have anticholinergic properties such as propantheline (Pro-Banthine), atropine, and dicyclomine (Bentyl) can also delay the entrance of drugs into the intestine from the stomach, resulting in a slower rate of absorption and a delay in the time to onset of action (4,7). Other medications that can cause the same effect are tricyclic antidepressants and low-potency neuroleptics (4). Some of the medications shown to be affected by changes in transit time and gastric emptying are lithium (9), L-dopa (10), chlordiazepoxide (Librium) (11), diazepam (Valium) (12), and chlorpromazine (Thorazine) (13,14). With all four of these medications, the overall results are decreased absorption and a slower time to onset. In patients with gastroparesis, some benzodiazepines may take up to 5 hours to reach peak effect. Both diazepam and flurazepam (Dalmane) are somewhat different in that they have a more rapid absorption than other benzodiazepines, with an overall peak effect occurring within one hour of oral administration. Thus, using benzodiazepines with rapid absorption in patients with gastroparesis can overcome the effect of delayed intestinal transit times (15).

Other reasons for decreased absorption may include decreases in blood flow and the transport mechanisms of the intestinal mucosa. Renal dysfunction can impair gastric mucosa transport by an unknown mechanism (6). Decreases in pulmonary function may affect absorption. As pulmonary status declines, cardiopulmonary work increases and shifts blood flow away from the splanic beds and gastrointestinal tracts. The overall effect of these changes is a decrease in drug uptake from the GI tract and peripheral tissues (16,17). Although these physiological changes may occur, the clinical relevance is unknown. The clinician needs to keep changes like these in mind should questions of absorption arise in a patient with these disease states.

A decreased transit time is often seen in patients with gastroenteritis, diarrheal disease, gastroenterostomy, duodenal ulcer, celiac disease, and stress. Medications such as metoclopramide (Reglan) or cisapride (Propulsid), which are promotility agents and are used for the treatment of gastroparesis, can move medications though the intestine faster by increasing the transit time. The effects of increased intestinal transit time and rapid gastric emptying on psychotropic medications has not been studied. The overall effect may be a decrease in absorption due to reduced contact of the drug with the intestinal mucosa. To date the only information available is on the absorption of sustained-release lithium preparations being decreased due to lack of contact with the small colon (18).

Once a drug is put into solution in the stomach and absorbed in the gastrointestinal tract, the amount of drug that reaches the systemic circulation may not be 100%. The bioavailability, or percentage of drug that does go into circulation, of most psychiatric drugs is variable and dependent of each chemical structure. The loss of drug as it passes through the organs of elimination such as the liver and gastrointestinal membranes is called the "first-pass effect" (2). If the metabolizing capability of the liver is great enough, then the bioavailability of the drug is low due the liver metabolizing a majority of the drug before it reaches systemic circulation. Drugs with a low first-pass effect are not metabolized to an appreciable amount before entering the circulation, thus more can be absorbed. The overall degree of drug availability, as stated earlier, is dependent on the chemical composition of the drug and intersubject variability, which depends on an individual's intrinsic metabolic capability and medical condition (7). In patients with conditions that shunt blood past hepatic sites of elimination, the availability of high–first-pass effect drugs is increased due to a reduction in the amount eliminated before it reaches systemic circulation. Specifically in cirrhosis, the normal blood flow though the liver is disrupted, and as pressure in the portal system increases collateral channels start to carry more flow. The result is a bypassing of the liver and a decreased amount of drug that is exposed to first-pass metabolism (6). Examples of an increased rate of drug absorption due to cirrhosis has been found with temazepam (Restoril) and alprazolam (Xanax) (19,20). Although these physiological changes would suggest that a majority of psychiatric medications experience similar increases in absorption, this has not been extensively studied. Clinically, each patient needs to be treated individually. Changes seen in patients with disease states, such as hepatitis, that may result in a shunting of blood flow from the liver need to be kept in mind to prevent potential medication side effects, or toxicity, which can result from increased absorption of the medication.

Distribution

The volume of distribution reflects the total amount of space in the systemic circulation and tissues that a drug can distribute and is defined in terms of the fluid from which it is measured (i.e., blood or plasma concentrations). It is a direct measure of the extent of distribution and rarely corresponds to a real volume such as plasma volume, extracellular water, or total body water (2). Drug distribution may be to the fluids and the tissues in the body, with tissue binding being so great that in some circumstances the volume of distribution may be several times the total body size. The volumes of distribution for a number of drugs are listed in Table 1. Medications that are lipid soluble have large volumes of distribution, while water-soluble medications have smaller ones

Table 1 Pharmacokinetics of Selective Psychotropic Medications

Parent drug	Protein bound (%)	Major metabolites	Half-life (hr)	Volume of distribution (liters/kg)
Benzodiazepines				
Oxazepam	97	Inactive glucuronide conjugation	5–13	0.6–2
Lorazepam	91	Inactive glucuronide conjugation	10–18	1.3
Alprazolam	70–80	α-Hydroxyalprazolam	12–15	1.1
Chloriazepoxide	47	Desmethylchlordiazepoxide	5–30	0.3
Diazepam	94–98	Desmethyldiazepam	20–50	1.1
Halazepam	>90	Desmethyldiazepam	14	NA
Prazepam	>90	Desmethyldiazepam	30–100	NA
Clorazepate	>90	Desmethyldiazepam	30–100	1.25–1.54
Clonazepam	47	7-Acetyl-amino derivatives	18–50	1.8–4
Temazepam	98	Inactive glucuronide conjugation	10–17	1.4
Flurazepam	97	N-Desalkylflurazepam	50–100	NA
Triazolam	89	α-Hydroxytriazolam	1.5–5.4	0.8–1.8
Estolazam	93	4-Hydroxyestazolam	10–24	NA
Midazolam	>95	O-Methylmidazolam	2.5	0.8–6.6
Quazepam	>95	2-Oxoquazepam	25–41	5
Antidepressants				
Amitriptyline	>90	Nortriptyline	9–25	6.4–36
Desipramine	>90	Hydroxydesipramine	14–62	78–168
Doxepin	80–85	Desmethyldoxepin	6–8	9–33
Imipramine	96	Desipramine	6–20	9.3–23
Maprotiline	88	Desmethylmaprotiline	51–58	16–32

	Absorption (%)	Metabolite		
Nortriptyline	93–95	Hydroxynortriptyline	18–28	21
Clomipramine	>90	Desmethyl clomipramine	15–62	9–25
Trazodone	85–95	m-chlorophenylpiperazine	4–9	0.8–1.5
Bupropion	82–88	Hydroxybupropion	14	19–21
Amoxapine	90	Hydroxyamoxapine	8.8–14	4600 L total
Fluoxetine	95	Norfluoxetine	26–220	12–42
Paroxetine	95	None	4–56	3–28
Sertraline	>97	Desmethylsertraline	26	20
Fluvoxamine	77	None	12–19	>5
Venlafaxine	30	O-Desmethylvenlafaxine	4	6–7
Nefazodone	>99	Hydroxynefazodone	2.7–10	0.22–0.87
Antipsychotics				
Chlorpromazine	91–99	Multiple	11–42	8–106
Thioridazine	>90	Mesoridazine	21	17.8
Haloperidol	90–92	Reduced haloperidol	10–36	20
Thiothixene	>90	NA	34	NA
Perphenazine	>90	Inactive sulfoxide	8.4–12	10–34
Fluphenazine	>90	Multiple	14–15	NA
Risperidone	90	9-Hydroxy-risperidone	20–30	NA
Clozapine	>90	Uncoagulated clozapine	5.5–33	NA
Olanzapine	>90	Glucuronide	27	NA
Mood stabilizers				
Lithium	0	Not metabolized	14–28	0.7–1
Valproic acid	80–90	Metabolized	8–17	0.19–0.23
Carbamazepine	75–90	Epoxide metabolite	12–55	0.59–2

NA: Value not available.
Source: Refs. 53, 60–62.

(6). The volume of distribution is dependent on age, sex, and weight and may vary in different disease states (6). Changes in vascular volume and tissue volume can alter the distribution of a drug (21). Some medical conditions in which volume changes can be seen include starvation, anorexia nervosa, cirrhosis with ascites, congestive heart failure with fluid retention, pregnancy, and renal impairment (4,6,22). In general, all of these conditions, aside from starvation and anorexia nervosa, are associated with an increase in the water compartment of the body. Thus, it may take more medication to reach therapeutic serum concentrations since the area in which the drugs are distributed is larger.

In starvation and anorexia nervosa, dehydration often occurs, which results in a reduction of total body water. Due to this change smaller doses of medication may be needed to reach acceptable serum concentrations, since the area in which the drug is distributed is decreased. Since the majority of psychotropic medications have very large volumes of distribution, changes produced by these disease states may not be clinically significant. The one exception to this is lithium. Lithium's volume of distribution closely follows total body water (6). These changes have been documented most closely in pregnant women, whose volume of distribution can double, thus doubling the amount of lithium needed to obtain the same steady-state serum concentrations. After delivery, this volume returns to normal and the dosage of lithium also needs to be decreased. If lithium is to be used during pregnancy, clinical guidelines for its use include monitoring of lithium serum concentrations to assure therapeutic levels, stopping the lithium prior to labor, and then restarting the lithium after childbirth at the original dose (23). The use of lithium in either congestive heart failure or cirrhosis with ascites is not well studied, but due to possible changes in volume of distribution, close monitoring of lithium serum concentrations to prevent lithium intoxication is warranted, especially in cases of acute fluid changes.

Hepatic disease can also affect the volume of distribution by increasing the amount of unbound drug within the serum. Within this volume of distribution, drugs are bound to plasma-binding proteins. The majority of psychotropic medications, except lithium, are highly protein bound (>88%) (4). Basic drugs bind to α_1-acid glycoprotein (AAGP), and acidic drugs bind to albumin (2). Generally changes in liver and renal function that cause alterations in protein binding will cause alterations in the amount of unbound drug in the serum. Often this is clinically important since the majority of the psychotropic medications are highly protein bound, and the unbound drug is the percentage of drug that is pharmacologically active. Thus, if a drug is 90% protein bound, changing the percentage bound to 80% would result in a doubling of the amount of unbound or active drug from 10 to 20%. This increase may result in an increase or worsening in incidence of adverse drug reactions or toxicity as well as allowing more drug to be available to act on receptors. Conversely, an increase in binding proteins may cause an opposite effect, and more drug may be required to produce a clinical effect.

Several disease states have been found to decrease serum-binding proteins. For example, in cirrhosis the liver produces fewer serum-binding proteins—primarily albumin. Increases in serum bilirubin can also compete with medications for binding sites. Both of these changes taken together can cause an increase in the percentage of drug that is unbound. In viral hepatitis, drugs that are highly metabolized may have a greater percentage of unbound drug with an extended half-life because the liver is not as efficient at eliminating drugs from the body (24,25). Renal dysfunction may also cause changes in protein binding, decreases in serum pH, lower production of serum protein, and endogenous competitive inhibition of protein binding (26). Other conditions that affect protein binding in a similar manner but to various degrees include cystic fibrosis, liver abscess, acute pancreatitis, malnutrition, protein-losing enteropathies, chronic inflammatory diseases, cancer, trauma, and surgery (4). Alternatively, AAGP can be elevated in diseases causing acute inflammation such as celiac disease or Crohn's disease (4).

Unfortunately, studies investigating the amount of bound and unbound drug for specific psychotropic medications used during medical illnesses are lacking. This lack of data leaves the clinician assuming that changes in protein binding will affect chemically similar medications in the same manner. The majority of psychotropic medications, except lithium, are all highly protein bound (>88%). The percentage of protein binding for each medication is listed in Table 1. The tricyclic antidepressants and some antipsychotics, such as haloperidol (Haldol), clozapine (Clozaril), and olanzapine (Zyprexa), have established therapeutic windows for efficacy, thus monitoring of blood levels may be warranted. The clinician needs to be cautioned that the serum level reported is a total level and assumes a standard percentage of unbound drug associated with this serum concentration. Thus, use of standard therapeutic drug monitoring does not reflect a percentage change in protein binding. For example, previous work has shown that in Crohn's disease, chlorpromazine levels are high due to an increased percentage of drug bound to serum proteins with the amount of free drug being unchanged (4). In response to these findings, dosage adjustment is not necessary since the amount of unbound drug is within the target range.

Metabolism

Three conditions determine the degree to which a drug undergoes hepatic metabolism: the rate of hepatic blood flow, the degree of enzyme capacity in the parenchyma, and the amount of protein binding of a particular agent. In general, it can be said that the liver transforms lipophilic drugs into more water-soluble compounds to facilitate elimination by the kidneys. Biotransformation by the liver occurs in two phases: phase I and phase II metabolism. Phase I metabolism is oxidative, reductive, or hydrolytic. The most important phase I enzyme system is the cytochrome P-450 system, located primarily in the hepatic smooth endoplasmic reticulum. The cytochrome P-450 system shows great variation, and metabolic rates may differ by a factor of 6 from individual to individual. Variations may be due to gender, race, or genetic differences. Probably the most widely studied cytochrome P-450s are IID6 (CYP2D6) and IIIA4 (CYP3A4). These enzymes may be more affected by medical illness such as acute viral hepatitis, alcoholic hepatitis, and active cirrhosis. Since these disorders have a major effect on the pericentral regions of the liver, where the cytochromes tend to be present, the metabolism of medications eliminated by these enzymes may be reduced.

In phase II metabolism, metabolites from the first phase may be conjugated with sugars, sulfates, or amino acids (6). The primary purpose of phase II metabolism is to render the parent drug or the metabolites produced from phase I metabolism more water soluble so that they can be excreted by the kidneys.

The extent to which a drug is metabolized by the liver also depends on the rate of drug delivery to the hepatic enzymes and the intrinsic capacity of the enzymes (4). If metabolism is dependent on drug delivery, then the rate-limiting step in this process is blood flow, since enzymes in the liver metabolize all the drug that it is presented with. Drugs metabolized in this manner have a high hepatic clearance. In the case of low hepatic clearance, metabolism is dependent on the amount of enzyme in the liver, and thus the enzyme's capacity is the rate-limiting step. Enzymes can become saturated with the drug faster than the blood delivers it to the liver, and the amount of drug metabolized per unit time does not increase (4). An exception to this is in severe hepatic dysfunction where accumulation of low hepatic clearances can occur due to decreases in the liver's enzyme levels. Some examples of high–hepatic clearance drugs are triazolam (Halcion), haloperidol, and tricyclic antidepressants. Low–hepatic clearance drugs include chlorpromazine and diazepam.

In addition, the activity of these enzymes can be induced or inhibited by other medications. External or environmental factors such as smoking and ethanol use can also affect the activity of these enzymes (27). Ethanol can act in several ways as a competitive inhibitor, a noncompetitive inhibitor, or an enhancer of drug metabolism. Chronically, ethanol can induce its own metabolism and the metabolism of other medications, since it induces the enzyme that it is metabolized by, cytochrome P-450IIE1 (CYP2E1). However, when consumed acutely, it can inhibit the metabolism of other drugs metabolized by this enzyme, thus increasing the serum concentrations of certain medications. (27). Smoking has been associated with decrease in the steady-state concentrations of many psychotropic medications (28–31). This effect is primarily due to the polyaromatic hydrocarbons that are present in cigarette smoke (27). Thus, taking into account whether a patient consumes ethanol acutely or chronically or smokes may influence the physician's decision on the amount of drug to use when treating their patient's psychiatric illness.

In disease states where the function of the liver is compromised, i.e., cirrhosis or hepatitis, phase I metabolism is usually impaired with little change in phase II metabolism. Drugs undergoing extensive phase I metabolism are poorly metabolized, while other medications that undergo primarily conjugative metabolism (phase II) are seemingly unaffected. Additionally the intrinsic clearance of the metabolizing enzymes may be decreased such that the differences in clearance rates between high and low clearance drugs is diminished. The primary reason for this is a reduction in the activity of the liver enzymes involved in the elimination of high-clearance drugs since blood flow does not change.

Examples of phase I metabolized benzodiazepines include all those listed in Table

1 except for lorazepam, temazepam, and oxazepam (Serax) (32–34). In hepatic dysfunction, the half-life of phase I metabolized benzodiazepines may be greater than 100 hours due to an accumulation of the active metabolite desmethyldiazepam. If a benzodiazepine other than the three mentioned above is used, the dose should be decreased by 50% since the clearance may be decreased by 33–60% (4,35).

Neuroleptics in themselves have been shown to cause liver dysfunction (36,37), and when they are given to patients with a predisposition for hepatic dysfunction elevated serum levels may develop or worsen (38). This has been associated with phenothiazine neuroleptics such as chlorpromazine, thioridazine (Mellaril), fluphenazine (Prolixin), perphenazine (Trilafon), and trifluorperazine (Stelazine). Due to this association some authors suggest avoiding these medications in patients with cholestatic jaundice (6). Patients with cirrhosis may have an increased sensitivity to the sedative effects of neuroleptics and whenever possible should be given lower doses (6). For neuroleptics in which serum concentration monitoring can be done, therapeutic drug monitoring of levels should be conducted to assure that the patient is getting the correct amount of drug (6). Additionally liver function enzymes should be checked for the first 2 months of therapy to assure no additional elevation in these laboratory values (39).

Generally, antidepressants are all highly metabolized by the liver, thus changes in their metabolism may cause an increase in serum concentration. This may not be clinically significant for the selective serotonin-reuptake inhibitors (SSRIs) and medications such as venlafaxine (Effexor) or nefazodone (Serzone), since no established therapeutic range has been found. Some of the tricyclic antidepressants (TCAs) do have therapeutic ranges, so therapeutic drug monitoring may be done to watch for toxicity. Although the pharmacokinetics of bupropion (Wellbutrin) have not shown significant alterations in hepatic dysfunction, the epileptogenic properties of this drug call for caution in hepatic dysfunction due to higher unbound percentages. Monoamine oxidase inhibitors (MAOIs), like some neuroleptics, have been associated with altered liver function and jaundice in normal subjects. Due to this and the fact that MAOI accumulation in hepatic dysfunction is unknown, the manufactures do not recommend their use in hepatic dysfunction (6).

The medications valproic acid (Depakote and Dapakene) and carbamazepine (Tegretol) are both highly protein-bound. Although no controlled clinical studies have investigated the effect of hepatic dysfunction on the drug, it is reasonable to assume that higher serum concentrations would be expected along with a decrease in the clearance. From this, it is recommended to reduce the dosage in this disease state (6). Valproic acid, on the other hand, has been shown to cause direct hepatotoxicity, with rare cases of hepatitis, and should be avoided in liver dysfunction (40). Should the drug be needed, then the dosage should be decreased, with blood level and liver function test monitoring performed (41).

Excretion

One of the primary measures of drug excretion is half-life. The half-life is defined as the time it takes for the medication's serum concentrations to decline by half. Clearance is also a measure of the rate of elimination and defines how efficiently the body can clear the waste and drug products from biological fluids (7). The units of measurement for clearance are volume per time. Both half-life and clearance are related to each other, in that the time course of a drug in the body depends on both of these parameters plus volume of distribution. Changes in one variable can cause changes in the other. Overall, the total rate of elimination of a medication from the body, or the total body clearance, depends on clearance rates from renal, hepatic, and other routes (i.e., biliary, pulmonary, etc.) of elimination all added together. The pharmacokinetic equation for this relationship is as follows (7):

$$CL \text{ (total)} = CL \text{ (renal)} + CL \text{ (hepatic)} + CL \text{ (other)}$$

For drugs that are hepatically eliminated as inactive metabolites, clearance is primarily dependent on hepatic function, and the half-life is an estimate of the amount of time it takes the liver to reduce the parent drug or metabolite's serum concentration by half. This example holds true for the majority of psychotropic medications except for lithium, which is not metabolized. For renally eliminated drugs, clearance is dependent on renal function with half-life estimating the time it takes for plasma concentrations to be reduced by half due to renal excretion of the drug. In the first example, the total body clearance is primarily dependent on hepatic clearance. In the second example, total body clearance is dependent on renal clearance. For medications that undergo both hepatic and renal elimination, both of these variables contribute to total body clearance. An example is the metabolism of a parent drug to an active metabolite that is renally excreted.

The majority of psychotropic medications are renally excreted after they are metabolized, except for lithium, which is entirely renally excreted and not metabolized. Serum creatinine (Scr) and blood urea nitrogen (BUN) are two laboratory tests that are indicators of general renal function or clearance. As renal function declines, the products from protein breakdown accumulate in the blood, causing an increase in BUN. Creatinine is a byproduct of muscle breakdown and will start to accumulate in the blood as renal function declines. Circulating levels of both of these indicators vary with age, muscle mass, diet, gender, etc., thus changes in Scr may also be indicative of changes in these factors rather than renal function (6). In clinical practice overall renal function can be estimated by using the Cockroft and Gault equation for measuring creatinine clearance and glomerular filtration rate (GFR) (42). In this equation ideal body weight is measured in kilograms, serum creatinine in mg/dl, and age in years. When using this equation for females, the calculated result must be multiplied by 0.85 to adjust for a reduced volume of distribution.

$$\text{Creatinine clearance (ml/min)} = \frac{[140 - \text{age (yr)}] \text{ IBW (kg)}}{72 \text{ [Scr(mg/dl)]}}$$

There are several limitations to this equation for the estimation of renal function (43). First, a patient's Scr must be at steady state. In situations where renal function may be rapidly changing, the Cockroft/Gault method may overestimate or underestimate renal function. Second, estimation of renal function by using creatinine clearance in patients on dialysis or in end-stage renal disease will cause the calculated values to overestimate renal function because the Scr and BUN are artificially eliminated from the body. A suitable alternative in both of these situations is to obtain a 24-hour urine collection for measurement of creatinine clearance. By monitoring Scr and creatinine clearance it can be determined if renal function has been acutely changing. Also, the actual values of GFR and overall renal functioning can be obtained. The use of calculated estimates may help guide dosing in lithium therapy based on renal function, as long as the limitations of this method are known.

For all patients on lithium therapy serum levels should guide drug dosing. Generally if the GFR is greater than 50 ml/min, no adjustment in dosage is needed. If GFR falls between 10–50 ml/min, then the dosage should be reduced by 25–50%, and if GFR falls to less then 10 ml/min, the dose should be reduced by 50–75% (44). Although no official guidelines for lithium use in dialysis patients exist, several authors have published their clinical experience (45,46). Most dialysis patients will only require a dose of 300–900 mg of lithium carbonate after dialysis. Since lithium is entirely excreted by the kidneys, no additional doses are usually required between dialysis sessions (45,46). The prescribing physician needs to check serum lithium levels between dialysis runs to be assured that the lithium is not accumulating. Predialysis lithium levels should be monitored and not exceed 0.92 mEq/liter. After dialysis the levels should be checked to confirm the removal of lithium during dialysis. The postdialysis dose of lithium may be expected to increase serum concentrations by 30% from levels obtained after the dialysis session (46).

As mentioned previously the majority of psychotropic medications, except lithium, are excreted by extrarenal metabolism, which is primarily hepatic. It should therefore be expected that little change in serum concentrations, or elimination, takes place when these drugs are used in renal dysfunction. An exception to this theory is the excretion of active metabolites that are renally cleared. Some of these metabolites are pharmacologically active, and accumulation due to renal dysfunction may lead to clinically significant effects secondary to competition with the parent drug for serum-binding protein or receptor sites on target tissues (6). Additionally some medications have metabolites, which have the potential to produce adverse drug reactions when accumulation occurs. An example is tricyclic antidepressants. Although the parent compounds do not accumulate in renal dysfunction, the hydroxylated metabolites, which are more cardiotoxic, may. In renal dysfunction, the plasma concentrations of these metabolites may be markedly increased and cause potential cardiac problems (47). Additionally, most benzodiazepines have active metabolites, which can accumulate in renal failure. The problem with accumulation of benzodiazepines is that the half-life of these compounds may exceed 100 hours. Exceptions include lorazepam, temazepam, and oxazepam, which are not metabolized to active compounds. Similar to benzodiazepine use in hepatic dysfunction, it may be more prudent to use those benzodiazepines not metabolized to active compounds in patients with renal dysfunction. In patients with creatinine clearances less than 10 ml/min, the dosage of lorazepam should be reduced by 50% and the dosage of oxazepam should be reduced by 25%. No other changes in dosing schedule are required (44). All patients should be monitored for signs of sedation, altered mental status, and other signs of benzodiazepine intoxication, since the signs and symptoms are similar to uremic encephalopathy (6).

No formal pharmacokinetic studies on neuroleptics have been conducted in renal dysfunction. In general, no dosage adjustment is needed due to their extensive metabolism, low production of renally excreted active metabolites, and large volume of distribution. Caution may be taken with haloperidol since its metabolite is somewhat pharmacologically active and may accumulate (48). In patients taking neuroleptics who experience adverse drug reactions such as extrapyramidal side effects, dystonic reactions, or anticholinergic side effects, dosage reduction should be taken into consideration.

Generally, the SSRIs, venlafaxine, nefazodone, and MAOIs do not show appreciable pharmacokinetic changes in renal failure (44,49–52). Of note is a study by Doyle et al. (53), which found an increase in paroxetine (Paxil) serum concentrations with decreasing renal function, even though individual drug concentrations varied significantly. Until future studies can clarify paroxetine's pharmacokinetics in renal dysfunction, the dose should be decreased in end-stage renal disease. Other antidepressants such as trazodone (Desyrel) and bupropion have also been poorly studied (22), but the manufactures of bupropion recommend reducing the dose due to potential accumulation of metabolites, which may cause an increased potential for seizures. Monoamine oxidase inhibitors are another class of antidepressants that have been poorly studied, however, the incidence of orthostatic hypotension may be increased when used in renal failure patients (22).

Carbamazepine and valproic acid are primarily eliminated hepatically. Although valproic acid has no known active metabolites, carbamazepine does. It has been suggested that the dose of carbamazepine be decreased by 25% when used in patients with GFRs less than 10 ml/min (44). No guidelines are available for valproic acid. Routine therapeutic drug monitoring of both medications should help guide therapy, with dosage reduction being considered in patients experiencing adverse drug reactions.

Finally, the possibility of renal failure in the presence of or due to hepatic failure needs to be discussed. In patients with hepatic failure the potential for the hepatorenal syndrome to occur exists, so clinicians need to be cautioned that the amount of medications used may need to be reduced due to coexisting hepatic and renal dysfunction.

Toxicity

Toxicity, in general, from any psychotropic medication can occur if serum concentrations are too high. In the medically ill, accumulation may be due to changes in absorption, first-pass elimination, protein binding, volume of distribution, hepatic elimination, and renal excretion. Toxicity can be present in many forms, but the most commonly seen manifestation of toxicity in this population is increased somnolence. Since most psychiatric medications are extensively metabolized, the greatest amount of sedation is often seen in patients with the most severe liver dysfunction or with a prior history of encephalopathy (4). Other common adverse reactions associated with psychotropic medications are often dose or blood concentration related. Despite the usage of "typical" doses, further reductions may be necessary since higher blood concentrations of these medications may be produced by pharmacokinetic changes. The phenothiazines are associated with causing hepatotoxicity, cirrhosis, and jaundice, thus potentially predisposing patients to hepatic dysfunction. The clinical findings usually include fever, chills, nausea, epigastric pain, right upper quadrant pain, and malaise. Laboratory findings include elevated alkaline phosphatase and conjugated bilirubin with mild elevations in asparate and alanine aminotransferases. Although preexisting liver disease has not been associated with an increased risk, cautious use of these agents in hepatic dysfunction is recommended. Hepatic function may return to normal with drug continuation but often may not resolve until the offending agent is removed (54).

In cases of lithium neurotoxicity associated with therapeutic lithium serum concentrations, the populations most at risk are patients with an organic or psychotic diagnosis (55,56). Often this is manifest by poor memory, poor concentration, distractibility, and impaired judgment. Additionally, abnormal movements such as ataxia and dysarthria may occur. In renal dysfunction the risk of lithium intoxication is several fold greater if serum concentrations are not monitored. Prudent use of lithium, along with careful monitoring, can prevent any potential situations in which intoxication can occur.

The medically ill population may also be at a higher risk of experiencing adverse drug reactions at "typical" dosages due to the changes in pharmacokinetics. This may be seen if protein binding is altered or metabolism is reduced. Many of the psychotropic medications, as well as medications used for medical illness, have anticholinergic side effects and may produce intoxication when used concomitantly. Signs of anticholinergic intoxication include disorientation, confusion, recent memory loss, agitation, dysarthria, incoherent speech, push of speech, visual hallucinations, delusions, ataxia, paranoia, anxiety, and coma (57). It has been shown in impaired elderly subjects that addition of anticholinergic medication may exacerbate preexisting baseline deficits (58). In a study of nursing home patients by Tollefson et al. (59), Mini-Mental Status Exam (MMSE) scores increased when reductions in the amount of medication with anticholinergic effects were instituted. Although the change in MMSE scores produced by medication discontinuation or alteration was not statistically significant, the authors caution against polypharmacy, particularly for medications with additive anticholinergic effects.

SUMMARY

The internal medicine/psychiatry population is a very diverse and complicated group. In addition to understanding their psychiatric problems, knowledge about their medical illness is essential to prevent toxicity from and adverse reactions to medications. Changes in the pharmacokinetics of psychotropic drugs may result from changes in medical conditions and must be considered when prescribing or recommending medication in this population. The reason for alterations in a medication's pharmacokinetics often is not confined to one specific change. For any disease state many factors play a role in altering the pharmacokinetics of medications. Since the medical literature regarding specific pharmacokinetic changes is relatively sparse, the clinician is encouraged to use such medications with prudence and to adjust dosages when clinically warranted by the situation. Subsequently, any medical condition can cause a whole assortment of pharmacokinetic changes. Taking this into account along with the fact that patients can show great variation in individual clinical responses to these medications requires that monitoring be done on a case-by-case basis.

REFERENCES

1. Stoudemire A, Moran MG, Fogel BS. Psychotropic drug use in the medically ill: Part I. Psychosomatics 1990; 31:377–391.
2. Rowland M, Tozer TN. Clinical Pharmacokinetics. 2nd ed. Philadelphia: Lea and Febiger, 1989.
3. Younkers KA, Kando JC, Cole JO, Blumenthal S. Gender differences in pharmacokinetics and pharmacodynamics of psychotropic medication. Am J Psychiatry 1992; 149:587–595.
4. Leipzig SM. Psychopharmacology in patients with hepatic and gastrointestinal disease. Int J Psychiatry Med 1990; 20:109–139.
5. Grossman MI, Krisner JB, Gillespie IA. Basal and histalog stimulated gastric secretion in control subjects and in patients with peptic ulcer or gastric cancer. Gastroenterology 1963; 45:14–26.
6. Rubey RN, Lydiard RB. Psychopharmacology in the medically ill: general principles. Adv Psychosomat Med 1994; 21:1–27.
7. Katzung BG. Basic and Clinical Pharmacology. 4th ed. Stamford, CT: Appleton and Lange, 1989.
8. Greenberger NJ, Isselbacher KJ. Disorders of absorption. In: Isselbacher KJ, Braunwald E, Wilson JD, Martin JB, Fauci AS, Kasper DL, eds. Harrison's Principles of Internal Medicine. 13th ed. New York: McGraw-Hill, 1994:1386–1403.
9. Crammer JL, Rosser RM, Crance G. Blood levels and management of lithium treatment. Br Med J 1974; 3:650–654.
10. Morgan JP, Rivera-Calimlim L, Messiha F, Sundaresan PR, Trabert N. Imipramine-mediated interference with levodopa absorption from the gastrointestinal tract in man. Neurology 1975; 25:1029–1034.
11. Greenblatt DJ, Shader RI, Harmantz JS, Franke K, Koch-Weser J. Absorption rate, blood concentration, and early response to oral chlordiazepoxide. Am J Psychiatry 1977; 134: 559–562.
12. Greenblatt DJ, Allen MD, McLaughlin DS, MacLaughlin DS, Harmatz JS, Shader RI. Diazepam absorption: effect of antacids and food. Clin Pharmacol Ther 1978; 24:600–609.

13. Fann WE, David JM, Janowsky DS, Sekerke HJ, Schmidt DM. Chlorpromazine: effects of antacids on its gastrointestinal absorption. J Clin Pharmacol 1973; 13:388–390.
14. Forrest FM, Forrest IS, Serva MT. Modification of chlorpromazine metabolism by some other drugs frequently administered to psychiatric patients. Biol Psych 1970; 2:53–58.
15. Abernathy DR, Greenblatt DJ, Shader RI. Benzodiazepine hypnotic metabolism: drug interactions and clinical implications. Acta Psychiatra Scand 1986; 332(suppl):32–38.
16. Watson CD. Adjustment of medications in pulmonary failure. In: Chernow C, eds. The Pharmacologic Approach to the Critcally ill patient. Baltimore: Williams & Wilkins, 1988: 112–130.
17. Hedley-Whyte J, Gurgess GE, Feeley T. Trauma and respiratory failure. In: Applied Physiology of Respiratory Care. Boston: Little, Brown, 1976.
18. Ehrlich BE, Diamond JM. Lithium absorption: implications for sustained-release lithium preparations (letter). Lancet 1983; i:306.
19. Ochs HR, Greenblatt DR, Verburg-Ochs B, Maltis R. Temazepam clearance unaltered in cirrhosis. Am J Gastroenterol 1986; 81:80–84.
20. Juhl RP, Van Thiel DH, Dihert LW, Smith RB. Alprazolam pharmacokinetics in alcoholic liver disease. J Clin Pharmacol 1984; 24:113–119.
21. Benet LZ, Sheiner LB. Pharmacokinetics: the dynamics of drug absorption, distribution and elimination. In: Gillman AG, Goodman LS, eds. The Pharmacological Basis of Therapeutics. New York: Macmillan, 1985:3–34.
22. Levy NB. Psychopharmacology in patients with renal failure. Int J Psychiatry Med 1990; 20:325–334.
23. Ward ME, Musa MN, Bailey L. Clinical pharmacokinetics of lithium. J Clin Pharmacol 1994; 34:280–285.
24. Farrell GC, Cooksley WGE, Powell LW. Drug metabolism in liver disease: activity of hepatic microsomal metabolizing enzymes. Clin Pharmacol Ther 1979; 26:483–492.
25. Schoene B, Fleschmann RA, Remmer H. Determination of drug metabolizing enzymes in needle biopsies of human liver. Eur J Clin Pharmacol 1972; 4:65–73.
26. Grossman SH, Davis DD, Kitchell BB, Shand DG, Routledge PA. Diazepam and lidocaine plasma protein biding in renal disease. Clin Pharmacol Ther 1982; (Mar):350–356.
27. Shoaf SE, Linnoila M. Interaction of ethanol and smoking of the pharmacokinetics and pharmacodynamics of psychotropic medications. Psychopharmacol Bull 1991; 27:577–594.
28. Gouezo F, Ropo PP, Viala A. Influence du sexe et du tabagisme sur les concentrations plasmatiques de la clomipramine, de l'amitriptylines et de leurs metabolites demethles. J Toxicol Clin Exp 1988; 8:39–46.
29. John VA, Luscombe DK, Kemp H. Effects of age, cigarette smoking and the oral contraceptive on the pharmacokinetics of clomipramine and its desmethyl metabolite during chronic dosing. J Int Med Res 1980; 8 (suppl 3):88–95.
30. Perel J, Hurwic M, Kanzler MB. Pharmacodynamics of impramine in depressed patients. Psychopharmacol Bull 1975; 114:16–18.
31. Sutfin TA, Perini GI, Molnar G, Jusko WJ. Multiple-dose pharmacokinetics of imipramine and its major active and conjugated metabolites in depressed patients. J Clin Psychopharmacol 1988; 8:48–53.
32. Shull JH, Wilkinson GR, Johnson R, Schenker S. Normal disposition of oxazapem in acute viral hepatitis and cirrhosis. Ann Intern Med 1976; 84:420–425.
33. Kraus JW, Desmond PV, Marshall JP, Johnson RF, Schenker S, Wilkinson GR. Effects

of aging and liver diseases on disposition of lorazepam. Clin Pharmacol Ther 1978; 24: 411–419.

34. Patwardhan R, Johnson R, Sheehan J, Desmond P, Wilkinson G, Hoyumpa A, Brranch R, Schenker S. Morphine metabolism in cirrhosis. Gastroenterology 1981; 80:1344.

35. Williams RL, Mamelock RD. Hepatic disease and drug pharmacokinetics. Clin Pharmacokinet 1980; 5:528–547.

36. Ishak KG, Irey NS. Hepatic injury associated with the phenothiazines. Arch Pathol 1972; 93:283–304.

37. Fuller CM, Yasinger S, Donlon P, Imperato TJ, Ruebner B. Haloperidol-induced liver disease. West J Med 1977; 127:515–518.

38. Alexander GJ, Machiz S, Alexander RB. Phenothiazine tranquilizers: effect of prolonged intake. Adv Exp Med Biol 1972; 27:151–160.

39. Levinson DF, Simpson GM. Serous nonextrapyramidal adverse effects of neuroleptics: sudden death, agranulocytosis, and hepatotoxicity. In: Meltzer TH, ed. Psychopharmacology: The Third Generation of Progress. New York: Raven Press, 1987:1431–1436.

40. Hyman SE, Arana GW. Handbook of Psychiatric Drug Therapy. Boston: Little, Brown, 1987.

41. Arns PA, Wedlund PJ, Branch RA. Adjustment of medications in liver failure. In: Chernow C, ed. The Pharmacologic Approach to the Critically Ill Patient. Baltimore: Williams & Wilkins, 1988:47–68.

42. Cockroft DW, Gault MH. Prediction of creatinine clearance from serum creatinine. Nephron 1976; 16:31–41.

43. Matzke GR and Millikin SP. Influence of renal function and dialysis of drug disposition. In: Evans WE, Schentag JJ, and Jusko WJ, eds. Applied Pharmacokinetics: Principles of Therapeutic Drug Monitoring. Vancouver: Applied Therapeutics, 1992.

44. Bennett WA, Aronoff GR, Morrison G, Golpher TA, Pulliam J, Wolfson M, Singer I. Drug prescribing in renal failure: dosing guidelines for adults. Am J Kid Dis 1983; 3:155–183.

45. Lydiard RB, Gelenberg AJ. Hazards and adverse effects of lithium. Ann Rev Med 1982; 33:327–344.

46. Port FK, Kroll PD, Rosenzweig J. Lithium therapy during maintenance hemodialysis. Psychosomatics 1977; 20:130–132.

47. Stoudemire A, Morgan MG, Fogel BS. Psychotropic drug use in the medically ill: Part I. Psychosomatatics 1990; 31:377–391.

48. Sramek JJ, Potkin SG, Hahn R. Neuroleptic plasma concentrations and clinical response: in search of a therapeutic window. DICP 1988; 22:373–380.

49. Bergstrom RF, Beasley CM, and Levey NB. Fluoxetine pharmacokinetics after daily doses of 20mg fluoxetine in patients with severly impaired renal function. Pharm Res 1991; 8(suppl 10):294.

50. Aronoff FR, Bergstrom RF, Pottraz ST. Fluoxetine kinetics and protein binding in normal and impaired renal function. Clin Pharmacol Ther 1984; 36:138–144.

51. Ellingrod VL and Perry PJ. Venlafaxine: a heterocyclic antidepressant. Am J Hosp Pharm 1994; 51:3033–3046.

52. Ellingrod VL, Perry PJ. Nefazodone: a new antidepressant. Am J Health-Syst Pharm 1995; 52:2799–2812.

53. Doyle CD, Laher M, Kelly JG. The pharmacokinetics of paroxetine in renal impairment. Acta Psychiatr Scand 1988; 80 (suppl 350):39–90.

54. Perry PJ, Alexander B, Liskow BI. PDH: Psychotropic Drug Handbook. 6th ed. Cincinnati: Harvey Whitney, 1991.
55. Shopsin B, Johnson G, Gershon S. Neurotoxicity with lithium: differential drug responsiveness. Int Pharmacopsychiatry 1970; 5:170–182.
56. Tucker GJ, Detre T, Harrow M et al. Behavior and symptoms of psychiatric patients and the EEG. Arch Gen Psychiatry 1965; 12:278–286.
57. Shader RI, Greenblatt DJ. Beladonna alkaloids and synethetic anticholinergics; uses and toxicity. In: Shader RI, ed. Psychiatric Complications of Medical Drugs. New York: Raven Press, 1972:102–147.
58. Agnoli A, Martucci N, Manna V, et al. Effect of cholinergic and anticholinergic drugs on short-term memory in Alzheimer's dementia: a neuropsychological and computerized electroencephalographic study. Clin Neuropharmacol 1983; 6:311–323.
59. Tollefson GD, Montague-Clouse J, Lancaster SP. The relationship of serum anticholinergic activity to menal status performance in an enderly nursing home population. J Neuropsychiatry Clin Neurosci 1991; 3:314–319.
60. Drug Facts and Comparisons. St. Louis: J. B. Lippincott Co., 1990.
61. Drugdex Information System. Vol. 91. Denver: Micromedex, 1985–1998.
62. Lacy C, Armstrom LL, Lipsy RJ, Lance LL. American Pharmaceutical Association, Drug Information Handbook. Hudson: Lexi-Comp, 1993.

23

Serum Level–Monitoring Strategies for Antipsychotics, Antidepressants, and Antimanic Agents

Paul J. Perry
University of Iowa College of Medicine and
University of Iowa College of Pharmacy

Kristine A. Bever
University of Iowa College of Pharmacy
Iowa City, Iowa

Bruce Alexander
Department of Veterans Affairs Medical Center
Iowa City, Iowa

Therapeutic drug monitoring of psychotropic drugs has clinical utility for several reasons. Interindividual pharmacokinetic variation usually makes it unrealistic to dose patients on the basis of body weight. Excessively high drug levels may be associated with clinical deterioration of the patient because of drug toxicity. Additionally, plasma level monitoring may help assure compliance and may reduce medication defaulting because of adverse effects.

There is support for the use of blood levels to monitor the antipsychotics haloperidol, clozapine, and olanzapine. Although the utility of using tricyclic antidepressant (TCA) blood levels is well documented, the value of monitoring selective serotonin-reuptake inhibitors (SSRIs) is doubtful. Among the antimanic agents it is clear that lithium must be closely monitored from an efficacy and adverse effect standpoint, while it is less clear of the significance of blood level measurements for carbamazepine and valproate.

ANTIPSYCHOTICS

Blood Levels and Therapeutic Response

For most clinicians, establishing the effective dose of an antipsychotic is largely dependent on trial and error. However, blood level monitoring in the management of schizophrenia is clinically useful for several antipsychotics. Most antipsychotic blood level versus therapeutic response studies were performed using patients with schizophrenia.

Most laboratories measuring antipsychotic concentrations use gas-liquid chromatography or high-performance liquid chromatography (1,2). Theoretically, the dopamine receptor assay technique detects the parent compound and all metabolites that compete with the dopamine receptor. This technique would separate active from nonactive antipsychotic metabolites. Early research suggested this assay would be a better measure of antipsychotic effect. However, most studies using the receptor assay have failed to demonstrate a relationship between therapeutic response and antipsychotic "concentrations" measured by this technique. The determination of antipsychotic concentrations in red blood cells, cerebrospinal fluid, or free (i.e., unbound) levels are of no clinical benefit (2).

Using receiver operating characteristics (ROCs) curves as an analytic tool for a meta-analysis of the antipsychotic blood level literature, work done in our laboratory concluded that there was compelling evidence to support the use of blood level data recommendations for haloperidol, clozapine, and olanzapine.

For typical antipsychotics, present data allows for a general recommendation for routine blood level monitoring and subsequent dosage adjustment only for haloperidol (3–5). A meta-analysis of seven haloperidol studies concluded that the therapeutic range was 5–18 ng/ml (6). Patients who fail a 6-week trial of haloperidol within this therapeutic range should be considered for an alternative agent.

Patients that fail a trial with a typical antipsychotic are often considered for treatment with an atypical or novel antipsychotic, such as risperidone, olanzapine, or clozapine. Of these three drugs, therapeutic response to plasma concentration correlation relationships has only been demonstrated for clozapine and olanzapine.

An early recommended therapeutic plasma concentration for clozapine was ≥350 ng/ml (7). This recommendation was based on the Brief Psychiatric Rating Scale (BPRS), which is a nonspecific rating scale for schizophrenia. Subsequently, the data were reanalyzed using the Scale for the Assessment of Positive Symptoms (SAPS) and Scale for the Assessment of Negative Symptoms (SANS). These two validated scales were designed to specifically assess the positive and negative symptoms of schizophrenia (8,9). The recommendation of ≥504 ng/ml is based on the SAPS/SANS, whereas the BPRS suggested a lower limit of 397 ng/ml for a therapeutic response to clozapine (10). The SAPS/SANS recommendation produced somewhat better sensitivity than the BPRS. The clozapine serum level recommendation has been replicated by three other studies (11–13).

Olanzapine was used in 79 inpatients with schizophrenia treated with fixed doses of 1 mg/day or 10 mg/day for up to 6 weeks (14). ROC curve analyses of the Brief

Psychiatric Rating Scale (BPRS) and the Positive and Negative Syndrome Scale (PANSS) data suggested a therapeutic threshold concentration of 9 ng/ml. According to the BPRS scores, 45% of the patients with olanzapine plasma concentrations of ≥9.3 responded, while only 13% of the patients with concentrations outside this range responded.

The clinical interpretation of the above blood level data suggests a three-step treatment algorithm for the treatment of the acutely ill schizophrenic patient:

1. Haloperidol for 6–12 weeks at a dose that achieves a blood level of 5–18 ng/ml

If the patient is haloperidol refractory or cannot tolerate the extrapyramidal adverse effects of haloperidol, then

2. Olanzapine for 6–12 weeks at a dose that achieves a blood level of >9 ng/ml

If the patient is olanzapine nonresponsive, then

3. Clozapine for 16 weeks at a dose that achieves a blood level of ≥504 ng/ml

The recommended sampling time for patients receiving oral antipsychotics should be 12–24 hours after the last dose. Subsequent blood levels should be obtained at the same sampling time. The patient's dose should be fixed for at least one week prior to sampling (for decanoate 3 months) (4). This recommendation will aid in the interpretation of subsequent antipsychotic levels. At steady state, increases or decreases in the dose will result in similar proportional changes in blood level. Importantly, relevant blood level information cannot be elicited if the patient is receiving more than one antipsychotic concurrently.

Maintenance Therapy

A review of five studies that lasted more than 9 months reported noncompliance with oral antipsychotics to average 33% (15,16). Since constant drug intake is important in preventing relapse of symptoms and rehospitalization, long-acting parenteral antipsychotics or depot antipsychotics have been recommended for patients who are repeatedly noncompliant with oral medication. Six studies have reported that depot antipsychotics significantly reduced the relapse rate compared to oral antipsychotics by an average of 16% (17). It is probable that the positive effect of depot antipsychotics compared to oral dosage forms is greater; however, many eligible patients that would benefit from a constant intake of medication do not consent to be studied because their compliance would be monitored. Additionally, significant numbers of patients default on their antipsychotic medication because of experiencing extrapyramidal side effects (e.g., akathisia, parkinsonism). However, these problems might be minimized by judicious blood level monitoring of the depot antipsychotic haloperidol.

A review of six studies indicated that the haloperidol decanoate maintenance dose ranged from 50 to 150 mg every month (18). One study reported average doses of 225 mg monthly (19). However, haloperidol decanoate monthly maintenance doses of 200, 100, 50, and 25 mg were reported to have relapse rates of 15, 23, 25, and 60%, respectively (17). Although a 200-mg monthly dose was associated with the lowest relapse rate, almost 75% of patients treated with 50 and 100 mg per month did not relapse. The important point is that 50–100 mg/month doses of haloperidol are predicted to produce steady-state levels in the range of 1.8–3.6 ng/ml. Obviously, these levels are well below the recommended therapeutic range of 5–18 ng/ml recommended in acutely ill patients with schizophrenia. Additionally, these concentrations are below the average haloperidol level associated with the development of slight hypokinesia-rigidity of 4.2 ± 2.4 mg/day (20). Thus, it can be argued that many patients with schizophrenia treated long term can be successfully maintained on the haloperidol doses that produce blood levels not associated with extrapyramidal side effects.

It has been recommended that after 6 months in the community approximately half of schizophrenic patients can have their maintenance dose reduced significantly. Twelve months after hospital discharge it was estimated that two thirds of the patients who had survived free of relapse required no more than half their dose at the time of discharge (21). This finding has been replicated in 51 stable schizophrenic outpatients. Fifty-three percent had levels at or below 5 ng/ml, whereas only 16% had levels greater than 17 ng/ml, the putative upper limit for acute treatment (22). Thus, continuous tapering of the depot neuroleptics is possible for many chronic schizophrenic patients

Table 1   Projected Plasma Steady-State Haloperidol Plasma
Concentrations Expected from Haloperidol Decanoate

Haloperidol decanoate (mg/4 weeks)	Haloperidol concentration, month 1 (ng/ml)	Haloperidol concentration, month 3 (ng/ml)
50	1.1	1.8
100	2.2	3.6
150	3.3	5.5
200	4.5	7.5
250	5.7	9.4
300	6.9	11.4
350	8.1	13.4
400	9.3	15.4

A patient's steady-state haloperidol serum level would be determined on oral drug. Using Table 1, a loading dose of haloperidol decanoate could be chosen based on the month 3 serum level. The corresponding maintenance dose could be determined by finding the matching haloperidol serum level in the month 1 column.

with the two distinct advantages of increased compliance being coupled with decreased extrapyramidal side effects.

The conversion of patients from oral haloperidol to the depot form may lead to problems if the differences in half-life of the two formulations are not considered. Steady-state serum concentrations of the oral and depot forms will be achieved after approximately 5 days and 3 months of continuous dosing, respectively. Conversely, drug serum concentrations will be close to zero after 5 days and 3 months, respectively. Thus, the patient has a risk of relapsing if he or she is directly switched from an oral to depot haloperidol formulation. This problem can be circumvented by applying the data of Reyntgens et al. (19), who measured plasma haloperidol concentrations in 181 chronic schizophrenic inpatients who received haloperidol decanoate injections every 4 weeks. It was assumed that steady-state levels had been reached after three injections, and concentrations were measured just prior to the next injection, (i.e., day 28). Using this data, Perry and Alexander (23) constructed Table 1, which presents the probable steady-state plasma haloperidol concentrations resulting from differing doses of haloperidol decanoate after the first dose and after three doses given on a 28-day schedule.

Prospective Dosing

Prospective dosing models using a simple nonpharmacokinetic approach have been developed for haloperidol, olanzapine, and clozapine.

Previous data for haloperidol suggested the possibility that haloperidol daily dosing requirements may be confounded by smoking (24). Multiple linear regression analysis showed a significant interaction between the variables of smoking and dose when the data was curve-fitted as a log-log function (24). The haloperidol plasma concentration to dose relationship was best described by the following equations for nonsmokers [Eq. (1)] and for smokers [Eq. (2)]:

$$\text{Haloperidol (ng/ml)} = e^{[0.467 \, * \, \ln(\text{dose}) + 3.397]} \tag{1}$$

$$\text{Haloperidol (ng/ml)} = e^{[1.088 \, * \, \ln(\text{dose}) + 3.716]} \tag{2}$$

The two equations explained 59% of the variance between haloperidol steady-state concentrations and the dose of haloperidol. The two dosing functions are presented in Figure 1. For example, to achieve a steady-state blood level of 10 ng/ml, a smoking patient would require a dose of approximately 0.28 mg/kg/day, whereas a nonsmoking patient would require a dose of only 0.1 mg/kg/day.

The clearance of olanzapine is approximately 30% higher in men than in women, 40% higher in those who smoke than in those who do not smoke, and 30% higher in the young than in the elderly. Dosing adjustments based on gender and smoking status should not be needed (25). However, patients who are debilitated, have a predisposition to hypotensive reactions, or exhibit factors that may result in slower metabolism (e.g., nonsmoking females ≥65 years of age) should be started on 5 mg/day and dose escalation should be done with caution (25). Based on clearance differences in

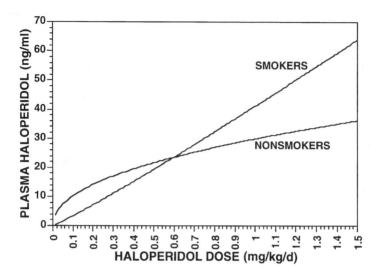

Figure 1 Haloperidol plasma concentration-to-dose relationship using linear scaling, where for nonsmokers [HLP] (ng/ml) = $e^{[0.467 \, * \, \ln(dose) \, + \, 3.397]}$ and for smokers [HLP](ng/ml) = $e^{[1.088 \, * \, \ln(dose) \, + \, 3.716]}$.

the olanzapine versus placebo and haloperidol study (HGAD study), which involved schizophrenic patients 18–65 years of age, there was a 37% increase in clearance in male smokers compared to male nonsmokers versus a 48% increase in the clearance of women smokers versus nonsmokers. If one compares changes in doses reflecting this increase in clearance, then the difference between male smokers and nonsmokers would be an increase of 6 mg/day or 16 mg/day (10 mg/day being the average daily dose), whereas the difference between females would be an increase of 9 mg/day or 19 mg/day (10 mg/day being the average daily dose).

Haring et al. (26), analyzing data from 148 patients receiving daily clozapine doses between 12.5 and 700 mg, found that the independent variables of weight, age, smoking, dose, and sex explained approximately 58% of the variance of clozapine plasma levels. Unfortunately, they did not supply the multiple-regression coefficients for these variables to describe this association. We attempted to replicate their observations in a series of 71 clozapine patients in order to generate a clozapine dosing nomogram to predict steady-state plasma clozapine concentrations (27). Stepwise multiple linear regression analysis was used to examine the relationship between the plasma clozapine concentration and the independent variables of gender, smoking status, age, and dose. The dosing model that optimally predicted steady-state clozapine plasma concentrations included the following variables: dose (mg/day), smoking (yes = 0; no = 1), gender, and dose-gender interaction. The model explained 47% of the variance

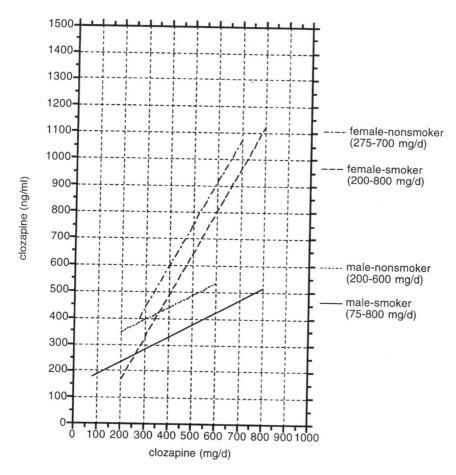

Figure 2 Clozapine dosing nomogram.

in the clozapine concentrations. The following equations describe the clozapine plasma concentration to dose relationship for males [Eq. (3)] and females [Eq. (4)]:

$$\text{Clozapine (ng/ml)} = 111 \text{ (smoke)} + 0.464 \text{ (dose)} + 145 \qquad (3)$$

$$\text{Clozapine (ng/ml)} = 111 \text{ (smoke)} + 1.590 \text{ (dose)} - 149 \qquad (4)$$

Thus, for a 500 mg/day dose a smoking male patient is predicted to have a steady-state clozapine plasma concentration of 377 ng/ml, whereas a smoking female patient would have a concentration of 646 ng/ml. For nonsmoking patients, a 500 mg/day dose in a male patient is predicted to have a steady-state clozapine plasma concentration of 488 ng/ml, whereas a female patient is predicted to have a concentration of approximately 757 ng/ml. Figure 2 illustrates the predicted clozapine plasma concentrations for the clozapine dose ranges surveyed by the data for each group.

ANTIDEPRESSANTS

Tricyclic Antidepressants

Perry et al. (28) performed a meta-analysis of the TCA blood level literature using ROC curves as the primary statistical tool. Sufficient data was available from multiple studies to examine the relationship between therapeutic response and blood levels for nortriptyline, desipramine, amitriptyline, and imipramine. For nortriptyline, a significant curvilinear relationship between therapeutic response and nortriptyline was observed in the range of 53–148 ng/ml. The sensitivity and specificity for the nortriptyline therapeutic window were 78% and 61%, respectively. The response rate within the therapeutic range was 66% versus 26% outside the therapeutic range. For desipramine, a significant linear relationship between therapeutic response and desipramine plasma concentration was observed. The threshold plasma concentration for therapeutic response was 116 ng/ml. The sensitivity and specificity for the desipramine threshold blood level were 81% and 59%, respectively. The response rate above the threshold level was 51% versus 15% below the therapeutic threshold concentration. For imipramine, a significant curvilinear relationship between therapeutic response and total imipramine (imipramine + desipramine) plasma concentration was observed between 175 and 350 ng/ml. The sensitivity and specificity for the total imipramine plasma concentrations were 52% and 74%, respectively. The response rate within the therapeutic range was 67% versus 39% outside the therapeutic range. For amitriptyline, a significant curvilinear relationship between therapeutic response and total amitriptyline (amitriptyline + nortriptyline) plasma concentration was observed between 93 and 140 ng/ml. The sensitivity and specificity for the total amitriptyline plasma concentrations were 37% and 80%, respectively. The response rate within the therapeutic range was 50% versus 30% outside the therapeutic range. A summary of these data are presented in Table 2.

Table 2 TCA Response Rates in and out of the Suggested Therapeutic Concentrations

Drug	Therapeutic range (ng/ml)	Response rate (in vs. out)
Nortriptyline	58–148	66% vs. 26%
Desipramine	>116	51% vs. 15%
Imipramine	175–350	67% vs. 39%
Amitriptyline	93–140	50% vs. 30%

Prospective Dosing

There is a linear relationship between a test dose plasma concentration and steady-state concentration for the TCA nortriptyline (29). The nortriptyline dosing nomogram in Figure 3 can be utilized to dose patients. The only information required to predict steady-state doses for maintenance doses of 50–150 mg/day using the nomogram is a plasma nortriptyline concentration measured 24 hours following the administration of

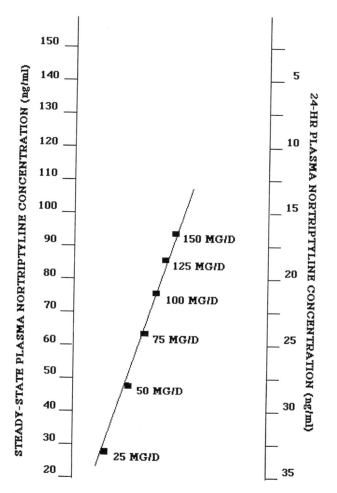

Figure 3   Nortriptyline dosing nomogram for predicting steady-state plasma concentrations for 25–150 mg/d maintenance doses following a 100-mg nortriptyline test dose and subsequent measurement of the 24-hour plasma nortriptyline concentration. The 150 mg/d dose should not be exceeded, because the relationship between nortriptyline plasma concentrations and maintenance doses may not be linear at higher doses.

a 100-mg test dose. The only caveat regarding the use of the nomogram is that a dose of 150 mg/day should not be exceeded because the relationship of nortriptyline plasma concentrations and maintenance doses may not be linear at higher doses.

Selective Serotonin-Reuptake Inhibitors

Fluoxetine, fluvoxamine, and paroxetine exhibit nonlinear pharmacokinetics, i.e., doubling the dose may triple or quadruple the plasma concentration. Unlike the other three SSRIs, sertraline exhibits linear pharmacokinetics, i.e., doubling the dose doubles the plasma concentration.

The elimination half-life of fluoxetine ranges from 26 to 220 hours with a mean of 84 hours, while the half-life of its active metabolite norfluoxetine ranges from 77 to 235 hours with a mean of 146 hours (30). Therefore, 6–7 weeks may be required before steady-state serum concentrations are reached. Likewise the same period of time is required to wash out the drug in nonresponding patients. Four fluoxetine studies have investigated the relationship between blood levels and therapeutic response (31–34). Two of the studies were unable to find any relationship (31,32). However, one observed a negative correlation between norfluoxetine concentrations and therapeutic response (33), while another noted that patients with high ratios of fluoxetine to norfluoxetine were more likely to respond than patients with low ratios (34).

The elimination half-life of paroxetine ranges between 7 and 37 hours (30). Plasma paroxetine concentrations were measured in 94 depressed patients. Steady-state concentrations ranged from 1 to 190 ng/ml, with 90% of the responders and nonresponders having plasma concentrations of <110 ng/ml. No correlation was found between clinical response or adverse effects and the drug concentrations in the plasma (35).

The mean elimination half-life of sertraline is 26 hours, while its less active (5–10 times) demethylated metabolite's mean half-life is 66 hours (30). No studies are currently available examining the relationship of sertraline blood levels to therapeutic response.

The mean elimination half-life of fluvoxamine in depressed patients is 23 hours (30). There is one unreplicated study that found that steady state fluvoxamine plasma concentrations between 160-200 ng/ml were more likely to be associated with a beneficial clinical response (36).

Monoamine Oxidase Inhibitors

Dosing of monoamine oxidase–inhibiting antidepressants has been therapeutically monitored by estimating the degree of monoamine oxidase (MAO) enzyme inhibition. Two studies support the validity of this practice. Ravaris et al. (37) found that the antidepressant phenelzine was more effective at 60 mg/day than either 30 mg/day or placebo according to the Hamilton Rating Scale for Depression (HRSD). The median MAO activity decrease in the phenelzine 60 mg/day group was 87% (45–98%) versus 61% (31–91%) in the phenelzine 30 mg/day group. The authors concluded that to achieve an antidepressant response with phenelzine of >80% inhibition of platelet MAO is required. To achieve this they recommend a phenelzine dose of 1 mg/kg/day. By measuring platelet MAO activity, Grasso et al. (38) concluded that 80% MAO inhibition can be achieved with a tranylcypromine dose of 0.7 mg/kg/day. An adequate therapeutic trial of a monoamine oxidase inhibitor (MAOI) lasts 6 weeks. Two weeks of therapy are required before the maximum MAO inhibitory effect of phenelzine 30 mg/day is reached, and 4 weeks are required for a dose of 60 mg/day (39).

ANTIMANICS

Lithium

Acute Mania

Prien et al. (40) studied the relationship between serum lithium concentrations and clinical response in acutely manic patients treated with lithium for 3 weeks. Patients with concentrations exceeding 1.4 mEq/liter experienced no greater improvement in their manic symptoms than patients with lower serum lithium concentrations. Although a few of the most ill patients showed either improvement or complete remission with serum concentrations above 1.4 mEq/liter, a similar proportion of very ill patients responded to serum concentrations below 1.4 mEq/liter while experiencing considerably fewer adverse drug reactions (ADRs). None of the patients with serum lithium concentrations below 0.9 mEq/liter experienced a complete remission. Of the mildly active patients with concentrations above 0.9 mEq/liter the failure and remission rates were 15% and 40%, respectively, while for patients with concentrations below 0.9 mEq/liter the respective failure and remission rates were 33% and 0%. Thus, it was concluded that a serum concentration 0.9–1.4 mEq/liter is required for treating acute mania. To achieve this therapeutic range, interindividual variability is quite large such that patients cannot be prospectively dosed simply on a mg/kg/day basis to achieve this therapeutic range.

Manic patients in the midst of an acute episode require and tolerate higher lithium doses due to an increased lithium clearance (41). These levels may not be tolerated once the manic episode begins to abate. Therefore, frequent lithium levels, normally drawn twice weekly, are required in the treatment of an acute manic episode because of the possibility of a rapid rise in lithium levels as the episode begins to resolve.

Prophylaxis

The ideal prophylactic serum lithium concentration is a question of considerable debate. Originally, most clinicians recommended a concentration range of 0.8–1.2 mEq/liter. However, data from both Hullin (42) and Coppen et al. (43) suggested that lower serum lithium concentrations were as effective. Utilizing a divided daily dosing schedule, Hullin (42) found that affective illness relapse rates were the same for patients with lithium doses producing lithium concentrations above 0.6 mEq/liter, as were the relapse rates of patients with concentrations between 0.4 to 0.6 mEq/liter. However, concentrations below 0.4 mEq/liter were associated with increased relapse rates. Coppen et al. (43) studied the effect of lowering the serum lithium concentration in 72 patients with recurrent affective illness. The patients were randomly allocated to one of three lithium concentration groups: 0.8–1.2, 0.6–0.79, or 0.45–0.59 mEq/liter. Patients were followed for at least one year. Interestingly, the patients who experienced the greatest decrease in affective illness morbidity were the patients with the lowest serum lithium concentration. No change in affective illness morbidity was observed in the group where the lithium dose was not altered. Abou-Saleh and Coppen (44) randomly allocated 90 bipolar and unipolar patients with recurrent affective illness to one of three lithium concentration groups: >0.79, 0.6–0.79, or 0.45–0.59 mEq/liter. Patients were followed for one year. There were no differences among the three groups with respect to dose and affective morbidity. Older patients (>59 years) experienced a worse outcome following dosage reduction. The low-level group had significantly less tremor, a decrease rather than an increase in weight, reduced polyuria (i.e., output), and lower TSH levels. Gelenberg et al. (45) followed 94 bipolar patients whose lithium concentrations were adjusted to a range of 0.8–1.0 or 0.4–0.6 mEq/liter. The relapse rate in the high-level group was only 13%, whereas the rate was 2.6 times higher (38%) in the low-dose group. Unlike the Abou-Saleh study, the authors did not take into account the effect age in an attempt to explain the discrepancy. Although controlled for, the authors also found that a greater number of prior episodes, a prior manic episode, and a shorter length of remission before intake contributed to a two- to threefold increase in risk of relapse. However, he did not control for polarity of the index episode. Maj (46) demonstrated that patients with an index episode of depression do worse on lithium prophylaxis than patients whose index episode is mania. Additionally, our own intent-to-treat analysis showed a 53% relapse rate in the low-dose group and a 32% relapse rate in the standard-dose group. This finding was not significant (Fisher's exact test, $p = 0.06$). Overall, these data suggest that serum lithium concentrations of 0.4–0.6 mEq/liter on a divided daily dose schedule or 0.45–0.59 mEq/liter on a single daily dose schedule are appropriate in the prophylactic treatment of affectively ill patients, although higher concentrations are required in the elderly. A reasonable clinical strategy would be to instruct patients that because they may be at higher risk of relapse at lower concentrations, they should increase their dose by 1.5 times at the first signs of any manic or depressive symptoms and then slowly taper downward to the lower concentration several months after the symptoms resolve. This is an important part of patient education as the Gelenberg data were later reanalyzed and it was found that the occurrence of subsyndromal symptoms of affective illness increased the risk of relapse fourfold regardless of the lithium level (47).

Lithium Prospective Dosing—Pharmacokinetic Method

Like nortriptyline, a linear relationship exists between lithium concentration in serum or plasma at steady state and a single lithium concentration at some time after a dose of lithium carbonate. Perry et al. (48) found that when the steady-state lithium serum concentrations observed at 12 hours postdose were retrospectively adjusted to an 1800 mg/day lithium maintenance dose, the following straight-line equation was derived

$$Css_{12h} = 0.13 + 3.3 \ (C^*24) \tag{5}$$

where C is the steady-state lithium concentration at 12 hours postdose for an 1800 mg/day dose and C_{24h} is the 24-hour serum lithium concentration following an initial 1200-mg dose. The dosing nomogram in Figure 4 can be utilized in place of the equation.

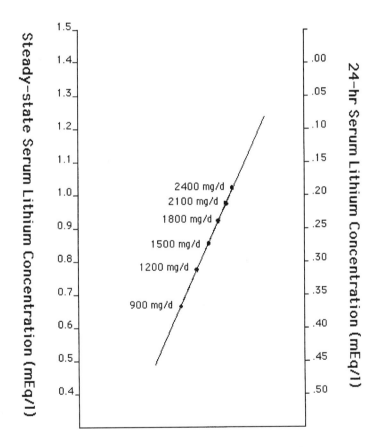

Figure 4 Lithium dosing nomogram for predicting steady-state serum concentrations for 900–2400 mg/d maintenance doses following a 1200-mg lithium carbonate test dose and subsequent measurement of the 24-hour serum lithium concentration.

Lithium Prospective Dosing—Nonpharmacokinetic Method

Zetin et al. (49), utilizing stepwise multiple linear regression analysis, derived a mathematical formula for determining a lithium dose based on a number of dependent variables. The regression model is presented in the following equation:

$$\text{Dose} = 746.83 \text{ (level)} + 92.01 \text{ (status)} - 74.73 \text{ (TCA)}$$
$$- 10.08 \text{ (age)} + 147.8 \text{ (sex)} + 5.95 \text{ (weight)} + 486.8 \tag{6}$$

where dose is expressed in milligrams per day, level is the desired lithium concentration in mEq/liter, status is zero if an outpatient and one if an inpatient, TCA is one for concomitant antidepressant use or zero for no antidepressant use, age is in years, sex is zero for females and one for males, and weight is in kg. The coefficient of variation (r^2) for the equation was 0.45. Unfortunately, the model was constructed incorrectly in that the true dependent variable, lithium level, was treated as an independent variable while dose should be an independent variable. Eq. (6) indicates that dose is a function of blood level while in reality lithium level is a function of dose. To investigate the effect of improperly assigning variables, we constructed a similar dosing model in bipolar patients using valproate. When valproate serum concentration was an independent variable with smoking and serum albumin concentration, r^2 was 0.43, whereas in the regression analysis when correctly treated as a dependent variable, r^2 was 0.13.

Lesar et al. (50) also utilized multiple linear regression analysis to derive a lithium-dosing equation. Their multiple regression model requiring a laboratory value, i.e., serum creatinine for a creatinine clearance determination, was defined by the following equation:

$$\text{Dose} = 9.56 - 1.19 \text{ (sex)} + 0.064 \text{ (weight, kg)} - 0.021 \text{ (age, years)}$$
$$- 2.73 \text{ (depression)} + 2.26 \text{ (state)} + 0.035(\text{Cl}_{cr}) \tag{7}$$

where the sex is 1 for males and 2 for females, depression is 1 for absence and 2 for presence and/or tricyclic antidepressant use, state is coded 1 for acute and 2 for non-acute symptoms, and Cl_{cr} is the creatinine clearance calculated by the Cockroft-Gault equation (51) presented in the following equation:

$$\text{Cl}_{cr} = \frac{(140 - \text{age})(\text{weight, kg})}{(72)(\text{serum creatinine})} \tag{8}$$

The resulting coefficient of variation (r^2) was 0.45 ($p < 0.05$). As in Eq. (6), the author treated lithium dose as a dependent variable rather than an independent variable. Since both of these nonpharmacokinetic dosing equations—if constructed correctly—predict less than 45% of the variance in the steady-state lithium concentration, their clinical utility is debatable.

Carbamazepine

Acute Treatment—Mania and Depression

A correlation between carbamazepine plasma concentrations and response of affective symptoms has not been demonstrated (52). Although one report found a correlation between the 10,11-epoxide metabolite and improvement in affective symptoms, this has not been replicated (53). The 10,11-epoxide metabolite is not routinely measured by commercial laboratories. It has been recommended that a nonresponding patient's carbamazepine dose be increased until initial adverse effects occur (52). This usually occurs with levels of 10–12 mg/ml.

Maintenance Treatment

There is no accepted therapeutic range for carbamazepine in the maintenance treatment of affective disorders (52). One maintenance study in bipolar patients reported that a carbamazepine plasma concentration of 4–7 mg/ml (mean 5.7) was effective in the majority of patients (54). A more recent 2-year open study reported no difference in prophylactic efficacy between carbamazepine 3.5–5.9 µg/ml versus 6.6–9.4 µg/ml and lithium 0.6–0.8 mEq/liter in patients with bipolar illness (55). However, in unipolar patients carbamazepine 3.5–5.9 µg/ml was ineffective in reducing the number of depressive episodes. More therapeutic response studies need to be performed with carbamazapine and its metabolite.

Valproic Acid

A therapeutic range for valproate in the acute or maintenance treatment of affective disorders has not been established (56–58). Many uncontrolled reports recommend levels between 50 and 150 µg/ml. A recent open trial reported that valproate levels in the range of 76–125 µg/ml (i.e., high-level group) were more effective in reducing manic symptoms in bipolar patients than levels of 25–75 µg/ml (low-level group) (59). However, in patients with schizophrenia positive symptom scores improved in both the low- and high-level groups, while overall BPRS scores improved with lower serum levels. In a blinded, controlled trial serum valproate levels >45 µg/ml were reported to reduce manic symptoms more than levels ≤ 44 µg/ml at a 5-day rating period (60). Unfortunately, valproate doses were only fixed for the first 5 days of the study; thereafter doses were adjusted "as clinically indicated." More fixed-dose studies need to be performed to determine a therapeutic range, if any, for valproate in affective and psychotic disorders.

SUMMARY

Therapeutic drug monitoring of psychotropic drugs using blood level data benefits patients in three ways. It facilitates dosing such that patients are receiving doses that have the greatest likelihood of producing a therapeutic effect. It avoids excessively high drug concentrations that are associated with patients experiencing more adverse effects, toxicity, and clinical deterioration. Finally, plasma level monitoring assures compliance and reduces medication defaulting because of unacceptable or intolerable adverse effects.

Significant correlation between therapeutic response and plasma concentration is the exception rather than the rule among psychotropic drugs. Among the typical antipsychotics, only haloperidol has demonstrated a reproducible correlation between clinical response and drug plasma concentration, while among the atypical antipsychotics this observation is only true of clozapine. Initial data suggest that olanzapine holds promise as an additional atypical antipsychotic for which therapeutic drug monitoring will be feasible. Although the utility of TCA plasma concentrations is well established, the value of monitoring SSRIs is equivocal. The more complicated dose-dependent pharmacokinetics of all of the SSRIs except sertraline quite likely contribute to this problem. Of the mood stabilizers, it is obvious that lithium must be closely monitored from an efficacy and toxicity standpoint. However, the value of measuring carbamazepine and valproate plasma concentrations is far less apparent.

REFERENCES

1. Jolly AG, Hirsch SR, McRink A, Manchanda R. Trial of brief intermittent neuroleptic prophylaxis for selected schizophrenic outpatients: clinical outcome at one year. Br Med J 1989; 298:985–991.
2. Garver DL. Neuroleptic drug levels and antipsychotic effects: a difficult correlation; potential advantage of free (or derivative) versus total plasma levels. J Clin Psychopharmacol 1989; 9:277–281.
3. Carpenter WT, Heinrichs DW, Hanlan TE. A comparative trial of pharmacologic strategies in schizophrenia. Am J Psychiatry 1987; 144:1466–1470.
4. Preskorn SH, Burke MJ, Fast GA. Therapeutic drug monitoring. Psychiatr Clin North Am 1993; 16:611–645.
5. Palao DJ, Arauxo A, Brunet M, Bernardo M, Haro JM, Ferrer J, Gonzalez-Monclus E. Haloperidol: therapeutic window in schizophrenia. J Clin Psychopharmacol 1994; 14:303–310.
6. Perry PJ, Smith DA. Neuroleptic plasma concentrations: an estimate of their sensitivity and specificity as predictors of response. In: Marder S, Davis J, eds. The Clinical Use of Neuroleptic Plasma Levels. Washington, DC: American Psychiatric Press, 1992:113–136.
7. Perry PJ, Miller DD, Arndt SV, Cadoret RJ. Clozapine and norclozapine plasma concentrations and clinical response in treatment-refractory schizophrenics. Am J Psychiatry 1991; 148:231–235.
8. Andreasen NC. The Scale for the Assessment of Negative Symptoms (SANS). Iowa City: University of Iowa, 1983.
9. Andreasen NC. The Scale for the Assessment of Positive Symptoms (SAPS). Iowa City: University of Iowa, 1984.
10. Perry PJ, Miller DD. Clinical use of clozapine plasma concentrations. In: Marder S, Davis J, eds. The Clinical Use of Neuroleptic Plasma Levels. Washington, DC: American Psychiatric Press, 1992:85–100.
11. Hasegawa M, Gutierrez-Esteinou R, Way L, Meltzer HY. Relationship between clinical efficacy and clozapine concentrations in plasma in schizophrenia: effect of smoking. J Clin Psychopharmacol 1993; 13:383–390.
12. Potkin SG, Bera R, Gulasekaram B, Costa J, Hayes S, Jin Y, Richmond G, Carreon D,

Sitanggan K, Gerber B, Telford J, Plon L, Plon H, Park L, Chang YJ, Oldroyd J, Cooper TB. Plasma clozapine concentrations predict clinical response in treatment-resistant schizophrenia. J Clin Psychiatry 1994; 55(suppl B):133–136.

13. Kronig MH, Munne RA, Szymanski S, Safferman AZ, Pollack S, Cooper T, Kane JM, Lieberman JA. Plasma clozapine levels and clinical response for treatment-refractory schizophrenic patients. Am J Psychiatry 1995; 152:179–182.

14. Perry PJ, Sanger T, Beasley C. Olanzapine plasma concentrations and clinical response in acutely ill schizophrenics. J Clin Psychopharmacol 1997; 17:472–477.

15. Groves JE, Mandel MR. The long-acting phenothiazines. Arch Gen Psychiatry 1975; 32: 893–900.

16. Kane JM. Depot neuroleptic therapy. Today's Ther Trends 1993; 11:93–102.

17. Davis JM, Kane JM, Marder SR, Brauzer B, Gierl B, Schooler N, Casey DE, Hassan M. Dose response of prophylactic antipsychotics. J Clin Psychiatry 1993; 54(suppl):24–30.

18. Beresford R, Ward A. Haloperidol decanoate: a preliminary review of its pharmacodynamic and pharmacokinetic properties and therapeutic use in psychosis. Drugs 1987; 33:31–49.

19. Reyntgens AJM, Heykants JJP, Woestenborghs RJH, Gelders YG, Aerts TJL. Pharmacokinetics of haloperidol decanoate. Int Pharmacopsychiatr 1982; 17:238–246.

20. McEvoy JP, Stiller RL, Farr R. Plasma haloperidol levels drawn at neuroleptic threshold doses: a pilot study. J Clin Psychopharmacol 1986; 6:133–138.

21. Johnson DAW. Observations on the dose regimen of fluphenazine decanoate in maintenance therapy of schizophrenia. Br J Psychiatry 1975; 126:457–461.

22. Garvey M, Wakefield DS, Perry P, Dysken M, Mcgraw R, Laughlin P, Jordan W. Assessment of prophylactic haloperidol plasma levels in stable outpatient schizophrenics. Ann Clin Psychiatry 1992; 4:121–126.

23. Perry PJ, Alexander B. Switching haloperidol from oral to im depot formulation (letter). DICP Ann Pharmacother 1991; 25:1270–1271.

24. Perry PJ, Miller DD, Arndt SV, Holman TL. Haloperidol dosing requirements: the contribution of smoking and non-linear pharmacokinetics. J Clin Psychopharmacol 1993; 13: 46–51.

25. Eli Lilly Company. Zyprexa package insert. Indianapolis, IN, September 1996.

26. Haring C, Meise U, Humpel C, Saria A, Fleischhacker WW, Hinterhuber H. Dose-related plasma levels of clozapine: influence of smoking behavior, sex and age. Psychopharmacology 1989; 99:S38–40.

27. Perry PJ, Bever KB, Arndt S, Combs M. Relationship between patient variables and plasma clozapine concentrations: a dosing nomogram. Biol Psychiatry. In press.

28. Perry PJ, Zeilmann C, Arndt S. Tricyclic antidepressant concentrations in plasma: an estimate of their sensitivity and specificity as a predictor of response. J Clin Psychopharmacol 1994; 14:230–240.

29. Perry PJ, Browne JL, Alexander B, Tsuang MT, Sherman AD, Dunner FJ. Two prospective dosing methods for nortriptyline. Clin Pharmacokinet 1984; 9:555–563.

30. DeVane CL, Jarecke CR. Cyclic antidepressants. In: Evans WE, Schoentag JJ, Jusko WJ, eds. Applied Pharmacokinetics. Principles of Therapeutic Drug Monitoring. San Francisco: Applied Therapeutics, 1992:1–34.

31. Kelly MW, Perry PJ, Holstad SG, Garver MJ. Serum fluoxetine and norfluoxetine concentrations and antidepressant response. Ther Drug Monit 1989; 11:165–170.

32. Beasley CM Jr, Bosomworth JC, Wernicke JF. Fluoxetine: relationships among dose, re-

sponse, adverse events, and plasma concentrations in the treatment of depression. Psychopharmacol Bull 1990; 26:18–24.

33. Montgomery SA, Baldwin D, Shah A, Green M, Fineberg N, Montgomery D. Plasma-level response relationships with fluoxetine and zimelidine. Clin Neuropharmacol 1990; 13(1, suppl):S71–75.

34. Tyrer SP, Marshall EP, Griffiths, HW. The relationship between response to fluoxetine, plasma drug levels, imipramine binding to platelet membranes and whole-blood 5-HT. Prog Neuropsychopharmacol Biol Psychiatry 1990; 14:797–805.

35. Tasker TCG, Kaye CM, Zussman BD, Link CGG. Paroxetine plasma levels: lack of correlation with efficacy or adverse effects. Acta Psychiatr Scand 1989; 80(suppl 350):152–155.

36. Nathan RS, Perel JM, Pollock BG, Kupfer DJ. The role of neuropharmacologic selectivity in antidepressant action: fluvoxamine versus desipramine. J Clin Psychiatry 1990; 51:367–372.

37. Ravaris CL, Nies A, Robinson DS, Ives JO, Lamborn KR, Korson L. A multiple-dose controlled study of phenelzine in depression-anxiety states. Arch Gen Psychiatry 1976; 33:347–350.

38. Grasso RA, Perry PJ, Sherman AD. Relationship between tranylcypromine dose and MAO inhibition (letter). DICP, Ann Pharmacother 1991; 25:99–100.

39. Robinson DS, Nies A, Ravaris CL, Ives JO, Bartlett D. Clinical pharmacology of phenelzine and amitriptyline. Arch Gen Psychiatry 1978; 35:629–635.

40. Prien RF, Caffey EM, Klett CJ. Relationship between serum lithium level and clinical response in acute mania treated with lithium. Br J Psychiatry 1971; 120:409–414.

41. Smith DF, Shimizu M. Effect of posture on renal lithium clearance. Clin Sci Mol Med 1976; 51:103–105.

42. Hullin RP. Minimum effective plasma lithium levels for long-term preventive treatment of recurrent affective disorders. In: Copper TB, Gershon S, Kline NS, et al., eds. Lithium: Controversies and Unresolved Issues. Amsterdam: Excerpta Medica, 1979:333–334.

43. Coppen A, Abou-Saleh M, Milln P, Wood K. Decreasing lithium dosage reduces morbidity and side effects during prophylaxis. J Affect Disord 1983; 5:353–362.

44. Abou-Saleh MT, Coppen A. The efficacy of low-dose lithium: clinical, psychological, and biological correlates. J Psychiatr Res 1989; 23:157–162.

45. Gelenberg AJ, Kane JM, Keller MB, Lavori P, Rosenbaum JF, Cole K, Lavelle J. Comparison of standard and low serum levels of lithium for maintenance treatment of bipolar disorder. N Engl J Med 1989; 321:1489–1493.

46. Maj M. Clinical prediction of response to lithium prophylaxis in bipolar patients: the importance of the previous pattern of course of the illness. Clinical Neuropharmacol 1990; 13(suppl):66–70.

47. Keller MB, Lavori PW, Kane JM, Gelenberg AJ, Rosenbaum JF, Walzer EA, Baker LA. Subsyndromal symptoms in bipolar disorder: a comparison of standard and low serum levels of lithium. Arch Gen Psychiatry 1992; 49:371–376.

48. Perry PJ, Alexander B, Prince RA, Dunner FJ. A single point dosing protocol for predicting steady state lithium levels. Br J Psychiatry 1986; 148:401–405.

49. Zetin M, Garber D, DeAntonio M, Schlegel A, Feureisen S, Fieve R, Jewett C, Reus V, Huey LY. Prediction of lithium dose: a mathematical alternative to the test dose method. J Clin Psychiatry 1986; 47:175–178.

50. Lesar TS, Tollefson GK, Koch M. Relationship between patient variables and lithium dosage requirements. J Clin Psychiatry 1985; 46:133–136.

51. Cockcroft DW, Gault MH. Prediction of creatinine clearance from serum creatinine. Nephron 1976; 16:31–47.

52. Ballenger JC. The clinical use of carbamazepine in affective disorders. J Clin Psychiatry 1988; 49(suppl 4):13–19.

53. Post RM, Uhde TW, Ballenger JC, Chatterji DC, Greene RF, Bunney WE. Carbamazepine and its 10,11-epoxide metabolite in plasma in CSF: relationship to antidepressant response. Arch Gen Psychiatry 1983; 40:673–676.

54. Stuppaeck C, Barnas C, Miller C, Schwitzer J, Fleischhacker WW. Carbamazepine in the prophylaxis of mood disorders. J Clin Psychopharmacol 1990; 10:39–42.

55. Simhandl C, Denk E, Thau K. The comparative efficacy of carbamazepine low and high serum level and lithium carbonate in the prophylaxis of affective disorders. J Affect Disord 1993; 28:221–231.

56. Janicak PG. The relevance of clinical pharmacokinetics and therapeutic drug monitoring: anticonvulsant mood stabilizers and antipsychotics. J Clin Psychiatry 1993; 54(suppl 9): 35–41.

57. McElroy SL, Keck PE. Treatment guidelines for valproate in bipolar and schizoaffective disorders. Can J Psychiatry 1993; 38(suppl 2):S62–S66.

58. Keck PE, McElroy SL, Tugrul KC, et al. Valproate oral loading in the treatment of acute mania. J Clin Psychiatry 1993; 54:305–308.

59. Ellenor G, Lohr JB, Ito M, Dishman B, Gammariello A. The comparative efficacy of divalproex low and high serum level in bipolar disorder and schizophrenia (abstr). Psychopharmacol Bull 1995; 31:563.

60. Bowden CL, Janicak PG, Orsulak P, Swann AC, Davis JM, Calabrese JR, Goodnick P, Small JG, Rush AJ, Kimmel SE, Risch SC, Morris DD. Relation of serum valproate concentration to response in mania. Am J Psychiatry 1996; 153:765–770.

24

Effects of Aging on Psychotropic Efficacy and Toxicity

Susan K. Schultz and Del D. Miller
University of Iowa College of Medicine
Iowa City, Iowa

PSYCHOTROPIC DRUGS AND THE AGING PROCESS

It is often remarked that the segment of the population over the age of 65 is increasing more rapidly than ever before, with the most dramatic rate of increase occurring in the over 85-year-old group. Additionally, older adults account for the majority of prescription and nonprescription drug use in the United States, a substantial portion of which is utilized for the treatment of various psychiatric disturbances. This highlights the need for clinicians in all disciplines to be aware of the special considerations for psychotropic medication use in the elderly. The impact of "age effects" on psychotropic efficacy and toxicity is a broad topic when one considers the many potential age-related physiological changes and comorbid medical illnesses. Each of these factors may influence distribution, response, and metabolism of psychotropic medications. To further complicate the picture, one must remain cognizant of the tremendous heterogeneity among individuals in aging. The clinician is therefore challenged to avoid complacency or fixed prescribing patterns applied generically to the elderly population.

PHYSIOLOGICAL CHANGES ASSOCIATED WITH NORMAL AGING

A number of physiological factors contribute to the frequent observation that older patients are more sensitive to the effects of psychotropic medications and more vulnerable to toxicity from these drugs. Age-related physiological changes relevant to pharmacological effects occur in nearly all organ systems. These changes include decreased cardiac output, decreased global and cerebral blood flow, as well as decrements in renal function, enzyme activity, and responsiveness of receptors (Table 1). Additionally, factors such as diet, stress, environment, level of physical activity, comorbid illnesses, and tobacco and alcohol abuse may further diminish the likelihood of proper utilization and efficacy of psychotropic agents. This portion of the chapter will review some of the main biological changes associated with normal aging.

Fundamental to the bioavailability of oral medications is the absorptive capability of the upper gastrointestinal system. The ability of the older individual to adequately absorb psychotropic agents has been evaluated in a number of studies. Overall, it has been shown that in terms of gastric emptying and intestinal absorption, only minimal

Table 1 Biological Changes Associated with Normal Aging

Body composition
 Decreased muscle mass
 Increased body fat with redistribution of fat to visceral regions
 Decreased total body water
 Decreased skeletal bone mineralization
Cardiovascular and respiratory system
 Decreased lung capacity likely secondary to fibrosis and environmental factors
 Decreased cardiac output and vascular compliance
 Decreased α_2-adrenergic modulation of adrenergic tone
 Decreased baroreceptor responsiveness
 Increased diastolic and systolic blood pressure
Gastrointestinal system
 Decreased gastric secretions
 Mildly decreased mesenteric and splanchnic blood flow
 Decreased hepatic blood flow with decreased liver mass
 Decreased miscrosomal enzyme activity, i.e., decreased biotransformation of substances to a
  water-soluble state for renal excretion
 Increased colonic transit time through large bowel
Renal system
 Decreased blood flow to kidneys
 Reduction in glomerular filtration rate by approximately half
 Increased production of erythropoietin to compensate for decline in production of
  erythroid precursors in bone marrow
 Decreased sodium-regulating capacity
Nervous system
 Decreased choline uptake in the presynaptic nerve terminals for the production of
  acetylcholine
 Decreased binding of acetylcholine to cholinergic receptors
 Decreased dopamine production likely due to decrement in dopa decarboxylase activity
 Decreased noradrenergic receptor activity in central nervous system with increased
  peripheral levels of norepinephrine

and clinically nonsignificant changes occur in the absence of gastrointestinal pathology (1). There is a decrease in gastric acid secretion with age as well as a reduction in gastric emptying rate and gastrointestinal blood flow. However, in general, changes in gastrointestinal absorption with age do not have a clinically significant impact on drug absorption. Decrements in intestinal motility with age primarily involve the large bowel and do not affect drug absorption but may make the older individual more vulnerable to the side effect of constipation.

In terms of overall body composition, normal aging is associated with a gradual increase in the ratio of body fat to lean muscle beginning in middle adulthood. By late life, there is a significant reduction in lean muscle mass, a reduction in total body water, and an increase in body fat (2). This may be clinically relevant to the distribution of lipid-soluble psychotropic agents such as antipsychotic medications. This expanded fat volume contributes to a longer half-life of lipid-soluble agents through greater disposition of drug (3). Further, the wider distribution of drug into peripheral tissues may have the effect of relatively less drug availability in the central nervous system (CNS). Thus, there may be a *decrement* in initial CNS effects of a psychotropic agent. However, the expanded volume of distribution in the face of slow elimination (particularly seen in agents with long half-lives, such as diazepam) may create a cumulative effect of prolonged drug activity. Clinically these physiological changes may result in a longer period of time necessary to achieve a therapeutic effect and also a longer period of time to clear from any toxic effects. Lithium carbonate is one exception to this circumstance due to its water-soluble property.

Lithium is the exception in yet another circumstance affected by aging. Virtually all other psychotropic agents are protein-bound, most notably benzodiazepines and anticonvulsants. The extent of available plasma albumin available for binding is inversely related to the amount of free drug available to exert its pharmacological effect. Due to the decrement in plasma albumin, particularly in late-late life, there may be a significantly greater percentage of available free drug per unit dose in the elderly individual. This concurs with the typical advice to the clinician to start at lower doses and titrate to a minimum therapeutic level. The medically compromised individual is at a greater risk for drug toxicity due to the effect of chronic medical illnesses further decreasing serum albumin concentration. However, the extent to which protein binding impacts on drug effects is dependent on a number of clinical variables. For example, an increase in α_1-acid glycoprotein occurs in *acute* medical conditions and may serve to *increase* the proportion of protein-bound drug. This highlights the importance of individualizing treatment depending on each clinical scenario.

In terms of organ systems most closely related to drug metabolism, the two major sites of metabolism/excretion, i.e., the liver and kidneys, are both affected by aging. The kidneys appear to be more measurably affected, largely due to age-related changes in renal blood flow. Glomerular filtration rate declines approximately 50% in the average adult over a lifetime. Further, tubular secretion, diffusion, and reabsorption all demonstrate measurable decrements. The liver is also affected by a gradual reduction in blood flow with concomitant decrements in liver mass by late life (4). This is associated with a decrease in biotransformation by the cellular microsomal enzyme CYP2D6 isozyme responsible for the oxidation phase of the metabolic pathway (Phase I). Phase I involves the introduction of a polar group to the molecule being metabolized to facilitate renal excretion. As discussed later, there are a number of psychotropic agents such as the selective serotonin-reuptake inhibitors (SSRIs) that inhibit this pathway (4). Age-related changes in drug metabolism by the liver are thought to affect primarily the Phase I reactions (e.g., oxidation, demethylation, hydroxylation) as opposed to Phase II (conjugation) reactions. Liver function is particularly relevant to the safe administration of psychotropic agents, as the majority undergo hepatic metabolism.

In addition to the above physiological changes in the liver and kidney, increased vulnerability to adverse cognitive effects of medications represents a very important change in the CNS in the older individual. Age-related changes in the function of the CNS may lead to increased susceptibility of the elderly individual to adverse effects such as sedation, confusion, orthostatic hypotension, gait instability, and parkinsonian side effects (5). This vulnerability is likely related to decrements in the bioavailability of the catecholamines and indolamines (e.g., dopamine, norepinephrine, serotonin) as well as decrements in central cholinergic function. This relative loss of neurotransmitter availability may create receptor supersensitivity, accounting for the clinical observation that older individuals are more likely to manifest cognitive impairment or delirium with quantities of medication that would produce only sedation, for example, in younger adults. For this reason, it is extremely important to actively assess and document each patient's mental status (ideally using a quantitative scale or rating) before starting or switching psychotropic agents. At a minimum, some documentation regarding presence or absence of cognitive impairment is essential.

Subsequent sections of this chapter will deal with individual groups of psychotropic agents in terms of special considerations in the management of the elderly patient. As there are entire volumes devoted solely to geriatric psychopharmacology, by no means does this chapter intend to comprehensively cover each medication, but rather to highlight important issues for the clinician pertinent to the main psychotropic groups.

TRICYCLIC ANTIDEPRESSANTS

Tricyclic antidepressant medications have been the most consistently studied and extensively used treatment for major depression since their introduction more than 30 years ago. The efficacy of tricyclics has been repeatedly demonstrated through placebo-controlled trials, a number of which have examined their use in the depressed elderly. One such trial examining efficacy in the elderly demonstrated a 60% response rate with nortriptyline compared to 13% with placebo (6). A double-blind, placebo-controlled study involving subjects in the very old (80+) age group also demonstrated nortriptyline to be more effective than placebo (7). However, in this population the therapeutic trial may be limited by the inability to tolerate an adequate dose of medication. Due to the constellation of potential adverse effects with the tricyclics, the safety of their use in the medically compromised elderly patient has been appropriately examined in a number of studies. Fortunately the findings from this work are largely reassuring, demonstrating that these medications may be used safely and effectively.

The tricyclic antidepressant agents may be grouped into secondary amines (e.g., nortriptyline, desipramine) and tertiary amines (e.g., imipramine, amitriptyline). This distinction has clinical meaning, as tertiary amines impart greater anticholinergic effects (likely due to increased affinity for muscarinic and histaminic receptors) as well as greater sedative effects and orthostatic hypotension related to α-adrenergic antagonism (8). In contrast to the tertiary amines, the secondary amines are comparatively less problematic in the older population in terms of side effects. In general, when a tricyclic is the agent of choice, the use of the secondary amines is probably most advisable for the older patient in light of their more favorable side effect profile.

When tricyclic antidepressants are utilized in the elderly, attention to the cardiac status of the patient is necessary due to the potential for intraventricular conduction delay imparted by the medication as well as the α-adrenergic antagonism, creating a risk of hypotension. It has been shown that older persons with depressive illness are at greater risk for cardiac morbidity and mortality even in the absence of documented cardiac disease (9,10). These data suggest that the depressed elderly individual is already vulnerable to adverse cardiac events even without the added influences of antidepressant medication. However, it is important to note that tricyclic antidepressants have been demonstrated to be safely administered in patients with heart disease. Veith et al. demonstrated that imipramine was effective in the treatment of depression in post–myocardial infarction patients and reduced the rate of premature ventricular contractions in this group compared to placebo (11). This study demonstrated that the quinidine-like antiarrhythmic effects of tricyclics may be beneficial in the post–myocardial infarction population. However, in clinical situations such as cardiac patients with conduction defects, unstable congestive failure, and orthostatic hypotension, tricyclics must be monitored closely to allow safe administration (12). Specific circumstances where tricyclics may be of greater risk than benefit include second or third degree heart block, left bundle branch block, and significant QT prolongation. In the case of the cardiac patient, administration of tricyclics is best conducted in close consultation with the patient's cardiologist.

Both in the cardiac patient and the healthy elderly, orthostatic hypotension may result in tricyclic discontinuation. Age-related decrements in left ventricular ejection fraction represent an additional risk factor for the occurrence of orthostatic changes in the elderly (13). Orthostatic changes represent a potentially worrisome side effect for the elderly due to the risk of falling and associated fractures in a population already likely to experience greater gait instability at baseline compared to younger adults. Notably, in the study mentioned earlier involving the 80+ age group treated with nortriptyline, the most common reported adverse reaction was falling (7). Interestingly, a recent review of 70 adults over the age of 70 reported that patients treated with tricyclic antidepressants were no more likely to discontinue treatment due to side effects than patients treated with selective serotonin-reuptake inhibitors (SSRIs), although this study did not report specifically on falling or gait instability (14). Anticholinergic effects such as urinary retention, blurred vision, dry mouth, and constipation also may create problems in compliance with tricyclic regimens in the older patient. Cognitive impairment due to central anticholinergic effects further poses a potential risk of adverse events warranting careful clinical attention (15). Particularly in the context of a medically compromised patient, compounded anticholinergic effects from the addition of an antiemetic or an antihistaminic agent may result in overt anticholinergic delirium. The clinician must be continually alert to the possibility of additive anticholinergic effects through the use of multiple medications, which may together result in cognitive impairment.

Tricyclic antidepressants undergo hepatic metabolism, such that their use in patients with severe liver disease may require a dose reduction by as much as two thirds. The secondary amine nortriptyline has the advantage of defined therapeutic levels (50–150 ng/ml) such that serum level monitoring may be utilized. Importantly, these agents undergo oxidative metabolism through the cytochrome P450 2D6 system, so the clinician must be aware that medications inhibiting this system (most notably the SSRIs) may increase tricyclic levels. Additionally, some tricyclic metabolites must be excreted by the kidney, so patients with renal insufficiency or hemodialysis should be followed closely for the appearance of side effects with the use of serum levels to guide dosage adjustments.

Clearly the tricyclic antidepressants are not to be used without careful thought given to their potential adverse effects. The elderly patient requires at minimum a thorough physical examination, an EKG, and review of medical history for adverse cardiac events. In the context of careful management, the tricyclics represent a group of medications with a long history of safe and successful treatment of depression. In addition to affective syndromes, tricyclic antidepressants also may be used with varying degrees of success in the treatment of anxiety disorders, chronic pain syndromes, complicated bereavement, and anxiety related to posttraumatic stress disorder. In each of these syndromes and others, the use of tricyclics requires a careful pretreatment assessment and consistent follow-up.

SELECTIVE SEROTONIN-REUPTAKE INHIBITORS

At the time of their introduction in the United States approximately a decade ago, SSRIs appeared to offer substantial benefits for the elderly population in terms of efficacious treatment of depression without the adverse side effect profile of the tricyclics. Beginning with the availability of fluoxetine in 1988, SSRIs have been observed to be as efficacious as tricyclics in the treatment of major depression. The SSRIs as a group have the advantage of a lower risk of orthostatic hypotension, sedation, constipation, and other anticholinergic effects, although they do have a risk of gastrointestinal discomfort, headache, insomnia, and sexual dysfunction (16). Interestingly, there have been reports of treatment with fluoxetine improving orthostatic hypotension (17). It is of note, however, that the SSRI paroxetine has been observed to have anticholinergic effects comparable to the secondary amines of the tricyclic antidepressants (18). Additionally, the SSRIs may be associated with other adverse effects including akathisia, hyponatremia, and a serotonergic syndrome, although these are relatively scarce given the wide use of these medications (19,20).

The "serotonergic syndrome" is characterized by excess CNS serotonin receptor agonist activity. This syndrome has been seen particularly in the clinical situation where an SSRI is combined with a monoamine oxidase inhibitor (including the selective inhibitors) or with tryptophan or trazodone (21). This syndrome involves mental status changes resembling delirium, restlessness, agitation, myoclonus, hyperreflexia, diaphoresis, chills, tremor, gastrointestinal distress, ataxia, and headache. It is not clear whether the elderly are at increased risk for this syndrome, although it is intuitive that this may be the case due to a relative excess of peripheral norepinephrine in the elderly and greater vulnerability to the CNS effects of psychotropic agents. In the absence of an overt syndrome, the "activating" effects of the SSRIs may be described by the elderly patient as an uncomfortable restlessness or a beneficial increase in energy. Fluvoxamine was recently added to the list of SSRIs available in the United States with an indication for obsessive-compulsive disorder. It is likely to have a similar profile to the other SSRIs and as such should be fairly well tolerated in the elderly. Finally, citalopram is an SSRI available in Europe, which may have beneficial effects in the treatment of poststroke depression and behavioral symptoms of dementia (22).

While there is another chapter in this text specifically addressing drug-drug interactions, the potential interactions associated with the SSRIs are of enough clinical importance to address in this chapter at the risk of redundancy. SSRIs such as fluoxetine act as inhibitors of the hepatic cytochrome p450 2D6 enzyme pathway, resulting in a substantial increase in serum levels of other agents cleared by this pathway. This may impede the metabolism of tricyclic antidepressants, benzodiazepines, and antipsychotic medications. Paroxetine also inhibits the p450 2D6 enzyme, but less so than fluoxetine; sertraline appears to have even less inhibition capability, and fluvoxamine has the least of all, although it must be kept in mind that all of the SSRIs have this potential.

Overall, the SSRIs represent a safe and highly effective group of antidepressants of significant benefit to the elderly population. Compared to the tricyclics, the relative safety of the SSRIs in overdose has been one influential characteristic favoring their use. There is also growing experience in the use of SSRIs in the treatment of depressive symptoms in the context of Alzheimer's disease as well as in the treatment of obsessive-compulsive disorder and various anxiety disorders (23).

OTHER ANTIDEPRESSANT MEDICATIONS

Venlafaxine is a novel antidepressant medication in the class of the combination serotonin-norepinephrine uptake blockers. Like SSRIs and buproprion (discussed below), venlafaxine has the advantage of avoiding the anticholinergic, antihistaminic, and α-adrenergic antagonist effects. Venlafaxine is metabolized through the cytochrome p450 pathway. Early observations including one open-label trial involving geriatric subjects suggest that venlafaxine is well tolerated and beneficial for the treatment of depression in the elderly. The one potential problem with this medication is the reported side effect of elevation of diastolic blood pressure. The implications of this modest increase in blood pressure may be of clinical importance in elderly patients with vascular disease, particularly those with a history of cerebrovascular events.

Nefazodone is another newer antidepressant agent with a favorable side effect profile for use in the elderly. Like trazodone, nefazodone is considered an atypical serotonin uptake inhibitor with serotonin agonist effects as well as α-adrenergic and 5HT2 antagonist effects. Both nefazodone and trazodone have been demonstrated to have anxiolytic and antidepressant properties with a low likelihood of adverse events, making these agents beneficial for use in the elderly. Trazodone does have prominent sedative effects, making it perhaps a more useful agent for the treatment of insomnia. Often low-dose trazodone (50–75 mg) may be helpful for insomnia in patients who are otherwise responding to SSRI treatment of depression. Due to the hepatic clearance of nefazodone and trazodone, it is likely prudent to reduce the initial dose and titrate gradually, a good general rule for most agents discussed in this chapter.

Mirtazapine is a recently available antidepressant agent, which acts to increase noradrenergic activity as well as increase specific serotonergic activity at 5HT1a receptors (24). Mirtazapine appears to have the advantage of avoiding anticholinergic side effects, but it has been reported to cause occasional gastrointestinal disturbance, weight gain, increased appetite, sedation, and dry mouth (25). Meta-analysis of pooled data from placebo-controlled studies has shown that mirtazapine is as effective as amitriptyline in the treatment of depression (26). However, another controlled study of 115 elderly patients showed that both mirtazapine and amitriptyline were effective in decreasing global depression ratings, although amitriptyline was somewhat more effective on measures of cognitive disturbance and psychomotor retardation (27). Other work in nonelderly subjects has also suggested that tricyclic antidepressants may be preferable over mirtazapine (28), although the greater tolerability of mirtazapine may lead to more successful use in the older population (29).

Buproprion is an atypical agent with a fairly successful history of use in the elderly over the past several years. It is generally quite well tolerated in the elderly, and initial concern regarding potential for seizures appears to be an issue only at the high end of the dosage range and for individuals with preexisting risk for seizure activity. In contrast to the above agents, buproprion has a more centrally activating, stimulant-like quality, due to increased noradrenergic and dopaminergic activity. Because of the relative absence of antimuscarinic effects and lack of α-adrenergic blockade, buproprion lacks many of the hazardous anticholinergic and hypotensive effects of other agents. Buproprion further does not inhibit the cytochrome p450 system, so it may be used without the level of concern regarding interactions with and elevations of other medication levels. One slight drawback is its stimulant-like quality, which imparts a small risk of psychomotor agitation and insomnia. Overall buproprion is a well-tolerated and useful medication for the medically compromised older patient.

MONOAMINE OXIDASE INHIBITORS

Monoamine oxidase inhibitors (MAOIs) may be particularly beneficial in the treatment of atypical depression and may be utilized when other antidepressant trials have been unsuccessful. These medications act by inhibiting the metabolism of catecholamines in the presynaptic nerve terminals by monoamine oxidase. Monoamine oxidase A is found in the CNS as well as the gastrointestinal system and metabolizes norepinephrine, serotonin, dopamine, and tyramine. Monoamine oxidase B is found in the CNS as well as in the liver and on platelets; monoamine oxidase B metabolizes dopamine, tyramine, and phenylethylamine. The typical MAOIs used in the United States for antidepressant treatment include phenelzine and tranylcypromine, both of which are nonselective inhibitors. Selegiline is also available as a treatment for Parkinson's disease and is selective for MAO-B, although at antidepressant doses (30 mg/day) it acts as a nonselective inhibitor. Selegiline has further been shown to be useful in behavioral disturbances associated with Alzheimer's disease, which may be supported by the observation that monoamine oxidase activity is increased in the CNS and platelets of Alzheimer's patients. Interestingly, monoamine oxidase activity is also noted to increase with aging, suggesting that these agents may have a role in the treatment of the older patient for a number of reasons (30).

The MAOIs have been available for clinical use approximately as long as the tricyclic antidepressants, since their inadvertent discovery in the 1950s during investigational synthesis of antituberculosis agents. As a result they have a long history of demonstrated efficacy including use in the elderly. MAOIs have been observed to be as efficacious as the tricyclic agents (6), and much like the tricyclic agents their use may be rate-limited by the appearance of adverse side effects. Adverse events unique to the MAOIs include the risk of hypertensive crisis, which further curtails their use clinically despite their documented efficacious profile. While MAOIs avoid the majority of the anticholingeric effects of the other antidepressants, they do have a dose-related hypotensive effect that may be particularly problematic in the older patient. Optimizing intake of fluids may be helpful, and in some cases the addition of fludrocortisone may help minimize the orthostatic hypotensive effects.

The metabolism of the MAOIs is not clearly understood, nor is there any information regarding the utility of following serum levels. It has been reported, however, that elderly patients tend to have higher serum levels of phenelzine per unit dose when compared to younger patients (31). This is consistent with the typical clinical expectation of slower drug metabolism in the elderly and supports the approach of initial dose reduction and gradual upward titration.

Finally, the clinician must be aware of the difficulty in compliance for many elderly patients, which may be compounded in the case of MAOIs due to the added difficulty of maintaining a special tyramine-free diet. While the diet is not particularly restrictive and not difficult for the young adult to adhere to, in the elderly population the depressed individual is both more likely to be experiencing cognitive impairment and is more likely to experience a poor outcome in the face of a hypertensive event. For these reasons and because of the above side effects, MAOIs are not typically a first-line agent in the elderly population. This is probably unfortunate, because MAOIs such as phenelzine have been reported to be as effective as nortriptyline in the treatment of the depressed elderly (6).

PSYCHOSTIMULANTS

Methylphenidate and other stimulants such as dextroamphetamine have been clinically utilized in the frail medically compromised elderly as agents potentially helpful in stimulating appetite and improving psychomotor retardation and apathy. The most commonly used stimulant, methylphenidate, is metabolized by the hepatic microsomal enzymes. Adverse effects include agitation, insomnia, and occasionally anorexia related to the central stimulant effects, although interestingly in the context of depression these agents often serve to stimulate appetite. Preexisting hypertension may become more labile in the context of stimulant use, but overall these medications may be relatively safely used in the elderly patient.

Placebo-controlled trials supporting the use of stimulants in the elderly are lacking, and to further complicate the picture, the targeted population is often highly confounded by comorbid medical illness. The literature in this area is for the most part largely confined to case series and open trials. However, one double-blind, placebo-controlled crossover study compared methylphenidate to placebo in 16 patients with debilitating medical illnesses and major depressive disorder (32). In this study, 10 of the 16 patients demonstrated at least moderate improvement in depression ratings. Similarly, a review of 59 cancer patients treated with dextroamphetamine or methylphenidate demonstrated moderate to marked improvement in 73% and at least some improvement in an additional 10%. Improvement in appetite was also noted in 54% of patients in this study (33). Clinical reports further suggest that the psychostimulants may be helpful for poststroke patients, patients with frontal lobe abulia syndromes secondary to head trauma, and those with HIV dementia and/or depression (34). A comparison study of methyphenidate and nortriptyline in poststroke depression reported that the rapid onset of response with methylphenidate (2.4 days compared to 27 days for nortriptyline) was especially beneficial for this patient population (35). More work in this area will help to document the beneficial effects of these agents.

LITHIUM AND OTHER ANTIMANIC AGENTS

Lithium's water-soluble property distinguishes it from other psychotropic agents. The use of lithium for the treatment of mania was delayed until the 1970s due to earlier experiences of toxicity and death when lithium was used briefly as a dietary replacement for sodium chloride. Since its approval, lithium carbonate has been widely used in bipolar and unipolar affective syndromes, various behavioral disturbances, schizoaffective disorder, personality disturbances, alcoholism, and cluster headaches. Lithium's water-soluble property has implications for its administration in the elderly. The older patient has a lower volume of distribution for lithium due to the smaller total lean body mass and therefore smaller volume of total body water. Combined with gradual decreases in glomerular filtration rate with age, the titration of lithium must be monitored carefully, but this by no means precludes its use in the older patient. It has been shown that symptoms of bipolar disorder, particularly episodes of mania, do not tend to become less severe with age such that young-onset patients with bipolar illness typically continue to require mania prophylaxis into late life. In addition, new cases of mania arise among late-onset bipolar disorder patients, often in association with some type of CNS insult. Together these disorders create an ongoing need for both lithium prophylaxis and acute antimanic treatment, although other agents such as valproic acid (discussed later in this section) are also increasingly used as alternative or adjunctive agents.

Initiation of lithium in the elderly patient should involve a gradual upward titration with monitoring of levels. In addition to a thorough physical examination, preliminary evaluation should include an assessment of blood urea nitrogen, creatinine (including 24-hour creatinine clearance), thyroid function studies, complete blood count, and electrolyte measures. The addition of an electrocardiogram and evaluation of cardiac status is also important, as there have been studies suggesting an association between lithium use and the sick sinus syndrome and/or t-wave abnormalities on electrocardiogram. Further, elderly patients are often on diuretics, lanoxin, and other heart medications, which may affect fluid status and alter lithium excretion. Lithium side effects that the clinician should be alert to include confusion, polyuria, gastrointestinal complaints, fine resting tremor, and ataxia.

While lithium clearly has beneficial properties for the treatment of manic symptoms in the elderly, controlled studies to document its efficacy are lacking. Clinical reports suggest that the lower doses (e.g., serum levels of 0.3–0.6) may be effective in mania prophylaxis for the older adult. While there may be few placebo-controlled studies, the long history of successful use of lithium supports its effectiveness provided careful monitoring is implemented. In the elderly the occurrence of secondary mania in the context of toxic, metabolic, or infectious insults as well as trauma or stroke may be particularly difficult to treat. Due to the risk of confusional states associated with lithium, its use may be limited in this neurologically vulnerable group and other agents discussed below may be more advantageous.

Other agents used in the treatment of mania include carbamazepine and valproic acid. Among the elderly there are clinical reports suggesting that both of these agents may impart beneficial effects. Moreover, in the case of rapid-cycling episodes these agents may be more effective than lithium (36). For the older manic patient with evidence of neurodegeneration (e.g., nonspecific changes on electroencephalogram), the anticonvulsant agents intuitively seem to be a prudent choice, although controlled trials have yet to establish the role of these agents in the treatment of late-life mania. The use of carbamazepine requires attention to the fact that its metabolism is accelerated via hepatic enzyme induction within the first few weeks of treatment such that an initial therapeutic level may become subtherapeutic within the first month. For this reason, monitoring of levels is essential to establish the therapeutic dose following enzyme induction. Additionally, the white blood cell count and liver function tests should be assessed prior to initiation and again in follow-up. Potential side effects of carbamazepine that may be particularly problematic for the elderly include ataxia, diplopia, sedation, and confusion. In addition to its antimanic properties, carbamazepine has been reported in a case series of 15 patients to be useful in treatment of agitation in dementia syndromes in patients refractory to management with a neuroleptic (37). In this small sample two subjects discontinued treatment due to adverse effects including leukopenia, highlighting the importance of following white blood cell counts and liver enzymes periodically during carbamazepine treatment.

Valproic acid may be similarly advantageous as an adjunct or first-line treatment of late-life primary or secondary mania. A series of 35 subjects treated with valproic acid for late-life affective disorders reported clinical improvement in 62% at a mean serum level of 52.9 mg/liter (38). Case series have also supported the beneficial effects of valproic acid in treating behavioral disturbances associated with dementia. In one case series, four subjects improved at least partially in terms of symptoms of aggressive behavior when treated with valproic acid. Serum levels ranged in this report from 24 to 54 mg/liter. Sedation appeared to limit the ability to approach typical therapeutic levels of 50–100 mg/liter (39). Another case series of 10 patients with agitated dementia reported that 8 of the 10 showed a 50% reduction in agitated behaviors (40). Further work delineating the benefits of valproate in the treatment of various symptoms related to the dementia syndromes is likely to yield additional positive findings.

ANTIPSYCHOTIC MEDICATIONS

For the medications discussed above, typically the clinician makes a decision to begin treatment based on symptom criteria much in the same way whether the patient is an older or younger adult, with special attention to dosage and clinical assessment for the older patient. For the antipsychotic medications, however, the use and indications vary more substantially when applied to the older patient. This situation is due to the fact that psychosis in the elderly arises from a wide variety of underlying disorders and vulnerabilities. Psychosis in the elderly is much more often related to an organic syndrome (e.g., dementia, delirium, stroke, tumor, metabolic imbalances) than a primary psychotic disorder such as schizophrenia. Because of the fairly broad use of antipsychotics in a variety of disturbances in the elderly, the Omnibus Budget Reconciliation Act of 1987 (OBRA) mandated guidelines to implement more a consistent and regulated use of antipsychotic agents in long-term care facilities. According to OBRA, the indications for which these agents are considered appropriate in long-term care facilities include schizophrenia, schizoaffective disorder, delusional disorder, psychotic mood disorders, brief reactive psychosis, Tourette's syndrome, Huntington's disease, and organic mental syndromes such as dementia and delirium with associated agitated behaviors that are documented to represent a danger to self or others or to create an impairment in functional capacity. These guidelines further severely curtailed the prn use of antipsychotic medications (41).

Treatment of psychosis in the elderly may involve lower doses of antipsychotic medication for reasons of diminished metabolism due to age-related changes in liver function, increased available free drug secondary to decreases in albumin, and possibly receptor supersensitivity leading to enhanced effect of drugs. Furthermore, among patients with schizophrenia, positive psychotic symptoms may become less severe over time and therefore may require less medication for effective treatment (42). Available literature documents that the majority of patients with schizophrenia with onset in late life respond to typical antipsychotic agents in terms of symptomatic improvement (43). Similarly, among early-onset chronic schizophrenic patients who reach geriatric treatment, the typical agents have been shown to have beneficial effects (44). The straightforward treatment of exacerbation of schizophrenia remains the exception rather than the rule, however, as mentioned above, the majority of antipsychotic medication use in the elderly is geared toward the treatment of behavioral disturbances in patients with dementia syndromes.

Overall the use of antipsychotics in both schizophrenia and dementia syndromes in the elderly may be limited by the side effect profile. Antipsychotic medications as a group have been associated with orthostatic hypotension, akathisia, parkinsonism, dystonia (least problematic of the extrapyramidal side effects among the elderly), tardive dyskinesia, neuroleptic malignant syndrome, and seizures. Of these side effects, the elderly are particularly vulnerable to the anticholinergic side effects and orthostatic hypotension seen most prominently with the low-potency antipsychotic medications (e.g., chlorpromazine, thioridazine, clozapine).

Extrapyramidal side effects (EPS) may include akathisia, abnormal movements, and parkinsonism. Of these, the older patient is most vulnerable to experiencing parkinsonian symptoms of rigidity, tremor, and masked facies. Clozapine is one agent that avoids this difficulty, as it does not appear to be associated with EPS. However clozapine must be titrated upward very gradually due to prominent sedation and orthostatic hypotension. Clozapine further requires weekly monitoring of the white blood cell count due to the risk of agranulocytosis. This imposes an added complexity to treatment that may create compliance difficulties for the older patient. Additionally, although only a few milliliters of blood are necessary for determination of the white count, the blood draws may constitute a risk for anemia in an individual with other risk factors for iron deficiency. On the positive side, there are encouraging clinical observations suggesting that clozapine may be particularly efficacious in the elderly patient with psychosis and Parkinson's disease (45).

Clozapine has also been studied in terms of its effects on psychosis of multiple sources and behavioral disruption in geriatric inpatients. One study reported behavioral improvement in 20 patients on clozapine (average dose = 208 mg). In this study 3 of the 20 subjects developed leukopenia. Sedation and lethargy were noted to constitute the most common side effects (46). There have been other case series supporting the use of clozapine in mixed groups of patients with schizophrenia and dementia (47,48). In these series the doses were lower, as is often the case in groups comprised of dementia and other behavioral syndromes (6.25–37.5 mg/day) with side effects noted to include bradycardia, delirium, and falls (48). Dosing guidelines for clozapine therapy in geriatric patients with dementia and psychosis include an initial dose of 12.5 mg/day with a maximum of approximately 75 mg (49).

Olanzapine is another atypical agent that may be advantageous due to a relative absence of extrapyramidal side effects. Olanzapine has pharmacological properties similar to those of clozapine, but olanzapine may be more convenient to administer due to the lack of necessity of weekly white blood cell counts. The side effect profile of olanzapine appears relatively similar due to its α-adrenergic, 5HT2 and muscarinic receptor blockade (50), but olanzapine appears to cause less sedation and hypotension than clozapine. Future studies will be helpful in examining the role of olanzapine in the treatment of the elderly patient. Like clozapine, it is possible that olanzapine has promise for the treatment of Parkinson's disease with psychosis.

Risperidone is yet another newer agent with D2 and 5HT2 antagonist activity that has been employed in the treatment of psychosis in the elderly. Risperidone may be especially well tolerated due to its lack of anticholinergic properties and minimal sedative effects, as it resembles the side effect profile of typical high-potency agents but is distinguished by its effects on the serotonin system. This serotonin receptor antagonism likely contributes to the observation that risperidone may also have fewer extrapyramidal side effects than other high-potency agents.

Recent case series have suggested a potential benefit from the use of risperidone in the elderly with relatively few adverse effects. In one series, the records of 26 patients over age 65 with various psychotic disorders and comorbid medical illnesses who received risperidone were reviewed for degree of improvement and ability to tolerate the medication (51). The authors reported that 85% showed some degree of clinical improvement and that 73% remained on the drug (mean dose = 3.8 mg/day), suggesting that it was well tolerated. Similarly, an open-label trial of 10 patients ages 66–81 with chronic schizophrenia reported significant improvement in negative symptom scores and cognitive measures on risperidone titrated to a maximum of 6 mg/day without the emergence of significant extrapyramidal side effects (52). Two other case series reported on the use of risperidone in mixed groups of schizophrenia spectrum, bipolar disorder, and dementia patients. These reports supported a clinically improved outcome with improvement in behavior, positive and negative symptoms, and a relative lack of EPS. In one report involving 11 patients, only two discontinued treatment due to hypotension or dizziness (53,54).

When selecting an antipsychotic agent for use in behavioral disorders associated with dementia syndromes, one must weigh carefully the risk of increased cognitive impairment and other adverse effects associated with anticholinergic activity in this patient group. Schneider et al. conducted a meta-analysis of controlled trials of antipsychotic treatment in patients with Alzheimers disease and reported that only 18% received significant benefit from treatment (55). Once the syndrome has progressed to overt behavioral disturbance/agitation, patients with dementia are often refractory to medications of any type. They may have the best chance for improvement with a combination of therapeutic strategies involving both optimization of medication management and behavioral/structural interventions. When the risk of hypotension, falls, and delirium is taken into account, the decision to initiate antipsychotic treatment becomes complex, requiring a careful assessment of risks and benefits.

The risk of tardive dyskinesia in the elderly is yet another reason to weigh carefully the decision to use antipsychotics. Patients with schizophrenia as well as those with chronic affective disorders may have a predisposition to abnormal movements and are at greater risk for tardive dyskinesia simply due to the long duration of exposure to antipsychotic agents. However, tardive dyskinesia may occur in *any* older patient receiving dopamine antagonist medications for any reason. In fact, independent of diagnosis, age is the single greatest risk factor for the development of tardive dyskinesia. This has substantial implications for the elderly population without psychiatric diagnosis who may be receiving, for example, compazine as an antiemetic agent or metoclopramide for gastroparesis. It is possible that the use of the newer antipsychotic agents may help to decrease the rate of tardive dyskinesia. In addition to those mentioned above, many of the new agents under development may also be of substantial benefit in this regard as they also appear to have low likelihood of EPS. These agents include quetiapine and ziprasidone.

As with most psychotropic agents, the antipsychotic medications are metabolized by the liver and should be adjusted accordingly in the older patient and the patient with liver disease. In administering antipsychotics, one must be keenly aware that while antipsychotic medications may improve the symptomatic behaviors of a delirious patient, the source of the delirium must be aggressively pursued. Hallucinations, particularly visual and tactile, frequently accompany a delirious state. They must be recognized

Table 2   Recommended Dosage Ranges for the Use of Antipsychotic Medications in Dementia Syndromes

Medication	Initial dose (mg/day)	Maximum dose (mg/day)
Haloperidol	0.5	2–5
Thioridazine	10–25	50–100
Perphenazine	2	16–24
Thiothixene	0.5–1.0	10–15
Risperidone	0.5–1.0	4–6
Clozapine	12.5	75–100

Source: Ref. 67.

as such (symptoms of delirium) as opposed to the assumption that the patient has a primary psychotic disorder and treatment with an antipsychotic is sufficient. On the contrary, increasing the dose of antipsychotic in a patient with persistent hallucinations secondary to delirium could potentially worsen the delirium. Thus, the use of psychotropic agents in the medically compromised patient requires a constant balance between efficacy and toxicity (Table 2).

ANXIOLYTIC AGENTS

Benzodiazepines have been a mainstay of treatment of anxiety, insomnia, and agitation for many years, but they must be used with special attention in the elderly population. The treatment of sleep disturbance and anxiety syndromes represents a very broad area of clinical practice that has been undergoing increasing scrutiny by researchers. Further research in this area promises to be of substantial clinical benefit, as data from the Epidemiological Catchment Areas (ECA) studies have suggested that anxiety disorders represent the most prevalent source of psychiatric morbidity among the elderly population (56). Important considerations regarding the use of benzodiazepines involve the potential side effects of gait instability, disinhibition, and cognitive impairment resulting in an increased risk of falls or dangerous behaviors.

One of the primary considerations for the clinician in selecting among benzodiazepines is their wide variety of half-life durations and metabolite products. For very temporary treatment of insomnia, the use of medium half-life agents with no active metabolites is probably the most wise. Examples of these agents include lorazepam, temazepam, and oxazepam. Similarly, in the treatment of chronic anxiety syndromes, the use of agents with long half-lives (e.g., diazepam, chlordiazepoxide, clonazepam) may initially be beneficial symptomatically, but may result in accumulation of drug over time secondary to less efficient elimination in the elderly. The choice of benzodiazepine may be very important in the elderly, as one study showed that the selection of a long-acting agent was associated with a 70% increase in falls and hip fractures, while selection of a short-acting benzodiazepine was not associated with increased falls compared to the absence of benzodiazepine use (57). Additionally, the delay in metabolism of these agents with increasing age may be substantial, such that agents not typically considered to be of long half-life may have extensive effects. For example, in one study it was observed that the half-life of alprazolam was shown to be nearly twice as long in older compared to younger subjects such that the half-life exceeded 20 hours on average in the elderly group (58).

Perhaps the most worrisome adverse effects associated with the benzodiazepines are impairment in cognition and sensorium. This may result in agitation, confusion, anterograde amnesia, memory impairment, and impaired motor skills that may affect gait stability and driving safety. Even during in-hospital treatment, benzodiazepines account for a substantial degree of confusion. One study examined 418 subjects over the age of 59 hospitalized for a variety of medical indications without observed cognitive impairment at admission. They observed that within that group, benzodiazepine use was associated with 29% of cases of cognitive impairment occurring prospectively during the hospitalization (59). Another adverse clinical situation occurring during hospitalization is related to abrupt withdrawal or decrement in benzopdiazepine use resulting in withdrawal-induced delirium. This may easily occur in the elderly population, who may be inadvertently taking more medication than prescribed or may be afraid to report extensive use of medication to the clinician. The signs and symptoms of withdrawal include insomnia, restlessness, agitation, tremulousness, photophobia, psychosis, and seizures. Comorbid alcoholism may further complicate the clinical picture, and its recognition is of substantial importance. Benzodiazepine or alcohol withdrawal symptoms occurring during a medical hospitalization are unfortunately frequently missed or attributed to medical illness or postoperative delirium.

Aside from the potential adverse effects and withdrawal syndromes, the benzodiazepines remain extensively utilized for the treatment of sleep disturbance and anxiety disorders. However, a newer agent for the treatment of insomnia, zolpidem, has recently been available as a short-term hypnotic agent. Zolpidem is of the imidazopyridine class, related to the benzodiazepines but more selective for a subset of GABA receptors. This agent lacks some of the anxiolytic properties of the benzodiazepines and is therefore indicated primarily for the treatment of sleep disturbance. One study has shown the use of zolpidem 5–10 mg to be well tolerated in elderly patients without evidence of confusion or rebound insomnia. Furthermore, there was no evidence of withdrawal effects following discontinuation of treatment (60). Additional studies will help to clarify the role of this promising agent in the treatment of sleep disorders among the elderly.

Nonbenzodiazepine agents for the treatment of anxiety and agitation in the elderly are also of great clinical utility. Buspirone, a partial 5HT receptor agonist, is one such agent that has been available for the past decade. Due to its more favorable side effect profile, there have been a number of studies examining its efficacy for a variety of disorders in the geriatric population. One placebo-controlled study examined the impact of buspirone (mean dose 18 mg/day) on anxiety ratings over 4 weeks of randomly assigned treatment. A significant decrease in anxiety symptoms was noted in the active group compared to placebo (61). The side effect profile of buspirone avoids many of the problematic effects of the benzodiazepines, but does include occasional restlessness, gastrointestinal distress, headache, and dizziness, although these are not prominent in clinical practice. Potential indications for the use of buspirone in the elderly include agitated dementia, symptoms of Parkinson's disease, and geriatric depression (62).

CHOLINERGIC COGNITIVE ENHANCERS

There has been a burgeoning of research activity in recent years investigating potential agents for the treatment of Alzheimer's disease and related dementia syndromes. One avenue for these investigations involves the development of agents that increase cholinergic transmission through either augmentation of acetylcholine precursors, reduction of degradation activity, or direct agonist activity at acetylcholine receptors. Other strategies have involved investigations of agents that increase monoamine, indolamine, and GABA activity, although results have not been compelling to date.

Tacrine, a reversible cholinesterase inhibitor, serves to increase cholinergic transmission by inhibiting the degradation of acetylcholine. Tacrine has been shown to be of clinical benefit particularly early in the course of illness, although it dose not appear to change the course of the underlying neuropathology. It should be remembered that tacrine serves to increase the availability of acetylcholine, while the disease process itself involves progressive neuronal death, and at present there is no available treatment known to interrupt this process (some promising agents are noted in Table 3). Nonetheless, tacrine was the first agent of its kind to impart symptomatic improvement in measures of cognitive function (63,64).

Tacrine is metabolized extensively by the liver, including the cytochrome p450 enzymes. Importantly, the use of tacrine has also been associated with liver toxicity such that weekly serum transaminase monitoring is indicated. This appears to be a dose-related phenomenon that resolves typically with decrease or discontinuation of drug. Another cholinesterase inhibitor approved for the treatment of Alzheimer's disease, donepezil, does not appear to have the hepatotoxicity associated with tacrine. Donepezil appears to have similar clinical benefits as tacrine with the advantage of once-daily dosing. A multicenter double-blind study demonstrated improvement in cognitive measures in patients receiving donepezil 5 mg/day compared to patients receiving placebo and noted no more reported side effects than placebo (65).

In addition to cholinesterase inhibitors, other studies have investigated the use of the selective monoamine oxidase inhibitor selegiline in the treatment of dementia. One study recently completed involved a controlled trial of selegiline, α-tocopherol (vitamin E), and placebo in the treatment of Alzheimer's disease of moderate severity.

Table 3 Agents Proposed for Use in Alzheimer's Disease

Agent	Action	Potential Benefit
Tacrine Donepezil	Acetylcholinesterase inhibitor	Increases acetylcholine availability
Selegiline	Monoamine oxidase inhibitor, selective for MAO-B	Antioxidant activity and increases catecholamine activity
α-Tocopherol	Lipid-soluble antioxidant vitamin	Decreases free radical damage through inhibition of lipid peroxidase
Acetyl-carnitine	Neuroprotective agent via enhanced mitochondrial function	Decreases neuronal cell loss
Estrogen	Probable neuroprotective effects	Decreases neuronal cell loss
Milameline	Simulates function of acetylcholine	Increases cholinergic activity

The outcome measures in the study included death, institutionalization, loss of ability to perform activities of daily living, or a Clinical Dementia Scale (66) of 3 or less. Both selegiline and α-tocopherol slowed the progression to these outcome measures more than placebo (30). Selegiline acts to increase catecholamine levels and is also thought to act as an antioxidant and potentially interrupt neuronal damage. α-Tocopherol is also thought to minimize neuronal damage through free radical–scavenging effects, reducing oxidative damage. Studies such as this reflect the wide range of potential agents that may be implicated in the etiology of Alzheimer's, likely reflecting its multifactorial pathogenesis. Other agents on the horizon, in addition to antioxidants, include hormonal treatments (e.g., estrogen therapy), anti-inflammatory agents, and other neuroprotective agents (see Table 3 for overview).

SPECIAL CONSIDERATIONS FOR THE ELDERLY: CONCLUSION

Of key importance is the clinician's awareness of the age-related physiological changes affecting pharmacokinetic and pharmacodynamic activity, which must be kept in mind when psychotropic agents are dispensed to the older patient. However, this is only one small piece of the complicated picture in the diagnosis and treatment of psychiatric syndromes in the older individual. In late life there is a remarkable convergence of neurological syndromes with psychiatric and cognitive manifestations that challenge the diagnostician and highlight the importance of a thorough clinical history.

Particularly in the older psychotic individual, the acquisition of a thorough psychiatric history including outside informants is of paramount importance in determining appropriate treatment. An older patient presenting with psychosis with no *previous* psychiatric history is a very different case pathoetiologically compared to an individual with a history of schizophrenia presenting in exacerbation. Very careful attention must be paid to the possibility of a dementia syndrome or delirium secondary to any number of toxic, metabolic, or pathological processes. Treatment of the underlying process is critical in these situations, although psychotropic medications may have a role in symptomatic relief. In contrast, in the case of preexisting schizophrenia one must be highly vigilant for dementia or delirium but also fairly confident that once these are excluded, the solution will be achieved through optimizing treatment with antipsychotic medication. Moreover, in the realm of affective and anxiety syndromes, the overlap of these symptoms with acute and chronic medical illness further challenges the clinician diagnostically. Once the psychiatric history is ascertained and confounding medical problems are addressed, the elderly patient may benefit from an array of newer antidepressant and antipsychotic agents that are well tolerated and may be highly effective.

As the newer agents become available in increasing numbers, there is a tremendous need for controlled trials of these agents in the late-life syndromes. With the escalating numbers of individuals entering the old-old phase of life, the need for well-established treatment algorithms becomes more and more pressing. Fortunately substantial efforts are underway in this direction, and newer medications are offering tremendous promise for relief of symptoms that were once thought in many cases to be part of "just getting old."

REFERENCES

1. Geokas M, Conteas C, Majumdar A. The aging gastrointestinal tract, liver and pancrease. Clin Geriatr Med 1985; 1:177–206.
2. Kenney AR. Physiology of Aging: A Synopsis. Chicago: Year Book Medical, 1989.
3. Cadieux RJ. Geriatric psychopharmacology: a primary care challenge. Postgrad Med 1993; 93:285–288.
4. Leventhal EA. Biology of Aging. In: Sadavoy J, Lazarus L, Jarvik L, Grossberg G, eds. Comprehensive Review of Geriatric Psychiatry—II. Washington, DC: American Psychiatric Press, 1996.
5. Abernathy DR. Psychotropic drugs and the aging process: pharmacokinetics and pharmacodynamics. In: Salzman C, ed. Clinical Geriatric Psychiatry. New York: Williams and Wilkins, 1992:61–76.
6. Georgotas A, McCue RE, Hapworth W. Comparative efficacy and safety of MAOIs versus TCAs in treating depression in the elderly. Biol Psychiatry 1986; 21:1155–1166.
7. Katz IR, Simpson GM, Curtlik SM. Pharmacologic treatment of major depression for elderly patients in residential care settings. J Clin Psychiatry 1990; 51:41–47.
8. Richelson E. Pharmacology of antidepressant in use in the United States. J Clin Psychiatry 1982; 43:4–13.
9. Anda RJ, Williamson D, Jones D, et al. Depressed affect, hopelessness, and the risk of ischemic heart disease in a cohort of U.S. adults. Epidemiology 1993; 4:285–294.
10. Frasure-Smith N. In-hospital symptoms of psychological stress as predictors of long-term outcome after acute myocardial infarction in men. Am J Cardiol 1991; 67:121–127.
11. Veith RC, Raskind MA, Caldwell JH. Cardiovascular effects of the tricyclic antidepressants in depressed patients with chronic heart disease. N Engl J Med 1982; 306:954–959.
12. Giardina EG, Johnson LL, Vita J. Effect of imipramine and nortriptyline on left ventricular function and blood pressure in patients treated for arrhythmias. Am Heart J 1985; 909: 992–998.
13. Glassman AH, Bigger J, Giardina EV. Clinical characteristics of imipramine induced hypotension. Lancet 1979; ii:468–472.
14. Kamath M, Finkel S, Moran M. A retrospective chart review of antidepressant use, effectiveness, and adverse events in adults age 70 and older. Am J Geriatr Psychiatry 1996; 4: 167–172.
15. Tiller JWG. Antidepressants, alcohol and psychomotor performance. Acta Psychiatr Scand 1990; 360(suppl):13–17.
16. Rothschild A. Selective serotonin reuptake inhibitor induced sexual dysfunction: efficacy of a drug holiday. Am J Psychiatry 1995; 10:1514–1516.
17. Grubb B. Fluoxetine hydrochloride for the treatment of severe refractory orthostatic hypotension. Am J Med 1994; 97:366–368.
18. Hays DP, Renner J, Franson KL, et al. Use of the newer antidepressants in the elderly. Nursing Home Med 1997; 5:28–40.
19. Addler L, Angrist B. Paroxetine and akathisia. Biol Psychiatry 1995; 37:336–337.

20. Bluff D, Oji N. SIADH in a patient receiving sertraline [letter]. Ann Intern Med 1995; 123:811.

21. Reeves R. Serotonin syndrome produced by paroxetine and low-dose trazodone. Psychosomatics 1995; 36:159–160.

22. Pollock BG, Mulsant BH, Sweet R. An open pilot study of citalopram for behavioral disturbances of dementia. Am J Geriatr Psychiatry 1997; 5:70–78.

23. Volicer L. Treatment of depression in advanced alzheimers disease using sertraline. J Geriatr Psychiatry Neurol 1994; 7:227–229.

24. Stimmel GL, Dopheide JA, Stahl SM. Mirtazapine: an antidepressant with noradrenergic and specific serotonergic effects (review). Pharmacotherapy 1997; 17:10–21.

25. Montgomery SA. Safety of mirtazapine: a review. Int Clin Psychopharmacol 1995; 4:37–45.

26. Kasper S. Clinical efficacy of mirtazapine: a review of meta-analyses of pooled data (review). Int Clin Psychopharmacol 1995; 4:25–35.

27. Hoyberg OJ, Maragakis B, Mullin J, et al. A double-blind multicentre comparison of mirtazapine and amitriptyline in elderly depressed patients. Acta Psychiatr Scand 1996; 93:184–190.

28. Bruijn JA, Moleman P, Mulder PG, et al. A double-blind, fixed blood-level study comparing mirtazapine with imipramine in depressed in-patients. Psychopharmacology 1996; 127:231–237.

29. Marttila M, Jaaskelainen J, Jarvi R, et al. A double-blind study comparing the efficacy and tolerability of mirtazapine and doxepin in patients with major depression. Eur Neuropsychopharmacol 1995; 5:441–446.

30. Sano M, Ernesto D, Thomas RG. A controlled trial of selegiline, alpha-tocopherol, or both as treatment for Alzheimer's disease. N Engl J Med 1997; 336:1216–1222.

31. Robinson DS. Monoamine oxidase inhibitors and the elderly. In: Raskin A, Robinson D, Levine J, eds. Age and the Pharmacology of Psychoactive Drugs. New York: Elsevier, 1981: 149–161.

32. Wallace A. Double-blind placebo-controlled trial of methylphenidae in older depressed medically ill patients. Am J Psychiatry 1995; 152:929–931.

33. Olin J, Masand P. Psychostimulants for depression in the hospitalized cancer patient. Psychosomatics 1996; 37:57–62.

34. Rosenberg PB, Amend K, Hurwitz S. Methylphenidate in depressed medically ill patients. J Clin Psychiatry 1991; 52:263–267.

35. Lazarus LW, Moberg PJ, Langsley PR, Lingam VR. Methylphenidate and nortriptyline in the treatment of poststroke depression: a retrospective comparison. Arch Phys Med Rehab 1994; 75:403–406.

36. Bowden CL, Brugger AM, Swann AC. Efficacy of divalproes versus lithium and placebo in the treatment of mania: The Depakote Mania Study Group. JAMA 1994; 271:918–924.

37. Lemke MR. Effect of carbamazepine on agitation in Alheimer's inpatients refractory to neuroleptics. J Clin Psychiatry 1995; 56:354–357.

38. Kando JC, Tohen M, Castillo J, Zarate CA. The use of valproate in an elderly population with affective symptoms. J Clin Psychiatry 1996; 57:238–240.

39. Sandborn WD, Bendfeldt F, Handy R. Valproic acid for physically aggressive behavior in geriatric patients. Am J Geriatr Psychiatry 1995; 3:239–242.

40. Lott AD, McElroy SL, Keys MA. Valproate in the treatment of behavioral agitation in elderly patients with dementia. J Neuropsychiatry Clin Neurosci 1995; 7:314–319.

41. OBRA. Omnibus Reconciliation Act. P.L. 100–203 1987; 101 Stat.:1330.
42. Pfohl B, Winokur G. The evolution of symptoms in institutionalized hebephrenic/catatonic schizophrenics. Br J Psychiatry 1982; 141:567–572.
43. Jeste DV, Lacro JP, Gilbert PL, Kline J, Kline N. Treatment of late-life schizophrenia with neuroleptics. Schizophrenia Bull 1993; 19:817–830.
44. Tsuang MM, Lu LM, Stotsky BA, Cole JO. Haloperidol versus thioridazine for hospitalized psychogeriatric patients: double-blind study. J Am Geriatr Soc 1971; 19:593–600.
45. Rabey J. Low dose clozapine in the treatment of levodopa-induced mental disturbances in Parkinson's disease. Neurology 1995; 45:432–434.
46. Salzman C, Vaccaro B, Lieff J. Clozapine in older patients with psychosis and behavioral disruption. Am J Geriatr Psychiatry 1995; 3:26–33.
47. Frankenburg FR, Kalunian D. Clozapine in the elderly. J Geriatr Psychiatry Neurol 1994; 7:129–132.
48. Pitner JK, Mintzer JE, Pennypacker LC, Jackson CW. Efficacy and adverse effects of clozapine in four elderly psychotic patients. J Clin Psychiatry 1995; 56:180–185.
49. Borison R. The safety of antipsychotic therapy in geriatric patients. Curr Approaches Dementia 1996; 2:10–12.
50. Lamberti JS, Tariot P. Schizophrenia in nursing home patients. Psychiatr Ann 1995; 25:441–452.
51. Sajatovic M, Ramirez LF, Vernon L, Brescan D, Simon M, Jurjus G. Outcome of risperidone therapy in elderly patients with chronic psychosis. Int J Psychiatry Med 1996; 26:309–317.
52. Berman I, Merson A, Rachov-Pavlow J. Risperidone in elderly schizophrenic patients. Am J Geriatr Psychiatry 1996; 4:173–179.
53. Raheja RK, Bharwani I, Penetrante AE. Efficacy of risperidone for behavioral disorders in the elderly. J Geriatr Psychiatry Neurol 1995; 8:159–161.
54. Madhusoodanan S, Brenner R, Araugo L, Abaza A. Efficacy of risperidone treatment for psychoses associated with schizophenia, schizoaffective disorder, bipolar disorder or senile dementia in 11 geriatric patients. J Clin Psychiatry 1995; 56:514–518.
55. Schneider L, Pollock V, Lyness S. A metaanalysis of controlled trials of neuroleptic treatment in dementia. J Am Geriatr Assoc 1990; 38:553–563.
56. Sheikh JI, Salzman C. Anxiety in the elderly. Psychiatr Clin North Am 1995; 18:871–873.
57. Ray WA, Griffin MR. Benzodiazepines of long and short half-life and risk of hip fracture. JAMA 1989; 3303–3307.
58. Kroboth PD, McAuley JW, Smith RB. Alprazolam in the elderly: pharmacokinetics and pharmacodynamics during multiple dosing. Psychopharmacology 1990; 100:477–484.
59. Foy A, O'Connell D, Henry D. Benzodiazepine use as a cause of cognitive impairment in elderly hospital inpatients. J Gerontol 1995; 50:M99–106.
60. Roger M, Attali P, Coquelin JP. Multicenter, double-blind, controlled comparison of zolpidem and triazolam in elderly patients with insomnia. Clin Ther 1993; 15:127–136.
61. Bohm C, Robinson DS, Gammans RE. Buspirone therapy in anxious elderly patients: a controlled clinical trial. J Clin Psychopharmacol 1990; 10:47S–57S.
62. Goldberg RJ. The use of buspirone in geriatric patients. J Clin Psychiatry Monogr 1994; 12:31–35.
63. Smucker MD. Maximizing function in Alzheimers disease: What role for tacrine? Am Fam Physician 1996; 54:645–652.

64. Knapp MJ, Knopman DS, Solomon PR. A 30 week randomized controlled trial of high-dose tacrine in patients with Alzheimers disease. JAMA 1994; 271:985–991.
65. Roger SL, Friedhoff LT. The efficacy and safety of donepezil in patients with Alzheimer's disease: results of a US multicenter, double-blind, placebo-controlled trial. Dementia 1996; 7:293–202.
66. Morris JC. The Clinical Dementia Rating Scale: Current version and scoring rules. Neurology 1993; 11:2412–2414.
67. Rabins P. Practice Guidelines for the treatment of patients with Alzheimers disease and other dementias of late life. Am J Psychiatry 1997; 154(suppl):22.

25

Psychotropic Drug Interactions

C. Lindsay DeVane
Medical University of South Carolina
Charleston, South Carolina

Charles B. Nemeroff
Emory University School of Medicine
Atlanta, Georgia

INTRODUCTION

Medically ill patients are at risk to develop psychiatric co-morbidity. When the need arises for pharmacological treatment, this situation increases the potential for drug interactions with existing drug therapy. Drug interactions can occur in either direction; in other words the psychiatric treatment may influence existing medical treatment or previous drug treatment may alter the disposition and/or clinical effects of the psychiatric treatment. The possible consequences of drug interactions include a change in the intensity or duration of medical treatment, a change in adverse effects, or the appearance of new adverse effects. However, a few drug interactions have been documented to be helpful in achieving therapeutic objectives and to decrease the cost of medical treatment (1,2). Many drug interactions either have no effect or increase the variability in patient response to drugs. The clinical significance of a drug interaction depends upon the specific drugs involved, the dosage and length of medical and psychiatric drug treatment, the stability of the patient, and other factors.

Psychiatric drug treatment may continue for a relatively long period of time, so awareness and management of drug interactions is an important quality-of-life issue. The behavioral and cognitive symptoms that psychoactive drugs treat often return when either the medications are discontinued or the episodic nature of the disorder presents as an exacerbation of illness. Maintenance therapy for major psychiatric disorders may continue for years (3). Thus, medical treatment will frequently occur in the context of previously existing pharmacotherapy of mental disorders.

Several new drugs to treat psychiatric illness, especially in the antidepressant and antipsychotic classes, have become available recently for clinical use. When new drugs are introduced into practice, knowledge of their drug interactions is often incomplete. It is impractical to study all possible combinations of a new drug with those agents likely to be co-administered in the postmarketing period. Thus, the clinician must frequently rely on general principles to predict and manage drug interactions.

This chapter will review the background for understanding drug interactions and provide guidelines for their avoidance and management. The topic will be approached from the situation of a medically ill patient who requires treatment with a psychoactive drug. A previous review of this topic is available that considers in depth the pharmacokinetic and pharmacodynamic effects of pharmacotherapy on each psychotropic drug class (4). Pertinent considerations will be discussed for selecting drugs from individual psychoactive drug classes to minimize or avoid interactions with existing medical drug treatment. Recognized interactions that are frequently clinically significant will be reviewed.

CLASSIFICATION OF DRUG INTERACTIONS

Drug interactions are either pharmacodynamic, pharmacokinetic, or pharmaceutical. Some examples are listed in Table 1. Pharmaceutical interactions occur as a result of physical incompatibility of drugs, such as the precipitation of one drug by another from being mixed together in intravenous fluids of inappropriate pH. There are few examples of these types of interactions involving psychotropic drugs.

Pharmacodynamic Drug Interactions

A pharmacodynamic interaction is one that occurs when the pharmacological response of one drug is modified by another drug without the effect's being the result of a change in drug concentration. The mechanisms of these interactions usually involve some alteration of pharmacological effect at a site of drug action. These types of interactions may go unnoticed because the pharmacological effects of psychoactive drugs can be difficult to measure, especially changes in behavior or mental status. A pharmacodynamic interaction that modifies a medical treatment may be more dramatic. However, a slight change in blood pressure or pulse rate may go unnoticed. By their nature, pharmacodynamic interactions are not as easily documented as pharmacokinetic interactions. The latter can be quantified through serial measures of plasma drug concentrations before and after the addition of concurrent pharmacotherapy.

The pharmacological effects of some drugs may be enhanced by pharmacodynamic interactions. This is the expected outcome in combining different classes of antihypertensives or antiparkinsonism drugs. Many drugs produce sedation as either a primary effect or an unintended adverse event. Additive sedation can result from the combination of traditional antihistamines, many antidepressants and antipsychotics

Table 1 Mechanisms and Examples of Drug-Drug Interactions with Psychoactive Drugs

Mechanism	Examples
Pharmacodynamic interactions	
Increased response: additive receptor occupancy or similar pharmacological effects	Benzodiazepines and alcohol; monoamine oxidase inhibitors and L-tryptophan
Decreased response: receptor antagonism	Morphine and naloxone; midazolam and flumazanil
Pharmacokinetic interactions	
Altered absorption	Al/Mg antacids combined with various drugs decrease absorption rate
Altered metabolic clearance of one or more drugs	
Hepatic enzyme induction	Carbamazepine increases the synthesis of enzymes that metabolize oral contraceptives
Hepatic enzyme inhibition	Some antidepressants competitively inhibit the enzymes that metabolize tricyclic antidepressants and other cytochrome P450 substrates
Protein-binding displacement	Highly plasma protein–bound psychoactive drugs may potentially increase the free fractions of drugs, such as warfarin.
Altered renal clearance: increased or decreased glomerular filtration, renal tubular secretion or re-absorption	Probenecid and penicillin; indomethacin and lithium

with benzodiazepines or alcohol. For this reason, most patients are well advised not to drink alcohol when prescribed psychoactive drugs. An example of a food–drug interaction with a pharmacodynamic basis is the combination of a nonselective monoamine oxidase inhibitor with over-the-counter sympathomimetics or foods rich in tyramine. Because of differing mechanisms of action, overstimulation of the sympathetic nervous system can result in pressor effects on blood pressure. A final example is provided by the serotonin syndrome, the diagnosis of which is usually made from a history of combining drugs that have a serotonergic mechanism of action (5). Prominent symptoms thought to result from excessive serotonergic activity include hyperthermia, rigidity, myoclonus, and autonomic instability. In its worst form, this is a serious drug interaction and has sometimes been fatal. The most feared interaction involving the selective serotonin-reuptake inhibitors (SSRIs) is their combination with monoamine oxidase inhibitors. Because of the fear of such a pharmacodynamic interaction, SSRIs should not be used together with an MAOI or within 14 days of stopping an MAOI. Similarly, an MAOI should not be used within 14 days of stopping an SSRI or within 28 days of stopping fluoxetine because it is more slowly eliminated from the body than are other antidepressants.

Some pharmacodynamic interactions are useful for their therapeutic benefits. In the treatment of Parkinson's disease, the dopamine agonists, including ropinirole and pramipexole, have complementary effects on motor performance when given together with levodopa. Their combination may allow a reduction in the dosage of levodopa. A disappointing therapeutic response to the administration of an antidepressant has often been remedied with the addition of an adjunctive medication such as lithium, thyroid, pindolol (2), or another antidepressant. Receptor antagonists are employed in several fields of medicine to reverse the effects of previously administered agonists. This is the principle behind using naloxone, propranolol, and flumazanil to reverse the effects of opiates, catecholamines, and benzodiazepines at their respective receptor sites.

Pharmacokinetic Drug Interactions

A pharmacodynamic interaction is one that occurs when one drug changes the plasma or tissue concentration of another drug. However, many interactions of this type may be clinically insignificant unless the change in concentration alters the patient response to one or both drugs. The most frequent type of pharmacokinetic interaction occurs as a result in the change of renal or hepatic clearance, but a few important interactions involve other major components of drug disposition.

Interactions Involving Absorption

Relatively few interactions involving psychoactive drugs have been found to involve changes in drug absorption. Recently, interest in these types of interactions has been renewed with the recognition that cytochrome P450 enzymes in the gastrointestinal tract are active in the metabolism of some psychoactive drugs (6). The bulk of drug absorption following oral administration takes place in the small intestine. The rate and/or extent of drug absorption can be modified by an alteration in the gastric emptying rate, a change in the release characteristics of drug from its dosage form, a physical interference with drug absorption, or a change in gastric pH or membrane permeability. Antacids, nonabsorbable bulk laxatives, or cholestyramine may physically retard the rate or extent of drug absorption, or they may slow the rate of gastric emptying and thus delay absorption.

A reduction in the rate of drug absorption may or may not result in a clinically significant consequence, but a reduction in the extent of drug absorption is more likely to be significant. For example, cholestyramine, a nonabsorbable agent administered to lower serum cholesterol, can lower the oral bioavailability of several drugs, including digoxin, warfarin, propranolol, and valproate. This interaction can lead to a significant reduction in the pharmacological effects of these drugs. If administration of cholestyramine and valproate are spaced apart by 3 hours, then the effects on drug absorption are minimized (7). When an antipsychotic or antidepressant is prescribed for patients receiving chronic antacid therapy, a reduction in the rate of drug absorption will probably occur, but the extent of absorption is less likely to be diminished. In this situation, drug effects during chronic administration should be unaltered since the therapeutic effects from these drugs are minimally dependent on the absorption rate of single doses.

The gut wall is the site of significant drug metabolism because cytochrome (CYP) P450 enzymes, especially CYP3A4, are metabolically active in the endothelial wall (6). This metabolic ability can influence the total amount of drug and metabolite absorbed following oral drug administration. For some drugs, interference with this process results in drug interactions. CYP3A4 inhibitors, including erythromycin and ketoconazole, have been used to retard the presystemic elimination of cyclosporine and increase its systemic availability (8). This is an example of a beneficial interaction from inhibition of gut-wall metabolism. Naturally occurring compounds called flavonoids in grapefruit juice can inhibit intestinal CYP3A4 and increase the concentration of drugs that are substrates for this isozyme (9). A measurable but nonsignificant effect occurred when terfenadine was coadministered with grapefruit juice (10). Orange juice does not produce a similar effect on intestinal metabolism. Fresh-squeezed grapefruit juice has minimal effects compared with juice reconstituted from frozen concentrate.

Interactions Involving Distribution

The extent of drug binding to plasma and tissue proteins is a major factor controlling their distribution in the body (11). A change in drug distribution can occur by displacement from binding sites on plasma or tissue proteins, alterations in partitioning in various tissue components, or changes in circulation and perfusion of tissues. The most common mechanism involves a plasma protein–binding displacement of one drug by another. When a displacement interaction increases the amount of free or unbound drug, then more drug is available to produce pharmacological effects.

It should be noted that protein-binding displacement interactions are dependent on the route of administration and the clearance characteristics of the drugs involved. Several drug interactions are thought to occur through this mechanism, but the interaction may not be significant unless the binding displacement actually modifies a drug's dose–effect relationship. This type of interaction is most likely to be significant for high-clearance drugs administered intravenously. Few psychoactive drugs have these characteristics.

An example of a drug-displacement interaction is the effect on albumin binding by warfarin from coadministered salicylate analgesics. This is a transient interaction in which the increase in the plasma concentration of warfarin is partially offset by an increase in drug clearance. Nevertheless, even small changes in free-drug concentration are likely to be important for drugs for which there are only small differences between therapeutic concentration and the concentration at which adverse events occur.

The antidepressants and antipsychotics are highly plasma protein–bound (>95% in some cases). Overall, drug-binding displacement interactions have not been documented to be a prevalent problem with either the SSRIs or atypical antipsychotics. Within the class of SSRIs, the effects on warfarin may vary considerably, from a direct effect on metabolism by sertraline or fluvoxamine to a potential pharmacodynamic effect on platelet serotonin (12). The effects of psychoactive drugs combined with warfarin are summarized in Table 2.

The anticonvulsant mood stabilizers have been shown to alter plasma protein binding. Valproate can displace the plasma binding of diazepam, phenytoin, tolbutamide, and warfarin from their albumin binding sites (13). Valproate is also a nonspecific weak hepatic enzyme inhibitor (14) and can potentiate the actions of other drugs in a medical regimen.

Whenever psychoactive drugs are prescribed to patients already receiving drugs with a narrow therapeutic range—i.e., only a small difference in dose separates therapeutic from adverse effects (e.g. warfarin, oral hypoglycemics, antiarrhythmics)—then vigilance should be exercised to detect evidence for drug interactions and dosage titration should proceed slowly. Even though some drugs are known to interact, proper dosing may allow them to be safely used together.

Interactions Involving Metabolism or Elimination

The majority of drug interactions of concern from adding psychotropic drugs to medical treatment involve alterations of drug metabolism, which commonly occur as a result of enzyme induction or inhibition (15). The increased or decreased activity of enzymes can alter clearance with the result of decreased or increased plasma drug concentration. Several common enzyme inducers are recognized. Cigarette smoking, phenobarbital, rifampin, carbamazepine, and ethanol have well-documented effects. Their administration stimulates the synthesis of specific cytochrome or other enzymes. The possible outcome is a lower plasma drug concentration of drugs metabolized prominently by the induced enzyme, leading to a diminished or loss of effect (Table 3). For example, an inductive effect on CYP3A4 has been shown to enhance steroid metabolism and can lead to a loss of contraceptive effect (16). However, the effect is not immediate. Enzyme induction may occur over a period of days or weeks, and the loss of clinical effects during an interaction of this type may go unnoticed. The reverse situation should also be kept in mind. Whenever therapy with an enzyme inducer is stopped, plasma concentration of affected substrates may rise over the course of several days, possibly leading to increased pharmacological effects.

The most common enzyme inhibition interactions occur when two drugs are administered that are both substrates for the same metabolizing enzyme. In this situation, a competitive inhibition may occur in which one drug is cleared at the expense of the other, resulting in impaired drug clearance and a rise in drug concentration. Noncompetitive enzyme inhibition can also occur when one drug forms a complex with the enzyme, preventing it from metabolizing its usual substrates. The inhibitor does not necessarily have to be metabolized by that enzyme to cause an inhibition. An example is quinidine, which is a potent CYP2D6 inhibitor but is metabolized by

Table 2 Recommendations for Using Psychotropic Drugs in Medical Patients Requiring Anticoagulants

Drug	Effects	Recommendations
SSRI	Multiple case reports of adverse effects on hemostasis apart from any direct effect on anticoagulants: bruising, epistaxis, ecchymosis, heavy menstrual flow, rectal bleeding. These effects may result from platelet serotonin effect. Fluvoxamine inhibits warfarin metabolism potently; sertraline nonsignificantly; paroxetine, citalopram, fluoxetine have fewer inhibitory effects. Effects on heparin are unknown.	Use all SSRIs cautiously with warfarin; monitor bleeding indices. No pharmacokinetic interactions of warfarin and paroxetine or citalopram. Nonkinetic effects on bleeding may be dose-dependent; more caution needed when combined with aspirin or nonsteroidal anti-inflammatory drugs.
Antipsychotics	Clozapine effects on anticoagulants are unknown. Bleeding, pulmonary embolism, deep vein thrombosis reported in addition to high potential for bone-marrow suppression and agranulocytosis. No pharmacokinetic interaction of olanzapine with warfarin. No specific data for risperidone or quetiapine on warfarin, but metabolic effects are not expected and only infrequent reports of bleeding problems. Older reports of antiplatelet effects from phenothiazines.	Clozapine not recommended in patients with hemic/lymphatic-system disorders. Drugs of choice are low doses of olanzapine, or risperidone.
Mood stabilizers	Clotting abnormalities, thrombocytopenia, other hemic problems are risks of valproate. Aplastic anemia and agranulocytosis have been associated with carbamazepine, and protein-binding interactions with warfarin have been described. Gabapentin should not affect the disposition of warfarin but no specific data are available. Lamotrigine effects are unknown. Lithium causes a benign reversible granulocytosis. No pharmacokinetic interaction with warfarin.	Valproate and carbamazepine are not recommended. Little clinical experience to guide the use of gabapentin or lamotrigine. Cautious use with anticoagulants advised. Lithium appears to lack blood-coagulation problems in patients.

Table 3 Substrates, Inducers, and Inhibitors of Important Cytochrome P450 Enzymes

Enzyme	CYP1A2	CYP2C9	CYP2C19	CYP2D6	CYP3A4
Substrates	Acetominophen[a]	Dapsone	Clomipramine[a]	Alprenolol	Alprazolam
	Amitriptyline[a]	Diclofenac	Diazepam[a]	Amitriptyline[a]	Diazepam[a]
	Antipyrine	Fluvastatin	Imipramine[a]	Chlorpheniramine	Midazolam
	Caffeine	Ibuprofen	Mephenytoin	Clomipramine[a]	Triazolam
	Clozapine	Indomethacin	Moclobemide	Codeine[a]	Diltiazem
	Haloperidol[a]	Irbesartan	Omeprazole	Desipramine[a]	Felodipine
	Imipramine[a]	Losartan[a]	Phenytoin	Dextromethorphan[a]	Nicardipine
	Olanzapine[a]	Naproxen	Propranolol[a]	Encainide	Nifedipine
	Ondansetron	Piroxicam	Tolbutamide	Flecainide	Nitrendipine
	Phenacetin	Tenoxicam	Citalopram[a]	Fluoxetine[a]	Verapamil[a]
	Propafenone[a]	S-Warfarin		Haloperidol[a]	Cyclophosphamide[a]
	Propranolol[a]			Imipramine[a]	Tamoxifen
	Tacrine			Indoramin	Taxol
	Theophylline			Metoprolol	Vinblastine
	Verapamil[a]			Nortriptyline	Estradiol
	Ropinirole[a]			Ondansetron[a]	Cortisol
				Oxycodone	Testosterone
				Paroxetine	Amiodarone
				Propranolol[a]	Lidocaine
				Propafenone[a]	Lovastatin
				Mexiletene	Simvastatin
				Venlafaxine	Pravastatin
				Fenfluramine	Carbamazepine

Substrates					Cisapride, Cyclosporine, Erythromycin, Macrolide antibiotics, Terfenadine, Astemizole, Nefazodone, Quinidine, Methadone[a], Ritonavir, Indinavir, Saquinavir, Citalopram[a], Sildenafil, Ropinirole[a], Tolcapone[a]
Inducers	Cigarette smoking, Marijuana smoking, Omeprazole	Rifampin	Rifampin	None known	Rifampin, Steroids (cortisol, dexamethasone), Simvastatin
Inhibitors	Fluvoxamine (HP), Fluoroquinolones (HP), Cimetidine	Fluvastatin (MP), Fluvoxamine (MP), Valproate	Fluvoxamine (MP), Fluoxetine (MP), Sertraline, Valproate	Quinidine (HP), Fluoxetine (HP), Paroxetine (HP), Ritonavir (HP), Sertraline	Fluvoxamine (HP), Nefazodone (HP), Erythromycin (HP), Clarithromycin (HP), Cimetidine, Fluoxetine, Protease inhibitors, Grapefruit juice

[a] More than one P450 enzyme is known to be involved in the metabolism of these drugs. Many drugs are metabolized by several enzymes in parallel, although in most cases only one of these has been positively identified.

HP = High potency; MP = moderate potency.

CYP3A4 and not CYP2D6. Interactions involving hepatic enzyme inhibition are frequently characterized by a dose dependence (17). Higher doses of the inhibitor result in an interaction of greater magnitude.

Because only a few psychoactive drugs are cleared substantially by renal elimination, drug interactions of this type are infrequent with psychoactive drugs (4). Lithium and gabapentin, which are not metabolized, are the exceptions (18). Pramipexole, a new dopamine agonist used in the treatment of Parkinson's disease, is renally clear but may have its plasma concentration increased by cimetidine. The likely mechanism is an interference with the anionic transport system, which is responsible for the renal tubular secretion of pramipexole. The antidepressants, antipsychotics, and anxiolytics are highly metabolized drugs, with typically less than 5% of an administered dose being excreted in the urine in an unchanged form. Thus, there is little concern that they alter the renal elimination of drugs used to treat medical illness.

PREDICTION OF METABOLIC DRUG INTERACTIONS

The tools of molecular biology, particularly the polymerase chain reaction (PCR), have made it easier to sequence and clone enzyme structures. This capability has stimulated interest in the cytochrome P450 (CYP) hepatic enzyme system. Although this family of hepatic enzymes is but one of several responsible for the metabolism of xenobiotics, it has been estimated that over 80% of therapeutically useful drugs are metabolized in part by the P450 system (19–21). These enzymes play additional roles in the metabolism of some endogenous substrates, including prostaglandins and steroids. Related enzymes are divided into families and subfamilies according to their amino acid homology. Families share greater than 40% homology in their amino acid sequences while subfamilies share greater than 55% homology. CYP2C19 and CYP2D6 exist in a polymorphic form, meaning that a small percentage of the population possesses mutant genes that alter the activity of these enzymes, usually by diminishing or abolishing activity (22). Table 3 lists the most important CYP enzymes involved in psychiatric treatment of the medically ill along with some of their substrates, inducers, and inhibitors. This is an active research area and the information is continually being updated.

Metabolic interactions can be predicted quantitatively with in vitro methodology using liver slices, intact hepatocyte preparations, or microsomes (23). The results of in vitro investigations are used in the drug-development process to design further in vivo studies to investigate the clinical significance of potential interactions. With knowledge of the affinity of a drug for a particular cytochrome isozyme, it is possible to predict the likelihood of an interaction with a drug cleared through cytochrome-mediated metabolism. However, for many drugs there is incomplete knowledge of their isozyme-specific metabolism, and the values of affinity constants vary according to the specific methodology used for their generation.

Clinicians can use simple guidelines and a qualitative approach to the prediction of drug interactions. This will identify the combinations of drugs that should be used cautiously or avoided because of their potential to interact. A starting point is to recognize the common drugs listed as inhibitors or inducers in Table 3 for each of the major P450 enzymes. It should be remembered that any drug that is a substrate of a particular enzyme has the potential to competitively inhibit other substrates of that same enzyme. Other factors also moderate the potential for an interaction. A pharmacokinetic interaction that results in an increased or decreased drug concentration may not necessarily translate into clinically meaningful consequences. Minor changes in clearance, steady-state plasma concentration, or half-life will be most meaningful for drugs with narrow limits of tolerable concentrations.

Cytochrome P-450 1A2

Cytochrome 1A2 participates in the metabolism of several widely used drugs (Table 3). A genetic polymorphism is possible but has not been confirmed. A trimodal pattern of disposition has been noted in the metabolism of caffeine (24), but this finding could be the result of a highly variable enzyme activity.

Nonpsychiatric drugs metabolized by CYP1A2 include theophylline, aminophylline, and caffeine (Table 3) (20,25–28). It plays a partial role in the elimination of the J-adrenergic blocker propranolol. Other substrates include the traditional antipsychotic drug haloperidol and the newer atypical antipsychotics, clozapine and olanzapine (29). Tetrahydroacridinamine (tacrine) is hydroxylated by CYP1A2.

CYP1A2 can be both induced and inhibited by other drugs. It is induced by cigarette smoke, charcoal-broiled foods, and some cruciferous vegetables (e.g., brussels sprouts). The effect of cigarette smoking can be considerable; stopping or reducing smoking can be expected over the course of a few weeks to result in the return to baseline of CYP1A2 activity. A psychiatric inpatient who was receiving clozapine and quit smoking experienced a seizure during his stay (30). This was presumably due to the withdrawal of the inductive effect of smoking.

Inhibitors of CYP1A2 include fluvoxamine and ciprofloxacin. Interactions have been described with increases of theophylline and clozapine concentration when these drugs were used together (31,32). A specific interaction of fluvoxamine to avoid or manage relates to its ability to inhibit theophylline metabolism. Because the elevation of serum theophylline has been found to double, it is recommended that when this antidepressant is prescribed for a medically ill patient the patient's theophylline dose be reduced by one-third. Fluvoxamine, the most potent of the newer antidepressants in the ability to inhibit CYP1A2, is the only antidepressant of real concern in this regard. Other psychoactive drugs, including haloperidol, some tertiary amine tricyclic antidepressants, and olanzapine, are partially metabolized by CYP1A2, but their affinity for this enzyme does not appear to be great enough to inhibit the metabolism of other CYP1A2 substrates (29).

Cytochrome P450 2C9/19

The cytochrome P450 2C subfamily consists of several closely related enzymes. CYP2C9 and CYP2C19, the most important, constitute about 18% of the P450 content of the liver. A genetic polymorphism has been described for CYP2C19. Approximately 18% of Japanese and African-Americans are poor metabolizers of CYP2C19 substrates (23). A smaller percentage of Caucasians—about 3 to 5%—inherit the defective genetic alleles that code for this deficiency. Affected individuals can be expected to have higher than normal plasma concentrations of CYP2C19 substrates from the doses usually administered.

Drugs metabolized by CYP2C9 include tolbutamide, S-warfarin, ibuprofen, diclofenac, and naproxyn (20,25–28). Drugs metabolized by CYP2C19 include phenytoin, diazepam, and the tertiary amine tricyclic antidepressants (clomipramine, amitriptyline, and imipramine) (Table 3). Three of the newer antidepressants have sufficient affinity for CYP2C enzymes (sertraline, fluoxetine, fluvoxamine) to result in potentially significant interactions. Fluvoxamine is the most potent, and interactions have been described with the tricyclic antidepressants, warfarin, and diazepam. A measurable but clinically insignificant interaction occurs between sertraline and tolbutamide. Fluoxetine interactions with phenytoin have been described. Negative interactions with the psychotropic drugs and the nonsteroidal anti-inflammatory drugs (NSAIDs) have not been described.

Cytochrome P450 2D6

CYP2D6 has been the most extensively studied of the P450 enzymes. A genetic polymorphism has been well characterized, with 7 to 10% of Caucasians inheriting an autosomal recessively transmitted defective allele (26). Affected individuals lack sufficient functional enzyme to metabolize normally the CYP2D6 substrates listed in Table 3. They will have higher plasma drug concentrations and slower clearances of these drugs from usual doses (34,35).

Some β-adrenergic blockers are metabolized by CYP2D6 (propranolol, metoprolol, timolol) and other cardiovascular drugs (mexilitene, propafenone). The metabolic pathway of codeine to morphine is mediated by CYP2D6, and poor metabolizers will have diminished analgesic effects from its administration (20,25–28). Among the newer antidepressants, paroxetine, venlafaxine, and fluoxetine are partially metabolized by CYP2D6. The tertiary amine tricyclic antidepressants (clomipramine, amitriptyline, imipramine) are hydroxylated by CYP2D6.

CYP2D6 does not appear to be inducible. Coadministration of drugs that decrease the concentration of CYP2D6 probably have this effect by affecting other pathways of elimination or increasing hepatic blood flow.

The newer antidepressants vary in their potency to inhibit the metabolism of CYP2D6 substrates (20,26,36). Based on in vitro data, paroxetine is the most potent, but in vivo, paroxetine and fluoxetine appear to have a similar magnitude of inhibition, probably because the metabolite of fluoxetine, norfluoxetine, is also a CYP2D6 competitive inhibitor. Sertraline is not as potent an inhibitor of CYP2D6, but an occasional patient taking a tricyclic antidepressant who is administered sertraline will have a rise in tricyclic concentration to a clinically meaningful degree. The degree of inhibition and the clinical consequences will depend on the specific substrate inhibited, the dose of both substrate and inhibitor, and other factors such as severity of illness.

Cytochrome P450 3A4

Cytochrome 3A4 is the most prominent P450 enzyme. It constitutes 60% of the P450 present in the liver and 70% of the cytochrome enzymes in the gut wall. A high-capacity enzyme, it participates in the metabolism of the largest number of drugs used therapeutically (27). A genetic polymorphism has not been described for CYP3A4, although the expressed activity is broad. The activity also appears to change with age: it may peak during adolescence, stay relatively stable during most of adult life, and then show a gradual decline after age 70 years (37). Comparative rates of change in the activity of other specific P450s have not been well characterized.

The long list of nonpsychiatric drugs metabolized by CYP3A4 (Table 3) includes cardiovascular drugs (diltiazem, verapamil, nifedipine), alfentanil, tamoxifen, testosterone, cortisol, progesterone, ethinyl estadiol, cisapride, cyclosporine, terfenadine, astemizole, quinidine, and the protease inhibitors.

CYP3A4 is a steroid-inducible enzyme. Its induction can result from coadministration of rifampin, rifabutin, carbamazepine, dexamethasone, and phenobarbital (38). Inhibition of CYP3A4 substrates occurs potently with administration of several antidepressants. Nefazodone is the most potent, followed by fluvoxamine. At higher dosages, fluoxetine may be an important CYP3A4 inhibitor, but all the antidepressants are less potent than the azole antifungal drugs (e.g., ketoconazole) and the macrolide antibiotics (27,39,40). A recent report of the sudden death of a child receiving pimozide who was treated with clarithromycin is a case of suspected CYP3A4 interaction (41). Inhibition of terfenadine metabolism by ketoconazole, itraconazole, erythromycin, or clarithromycin poses a risk of cardiotoxicity from elevated concentrations of the parent drug. The noncardioactive metabolite of terfenadine, carboxyterfenadine, has been marketed as a nonsedating antihistamine. Either this drug or loratadine are strongly preferred if a psychoactive drug must be prescribed together with a nonsedating antihistamine.

USING SPECIFIC PSYCHOTROPIC DRUGS IN MEDICALLY ILL PATIENTS

Mood Stabilizers

The mood stabilizers are used primarily for psychiatric comorbidity when symptoms of acute mania are present and for the prevention of mania in patients with bipolar disorder. Lithium has been the standard for decades, but the list of available drugs for this purpose includes carbamazepine, valproate, and lamotrigine. The choice of a specific mood stabilizer in a medically ill patient will depend mostly on efficacy considerations, but should also take into account the potential for drug interactions.

Lithium has a very narrow therapeutic range of serum concentration associated with therapeutic effects. A concentration less than 50% above the therapeutic range may result in serious toxicity. Any condition that affects renal function may pose a risk of inducing lithium toxicity. Drugs that can reduce the clearance of lithium include thiazide diuretics, nonsteroidal anti-inflammatory drugs, and ACE inhibitors (18). Aspirin and sulindac appear not to be associated with any interaction. The initiation of lithium therapy in medical patients receiving any of these drugs may necessitate small initial doses and frequent serum lithium–concentration monitoring. Alternatively, lithium is not expected to influence the clearance of coadministered drugs. The relevance of drug interactions with lithium has recently been summarized (18).

Carbamazepine induces CYP3A4, which accounts for the autoinduction and decrease in plasma concentration several weeks following initiation of dosing. Other CYP3A4 substrates can be affected (Table 3), and decreases in several—e.g., cyclosporine (16)—have been noted in case reports and formal studies. Plasma-concentration measures of previous treatment with CYP3A4 substrates before initiation of psychotropic drug regimens may be useful to adjust doses.

Valproate is a mild enzyme inhibitor in addition to having the capacity to displace other drugs from their plasma protein–binding sites (13,14). The degree of interaction between valproate and specific CYP isozymes is unclear. Valproate has been shown to inhibit the metabolism of zidovudine (14) and affects the elimination of phenytoin and diazepam. An interaction with phenytoin may result from both an inhibition of metabolism by CYP2C9 and a protein-binding displacement reaction, increasing the concentration of unbound phenytoin. In contrast, valproate has no inhibitory effect on substrates of CYP2D6.

Lamotrigine has little apparent influence on the pharmacokinetics of other drugs. It is largely excreted renally and not metabolized by the CYP P450 system but undergoes glucuronidation. Lamotrigine may interact with carbamazepine, but this may be primarily pharmacodynamic rather than pharmacokinetic. It can increase the clearance of valproate but generally lacks the enzyme induction associated with carbamazepine.

Antidepressants

There is considerable comorbidity between depression and medical disorders. Treatment of depression syndromes in patients with cardiovascular disease, dementia, or neurological disease routinely includes the use of tricyclic or newer antidepressants. The currently available drugs come from several chemical classes. The tricyclics have been extensively used in the past, but they are being surpassed in popularity by the selective serotonin-reuptake inhibitors and other newer agents. Compared with the tricyclics, these drugs are better tolerated, lack anticholinergic side effects, and are generally nonlethal in overdose.

The tricyclics are metabolized by multiple P450 enzymes, including 1A2, 2C, 2D6, and 3A4. Amitriptyline, imipramine, and clomipramine are demethylated by CYP2C, CYP1A2, and possibly CYP3A4, and are hydroxylated by CYP2D6. Their elimination may be affected by inhibition of any of these pathways; however, there is incomplete evidence for the ability of the tricyclics to inhibit these enzymes resulting in significant metabolic interactions with other drugs. It is theoretically possible for any drug that is a substrate for a specific CYP enzyme to be a competitive inhibitor of the same enzyme. Therefore, desipramine and nortriptyline, for example, complete for metabolism with other CYP2D6 substrates (Table 3).

The SSRIs are metabolized by CYP2D6 and CYP3A4. Inhibition of their metabolism has not been a clinically significant problem as patients tolerate a broad range of plasma concentrations of these drugs and their concentrations have not been robustly related to clinical effect. These drugs have varying ability to inhibit cytochrome enzymes (Table 3). Fluvoxamine is a potent inhibitor of CYP1A2 with lesser effects on CYP2C and CYP3A4. Interactions have been described with clozapine, theophylline, diazepam, and alprazolam. Other substrates for the affected enzymes in Table 3 could presumably be inhibited. Paroxetine and fluoxetine are potent inhibitors of CYP2D6, while sertraline is only a mild inhibitor. In addition, fluoxetine has mild effects on CYP3A4 and CYP2C. Nefazodone, metabolized by CYP3A4, is also a potent inhibitor of CYP3A4, as shown by interactions with triazolam and alprazolam. It should be added to drug therapy regimens containing CYP3A4 substrates with recognition of the possibility of an inhibitory interaction (40). The remaining antidepressants—bupropion, citalopram, trazodone, venlafaxine, and mirtazapine—do not appear to have meaningful inhibitory effects on cytochrome enzymes.

Antipsychotics

The antipsychotic drugs are used in medically ill patients to treat psychotic symptoms arising from a variety of causes. These include schizophrenia, dementia of the Alzheimer's type, delirium from various causes, and other severe behavioral symptoms such as assaultiveness and aggression. The traditional antipsychotic drugs include the phenothiazines, thiothixene, molindone, and haloperidol. Due to their better tolerability profile, especially a lower propensity to cause extrapyramidal side effects, the atypical antipsychotics are favored for many patients requiring an antipsychotic drug.

The atypical antipsychotics consist of clozapine, risperidone, olanzapine, and quetiapine. Clozapine is reserved for use in patients who are treatment resistant or intolerant of the side effects from traditional antipsychotics, and its use must be monitored closely to detect and avoid agranulocytosis occurring in approximately 1% of recipients. Its drug interactions have been recently summarized (42). Clozapine is oxidized by CYP1A2 and CPY3A4, and its metabolism is subject to induction by cigarette smoking and inhibition by fluvoxamine and CYP3A4 inhibitors (Table 3). It is not expected to have effects on other co-administered drugs. Of particular concern is the addition of clozapine to medical regimens containing benzodiazepines because apparent pharmacodynamic interactions of unknown mechanism have occurred with severe respiratory depression.

Olanzapine is cleared in an analogous fashion to clozapine with additional pathways through non-P450 routes (29). Cigarette smoking will predictably lower its plasma concentration and possibly increase the need for a higher dosage. Olanzapine is unlikely to cause metabolic interactions of drugs metabolized by CYPs 1A2, 2C, 2D6, or 3A4. However, it may participate in pharmacodynamic interactions related to its sedative or dopamine antagonist effects.

Risperidone's elimination to its primary active metabolite, 9-hydroxy-risperidone, is mediated by CYP2D6. While concurrent therapy with SSRIs that inhibit CYP2D6, or the presence of the poor metabolizer genotype, will increase risperidone's plasma concentration and prolong its elimination half-life, the overall therapeutic effects appear to be unaltered. It lacks a documented effect on the metabolism of other drugs.

Quetiapine is cleared primarily by CYP3A4 (43). Phenytoin has been found to increase its plasma concentration and thioridazine to decrease its concentration. Other CYP3A4 interactions could be predicted to occur with specific inhibitors, but such interactions have not been described in the literature. Overall, while the elimination of the newer atypical antipsychotics are mediated to varying degrees by P-450 enzymes, these drugs apparently do not have sufficient affinity to cytochrome enzymes to result in inhibition or induction of other drugs.

Thioridazine, a phenothiazine antipsychotic, has been found to inhibit CYP2D6 in studies involving the concomitant use of antidepressants (44,45). It significantly increases plasma concentrations of trazodone, imipramine, and mianserin, all antidepressants partially metabolized by CYP2D6. Thus, it could be expected that the addition of thioridazine to a medical regimen including CYP2D6 substrates would result in metabolic drug interactions. Substantial documentation of cytochrome inhibition by other antipsychotics is not available.

Anxiolytics

A variety of comorbid anxiety disorders have been described in patients with medical disorders, including adjustment disorder with anxiety, panic disorder, and generalized anxiety disorder (46). The benzodiazepines, cyclic antidepressants, and buspirone are the drugs most frequently used for anxiety in both medical and psychiatric settings.

There is little evidence that the benzodiazepines, the major class of drugs used for antianxiety effects, have inductive or inhibitory effects on hepatic oxidizing enzymes. Their sedative effects, however, can be enhanced when combined with a medical regimen containing other drugs capable of causing depression of cognitive function, e.g., first-generation antihistamines and barbiturates.

The benzodiazepines are cleared primarily by oxidative metabolism and glucuronide conjugation. Oxazepam, lorazepam, and temazepam undergo conjugation followed by renal excretion. The other benzodiazepines are first oxidized by cytochrome enzymes except for clonazepam, which undergoes nitroreduction. Diazepam has received the most study, and its metabolism is mediated by CYP2C19 and CYP3A4 (47). The specific isozymes involved in the clearance of the other drugs are less certain. Thus, commonly used inhibitors such as cimetidine or the macrolide antibiotics and some SSRIs may impair the metabolism of several benzodiazepines and raise their plasma concentration.

Buspirone, a nonbenzodiazepine anxiolytic, is metabolized by unknown oxidizing enzymes. It is highly plasma protein bound (>95%) but does not displace other highly bound drugs (e.g., phenytoin, propranolol, and warfarin) from their binding sites. There is little evidence for metabolic interactions. A study in normal volunteers suggested that buspirone could inhibit the metabolism of haloperidol (a CYP1A2 and CYP2D6 substrate), but data obtained from schizophrenic patients in whom buspirone was added to a regimen of haloperidol produced no evidence of interference with drug metabolism (48).

GENERAL PRINCIPLES FOR AVOIDING AND MANAGING DRUG INTERACTIONS

The consequences of a drug interaction may be minimum or substantial depending upon several factors. These include the clinical state of the patient, the therapeutic ratio of the inhibited drug, and factors related to dosage such as length of treatment. For an elderly or debilitated patient, the likelihood that an interaction will have an impact on health or functioning is increased. A medically healthy young adult would be expected to suffer less significant consequences of an interaction compared to an unstable elderly patient. Interactions should always be viewed with an assessment of how cognition will be affected and if the goals of pharmacotherapy with existing therapy will need to be altered. Some general principles for avoiding or minimizing the impact of drug interactions are summarized in Table 4.

Drug interactions are most likely whenever therapy is stopped, started, or major dosage changes are made. It should be remembered that interactions are likely to be dose

Table 4 General Principles for Avoiding and Managing Drug Interactions

Space administration times to minimize competitive inhibition in the liver from drug's highest concentrations.
Select or change to a noninteracting drug.
Change the drug dose if an inducer or inhibitor is added to the treatment regimen.
Discontinue any unnecessary medications.
Practice therapeutic drug monitoring for drugs with a narrow range of effective or safe concentrations.
Initiate therapy with low doses. Most drug-drug interactions are dose dependent.
Monitor for problems. Crucial times are when drugs are started, stopped, or dosages changed.

dependent and that starting with a lower-than-normal initial dose will allow therapy to be titrated while monitoring the patient for evidence of an interaction. Also, choosing a psychoactive drug with a relatively short elimination half-life will facilitate the treatment of an interaction if it is necessary to discontinue the psychoactive drug. For drugs that have a defined therapeutic plasma concentration associated with therapeutic effects (theophylline, anticonvulsants), monitoring of blood levels during dosage titration may be especially helpful. Finally, extra attention should be paid to patient reports of drug effects for potential evidence of increased intensity of side effects or the appearance of new side effects.

It should be remembered that drug interactions can result from the pharmacological effects of nonprescription drugs (e.g., cimetidine). Many patients take over-the-counter preparations or medications prescribed to another family member or friend. A complete medication history can be helpful in investigating the cause of a suspected drug interaction. A sudden change in compliance with a prescribed dosage regimen can alter the pharmacodynamic effects of drugs. Fortunately, most drugs have reasonable therapeutic indices so that minor alterations in plasma concentration or half-life do not translate into untoward effects. Keeping the principles of drug interactions in mind and following general guidelines for management (see Table 4) should help minimize the impact of unpredictable or unavoidable drug interactions.

REFERENCES

1. Smith CL, Hampton EM, Pederson JA, Pennington LR, Bourne DW. Clinical and medicoeconomic impact of the cyclosporine-diltiazem interaction in renal transplant recipients. Pharmacotherapy 1994; 14:471–481.
2. Tome MB, Isaac MT, Harte R, Holland C. Paroxetine and pindolol: a randomized trial of serotonergic autoreceptor blockade in the reduction of antidepressant latency. Int Clin Psychopharmacol 1997; 12:81–89.
3. Hirschfeld RM, Schatzberg AF. Long-term management of depression. Am J Med 1994; 97(6A):33S–38S.
4. DeVane CL, Nemeroff CB. Psychotropic drug interactions. Primary Psychiatry 1998; 5: 36–70.
5. Sternbach HS. The serotonin syndrome. Am J Psychiatry 1991; 148:705–713.
6. Kolars JC, Schmiedlin-Ren P, Schuetz JD, Fang C, Watkins PB: Identification of rifampin-inducible P450IIIA4 (CYP3A4) in human small bowel enterocytes. J Clin Invest 1992; 90:1871–1878.
7. Malloy MJ, Ravis R, Pennell AT, Diskin CJ. Effect of cholestyramine on single dose valproate pharmacokinetics. Int J Clin Pharmacol Ther 1996; 34:208–211.
8. Gomez DY, Wacher VJ, Tomlanovich SJ, Hebert MF, Benet LZ. The effects of ketoconazole on the intestinal metabolism and bioavailability of cyclosporine. Clin Pharmacol Ther 1995; 58:15–19.
9. Fuhr U, Kummert AL. The fate of naringin in humans: A key to grapefruit juice-drug interactions? Clin Pharmacol Ther 1995; 58:365–373.

10. Rau SE, Bend JR, Arnold MO, Tran LT, Spence JD, Bailey DG. Grapefruit juice–terfena-dine single-dose interaction: magnitude, mechanism, and relevance. Clin Pharmacol Ther 1997; 61:401–409.

11. Wilkinson GR. Plasma and tissue binding considerations in drug disposition. Drug Metab Rev 1983; 14:427.

12. Apseloff G, Wilner KD, Gerber N, Tremaine LM. Effect of sertraline on protein binding of warfarin. Clin Pharmacokinet 1997; 32 (suppl 1):37–42.

13. Wong SL, Cavanaugh J, Shi H, Awni WM, Granneman GR. Effects of divalproex sodium on amitriptyline and nortriptyline pharmacokinetics. Clin Pharmacol Ther 1996; 60:48–53.

14. Akula SK, Rege AB, Dreisbach AW, Dejace PM, Lertora JJ. Valproic acid increases cerebro-spinal fluid zidovudine levels in a patient with AIDS. Am J Med Sci 1997; 313:244–246.

15. DeVane CL. Principles of pharmacokinetics and pharmacodynamics. In: Schatzberg AF, Nemeroff CB, eds. American Psychiatric Press Textbook of Psychopharmacology. 2d ed. Washington, DC: American Psychiatric Press, 1998:155–169.

16. Spina E, Pisani F, Perucca E. Clinically significant pharmacokinetic drug interactions with carbamazepine. An update. Clin Pharmacokinet 1996; 31:198–214.

17. DeVane CL. Clinical implications of dose-dependent cytochrome P-450 drug-drug interac-tions with antidepressants. Human Psychopharmacol 1998; 13:329–336.

18. Finley PR, Warner MD, Peabody CA. Clinical relevance of drug interactions with lithium. Clin Pharmacokinet 1995; 29:172–191.

19. Wrighton SA, Stevens JC. The human hepatic cytochromes P450 involved in drug metabo-lism. Crit Rev Toxicol 1992; 22:1–21.

20. Nemeroff CB, DeVane CL, Pollock BG. Antidepressants and the cytochrome P450 system. Am J Psychiatry 1996; 153:311–320.

21. Harvey AT, Preskorn SH. Cytochrome P450 enzymes: interpretation of their interactions with selective serotonin reuptake inhibitors. Part I. J Clin Psychopharmacol 1996; 16:273–285.

22. Meyer UA, Zanger UM, Grant D, Blum M. Genetic polymorphisms of drug metabolism. Adv Drug Res 1990; 19:197–241.

23. Bertz RJ, Granneman GR. Use of in vitro and in vivo data to estimate the likelihood of metabolic pharmacokinetic interactions. Clin Pharmacokinet 1997; 32:210–258.

24. Butler MA, Lang NP, Young JF, Caporaso NE, Vincis P, Hayes RB, Teitel CH, Massengil JP, Lawsen MF, Kadlubar FF. Determination of CYP1A2 and NAT2 phenotypes in human populations by analysis of caffeine urinary metabolites. Pharmacogenetics 1992; 2:116–127.

25. Brosen K. Recent developments in hepatic drug oxidation implications for clinical pharma-cokinetics. Clin Pharmacokinet 1990; 18:220–239.

26. Ereshefsky L, Riesenman C, Lam YW. Antidepressant drug interactions and the cyto-chrome P450 system: the role of cytochrome P450 2D6. Clin Pharmacokinet 1995; 29(suppl 1):10–19.

27. Ketter TA, Flockhart DA, Post RM, et al. The emerging role of cytochrome P450 3A in psychopharmacology. J Clin Psychopharmacol 1995; 15:387–398.

28. Michalets EL. Update: clinically significant cytochrome P-450 interactions. Pharmacother-apy. 1998; 18:84–112.

29. Ereshefsky L. Pharmacokinetics and drug interactions: update for new antipsychotics. J Clin Psychiatry 1996; 57 (suppl 11):12–15.

30. McCarthy R. Seizure following smoking cessation in a clozapine responder. Pharmacopsychiatry 1994; 27:210–211.

31. Brosen K, Skjelbo E, Rasmussen BB, Poulsen HE, Loft S. Fluvoxamine is a potent inhibitor of cytochrome P4501A2. Biochem Pharmacol 1993; 45:1211–1214.

32. Brouwers JR. Drug interactions with quinolone antibacterials. Drug Safety 1992; 4:268–281.

33. Wilkinson GR, Guengerich FP, Branch RA. Genetic polymorphism of S-mephenytoin hydroxylation. Pharmacol Ther 1989; 43:53–76.

34. von Moltke LL, Greenblatt DJ, Cotreau-Bibbo MM, et al. Inhibition of desipramine hydroxylation in vitro by serotonin-reuptake-inhibitor antidepressants, and by quinidine and ketoconazole: a model system to predict drug interactions in vivo. J Pharmacol Exp Ther 1994; 268:1278–1283.

35. Bergstrom RF, Peyton AL, Lemberger L, et al. Quantification and mechanism of the fluoxetine and tricyclic antidepressant interaction. Clin Pharmacol Ther 1992; 51: 239–248.

36. Preskorn SH, Alderman J, Chung M, et al. Pharmacokinetics of desipramine coadministered with sertraline or fluoxetine. J Clin Psychopharmacol 1994; 14:90–98.

37. Korinthenberg R, Haug C, Hannak D. The metabolization of carbamazepine to CBZ-10, 11-epoxide in children from the newborn age to adolescence. Neuropediatrics 1994; 25: 214–216.

38. Backman JT, Olkkola KT, Neuvonen PJ. Rifampin drastically reduces plasma concentrations and effects of oral midazolam. Clin Pharmacol Ther 1996; 59:7–13.

39. Honig PK, Wortham DC, Zamani K, Conner DP, Mullin JC, Aantilena LR. Terfenadine-ketoconazole interaction: pharmacokinetic and electrocardiographic consequences. JAMA 1993; 269:1513–1518.

40. Barbhaiya RH, Shukla UA, Kroboth PD, Greene DS. Coadministration of nefazodone and benzodiazepines: II. A pharmacokinetic interaction study with triazolam. J Clin Psychopharmacol 1995; 15:320–326.

41. Flockhart DA, Richard E, Woosley RL, Pearle PL Drici M-D. A metabolic interaction between clarithromycin and pimozide may result in cardiac toxicity (abstr). Clin Pharmacol Ther 1996; 59:189.

42. Edge SC, Markowitz JS, DeVane CL. Clozapine drug-drug interactions: a review of the literature. Hum Psychopharmacol 1997; 12:5–20.

43. Thyrum PT, Fabre LF, Wong YWJ, Ewing BJ, Yeh C. Multiple dose pharmacokinetics of ICI 204,636 in schizophrenia men and women (abstr). Psychopharmacol Bull 1996; 32:525A.

44. Yasui N, Tybring G, Otani K, et al. Effects of thioridazine, an inhibitor of CYP2D6, on the steady-state plasma concentrations of the enantiomers of mianserin and its active metabolite, desmethylmianserin, in depressed japanese patients. Pharmacogenetics 1997; 369–374.

45. Maynard GL, Soni P. Thioridazine interferences with imipramine metabolism and measurement. Ther Drug Monitor 1996; 18:729–731.

46. Stoudemire A. Epidemiology and psychopharmacology of anxiety in medical patients. J Clin Psychiatry 1996; 57 (suppl 7):64–72.

47. Schmider J, Greenblatt DG, von Moltke LL, Shader LI. Relationship of in vitro data on drug metabolism to in vivo pharmacokinetics and drug interactions: Implications for diazepam disposition in humans. J Clin Psychopharmacol 1996; 16:267–272.
48. Huang HF, Jann MW, Wei FC, et al. Lack of pharmacokinetic interaction between buspirone and haloperidol in patients with schizophrenia. J Clin Pharmacol 1996; 36:963–969.

Index

Page numbers in *italics* indicate figures. Page numbers followed by "t" indicate tables.

About the Editors

Robert G. Robinson is the Paul W. Penningroth Professor of Psychiatry and Head of the Department of Psychiatry at the University of Iowa College of Medicine, Iowa City, Iowa. He is the author or coauthor of more than 420 abstracts, book chapters, and journal articles, as well as the author of the *Neuropsychiatry of Stroke* and the co-editor of *Depression and Coexisting Disease* (with P. V. Rabins) and *Depression in Neurologic Disease* (with S. E. Starkstein). He is certified by the National Board of Medical Examiners and the American Board of Neurology and Psychiatry in Psychiatry and Geriatric Psychiatry. He is Executive Director of the American Neuropsychiatric Association and a Fellow of the American College of Neuropsychopharmacology, the American Psychiatric Association, and the Stroke Council of the American Heart Association. He is also a member of the editorial boards of seven different journals and has been a guest editor of *Depression* and *Neurocase.* Dr. Robinson received the B.S. degree (1967) in engineering physics from Cornell University, Ithaca, New York, and the M.D. degree (1971) from Cornell University Medical College, New York, N.Y.

William R. Yates is a Professor of Psychiatry and Family Practice and the Chair of the Department of Psychiatry at the University of Oklahoma Health Sciences Center, Tulsa. The author or coauthor of many articles in peer-reviewed journals, he has conducted research on alcoholism for the National Institutes of Health and on bulimia, depression, and other disorders for pharmaceutical companies such as Eli Lilly, Upjohn, and Ciba-Geigy. He is a Fellow of the Academy of Psychosomatic Medicine and a member of the American Society of Clinical Psychopharmacology, the Society of Biological Psychiatry, and the American Psychiatric Association, among others. Dr. Yates received the B.A. degree (1974) in chemistry from Dana College, Blair, Nebraska, and the M.D. degree (1977) from the University of Nebraska–Lincoln. He is also the recipient of the M.S. degree (1986) in Preventive Medicine from the University of Iowa, Iowa City.